The GALE
ENCYCLOPEDIA of
SURGERY AND
MEDICAL TESTS

SECOND EDITION

The GALE ENCYCLOPEDIA of SURGERY AND MEDICAL TESTS

SECOND EDITION

VOLUME

2

D–K

BRIGHAM NARINS, EDITOR

GALE
CENGAGE Learning

Detroit • New York • San Francisco • New Haven, Conn • Waterville, Maine • London

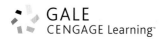

Gale Encyclopedia of Surgery and Medical Tests, Second Edition

Project Editor: Brigham Narins

Editorial: Donna Batten, Amy Kwolek, Jeffrey Wilson

Product Manager: Kate Hanley

Editorial Support Services: Andrea Lopeman

Indexing Services: Katherine Jensen, Indexes, etc.

Rights Acquisition and Management: Margaret Chamberlain-Gaston, Kelly A. Quin, and Robyn V. Young

Composition: Evi Abou-El-Seoud

Manufacturing: Wendy Blurton

Imaging: Lezlie Light

Product Design: Pam Galbreath

For product information and technology assistance, contact us at **Gale Customer Support, 1-800-877-4253.**
For permission to use material from this text or product, submit all requests online at **www.cengage.com/permissions.**
Further permissions questions can be emailed to **permissionrequest@cengage.com**

While every effort has been made to ensure the reliability of the information presented in this publication, Gale, a part of Cengage Learning, does not guarantee the accuracy of the data contained herein. Gale accepts no payment for listing; and inclusion in the publication of any organization, agency, institution, publication, service, or individual does not imply endorsement of the editors or publisher. Errors brought to the attention of the publisher and verified to the satisfaction of the publisher will be corrected in future editions.

Library of Congress Cataloging-in-Publication Data

The Gale encyclopedia of surgery and medical tests : a guide for patients and caregivers / Brigham Narins, editor. -- 2nd ed.
    p. cm.
    Includes bibliographical references and index.
    ISBN-13: 978-1-4144-4884-8 (set : alk. paper)
    ISBN-13: 978-1-4144-4885-5 (vol. 1 : alk. paper)
    ISBN-13: 978-1-4144-4886-2 (vol. 2 : alk. paper)
    ISBN-13: 978-1-4144-4887-9 (vol. 3 : alk. paper)
    [etc.]
        1. Surgery--Encyclopedias. 2. Diagnosis--Encyclopedias. I. Narins, Brigham, 1962-.

RD17.G342 2008
617.003--dc22   2008020207

Gale
27500 Drake Rd.
Farmington Hills, MI, 48331-3535

ISBN-13: 978-1-4144-4884-8 (set)   ISBN-10: 1-4144-4884-8 (set)
ISBN-13: 978-1-4144-4885-5 (vol. 1)   ISBN-10: 1-4144-4885-6 (vol. 1)
ISBN-13: 978-1-4144-4886-2 (vol. 2   ISBN-10: 1-4144-4886-4 (vol. 2)
ISBN-13: 978-1-4144-4887-9 (vol. 3)   ISBN-10: 1-4144-4887-2 (vol. 3)
ISBN-13: 978-1-4144-4888-6 (vol. 4)   ISBN-10: 1-4144-4888-0 (vol. 4)

This title is also available as an e-book.
ISBN-13: 978-1-4144-4889-3 ISBN-10: 1-4144-4889-9
Contact your Gale, Cengage Learning sales representative for ordering information.

Printed in China
1 2 3 4 5 6 7 12 11 10 09 08

CONTENTS

List of Entries vii

List of Entries by Body System xiii

Introduction... xix

Advisory Board... xxi

Contributors xxiii

Entries

Volume 1: A-C.. 1

Volume 2: D-K 465

Volume 3: L-P 915

Volume 4: Q-Z 1355

Organizations... 1771

Glossary 1785

General Index 1865

LIST OF ENTRIES

A

Abdominal ultrasound
Abdominal wall defect repair
Abdominoplasty
ABO blood typing
Abortion, induced
Abscess incision and drainage
Acetaminophen
Adenoidectomy
Admission to the hospital
Adrenalectomy
Adrenergic drugs
Adult day care
Alanine aminotransferase test
Albumin Test, Blood
Ambulatory surgery centers
Amniocentesis
Amputation
Anaerobic bacteria culture
Analgesics
Analgesics, opioid
Anesthesia evaluation
Anesthesia, general
Anesthesia, local
Anesthesiologist's role
Angiography
Angioplasty
Anterior temporal lobectomy
Antianxiety drugs
Antibiotics
Antibiotics, topical
Antibody tests, immunoglobulins
Anticoagulant and antiplatelet
  drugs

Antihypertensive drugs
Antinausea drugs
Antiseptics
Antrectomy
Aortic aneurysm repair
Aortic valve replacement
Appendectomy
Arterial blood gases (ABG)
Arteriovenous fistula
Arthrography
Arthroplasty
Arthroscopic surgery
Artificial sphincter insertion
Aseptic technique
Aspartate aminotransferase test
Aspirin
Autologous blood donation
Axillary dissection

B

Balloon valvuloplasty
Bandages and dressings
Bankart procedure
Barbiturates
Barium enema
Bedsores
Biliary stenting
Biofeedback
Bispectral index
Bladder augmentation
Blepharoplasty
Blood Ca (calcium) level
Blood carbon dioxide level

Blood culture
Blood donation and registry
Blood phosphate level
Blood potassium level
Blood pressure measurement
Blood salvage
Blood sodium level
Blood type test
Blood urea nitrogen test
Bloodless surgery
Body temperature
Bone grafting
Bone marrow aspiration and
  biopsy
Bone marrow transplantation
Bone x rays
Bowel preparation
Bowel resection
Bowel resection, small intestine
Breast biopsy
Breast implants
Breast reconstruction
Breast reduction
Bronchoscopy
BUN-creatinine ratio
Bunionectomy

C

Cardiac catheterization
Cardiac event monitor
Cardiac marker tests
Cardiac monitor
Cardiopulmonary resuscitation

Cardioversion
Carotid endarterectomy
Carpal tunnel release
Catheterization, female
Catheterization, male
Cephalosporins
Cerebral aneurysm repair
Cerebrospinal fluid (CSF) analysis
Cervical cerclage
Cervical cryotherapy
Cesarean section
Chemistry screen
Chest tube insertion
Chest x ray
Cholecystectomy
Cholesterol and triglyceride tests
Circumcision
Cleft lip repair
Closures: stitches, staples, and glue
Club foot repair
Cochlear implants
Collagen periurethral injection
Colonic stent
Colonoscopy
Colorectal surgery
Colostomy
Colporrhaphy
Colposcopy
Colpotomy
Complete blood count
Cone biopsy
Corneal transplantation
Coronary artery bypass graft surgery
Coronary stenting
Corpus callosotomy
Corticosteroids
Craniofacial reconstruction
Craniotomy
Creatine phosphokinase (CPK)
Cricothyroidotomy
Cryotherapy
Cryotherapy for cataracts
CT scans
Curettage and electrosurgery

Cyclocryotherapy
Cystectomy
Cystocele repair
Cystoscopy

D

Death and dying
Debridement
Deep brain stimulation
Defecography
Defibrillation
Dental implants
Dermabrasion
Dilatation and curettage
Discharge from the hospital
Disk removal
Diuretics
Diverticulitis
Do not resuscitate (DNR) order
Drug-resistant organisms

E

Ear, nose, and throat surgery
Echocardiography
Elective surgery
Electrocardiogram
Electrocardiography
Electroencephalography
Electrolyte tests
Electrophysiology study of the heart
Emergency surgery
Endolymphatic shunt
Endoscopic retrograde cholangiopancreatography
Endoscopic sinus surgery
Endoscopic ultrasound
Endotracheal intubation
Endovascular stent surgery
Enhanced external counterpulsation
Enucleation, eye
Epidural therapy
Episiotomy

Erythromycins
Esophageal atresia repair
Esophageal function tests
Esophageal resection
Esophagogastrectomy
Esophagogastroduodenoscopy
Essential surgery
Exenteration
Exercise
Extracapsular cataract extraction
Eye muscle surgery

F

Face lift
Fallopian tube implants
Fasciotomy
Femoral hernia repair
Fetal surgery
Fetoscopy
Fibrin sealants
Finding a surgeon
Finger reattachment
Fluoroquinolones
Forehead lift
Fracture repair

G

Gallstone removal
Ganglion cyst removal
Gastrectomy
Gastric acid inhibitors
Gastric bypass
Gastroduodenostomy
Gastroenterologic surgery
Gastroesophageal reflux scan
Gastroesophageal reflux surgery
Gastrostomy
General surgery
Gingivectomy
Glossectomy
Glucose tests
Goniotomy

H

Hair transplantation
Hammer, claw, and mallet toe
 surgery
Hand surgery
Health care proxy
Health history
Health Maintenance
 Organization (HMO)
Heart surgery for congenital
 defects
Heart transplantation
Heart-lung machines
Heart-lung transplantation
Heller myotomy
Hemangioma excision
Hematocrit
Hemispherectomy
Hemoglobin test
Hemoperfusion
Hemorrhoidectomy
Hepatectomy
Hiatal hernia
HIDA Scan
Hip osteotomy
Hip replacement
Hip revision surgery
Home care
Hospice
Hospital services
Hospital-acquired infections
Human leukocyte antigen test
Hydrocelectomy
Hypophysectomy
Hypospadias repair
Hysterectomy
Hysteroscopy

I

Ileal conduit surgery
Ileoanal anastomosis
Ileoanal reservoir surgery
Ileostomy
Immunoassay tests

Immunologic therapies
Immunosuppressant drugs
Implantable cardioverter-
 defibrillator
In vitro fertilization
Incision care
Incisional hernia repair
Informed consent
Inguinal hernia repair
Intensive care unit
Intensive care unit equipment
Intestinal obstruction repair
Intra-Operative Parathyroid
 Hormone Measurement
Intravenous rehydration
Intussusception reduction
Iridectomy
Islet cell transplantation

K

Kidney dialysis
Kidney function tests
Kidney transplantation
Knee arthroscopic surgery
Knee osteotomy
Knee replacement
Knee revision surgery
Kneecap removal

L

Laceration repair
Laminectomy
Laparoscopy
Laparoscopy for endometriosis
Laparotomy, exploratory
Laryngectomy
Laser in-situ keratomileusis
 (LASIK)
Laser iridotomy
Laser posterior capsulotomy
Laser skin resurfacing
Laser surgery
Laxatives

LDL cholesterol test
Leg lengthening or shortening
Length of hospital stay
Limb salvage
Lipid profile
Lipid tests
Liposuction
Lithotripsy
Liver biopsy
Liver function tests
Liver transplantation
Living will
Lobectomy, pulmonary
Long-term care insurance
Lumpectomy
Lung biopsy
Lung transplantation
Lymphadenectomy

M

Magnetic resonance angiogram
Magnetic resonance imaging
Magnetic resonance venogram
Mammography
Managed care plans
Mantoux test
Mastectomy
Mastoidectomy
Maze procedure for atrial
 fibrillation
Mechanical circulation support
Mechanical ventilation
Meckel's diverticulectomy
Mediastinoscopy
Medicaid
Medical charts
Medical co-morbidities
Medical errors
Medicare
Medication Monitoring
Meningocele repair
Mental health assessment
Mentoplasty
Microsurgery

Minimally invasive heart surgery
Mitral valve repair
Mitral valve replacement
Modified radical mastectomy
Mohs surgery
Multiple-gated acquisition (MUGA) scan
Muscle relaxants
Myelography
Myocardial resection
Myomectomy
Myringotomy and ear tubes

N

Necessary surgery
Needle bladder neck suspension
Negative pressure rooms
Nephrectomy
Nephrolithotomy, percutaneous
Nephrostomy
Neurosurgery
Nonsteroidal anti-inflammatory drugs
Nursing homes

O

Obstetric and gynecologic surgery
Omphalocele repair
Oophorectomy
Open prostatectomy
Operating room
Ophthalmologic surgery
Ophthalmoscopy
Oral glucose tolerance test
Orchiectomy
Orchiopexy
Orthopedic surgery
Otoplasty
Outpatient surgery
Oxygen therapy

P

Pacemakers
Pain management
Pallidotomy
Pancreas transplantation
Pancreatectomy
Paracentesis
Parathyroidectomy
Parentage testing
Parotidectomy
Partial thromboplastin time
Patent urachus repair
Patient confidentiality
Patient rights
Patient-controlled analgesia
Pectus excavatum repair
Pediatric concerns
Pediatric surgery
Pelvic ultrasound
Penile prostheses
Pericardiocentesis
Peripheral endarterectomy
Peripheral vascular bypass surgery
Peritoneovenous shunt
pH monitoring
Phacoemulsification for cataracts
Pharyngectomy
Phlebography
Phlebotomy
Photocoagulation therapy
Photorefractive keratectomy (PRK)
Physical examination
Planning a hospital stay
Plastic, reconstructive, and cosmetic surgery
Pneumonectomy
Portal vein bypass
Positron emission tomography (PET)
Postoperative care
Post-surgical infections
Post-surgical pain
Power of attorney
Preoperative care
Preparing for surgery

Presurgical testing
Private insurance plans
Prophylaxis, antibiotic
Prothrombin time
Proton pump inhibitors
Pulse oximeter
Pyloroplasty

Q

Quadrantectomy

R

Radical neck dissection
Recovery at home
Recovery room
Rectal prolapse repair
Rectal resection
Red blood cell indices
Reoperation
Retinal cryopexy
Retropubic suspension
Rh blood typing
Rheumatoid factor testing
Rhinoplasty
Rhizotomy
Robot-assisted surgery
Root canal treatment
Rotator cuff repair

S

Sacral nerve stimulation
Salpingo-oophorectomy
Salpingostomy
Scar revision surgery
Scleral buckling
Sclerostomy
Sclerotherapy for esophageal varices
Sclerotherapy for varicose veins
Scopolamine patch
Second opinion
Second-look surgery
Sedation, conscious

Sedimentation rate
Segmentectomy
Sentinel lymph node biopsy
Septoplasty
Serum chloride level
Serum creatinine level
Serum glucose level
Sestamibi scan
Sex reassignment surgery
Shoulder joint replacement
Shoulder resection arthroplasty
Sigmoidoscopy
Simple mastectomy
Skin grafting
Skull x rays
Sling procedure
Smoking cessation
Snoring surgery
Sphygmomanometer
Spinal fusion
Spinal instrumentation
Spirometry tests
Splenectomy
Stapedectomy
Stereotactic radiosurgery
Stethoscope
Stress test
Sulfonamides
Surgical instruments
Surgical mesh
Surgical oncology
Surgical risk
Surgical team
Surgical training
Surgical triage
Sympathectomy
Syringe and needle

T

Talking to the doctor
Tarsorrhaphy
Telesurgery
Temperature measurement
Tendon repair
Tenotomy
Tetracyclines
Thermometer
Thoracic surgery
Thoracotomy
Thrombolytic therapy
Thyroidectomy
Tonsillectomy
Tooth extraction
Tooth replantation
Trabeculectomy
Tracheotomy
Traction
Transfusion
Transplant surgery
Transurethral bladder resection
Transurethral resection of the prostate
Trocars
Tubal ligation
Tube enterostomy
Tube-shunt surgery
Tumor marker tests
Tumor removal
Tympanoplasty
Type and screen

U

Ultrasound
Umbilical hernia repair

Upper GI exam
Ureteral stenting
Ureterosigmoidoscopy
Ureterostomy, cutaneous
Urinalysis
Urinary anti-infectives
Urine culture
Urologic surgery
Uterine stimulants

V

Vagal nerve stimulation
Vagotomy
Vascular surgery
Vasectomy
Vasovasostomy
Vein ligation and stripping
Venous thrombosis prevention
Ventricular assist device
Ventricular shunt
Vertical banded gastroplasty
Vital signs

W

Webbed finger or toe repair
Weight management
Whipple procedure
White blood cell count and differential
Wound care
Wound culture
Wrist replacement

LIST OF ENTRIES BY BODY SYSTEM

Cardiovascular

Angiography
Angioplasty
Aortic aneurysm repair
Aortic valve replacement
Arteriovenous fistula
Balloon valvuloplasty
Cardiac catheterization
Cardiac event monitor
Cardiac marker tests
Cardiac monitor
Cardiopulmonary resuscitation
Cardioversion
Carotid endarterectomy
Coronary artery bypass graft
  surgery
Coronary stenting
Defibrillation
Echocardiography
Electrocardiogram
Electrocardiography
Electrophysiology study of the
  heart
Endovascular stent surgery
Femoral hernia repair
Heart surgery for congenital
  defects
Heart transplantation
Heart-lung machines
Heart-lung transplantation
Hemangioma excision
Implantable cardioverter-
  defibrillator
Magnetic resonance angiogram

Magnetic resonance venogram
Maze procedure for atrial
  fibrillation
Mechanical circulation support
Minimally invasive heart surgery
Mitral valve repair
Mitral valve replacement
Multiple-gated acquisition
  (MUGA) scan
Myocardial resection
Pacemakers
Pericardiocentesis
Peripheral endarterectomy
Peripheral vascular bypass
  surgery
Portal vein bypass
Sclerotherapy for varicose veins
Stress test
Vascular surgery
Vein ligation and stripping
Venous thrombosis prevention
Ventricular assist device
Ventricular shunt

Endocrine

Adenoidectomy
Adrenalectomy
Endoscopic retrograde
  cholangiopancreatography
Hypophysectomy
Intra-Operative Parathyroid
  Hormone Measurement
Islet cell transplantation
Oral glucose tolerance test

Pancreas transplantation
Pancreatectomy
Parathyroidectomy
Sestamibi scan
Thyroidectomy
Whipple procedure

Gastrointestinal

Antrectomy
Appendectomy
Artificial sphincter insertion
Barium enema
Biliary stenting
Bowel preparation
Bowel resection
Bowel resection, small intestine
Cholecystectomy
Colonic stent
Colonoscopy
Colorectal surgery
Colostomy
Defecography
Diverticulitis
Endoscopic ultrasound
Esophageal atresia repair
Esophageal function tests
Esophageal resection
Esophagogastrectomy
Esophagogastroduodenoscopy
Gastrectomy
Gastric acid inhibitors
Gastric bypass
Gastroduodenostomy

Gastroenterologic surgery

Gastroesophageal reflux scan

Gastroesophageal reflux surgery

Gastrostomy

Glossectomy

Heller myotomy

Hemorrhoidectomy

Hepatectomy

HIDA Scan

Ileoanal anastomosis

Ileoanal reservoir surgery

Ileostomy

Intestinal obstruction repair

Intussusception reduction

Liver biopsy

Liver transplantation

Laxatives

Parotidectomy

Pyloroplasty

Rectal prolapse repair

Rectal resection

Sclerotherapy for esophageal varices

Sigmoidoscopy

Tube enterostomy

Upper GI exam

Vagotomy

Vertical banded gastroplasty

Hematological

ABO blood typing

Alanine aminotransferase test

Albumin Test, Blood

Anticoagulant and antiplatelet drugs

Arterial blood gases (ABG)

Aspartate aminotransferase test

Autologous blood donation

Blood Ca (calcium) level

Blood carbon dioxide level

Blood culture

Blood donation and registry

Bloodless surgery

Blood phosphate level

Blood potassium level

Blood pressure measurement

Blood salvage

Blood sodium level

Blood type test

Blood urea nitrogen test

Bone marrow aspiration and biopsy

Bone marrow transplantation

BUN-creatinine ratio

Chemistry screen

Cholesterol and triglyceride tests

Complete blood count

Creatine phosphokinase (CPK)

Electrolyte tests

Enhanced external counterpulsation

Hematocrit

Hemoglobin test

Hemoperfusion

Human leukocyte antigen test

LDL cholesterol test

Lipid profile

Lipid tests

Liver function tests

Meckel's diverticulectomy

Partial thromboplastin time

Phlebography

Phlebotomy

Photocoagulation therapy

Prothrombin time

Pulse oximeter

Red blood cell indices

Rh blood typing

Rheumatoid factor testing

Sedimentation rate

Serum chloride level

Serum creatinine level

Serum glucose level

Sphygmomanometer

Thrombolytic therapy

Transfusion

Type and screen

White blood cell count and differential

Integumentary

Bedsores

Blepharoplasty

Cleft lip repair

Debridement

Dermabrasion

Face lift

Fasciotomy

Forehead lift

Laceration repair

Laser skin resurfacing

Mohs surgery

Skin grafting

Webbed finger or toe repair

Musculoskeletal

Abdominal wall defect repair

Abdominoplasty

Amputation

Arthrography

Arthroplasty

Arthroscopic surgery

Bankart procedure

Bone grafting

Bone x rays

Bunionectomy

Club foot repair

Craniofacial reconstruction

Disk removal

Eye muscle surgery

Finger reattachment

Fracture repair

Ganglion cyst removal

Hammer, claw, and mallet toe surgery

Hand surgery

Hiatal hernia

Hip osteotomy

Hip replacement

Hip revision surgery

Incisional hernia repair
Inguinal hernia repair
Knee arthroscopic surgery
Knee osteotomy
Knee replacement
Knee revision surgery
Kneecap removal
Laminectomy
Leg lengthening or shortening
Limb salvage
Mastoidectomy
Mentoplasty
Orthopedic surgery
Pectus excavatum repair
Rotator cuff repair
Shoulder joint replacement
Shoulder resection arthroplasty
Skull x rays
Spinal fusion
Spinal instrumentation
Tendon repair
Tenotomy
Traction
Umbilical hernia repair
Wrist replacement

Neurological

Anterior temporal lobectomy
Bispectral index
Carpal tunnel release
Cerebral aneurysm repair
Cerebrospinal fluid (CSF)
  analysis
Corpus callosotomy
Craniotomy
Deep brain stimulation
Electroencephalography
Hemispherectomy
Meningocele repair
Myelography
Neurosurgery
Pallidotomy
Rhizotomy
Stereotactic radiosurgery
Sympathectomy
Vagal nerve stimulation

Reproductive, Female

Abortion, induced
Amniocentesis
Breast biopsy
Breast implants
Breast reconstruction
Breast reduction
Cervical cerclage
Cervical cryotherapy
Cesarean section
Colporrhaphy
Colposcopy
Colpotomy
Cone biopsy
Dilatation and curettage
Episiotomy
Fallopian tube implants
Fetal surgery
Fetoscopy
Hysterectomy
Hysteroscopy
In vitro fertilization
Laparoscopy for endometriosis
Lumpectomy
Mammography
Mastectomy
Modified radical mastectomy
Myomectomy
Obstetric and gynecologic surgery
Oophorectomy
Quadrantectomy
Salpingo-oophorectomy
Salpingostomy
Simple mastectomy
Tubal ligation
Uterine stimulants

Reproductive, Male

Circumcision
Hydrocelectomy
Hypospadias repair

Open prostatectomy
Orchiectomy
Orchiopexy
Penile prostheses
Transurethral resection of the
  prostate
Vasectomy
Vasovasostomy

Respiratory

Bronchoscopy
Chest tube insertion
Cricothyroidotomy
Endoscopic sinus surgery
Endotracheal intubation
Laryngectomy
Lobectomy, pulmonary
Lung biopsy
Lung transplantation
Mantoux test
Mechanical ventilation
Mediastinoscopy
Pharyngectomy
Pneumonectomy
Septoplasty
Snoring surgery
Spirometry tests
Tracheotomy

Sensory

Cochlear implants
Corneal transplantation
Cryotherapy for cataracts
Cyclocryotherapy
Endolymphatic shunt
Enucleation, eye
Extracapsular cataract extraction
Goniotomy
Iridectomy
Laser in-situ keratomileusis
  (LASIK)
Laser iridotomy
Laser posterior capsulotomy
Myringotomy and ear tubes

Ophthalmologic surgery
Ophthalmoscopy
Otoplasty
Phacoemulsification for
  cataracts
Photorefractive keratectomy
  (PRK)
Retinal cryopexy
Scleral buckling
Sclerostomy
Stapedectomy
Tarsorrhaphy
Trabeculectomy
Tube-shunt surgery
Tympanoplasty

Urinary

Bladder augmentation
Catheterization, female
Catheterization, male
Collagen periurethral injection
Cystectomy
Cystocele repair
Cystoscopy
Gallstone removal
Ileal conduit surgery
Kidney dialysis
Kidney function tests
Kidney transplantation
Lithotripsy
Needle bladder neck suspension
Nephrectomy
Nephrolithotomy, percutaneous
Nephrostomy
Patent urachus repair
Retropubic suspension
Sacral nerve stimulation
Sling procedure
Transurethral bladder
  resection
Ureteral stenting
Ureterosigmoidoscopy
Ureterostomy, cutaneous
Urinalysis
Urinary anti-infectives

Urine culture
Urologic surgery

Other Surgeries

Abscess incision and drainage
Axillary dissection
Curettage and electrosurgery
Ear, nose, and throat surgery
Elective surgery
Emergency surgery
Essential surgery
Exenteration
General surgery
Gingivectomy
Laparoscopy
Laparotomy, exploratory
Laser surgery
Lymphadenectomy
Microsurgery
Necessary surgery
Omphalocele repair
Outpatient surgery
Pediatric surgery
Plastic, reconstructive, and
  cosmetic surgery
Radical neck dissection
Rhinoplasty
Robot-assisted surgery
Root canal treatment
Scar revision surgery
Second-look surgery
Segmentectomy
Sex reassignment surgery
Splenectomy
Telesurgery
Thoracic surgery
Thoracotomy
Tonsillectomy
Tooth extraction
Tooth replantation
Trabeculectomy
Transplant surgery
Tumor removal

Other Tests & Procedures

Abdominal ultrasound
Anaerobic bacteria culture
Antibody tests, immunoglobulins
Biofeedback
Chest x ray
Cryotherapy
CT scans
Dental implants
Epidural therapy
Glucose tests
Hair transplantation
Immunoassay tests
Immunologic therapies
Intravenous rehydration
Liposuction
Magnetic resonance imaging
Medication Monitoring
Mental health assessment
Oxygen therapy
Paracentesis
Parentage testing
Pelvic ultrasound
Peritoneovenous shunt
pH monitoring
Physical examination
Positron emission tomography
  (PET)
Sentinel lymph node biopsy
Temperature measurement
Tumor marker tests
Ultrasound
Weight management

Drugs

Acetaminophen
Adrenergic drugs
Analgesics
Analgesics, opioid
Anesthesia evaluation
Anesthesia, general
Anesthesia, local

Antianxiety drugs
Antibiotics
Antibiotics, topical
Antihypertensive drugs
Antinausea drugs
Antiseptics
Aspirin
Barbiturates
Cephalosporins
Corticosteroids
Diuretics
Erythromycins
Fluoroquinolones
Immunosuppressant drugs
Muscle relaxants
Nonsteroidal anti-inflammatory drugs
Prophylaxis, antibiotic
Proton pump inhibitors
Scopolamine patch
Sedation, conscious
Sulfonamides
Tetracyclines

Related Issues & Topics

Admission to the hospital
Adult day care
Ambulatory surgery centers
Anesthesiologist's role
Aseptic technique
Bandages and dressings
Body temperature

Closures: stitches, staples, and glue
Death and dying
Discharge from the hospital
Do not resuscitate (DNR) order
Drug-resistant organisms
Exercise
Fibrin sealants
Finding a surgeon
Health care proxy
Health history
Health Maintenance Organization (HMO)Home care
Hospice
Hospital services
Hospital-acquired infections
Incision care
Informed consent
Intensive care unit
Intensive care unit equipment
Length of hospital stay
Living will
Long-term care insurance
Managed care plans
Medicaid
Medical charts
Medical co-morbidities
Medical errors
Medicare
Medication Monitoring
Mental health assessment
Negative pressure rooms
Nursing homes
Operating room

Pain management
Patient confidentiality
Patient rights
Patient-controlled analgesia
Pediatric concerns
Planning a hospital stay
Postoperative care
Post-surgical infections
Post-surgical pain
Power of attorney
Preoperative care
Preparing for surgery
Presurgical testing
Private insurance plans
Recovery at home
Recovery room
Reoperation
Second opinion
Smoking cessation
Stethoscope
Surgical instruments
Surgical mesh
Surgical oncology
Surgical risk
Surgical team
Surgical training
Surgical triage
Syringe and needle
Talking to the doctor
Thermometer
Trocars
Vital signs
Wound care
Wound culture

PLEASE READ—IMPORTANT INFORMATION

The *Gale Encyclopedia of Surgery and Medical Tests, 2nd Edition* is a health reference product designed to inform and educate readers about a wide variety of surgeries, tests, diseases and conditions, treatments and drugs, equipment, and other issues associated with surgical and medical practice. Cengage Learning believes the product to be comprehensive, but not necessarily definitive. It is intended to supplement, not replace, consultation with physicians or other healthcare practitioners. While Cengage Learning has made substantial efforts to provide information that is accurate, comprehensive, and up-to-date, Cengage Learning makes no representations or warranties of any kind, including without limitation, warranties of merchantability or fitness for a particular purpose, nor does it guarantee the accuracy, comprehensiveness, or timeliness of the information contained in this product. Readers should be aware that the universe of medical knowledge is constantly growing and changing, and that differences of opinion exist among authorities. Readers are also advised to seek professional diagnosis and treatment for any medical condition, and to discuss information obtained from this book with their healthcare provider.

INTRODUCTION

The *Gale Encyclopedia of Surgery and Medical Tests, 2nd Edition* is a unique and invaluable source of information. This collection of 535 entries provides in-depth coverage of various issues related to surgery, medical tests, diseases and conditions, hospitalization, and general health care. These entries generally follow a standard format, including a definition, purpose, demographics, description, diagnosis/preparation, aftercare, precautions, risks, side effects, interactions, morbidity and mortality rates, alternatives, normal results, questions to ask your doctor, and information about who performs the procedures and where they are performed. Topics of a more general nature related to surgical hospitalization and medical testing round out the set. Examples of this coverage include entries on Adult day care, Ambulatory surgery centers, Death and dying, Discharge from the hospital, Do not resuscitate (DNR) order, Exercise, Finding a surgeon, Hospice, Hospital services, Informed consent, Living will, Long-term care insurance, Managed care plans, Medicaid, Medicare, Patient rights, Planning a hospital stay, Power of attorney, Private insurance plans, Second opinion, Talking to the doctor, and others.

Scope

The *Gale Encyclopedia of Surgery and Medical Tests, 2nd Edition* covers a wide variety of topics relevant to the user. Entries follow a standardized format that provides information at a glance. Rubrics include the following (not every entry will make use of all of them):

- Definition
- Description
- Purpose
- Demographics
- Diagnosis/preparation
- Aftercare
- Precautions
- Risks
- Side effects
- Interactions
- Morbidity and mortality rates
- Alternatives
- Normal results
- "Questions to ask the doctor"
- "Who performs the procedure and where is it performed?"
- Resources
- Key Terms

Inclusion criteria

A preliminary list of topics was compiled from a wide variety of sources, including health reference books, general medical encyclopedias, and consumer health guides. The advisory board evaluated the topics and made suggestions for inclusion. Final selection of topics to include was made by the advisory board in conjunction with the editor.

About the contributors

The essays were compiled by experienced medical writers, including medical doctors, pharmacists, and registered nurses. The advisers reviewed the completed essays to ensure that they are appropriate, up-to-date, and accurate.

How to use this book

The *Gale Encyclopedia of Surgery and Medical Tests, 2nd Edition* has been designed with ready reference in mind.

- Straight **alphabetical arrangement** of topics allows users to locate information quickly.

- **Bold-faced terms** within entries direct the reader to related articles.

- **Cross-references** placed throughout the encyclopedia direct readers from alternate names and related topics to entries.

- A list of **Key terms** is provided where appropriate to define terms or concepts that may be unfamiliar to the user. A **glossary** of key terms in the back of the fourth volume contains a concise list of terms arranged alphabetically.

- The **Resources** section directs readers to additional sources of information on a topic.

- Valuable **contact information** for health organizations is included with most entries. An Appendix of **organizations** in the back of the fourth volume contains an extensive list of organizations arranged alphabetically.

- A comprehensive **general index** guides readers to significant topics mentioned in the text.

Graphics

The *Gale Encyclopedia of Surgery and Medical Tests, 2nd Edition* is also enhanced by color photographs, illustrations, and tables.

Acknowledgements

The editor wishes to thank all of the people who contributed to this encyclopedia. There are too many names to list here, so the reader is urged to review the Advisory board and Contributors pages for the list of writers, physicians, and health-care experts to whom he is indebted. Special thanks must go to Rosalyn Carson-DeWitt for all the writing, updating, and advising she did; the project could not have been completed without her. L. Fleming Fallon provided invaluable assistance at every step of the way; his writing, advice, and good humor made this project a pleasure. Laurie Cataldo's expertise in so many areas helped make this book as good as it is. And Maria Basile provided not only many beautifully written entries, but she performed some last-minute review work for which the editor is most grateful. To all of you, my deepest thanks.

ADVISORS

A number of experts in the medical community provided invaluable assistance in the formulation of this encyclopedia. Our advisory board performed a myriad of duties, from defining the scope of coverage to reviewing individual entries for accuracy and accessibility. The editor would like to express his appreciation to them.

Rosalyn Carson-DeWitt, MD
Medical Writer
Durham, NC

Laura Jean Cataldo, RN, EdD
Nurse, Medical Consultant,
*   Educator*
Germantown, MD

L. Fleming Fallon, Jr, MD, DrPH
Professor of Public Health

Bowling Green State University
Bowling Green, OH

Chitra Venkatasubramanian, MD
Clinical Assistant Professor,
*   Neurology and Neurological*
*   Sciences*
Stanford University School of
    Medicine
Palo Alto, CA

CONTRIBUTORS

Laurie Barclay, MD
Neurological Consulting
  Services
Tampa, FL

Jeanine Barone
Nutritionist, Exercise Physiologist
New York, NY

Julia Barrett
Science Writer
Madison, WI

Donald G. Barstow, RN
Clinical Nurse Specialist
Oklahoma City, OK

Maria Basile, PhD
Neuropharmacologist
Roselle, NJ

Mary Bekker
Medical Writer
Willow Grove, PA

**Mark A. Best, MD, MPH,
  MBA**
Associate Professor of Pathology
St. Matthew's University
Grand Cayman, BWI

Randall J. Blazic, MD, DDS
Oral and Maxillofacial Surgeon
Goodyear, AZ

Robert Bockstiegel
Medical Writer
Portland, OR

Maggie Boleyn, RN, BSN
Medical Writer
Oak Park, MN

Susan Joanne Cadwallader
Medical Writer
Cedarburg, WI

Diane M. Calabrese
*Medical Sciences and Technology
  Writer*
Silver Spring, MD

Richard H. Camer
Editor
International Medical News Group
Silver Spring, MD

Rosalyn Carson-DeWitt, MD
Medical Writer
Durham, NC

Laura Jean Cataldo, RN, EdD
*Nurse, Medical Consultant,
  Educator*
Germantown, MD

Lisa Christenson, Ph.D.
Science Writer
Hamden, CT

Rhonda Cloos, RN
Medical Writer
Austin, TX

Constance Clyde
Medical Writer
Dana Point, CA

Angela M. Costello
Medical writer
Cleveland, OH

L. Lee Culvert, PhD
Health writer
Alna, ME

Tish Davidson, AM
Medical Writer
Fremont, CA

Lori De Milto
Medical Writer
Sicklerville, NJ

Victoria E. DeMoranville
Medical Writer
Lakeville, MA

Altha Roberts Edgren
Medical Writer
Medical Ink
St. Paul, MN

Lorraine K. Ehresman
Medical Writer
Northfield, Quebec, Canada

Abraham F. Ettaher, MD

**L. Fleming Fallon, Jr, MD,
  DrPH**
Professor of Public Health
Bowling Green State
  University
Bowling Green, OH

Paula Ford-Martin
Medical Writer
Warwick, RI

Janie F. Franz
Journalist
Grand Forks, ND

Rebecca J. Frey, PhD
Medical Writer
New Haven, CT

Debra Gordon
Medical Writer
Nazareth, PA

Jill Granger, MS
Sr. Research Associate
Dept. of Pathology
University of Michigan Medical
  Center
Ann Arbor, MI

Peter Gregutt
Medical Writer
Asheville, NC

Laith Farid Gulli, MD, MS
Consultant Psychotherapist in Private Practice
Lathrup Village, MI

Stephen John Hage, AAAS, RT(R), FAHRA
Medical Writer
Chatsworth, CA

Maureen Haggerty
Medical Writer
Ambler, PA

Robert Harr
Associate Professor and Chair
Department of Public and Allied Health
Bowling Green State University
Bowling Green, OH

Dan Harvey
Medical Writer
Wilmington, DE

Katherine Hauswirth, APRN
Medical Writer
Deep River, CT

Caroline A. Helwick
Medical Writer
New Orleans, LA

Lisette Hilton
Medical Writer
Boca Raton, FL

Fran Hodgkins
Medical Writer
Sparks, MD

René A. Jackson, RN
Medical Writer
Port Charlotte, FL

Nadine M. Jacobson, RN
Medical Writer
Takoma Park, MD

Randi B. Jenkins, BA
Copy Chief
Fission Communications
New York, NY

Michelle L. Johnson, MS, JD
Patent Attorney
ZymoGenetics, Inc.
Seattle, WA

Paul Johnson
Medical Writer
San Diego, CA

Cindy L. A. Jones, PhD
Biomedical Writer
Sagescript Communications
Lakewood, CO

Linda D. Jones, BA, PBT (ASCP)
Medical Writer
Asheboro, NY

Crystal H. Kaczkowski, MSc
Health writer
Chicago, IL

Beth A. Kapes
Medical Writer
Bay Village, OH

Mary Jeanne Krob, MD, FACS
Physician, writer
Pittsburgh, PA

Monique Laberge, PhD
Sr. Res. Investigator
Dept. of Biochemistry & Biophysics, School of Medicine
University of Pennsylvania
Philadelphia, PA

Richard H. Lampert
Senior Medical Editor
W.B. Saunders Co.
Philadelphia, PA

Renee Laux, MS
Medical Writer
Manlius, NY

Victor Leipzig, PhD
Biological Consultant
Huntington Beach, CA

Lorraine Lica, PhD
Medical Writer
San Diego, CA

John T. Lohr, PhD
Assistant Director, Biotechnology Center
Utah State University
Logan, UT

Jennifer Lee Losey, RN
Medical Writer
Madison Heights, MI

Nicole Mallory, MS, PA-C
Medical Student, Wayne State University
Detroit, MI

Jacqueline N. Martin, MS
Medical Writer
Albrightsville, PA

Nancy McKenzie, PhD
Public Health Consultant
Brooklyn, NY

Mercedes McLaughlin
Medical Writer
Phoenixville, CA

Miguel A. Melgar, MD, PhD
Neurosurgeon
New Orleans, LA

Christine Miner Minderovic, BS, RT, RDMS
Medical Writer
Ann Arbor, MI

Mark Mitchell, MD, MPH, MBA
Medical Writer
Bothell, WA

Alfredo Mori, MD, FACEM, FFAEM
Emergency Physician
The Alfred Hospital
Victoria, Australia

Bilal Nasser, MD, MS
Senior Medical Student, Wayne State University
Detroit, MI

Erika J. Norris
Medical Writer
Oak Harbor, WA

Teresa Norris, RN
Medical Writer
Ute Park, NM

Debra Novograd, BS, RT(R)(M)
Medical Writer
Royal Oak, MI

Jane E. Phillips, PhD
Medical Writer
Chapel Hill, NC

J. Ricker Polsdorfer, MD
Medical Writer
Phoenix, AZ

Elaine R. Proseus, MBA/TM, BSRT, RT(R)
Medical Writer
Farmington Hills, MI

Robert Ramirez, BS
Medical Student
University of Medicine & Dentistry of New Jersey
Stratford, NJ

Esther Csapo Rastegari, RN, BSN, EdM
Medical Writer
Holbrook, MA

Martha Reilly, OD
Clinical Optometrist, Medical Writer
Madison, WI

Toni Rizzo
Medical Writer
Salt Lake City, UT

Richard Robinson
Medical Writer
Sherborn, MA

Nancy Ross-Flanigan
Science Writer
Belleville, MI

Belinda Rowland, PhD
Medical Writer
Voorheesville, NY

Laura Ruth, PhD
Medical, Science, & Technology Writer
Los Angeles, CA

Uchechukwu Sampson, MD, MPH, MBA

Kausalya Santhanam, PhD
Technical Writer
Branford, CT

Joan M. Schonbeck
Medical Writer
Nursing
Massachusetts Department of Mental Health
Marlborough, MA

Stephanie Dionne Sherk
Medical Writer
University of Michigan
Ann Arbor, MI

Lee A. Shratter, MD
Consulting Radiologist
Kentfield, CA

Jennifer E. Sisk, MA
Medical Writer
Havertown, PA

Allison Joan Spiwak, MSBME
Circulation Technologist
The Ohio State University
Columbus, OH

Kurt Richard Sternlof
Science Writer
New Rochelle, NY

Margaret A Stockley, RGN
Medical Writer
Boxborough, MA

Dorothy Elinor Stonely
Medical Writer
Los Gatos, CA

Bethany Thivierge
Biotechnical Writer and Editor
Technicality Resources
Rockland, ME

Carol A. Turkington
Medical Writer
Lancaster, PA

Samuel D. Uretsky, PharmD
Medical Writer
Wantagh, NY

Chitra Venkatasubramanian, MD
Clinical Assistant Professor, Neurology and Neurological Sciences
Stanford University School of Medicine
Palo Alto, CA

Ellen S. Weber, MSN
Medical Writer
Fort Wayne, IN

Barbara Wexler
Medical Writer
Chatsworth, CA

Abby Wojahn, RN, BSN, CCRN
Medical Writer
Milwaukee, WI

Kathleen D. Wright, RN
Medical Writer
Delmar, DE

Mary Zoll, PhD
Science Writer
Newton Center, MA

Michael Zuck, PhD
Medical Writer
Boulder, CO

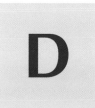

D

D & C *see* **Dilatation and curettage**

Death and dying

Definition

Death is the end of life, a permanent cessation of all vital functions. Dying refers to the body's preparation for death, which may be very short in the case of accidental death, or can last weeks or months in some patients such as those suffering from cancer.

Description

Risks of surgery

Specific risks vary from surgery to surgery and should be discussed with a physician. All surgeries and every administration of anesthesia have some risks; they are dependent upon many factors including the type of surgery and the medical condition of the patient. The patient should ask the anesthesiologist about any risks that may be associated with the anesthesia. Specific standards are set by the American Society of Anesthesiologists to enhance the safety and quality of anesthesia before surgery, basic methods of monitoring patients during surgery, and the best patient care during recovery.

Overwhelming data compiled in 2001 has confirmed that albumin is an effective marker of general nutrition; low albumin levels can increase the likelihood of post-surgery complications such as pneumonia, infection, and the inability to wean from a ventilator, by as much as 50%. In a national study of 54,000 surgery patients (average age of 61 years old), it was found that only one in five surgical patients were tested for low albumin before their operations.

In a study of 2,989 hospitalized patients admitted for more than one day, risk factors such as cholesterol levels (primarily low levels of high-density lipoprotein,

HDL) and low serum albumin were associated with in-hospital death, infection, and length of stay. During the study follow-up, 62 (2%) of the patients died, 382 (13%) developed a nosocomial infection, and 257 (9%) developed a surgical site infection.

The National Veterans Affairs Surgical Risk Study was conducted in 44 Veterans Affairs Medical Centers and included 87,078 major noncardiac operations performed under general, spinal, or epidural anesthesia. Patient risk factors predictive of postoperative death included serum albumin level, American Society of Anesthesia class, emergency operation, and 31 additional preoperative variables.

Other factors related to death during surgery are: increasing age, **emergency surgery**, and general postoperative complications including cardiac, renal, and pulmonary complications. Age-related changes in the immune system play a significant role in the increased risk of infection, decreased ability to fight diseases, and slower wound healing after surgery. An aging body is more susceptible to subsequent infections because of previous illness or surgery and the subsequent weakening of the immune system. The anti-inflammatory medications (e.g., to control conditions such as arthritis) that many older people take are also known to slow wound healing.

One study found that risk of death during **coronary artery bypass graft surgery** is associated with hospital volume, i.e., the number of surgeries performed. High volume hospitals had a lower mortality rate during surgery. Mortality decreased with increasing volume of surgeries performed (3.6% in low [less than 500 cases], 3% in moderate [500-1,000 cases], and 2% in high [over 1,000 cases] volume hospitals). Thus, the volume of surgeries performed may be an important consideration when selecting a hospital.

Complications of surgery

The most common complications to surgery that can prove fatal are infection, bleeding, and complications of anesthesia.

KEY TERMS

Anesthesia—Loss of sensation and usually of consciousness without loss of vital functions artificially produced by the administration of one or more agents that block the passage of pain impulses along nerve pathways to the brain.

Anesthesiologist—A physician specializing in administering anesthesia.

Electrocautery—The use of a low-voltage electrified probe used to remove tissue through cauterization (burning).

Endoscopic—Of, relating to, or performed by means of an endoscope or endoscopy.

Euthanasia—To bring about the death of another person who has an incurable disease or condition.

High-density lipoprotein—A cholesterol-poor, protein-rich lipoprotein of blood plasma correlated with reduced risk of atherosclerosis.

Nosocomial—Originating or taking place in a hospital.

Percutaneous—Effected or performed through the skin.

Serum albumin—A crystallizable albumin or mixture of albumins that normally constitutes more than half of the protein in blood serum and serves to maintain the osmotic pressure of the blood.

The Joint Commission's Board of Commissioners reviewed 64 cases related to operative and post-operative complications since the late 1990s. Of the events reviewed, 84% of the complications resulted in patient deaths, while 16% resulted in a serious injury. All of the cases occurred in acute care hospitals; cases directly related to medication errors or to the administration of anesthesia were excluded. Of these complications, 58% occurred during the postoperative procedure period, 23% during intra-operative procedures, 13% during post-anesthesia recovery, and 6% during anesthesia induction.

The following types of procedures were most frequently associated with these reported complications:

- endoscopy and/or interventional imaging
- catheter or tube insertion
- open abdominal surgery
- head and neck surgery
- thoracic surgery
- orthopedic surgery

Of the 64 cases reviewed, 90% occurred in relation to non-emergent (elective or scheduled) procedures. The most frequent complications by type of procedure included the following:

- Naso-gastric/feeding tube insertion into the trachea or a bronchus.
- Massive fluid overload from absorption of irrigation fluids during genito-urinary/gynecological procedures.
- Endoscopic procedures (including non-gastrointestinal procedures) with perforation of adjacent organs. Of all abdominal and thoracic endoscopic surgery, liver lacerations were among the most common complications.
- Central venous catheter insertion into an artery.
- Burns from electrocautery used with a flammable prep solution.
- Open orthopedic procedures associated with acute respiratory failure, including cardiac arrest in the operating room.
- Imaging-directed percutaneous biopsy or tube placement resulting in liver laceration, peritonitis, or respiratory arrest while temporarily off prescribed oxygen.

Complications associated with misplacement of tubes or catheters usually involved a failure to confirm the position of the tube or catheter, a failure to communicate the results of the confirmation procedure, or misinterpretation of the radiographic image by a non-radiologist.

Preparing for death or incapacitation legally

An advance directive is a way to allow caregivers to know a patient's wishes, should the patient become unable to make a medical decision. The hospital must be told about a patient's advance directive at the time of admission. Description of the type of care for different levels of illness should be in an advance directive. For instance, a patient may wish to have or not to have a certain type of care in the case of terminal or critical illness or unconsciousness. An advance directive will protect the patient's wishes in these matters.

A **living will** is one type of advance directive and may take effect when a patient has been deemed terminally ill. Terminal illness in general assumes a life span of six months or less. A living will allows a patient to outline treatment options without interference from an outside party.

A durable **power of attorney** for health care (DPA) is similar to a living will; however, it takes effect any time unconsciousness or inability to make informed medical decisions is present. A family member or friend is stipulated in the DPA to make medical decisions on behalf of the patient.

While both living wills and DPAs are legal in most states, there are some states that do not officially recognize these documents. However, they may still be used to guide families and doctors in treatment wishes.

Do-not-resuscitate (DNR) orders can be incorporated into an advance directive or by informing hospital staff. Unless instructions for a DNR are in effect, hospital staff will make every effort to help patients whose hearts have stopped or who have stopped breathing. DNR orders are recognized in all states and will be incorporated into a patient's medical chart if requested. Patients who benefit from a **DNR order** are those who have terminal or other debilitating illnesses. It is recommended that a patient who has not already been considered unable to make sound medical decisions discuss this option with his or her physician.

None of the above documents are complicated. They may be simple statements of desires for medical care options. If they are not completed by an attorney, they should be notarized and a copy should be given to the doctor, as well as to a trusted family member.

Mourning and grieving among cultures

The death of a loved one is a severe trauma, and the grief that follows is a natural and important part of life. No two people grieve exactly the same way, and cultural differences play a significant part in the grieving process. For many, however, the most immediate response is shock, numbness, and disbelief. Physical reactions may include shortness of breath, heart palpitations, sweating, and dizziness. At other times, there may be reactions such as loss of energy, sleeplessness or increase in sleep, changes in appetite, or stomach aches. Susceptibility to common illnesses, nightmares, and dreams about the deceased are not unusual during the grieving period.

Emotional reactions are as individual as physical reactions. A preoccupation with the image of the deceased, feelings of fear, hostility, apathy, emptiness, and even fear of one's own death, may occur. Depression, diminished sex drive, sadness, and anger at the deceased may occur. Bereavement may cause short- or long-term changes in the family unit and other relationships of the bereaved.

It is important for the bereaved to work through their feelings and not avoid their emotions. If emotions and feelings are not discussed with family members, friends, or primary support groups, then a therapist should be consulted to assist with the process.

Various cultures and religions view death in different manners and conduct mourning rituals according to their own traditions. In most cultures, visitors often come to express their condolences to the family and to bid farewell to the deceased. At times, funeral services are private. Various ethnic groups host a gathering after the funeral for those who attended. It is common for these events to become a celebration of the life of the deceased, which also helps the bereaved to begin the mourning process positively. Memories are often exchanged and toasts made in memory of the deceased. Knowing how much a loved one is cherished and remembered by friends and family is a comfort to those who experience the loss. Other methods of condolences include sending flowers to the home or the funeral parlor; sending a mass card, sending a donation to a charity that the family has chosen; or bringing a meal to the family during the weeks after the death.

Resources

BOOKS

Beauchamp, Daniel R., Mark B. Evers, Kenneth L. Mattox, Courtney M. Townsend, and David C. Sabiston, eds. *Sabiston Textbook of Surgery: The Biological Basis of Modern Surgical Practice.* 16th ed. London: W. B. Saunders Co., 2001.

Coberly, Margaret. *Sacred Passage: How to Provide Fearless, Compassionate Care for the Dying.* Boston: Shambhala Publications, 2002.

Heffner, John E., Ira R. Byock, and Lra Byock, eds. *Palliative and End-of-Life Pearls.* Philadelphia: Hanley and Belfus, Inc., 2002.

Kubler-Ross, Elisabeth, and David Kessler. *Life Lessons: Two Experts on Death and Dying Teach Us About the Mysteries of Life and Living.* New York: Scribner, 2000.

Soto, Gary. *The Afterlife.* Orlando, FL: Harcourt Children's Books, 2003.

Staton, Jana, Roger Shuy, and Ira Byock. *A Few Months to Live: Different Paths to Life's End* Baltimore, MD: Georgetown University Press, 2001.

Sweitzer, Bobbie Jean, ed. *Handbook of Preoperative Assessment and Management.* Philadelphia: Lippincott Williams & Wilkins, 2000.

PERIODICALS

Byock, Ira, and Steven H. Miles. "Hospice Benefits and Phase I Cancer Trials." *Annals of Internal Medicine* 138, no. 4 (February 2003): 335–337.

Smykowski, L., and W. Rodriguez. "The Post Anesthesia Care Unit Experience: A Family-centered Approach." *Journal of Nursing Care Quality* 18, no. 1 (January-March 2003): 5–15.

ORGANIZATIONS

American College of Physicians—American Society of Internal Medicine, 190 N. Independence Mall West, Philadelphia, PA 19106-1572. Washington Office: 2011 Pennsylvania Avenue NW, Suite 800, Washington, DC 20006-1837. (202) 261-4500 or (800) 338-2746. http://www.acponline.org.

Hospice Foundation of America, 2001 "S" Street, NW, Suite 300, Washington, DC 20009. (800) 854-3402 or (202) 638-5419. Fax: (202) 638-5312. Email: jon@hospice foundation.org. www.hospicefoundation.org.

Inter-Institutional Collaborating Network on End-of-Life Care (IICN). (415) 863-3045. http://www.growthhouse.org.

National Institutes of Health, 9000 Rockville Pike, Bethesda, MD 20892. (301) 496-4000. Email: NIHInfo@OD.NIH.GOV. http://www.nih.gov/.

Promoting Excellence in End of Life Care, RWJ Foundation National Program Office, c/o The Practical Ethics Center, The University of Montana, 1000 East Beckwith Avenue, Missoula, MT 59812. (406) 243-6601. Fax: (406) 243-6633. Email: excell@selway.umt.edu. http://www.promotingexcellence.org.

Washington Home Center for Palliative Care Studies(CPCS), 4200 Wisconsin Avenue, NW, 4th Floor, Washington, DC 20016. (202) 895-2625. Fax: (202) 966-5410. Email: info@medicaring.org. http://www.medicaring.org.

OTHER

American College of Physicians. "How to Help During the Final Weeks of Life." *ACP Home Care Guide for Advanced Cancer.* [cited March 2, 2003]. http://www.acponline.org/public/h_care/7-final.htm.

American College of Physicians. "What to Do Before and After the Moment of Death." *ACP Home Care Guide.* [cited March 2, 2003]. http://www.acponline.org/public/h_care/8-moment.htm.

Byock, Ira, M.D. *DyingWell.org.* [cited March 2, 2003]. http://www.dyingwell.org/default.htm.

Kubler-Ross, Elisabeth, and Carol Bilger. *On Death and Dying: What the Dying Have to Teach Doctors, Nurses, Clergy, and Their Own Family.* (Audio Cassette, Abridged edition.) New York: Audio Renaissance, 2000.

Jacqueline N. Martin, M.S.
Crystal H. Kaczkowski, M.Sc.

Debridement

Definition

Debridement is the process of removing dead (necrotic) tissue or foreign material from and around a wound to expose healthy tissue.

Purpose

An open wound or ulcer can not be properly evaluated until the dead tissue or foreign matter is removed. Wounds that contain necrotic and ischemic (low oxygen content) tissue take longer to close and heal. This is because necrotic tissue provides an ideal growth medium for bacteria, especially for *Bacteroides* spp. and *Clostridium perfringens* that causes the gas gangrene so feared in military medical practice. Though a wound may not necessarily be infected, the bacteria can cause inflammation and strain the body's ability to fight infection. Debridement is also used to treat pockets of pus called abscesses. Abscesses can develop into a general infection that may invade the bloodstream (sepsis) and lead to **amputation** and even **death**. Burned tissue or tissue exposed to corrosive substances tends to form a hard black crust, called an eschar, while deeper tissue remains moist and white, yellow and soft, or flimsy and inflamed. Eschars may also require debridement to promote healing.

Description

The four major debridement techniques are surgical, mechanical, chemical, and autolytic.

Surgical debridement

Surgical debridement (also known as sharp debridement) uses a scalpel, scissors, or other instrument to cut necrotic tissue from a wound. It is the quickest and most efficient method of debridement. It is the preferred method if there is rapidly developing inflammation of the body's connective tissues (cellulitis) or a more generalized infection (sepsis) that has entered the bloodstream. The physician starts by flushing the area with a saline (salt water) solution, and then applies a topical anesthetic or antalgic gel to the edges of the wound to minimize pain. Using forceps to grip the dead tissue, the physician cuts it away bit by bit with a scalpel or scissors. Sometimes it is necessary to leave some dead tissue behind rather than disturb living tissue. The physician may repeat the process again at another session.

Mechanical debridement

In mechanical debridement, a saline-moistened dressing is allowed to dry overnight and adhere to the dead tissue. When the dressing is removed, the dead tissue is pulled away too. This process is one of the oldest methods of debridement. It can be very painful because the dressing can adhere to living as well as nonliving tissue. Because mechanical debridement cannot select between good and bad tissue, it is an unacceptable debridement method for clean wounds where a new layer of healing cells is already developing.

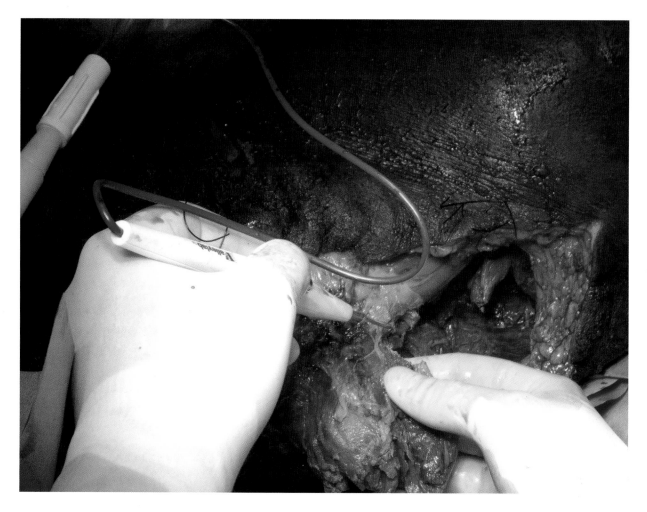

A surgeon using electrocautery to perform debridement of necrotic muscle. *(Barry Slaven, MD, PhD,/Phototake. Reproduced by permission.)*

Chemical debridement

Chemical debridement makes use of certain enzymes and other compounds to dissolve necrotic tissue. It is more selective than mechanical debridement. In fact, the body makes its own enzyme, collagenase, to break down collagen, one of the major building blocks of skin. A pharmaceutical version of collagenase is available and is highly effective as a debridement agent. As with other debridement techniques, the area first is flushed with saline. Any crust of dead tissue is etched in a cross-hatched pattern to allow the enzyme to penetrate. A topical antibiotic is also applied to prevent introducing infection into the bloodstream. A moist dressing is then placed over the wound.

Autolytic debridement

Autolytic debridement takes advantage of the body's own ability to dissolve dead tissue. The key to the technique is keeping the wound moist, which can be accomplished with a variety of **dressings**. These dressings help to trap wound fluid that contains growth factors, enzymes, and immune cells that promote wound healing. Autolytic debridement is more selective than any other debridement method, but it also takes the longest to work. It is inappropriate for wounds that have become infected.

Biological debridement

Maggot therapy is a form of biological debridement known since antiquity. The larvae of *Lucilia sericata* (greenbottle fly) are applied to the wound as these organisms can digest necrotic tissue and pathogenic bacteria. The method is rapid and selective, although patients are usually reluctant to submit to the procedure.

Diagnosis/Preparation

The physician or nurse will begin by assessing the need for debridement. The wound will be examined,

KEY TERMS

Abscess—A localized collection of pus buried in tissues or organs that may or may not discharge and usually results from an infectious process.

Anaerobic—Pertaining to a microorganism that either does not use oxygen or actually cannot live in the presence of oxygen.

Antalgic—Medication that alleviates pain.

Bacteroides—A family of anaerobic, rod-shaped bacteria. Its organisms are normal inhabitants of the oral, respiratory, intestinal, and urogenital cavities of humans, animals, and insects. Some species are infectious agents.

Eschar—A hardened dry crust that forms on skin exposed to burns or corrosive agents.

Gangrene—Death of tissue, usually in considerable mass and generally associated with loss of blood supply and followed by bacterial infection and decomposition.

Gas gangrene—A severe form of gangrene caused by *Clostridium* infection.

Hypoxia—Reduction of oxygen supply to tissues below physiological requirements despite adequate perfusion of the tissue by blood.

Ischemic—Tissue that has a low oxygen supply due to obstruction of the arterial blood supply or inadequate blood flow.

Necrotic—Affected with necrosis (cell death).

Pressure ulcer—Also known as a decubitus ulcer, pressure ulcers are open wounds that form whenever prolonged pressure is applied to skin covering bony outcrops of the body. Patients who are bedridden are at risk of developing pressure ulcers, commonly known as bedsores.

Sepsis—A severe systemic infection in which bacteria have entered the bloodstream.

WHO PERFORMS THE PROCEDURE AND WHERE IS IT PERFORMED?

Debridement is performed by physicians such as plastic surgeons, dermatologists or surgeons, depending on the condition requiring the procedure. General physicians and surgeons are all trained in debridement techniques and they usually perform debridement procedures. Nurses specializing in wound care are prepared to perform conservative sharp wound debridement once they have satisfactorily completed didactic and clinical instruction in the sharp debridement procedure from an accredited agency, wound management specialty course, or an approved course in debridement.

Surgical debridement is usually performed on an outpatient basis or at the bedside. If the target tissue is deep or close to another organ, however, or if the patient is experiencing extreme pain, the procedure may be done in an operating room.

---

frequently by inserting a gloved finger into the wound to estimate the depth of dead tissue and evaluate whether it lies close to other organs, bone, or important body features. The assessment addresses the following points:

- the nature of the necrotic or ischemic tissue and the best debridement procedure to follow
- the risk of spreading infection and the use of antibiotics
- the presence of underlying medical conditions causing the wound

- the extent of ischemia in the wound tissues
- the location of the wound in the body
- the type of pain management to be used during the procedure

Before surgical or mechanical debridement, the area may be flushed with a saline solution, and an antalgic cream or injection may be applied. If the antalgic cream is used, it is usually applied over the exposed area some 90 minutes before the procedure.

Aftercare

After surgical debridement, the wound is usually packed with a dry dressing for a day to control bleeding. Afterward, moist dressings are applied to promote wound healing. Moist dressings are also used after mechanical, chemical, and autolytic debridement. Many factors contribute to wound healing, which frequently can take considerable time. Debridement may need to be repeated.

Risks

It is possible that underlying tendons, blood vessels or other structures may be damaged during the examination of the wound and during surgical debridement. Surface bacteria may also be introduced deeper into the body, causing infection.

Normal results

Removal of dead tissue from pressure ulcers and other wounds speeds healing. Although these procedures cause some pain, they are generally well tolerated by patients and can be managed more aggressively. It is not uncommon to debride a wound again in a subsequent session.

Alternatives

Adjunctive therapies include electrotherapy and low laser irradiation. However, at present, insufficient research has been completed to recommend their general use.

Not all wounds need debridement. Sometimes it is better to leave a hardened crust of dead tissue (eschar), than to remove it and create an open wound, particularly if the crust is stable and the wound is not inflamed. Before performing debridement, the physician will take a medical history with attention to factors that might complicate healing, such as medications being taken and smoking. The physician will also note the cause of the wound and the ways it has been treated. Some ulcers and other wounds occur in places where blood flow is impaired, for example, the foot ulcers that can accompany diabetes mellitus. In such cases, the physician or nurse may decide not to debride the wound because blood flow may be insufficient for proper healing.

Resources

BOOKS

Falanga, V., and K. G. Harding, eds. *The Clinical Relevance of Wound Bed Preparation*. New York: Springer Verlag, 2002.

Harper, Michael S. *Debridement*. Berkeley, CA: Paradigm Press, 2001.

Maklebust, JoAnn and Mary Y. Sieggreen. *Pressure Ulcers: Guidelines for Prevention and Nursing Management*. 2nd ed. Springhouse, PA: Springhouse Corporation, 1996.

PERIODICALS

Dervin, G. F., I. G. Stiell, K. Rody, and J. Grabowski. "Effect of Arthroscopic Debridement for Osteoarthritis of the Knee on Health-Related Quality of Life." *The Journal of Bone and Joint Surgery (American)* 85-A (January 2003): 10–19.

Friberg, T. R., M. Ohji, J. J. Scherer, and Y. Tano. "Frequency of Epithelial Debridement During Diabetic Vitrectomy." *American Journal of Ophthalmology* 135 (April 2003): 553–554.

Reynolds, N., N. Cawrse, T. Burge, and J. Kenealy. "Debridement of a Mixed Partial and Full Thickness Burn With an Erbium: YAG Laser." *Burns* 29 (March 2003): 183–188.

Schirmer, B. D., A. D. Miller, and M. S. Miller. "Single Operative Debridement for Pancreatic Abscess." *Journal of Gastrointestinal Surgery* 7 (February 2003): 289.

Terzi, C., A. Bacakoglu, T. Unek, and M. H. Ozkan. "Chemical Necrotizing Fasciitis Due to Household Insecticide Injection: Is Immediate Radical Surgical Debridement Necessary?" *Human & Experimental Toxicology* 21 (December 2002): 687–690.

Wolff, H., and C. Hansson. "Larval Therapy—an Effective Method of Ulcer Debridement." *Clinical and Experimental Dermatology* 28 (March 2003): 134–137.

ORGANIZATIONS

American Academy of Wound Management. 1255 23rd St., NW, Washington, DC 20037. (202) 521-0368. http://www.aawm.org.

Wound Care Institute. 1100 N.E. 163rd Street, Suite #101, North Miami Beach, FL 33162. (305) 919-9192. <http://woundcare.org>.

OTHER

Moses, Scott. "Wound Debridement." *Family Practice Notebook*. February 12, 2003 [cited May 15, 2003]. http://www.fpnotebook.com/SUR12.htm.

"Types of Wound Debridement." Wound Care Information Network: Types of Wound Debridement. 2002 [cited May 15, 2003]. http://www.medicaledu.com/debridhp.htm.

Richard H. Camer
Monique Laberge, PhD

Decubitus ulcers *see* **Bedsores**

Deep brain stimulation

Definition

Deep brain stimulation (DBS) delivers a constant low electrical stimulation to a small region of the brain, through implanted electrodes connected to an implanted battery. It is used to partially restore

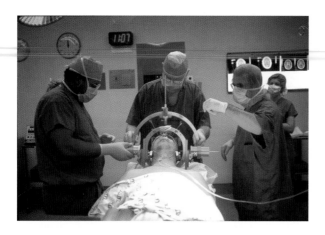

Deep brain stimulation. *(PHOTOTAKE Inc. / Alamy)*

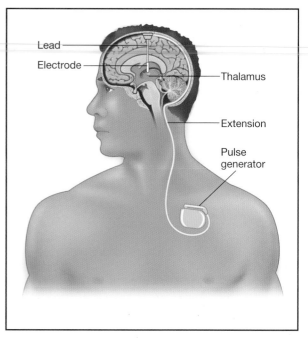

(Illustration by Electronic Illustrators Group.)

normal movements in Parkinson's disease, essential tremor, and dystonia.

Purpose

Parkinson's disease is due to degeneration of a group of cells called the substantia nigra. These cells interact with other brain regions to help control movement. The normal signals from the substantia nigra inhibit these other regions, and so when it degenerates, these regions become overactive. The electrical signals from the DBS electrodes mimic the inhibitory function of the substantia nigra, helping to restore more normal movements.

The substantia nigra normally releases the chemical dopamine, which exerts its inhibitory action on the globus pallidus interna (GPi) and the subthalamic nucleus (STN). For Parkinson's disease, deep brain stimulation is performed on these two centers. The target for DBS in dystonia is the GPi as well. Treatment of essential tremor usually targets the thalamus.

Each of these brain regions has two halves, which control movement on the opposite side of the body: right controls left, and left controls right. Unilateral DBS may be used if the symptoms are much more severe on one side. Bilateral DBS is used to treat symptoms on both sides.

Demographics

Parkinson's disease affects approximately one million Americans. The peak incidence is approximately age 62, but young-onset PD can occur as early as age 40. Because young-onset patients live with their disease for so many more years, they are more likely to become candidates for surgery than older-onset patients. In addition, younger patients tend to do better and suffer fewer adverse effects of surgery. Approximately 5% of older PD patients receive one form or another of PD

surgery. Many more develop the symptoms for which surgery may be effective, but either develop them at an advanced age, making surgery inadvisable, or decide the risks of surgery are not worth the potential benefit, or do not choose surgery for some other reason.

Essential tremor is more common than Parkinson's disease, but rarely becomes severe enough to require surgery. Dystonia is a very rare condition, and the number of patients who have received DBS as of 2003 is under 100.

Description

Deep brain stimulation relies on implanting a long thin electrode deep into the brain, through a hole in the top of the skull. In order to precisely locate the target area and to ensure the probe is precisely placed in the target, a "stereotactic frame" is used. This device is a rigid frame attached to the patient's head, providing an immobile three-dimensional coordinate system, which can be used to precisely track the location of the GPi or STN and the movement of the electrode.

For unilateral DBS, a single "burr hole" is made in the top of the skull. Bilateral DBS requires two holes. A strong topical anesthetic is used to numb the skin while this hole is drilled. Since there are no pain receptors in the brain, there is no need for deeper anesthetic. In addition, the patient must remain awake in order to report any sensory changes during the surgery. The electrode is placed very close to several important brain structures. Sensory changes during electrode placement may indicate the electrode is too close to one or more of these regions.

Once the burr hole is made, the surgeon inserts the electrode. Small electric currents from the electrode are used to more precisely locate the target. This is harmless, but may cause twitching, light flashes, or other sensations. A contrast dye may also be injected into the spinal fluid, which allows the surgeon to visualize the brain's structure using one or more imaging techniques. The patient will be asked to make various movements to assist in determining the location of the electrode.

The electrode is connected by a wire to an implanted pulse generator. This wire is placed under the scalp and skin. A small incision is made in the area of the collarbone, and the pulse generator is placed there. This portion of the procedure is performed under **general anesthesia**.

Diagnosis/Preparation

DBS for Parkinson's disease is considered as an option in a patient who is still responsive to levodopa (used to treat symptoms) but has developed motor complications. These include the rapid loss of benefit from a single dose (wearing off), unpredictable fluctuations in benefit (on-off), and uncontrolled abnormal movements (dyskinesias). Essential tremor patients who are candidates for surgery are those whose tremor is unsatisfactorily controlled by medications and whose tremor significantly impairs activities of daily living. Similar criteria apply for dystonia patients.

The patient who is a candidate for DBS discusses all the surgical options with his neurologist before deciding on deep brain stimulation. A full understanding of the risks and potential benefits must be understood before consenting to the surgery.

The patient will undergo a variety of medical tests, and one or more types of neuroimaging procedures, including MRI, CT scanning, **angiography** (imaging the brain's blood vessels) and ventriculography (imaging the brain's ventricles). On the day of the surgery, the stereotactic frame is fixed to the patient's head. A local anesthetic is used at the four sites where the frame's pins contact the head; there may nonetheless be some initial discomfort. A final MRI is done with the frame in place, to set the coordinates of the targeted area of the brain in relation to the frame.

The patient will receive a mild sedative to ease the anxiety of the procedure. Once the electrodes are positioned, the patient receives general anesthetic to implant the pulse generator.

WHO PERFORMS THE PROCEDURE AND WHERE IS IT PERFORMED?

Deep brain stimulation is performed by a neurosurgeon in a hospital.

Aftercare

The procedure is lengthy, and the patient will require a short hospital stay afterward to recover from the surgery. Following the procedure itself, the patient meets several times with the neurologist to adjust the stimulation. The pulse generator is programmable, and can be fine-tuned to the patient's particular needs. This can provide a higher degree of symptom relief than lesioning surgeries, but requires repeated visits to the neurologist. Pulse generator batteries must be replaced every three to five years. This is done with a small incision as an outpatient procedure. Since the generator is in the chest area, no additional brain surgery is required.

The patient's medications are adjusted after surgery, with a reduction in levodopa likely in most patients who receive DBS of the subthalamic nucleus.

Risks

Deep brain stimulation entails several risks. There are acute surgical risks, including hemorrhage and infection, and the risks of general anesthesia. The electrodes can be placed too close to other brain regions, which can lead to visual defects, speech problems, and other complications. These may be partially avoided by adjusting the stimulation settings after the procedure. Because a device is left implanted under the skin, there is the risk of breakage or malfunction, which requires surgical removal.

A patient with implanted electrodes must not receive diathermy therapy. Diathermy is the passage of radiowaves through the tissue to heat it, and is used as a physical therapy for muscle pain and other applications. Diathermy poses a risk of **death** in a patient with DBS electrodes.

Patients who are cognitively impaired may become more so after surgery, and cognitive impairment usually prevents a patient from undergoing surgery.

Normal results

Deep brain stimulation improves the movement disorder symptoms of Parkinson's disease by 25–75%, depending on the care of the placement and the ability to find the optimum settings. These improvements are seen most while off levodopa; DBS does little to improve the best response to levodopa treatment. Levodopa dose will likely be reduced, leading to a significant reduction in dyskinesias.

Morbidity and mortality rates

The rate of complications depends highly on the skill and experience of the **surgical team** performing the procedure. Rates from one of the most experienced teams, in a study of over 200 patients, were as follows.

Post-operative complications:

- asymptomatic intracranial bleed (10% of procedures)
- symptomatic intracranial bleed (2%)
- seizures (3%)
- headache (25%)
- infection (6%)

Device-related complications:

- lead replacements (9%)
- lead repositionings (8%)
- extension wire replacements (6%)
- implantable pulse generator replacements (17%), approximately half of which were due to malfunction

The risk of death is less than 1%.

Alternatives

Patients who are candidates for deep brain stimulation have usually been judged to require surgery for effective treatment of their symptoms. Other surgical alternatives for Parkinson's disease include **pallidotomy** and thalamotomy, which destroy brain tissue to achieve the same effect as the stimulation. Pallidotomy is rarely performed for Parkinson's disease, unless tremor is the only debilitating symptom. It is common in essential tremor. DBS for dystonia is the only really promising neurosurgical treatment for this condition. Some peripheral surgeries may be appropriate for selected patients.

Resources

BOOKS

Jahanshahi, M., and C. D. Marsden. *Parkinson's Disease: A Self-Help Guide.* New York: Demos Medical Press, 2000.

ORGANIZATIONS

National Parkinson's Disease Foundation. Bob Hope Parkinson Research Center, 1501 N.W. 9th Avenue, Bob Hope Road, Miami, FL 33136-1494. (305) 547-6666. (800) 327-4545. Fax: (305) 243-4403. http://www.parkinson.org.

WE MOVE, Worldwide Education and Awareness for Movement Disorders. 204 West 84th Street, New York, NY 10024. (800) 437-MOV2, Fax: (212) 875-8389. http://www.wemove.org.

Richard Robinson
Chitra Venkatasubramanian

Deep vein thrombosis *see* **Venous thrombosis prevention**

Defecography

Definition

Defecography is an imaging test in which x rays are taken of the rectum and anal canal during the course of defecation.

Purpose

Defecography is used to evaluate the muscles needed for bowel evacuation and the surrounding tissues. It is used during the evaluation of a number conditions, including:

- Intussusception
- **Rectal prolapse**
- Rectocele
- Enterocele
- Cystocele
- Vaginal prolapse
- Chronic constipation
- Fecal incontinence
- Anismus

Precautions

Patients must carefully follow directions regarding when to stop eating and drinking, and when to begin their bowel prep. Patients who are diabetic may

KEY TERMS

Anismus—Dysfunctional contraction or spasm of the muscle comprising the anal sphincter.

Constipation—Difficulty passing a bowel movement. May refer to infrequent passage of stool, or to a hard, dry stool requiring straining and physical effort in order to pass.

Cystocele—Sagging or bulging of the bladder through the front wall of the vagina.

Enterocele—Sagging or bulging of an area of the intestine into the vagina.

Fecal incontinence—Involuntary passage of stool.

Intussusception—Telescoping of one part of the intestine or the rectum into the neighboring part.

Rectal prolapse—Sagging or bulging of the lining of the rectum into the rectum or actually through and out of the anal opening.

Rectocele—Sagging or bulging of the rectum through the back wall of the vagina.

Vaginal prolapse—Weakening of the supportive tissues of the uterus and vagina, such that the uterus and cervix bulge into the vaginal canal, or even out through the vaginal opening.

need to talk to their physician about adjusting their insulin schedule in response to fasting.

Description

Patients who are undergoing defecography are asked to drink several glasses of water, along with a barium contrast solution, upon arrival at the testing site. An hour later, a barium paste will be inserted into the patient's rectum and (for women) into the vagina. Alternatively, some sites have an artificial stool preparation that can be used for this same purpose. The advantage of the artificial stool is in its greater textural similarity to natural stool.

The patient will be asked to sit on a special commode. The barium paste will show up on x rays taken with it in place. A variety of x-ray views will be taken while the patient is at rest, while they are squeezing the pelvic muscles, and while they are straining during evacuation of the barium paste from their rectum.

Preparations

The patient is usually asked to stop eating and drinking for the two hours before they are scheduled to have defecography. Two hours prior to the test, the patient may be asked to self-administer an enema. The enema is usually repeated fifteen minutes later.

Aftercare

After the test, patients are asked to drink extra water, in order to rid all of the barium from their system. Normal diet and activity can usually be resumed directly following completion of the test.

Risks

The greatest risk of this examination is one of embarrassment to the patient. Some patients find themselves unable to evacuate their bowels while under examination.

Normal results

This test assesses how quickly and completely the rectum is emptied, the angle of the anus and rectum (compared to known normal values of the anorectal angle), and the degree to which the perineum descends during straining. Structural abnormalities can also be demonstrated during defecography, including vaginal and/or rectal prolapse, intussusception, and recto-, enter-, and cystocele. Dysfunctional contraction of the anal sphincter can also be identified during defecography.

Resources

BOOKS

Feldman, M., et al. *Sleisenger & Fordtran's Gastrointestinal and Liver Disease*. 8th ed. St. Louis: Mosby, 2005.

PERIODICALS

Morgan, D. M. "Symptoms of anal incontinence and difficult defecation among women with prolapse." *American Journal of Obstetrics and Gynecology* 197 (November 2007): 509e1–6.

Rao, S. S. "Constipation: evaluation and treatment of colonic and anorectal motility disorders." *Gastroenterological Clinics of North America* 36 (September 2007): 687–711.

Rosalyn Carson-DeWitt, MD

Defibrillation

Definition

Defibrillation is a process in which an electrical device called a defibrillator sends an electric shock to the heart to stop an arrhythmia (irregular heartbeat), resulting in the return of a productive heart rhythm.

Purpose

Defibrillation is performed to correct life-threatening arrhythmias of the heart, including ventricular fibrillation and cardiac arrest. In cardiac emergencies it should be performed immediately after identifying that the patient is experiencing an arrhythmia, indicated by lack of pulse and unresponsiveness. If an **electrocardiogram** is available, the arrhythmia can be displayed visually for additional confirmation. In non-life threatening situations, a physician can use atrial defibrillation to treat atrial fibrillation or flutter.

Precautions

Defibrillation should not be performed on a patient who has a pulse or is alert, as this could cause a lethal heart rhythm disturbance or cardiac arrest. The paddles used in the procedure should not be placed on a woman's breasts or over an internal pacemaker.

Cardiac arrhythmias that prevent the heart from pumping blood to the body can cause irreversible damage to the major organs including the brain and heart. These arrhythmias include ventricular tachycardia, fibrillation, and cardiac arrest. About 10% of the ability to restart the heart is lost with every minute that the heart fibrillates. **Death** can occur in minutes unless a productive heart rhythm, able to generate a pulse, is restored through defibrillation. Because immediate defibrillation is crucial to the patient's survival, the American Heart Association has called for the integration of defibrillation into an effective emergency cardiac care system. The system should include early access, early **cardiopulmonary resuscitation**, early defibrillation, and early advanced cardiac care.

Defibrillators deliver a brief electric shock to the heart, which enables the heart's natural pacemaker to regain control and establish a productive heart rhythm. The defibrillator is an electronic device that includes defibrillator paddles and electrocardiogram monitoring.

During external defibrillation, the paddles are placed on the patient's chest, with a conducting gel ensuring good contact with the skin. When the heart can be visualized directly, during **thoracic surgery**, sterile internal paddles are applied directly to the heart. Direct contact with the patient is discontinued by all caregivers. If additional defibrillation is required, the paddles should be repositioned exactly to increase the likelihood of further shocks being effective in stopping the arrhythmia. The patient's pulse and/or electrocardiogram are continually monitored when defibrillation is not in progress. Medications to treat possible causes

KEY TERMS

Arrhythmia—A cardiac rhythm different then normal sinus rhythm with a rate outside of the range of 60–120 beats per minute for an adult patient.

Cardiac arrest—A condition in which the heart has no discernable electrical activity to stimulate contraction, therefore no blood is pumped.

Fibrillation—Very independent rapid contraction of cardiac muscle fibers producing no productive contraction, therefore no blood is pumped.

Intubation—Placing a tube into the lungs through the trachea to provide forced respiration.

Pacemaker—A surgically implanted electronic device that sends out electrical impulses to regulate a slow or erratic heartbeat.

of the abnormal heart rhythm may be administered. Defibrillation continues until the patient's condition stabilizes or the procedure is ordered to be discontinued.

Early defibrillators, about the size and weight of a car battery, were used primarily in ambulances and hospitals. The American Heart Association now advocates public access defibrillation; this calls for placing automated external defibrillators (AEDS) in police vehicles, airplanes, and at public events, etc. The AEDS are smaller, lighter, less expensive, and easier to use than the early defibrillators. They are computerized to provide simple, verbal instructions to the operator and to make it impossible to deliver a shock to a patient whose heart is not fibrillating. The placement of AEDs is likely to expand to many public locations.

Preparation

Once a patient is found in cardiac distress, without a pulse and non-responsive, and help is summoned, cardiopulmonary resuscitation (CPR) is begun and continued until the caregivers arrive and are able to provide defibrillation. Electrocardiogram leads are attached to the patient chest. Gel or paste is applied to the defibrillator paddles, or two gel pads are placed on the patient's chest. The caregivers verify lack of a pulse while visualizing the electrocardiogram, assure contact with the patient is discontinued, and deliver the electrical charge.

Atrial defibrillation is a treatment option that will be ordered for treatment of atrial fibrillation or flutter. The electrocardiogram will be monitored throughout the procedure. The paddles are placed on the patients chest with conducting gel to ensure good contact between the paddles and skin. If the heart can be visualized directly during thoracic surgery, the paddles will be applied directly to the heart. The defibrillator is programmed to recognize distinct components of the electrocardiogram and will only fire the electrical shock at the correct time. Again, all direct contact with the patient is discontinued prior to defibrillation.

Aftercare

After defibrillation, the patient's cardiac status, breathing, and **vital signs** are monitored with a **cardiac monitor**. Additional tests to measure cardiac damage will be performed, which can include a 12-lead electrocardiogram, a chest x-ray, and **cardiac catheterization**. Treatment options will be determined from the outcome of these procedures. The patient's skin is cleansed to remove gel and, if necessary, electrical burns are treated.

Risks

Skin burns from the defibrillator paddles are the most common complication of defibrillation. Other risks include injury to the heart muscle, abnormal heart rhythms, and blood clots.

Normal results

Defibrillation performed to treat life-threatening ventricular arrhythmias is most likely to be effective within the first five minutes, preventing brain injury and death by returning the heart to a productive rhythm able to produce a pulse. Patients will be transferred to a hospital critical care unit for additional monitoring, diagnosis, and treatment of the arrhythmia. Intubation may be required for respiratory distress. Medications to improve cardiac function and prevent additional arrhythmias, are frequently administered. Some cardiac function may be lost due to the actual defibrillation, but is also associated with the underlying disease.

Atrial defibrillation is successful at restoring cardiac output, alleviating shortness of breath, and decreasing the occurrence of clot formation in the atria.

Resources

BOOKS

Giuliani, E. R., et al., eds. "Arrhythmias." In *Mayo Clinic Practice of Cardiology*. 3rd ed. St. Louis: Mosby, 1996.

PERIODICALS

Bur, Andreas, et al. "Effects of Bystander First Aid, Defibrillation and Advanced Life Support on Neurological Outcome and Hospital Costs in Patients after Ventricular Fibrillation Cardiac Arrest." *Intensive Care Medicine* 27 (2001): 1474–1480.

Herlitz, J., et al. "Characteristics and Outcome Among Patients Suffering In-hospital Cardiac Arrest in Monitored and Non-monitored Areas." *Resuscitation* 48 (2001): 125–135.

Matarese, Leonard. "Police and AEDS: A Chance to Save Thousands of Lives Each Year." *Public Management* 79 (June 1997): 4.

"Medical Breakthroughs That Could Save Your Life." *Body Bulletin* (February 1998): 1.

"Upping the Odds of Survival." *Hospitals and Health Networks* 71 (June 5, 1997): 13.

ORGANIZATIONS

American Heart Association. 7320 Greenville Ave. Dallas, TX 75231. (214) 373-6300. http://www.americanheart.org

OTHER

"AARC Clinical Practice Guideline: Defibrillation During Resuscitation." *Respiratory Care* 40 (1995): 744–748. [cited May 2003]. http://www.hsc.missouri.edu/~shrp/rtwww/rcweb/aarc/ddrcpg.html

"Defibrillation." *American Heart Association*. [cited May 2003]. http://www.americanheart.org

Lori De Milto
Allison J. Spiwak, MSBME

Defibrillator, automatic *see* **Implantable cardioverter-defibrillator**

Dental implants

Definition

Dental implants are surgically fixed substitutes for roots of missing teeth. Embedded in the jawbone, they act as anchors for a replacement tooth, also known as a crown, or a full set of replacement teeth.

Purpose

The purpose of dental implant surgery is to position metallic anchors in the jawbone so that they can receive the replacement teeth and hold them in place. Dental implants should be considered as an option for replacing failing or missing teeth, and often provide more predictable results than bridgework, resin bonded bridges, or endodontic treatment.

Demographics

In 2000, the estimated number of dental implants placed in the United States was 910,000, and this number is expected to increase at a rate of about 18% per year through 2010. Dental implants are equally popular

Dental implants

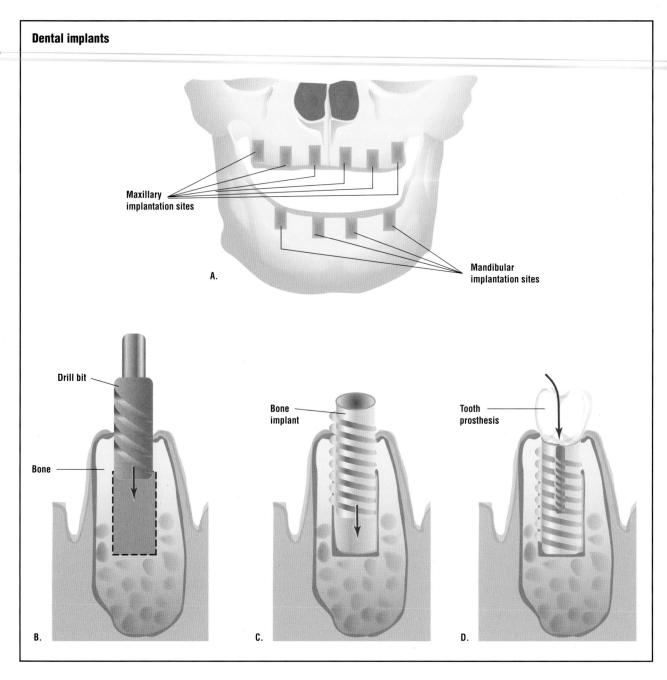

A. Maxillary implantation sites

Mandibular implantation sites

Drill bit

Bone

B.

Bone implant

C.

Tooth prosthesis

D.

A dental drill is used to make a hole for the implant in the jawbone (B). The bone implant is secured into the drilled hole (C), and the tooth prosthesis is built onto the implant (D). *(Illustration by GGS Information Services. Cengage Learning, Gale.)*

in Europe, especially in Germany where the procedure is reimbursed by the national healthcare system.

Description

By replacing a lost tooth with a dental implant, the overall health and function of the surrounding teeth is maintained. The implant can prevent tooth migration and loss of structure and will help avoid loss of bone from the jaw in that area. Further, implants reduce the impact of the lost tooth on surrounding teeth, as traditional bridge structures often require reduction (filing down) of the two flanking teeth to hold the bridge in place with a crown. Implanting avoids such alterations to the surrounding teeth when replacing a lost tooth.

KEY TERMS

Computed tomography (CT) scan—A method of imaging both hard and soft tissue of the body used in placement of dental implants that are not within the bone.

Crown—An artificial replacement tooth.

Endosteal implants—Dental implants that are placed within the bone.

Prosthetic tooth—The final tooth that is held in place by the dental implant anchor.

Resorbed—Absorbed by the body because of lack of function. This happens to the jawbone after tooth loss.

When replacing dentures, implants can provide even more benefits. Implants do not slip nor do they have the potential of limiting the diet to easily chewed foods as can happen with poorly fitting dentures. If appropriate, implants are the method most able to surgically restore one or more missing teeth to their original conditions.

Under **local anesthesia**, the first step for most implant procedures is the exposure of the bone where the implant is to be made. This is followed by placement of the implant into the exposed jawbone. Implants that are placed in the bone are called endosteal implants and are made of titanium or a titanium alloy because this metal does not adversely interact with biological tissue. After placement of the implant, a cover screw is put in and the wound is closed with **stitches** and allowed to heal. In general, placements in the lower jaw need to heal about three months, while placements in the upper jaw need to heal about six months.

After healing, in a second surgical procedure, the implant is uncovered, the cover screw is removed, and a healing abutment or a temporary crown is placed in the implant. Temporary crowns are generally used for esthetic reasons, when the implant is in a place that is visible. Both healing abutments and temporary crowns allow the tissue around the implant to be trained to grow around the final prosthetic tooth.

After about two months, the soft tissue will be healed enough to receive the final prosthetic tooth. Impressions are used to make custom abutments that take into account the neck morphology of the implant. The prosthetic tooth is sometimes attached to a gold cylinder that can be screwed into the abutment or it

WHO PERFORMS THIS PROCEDURE AND WHERE IS IT PERFORMED?

Implants can be done by dentists, periodontists, or oral surgeons. The procedure is done in the dental professional's office.

can be directly cemented onto the abutment. This multi-stage process, where the two surgical procedures are separated by a lengthy healing time, has proven to provide excellent stability in the final implant. Single-step surgical implants are available, but some stability of the final implant is often lost by eliminating the healing step.

Preparation/Diagnosis

At the first appointment, the dentist or oral surgeon performs a thorough examination to determine whether implants are appropriate to replace the missing teeth. Often, x rays are necessary to discover the state of the jawbone, particularly if the teeth have been lost for some time. This information is used to determine if implants are appropriate and, if so, what particular type of implant would be best for the clinical situation.

There are two solutions commonly used if the initial examination indicates that the bone in the area where the implant is to occur is too resorbed to support the implant. The first is **bone grafting**. This involves undergoing a procedure that moves bone from one place in the body to another to enlarge the bone structure at the implant site. Often, bone can be moved from one place in the mouth to another. Sometimes a graft from a donor, or an animal, or artificial bone can be used if bone from the patient is not available. Grafting usually is done four to eight months before the implant procedure to allow the graft a chance to heal before it is disturbed with the implant process.

A second solution is the use of subperiosteal implants that ride above the bone but beneath the gum. These types of implants are not placed in the bone. A computed tomography (CT) scan is commonly used to obtain a model of the bone structure and then the implant fixture is molded to precisely fit the bone model.

Risks

The greatest risk following the surgical procedures is that the implant will fail. For implants placed within the bone, most failures occur within the first year and then occur at a rate of less than 1% per year thereafter. Recent research has indicated that tobacco use by the patient and use of a single-stage implant procedure are two risk factors that increase failure rate.

Normal results

Overall, the success rate for all implants runs from 90–95%. Most failed implants can be replaced with a second attempt.

Resources

BOOKS

Babbush, Charles A. *As Good as New: A Consumer's Guide to Dental Implants.* Lyndhurst, OH: Dental Implant Center Press, 2004.

Misch, Carl E. *Contemporary Implant Dentistry.* St. Louis, MO: Mosby, 2007.

PERIODICALS

Bartlett, D. "Implants for Life? A Critical Review of Implant-supported Restorations." *Journal of Dentistry* 35 no.10 (2007): 768–7721.

ORGANIZATIONS

American Academy of Implant Dentistry. 211 E. Chicago Avenue, Suite 750, Chicago, IL 60611. (312) 335-1550, Fax: (312) 335-9090. http://www.aaid-implant.org (accessed March 11, 2008).

American Dental Association. 211 E. Chicago Ave. Chicago, IL 60611. (312) 440-2500, Fax: (312) 440-7494. http://www.ada.org (accessed March 11, 2008).

Michelle Johnson, MS, JD
Tish Davidson, A M

Dermabrasion

Definition

Dermabrasion is a procedure to improve the appearance of the skin, most commonly of the face. It involves the mechanical removal of the top layer, using a high-speed rotary wheel.

Purpose

Originally developed as a means of treating acne scars, dermabrasion can be used to treat many kinds of skin problems, including scars from other types of wounds, wrinkles, skin coloration abnormalities, and other more serious conditions such as rhinophyma, a disfiguring form of rosacea that affects the nose. Although the treatment is not a cure, in that the scar or other abnormality cannot be entirely removed, dermabrasion does soften the edges of the scar or other abnormality and can radically improve its appearance.

Dermabrasion is often used in combination with other **plastic surgery** techniques, such as chemical peels, excisions, punch grafting, and CO_2 laser resurfacing, to achieve an overall smoothing of various skin abnormalities, particularly of the face.

Demographics

Dermabrasion is a technique that has been used in dermatology for over 100 years. Although used much less often since the advent of laser resurfacing, dermabrasion continues to be a viable treatment that has been reported to have quicker healing times, similar rates of complications, and is more effective in eliminating some types of lesions, particularly surgical scars. According to the American Society for Aesthetic Plastic Surgery, there were about 30,604 dermabrasion procedures performed in 2006.

Description

Dermabrasion is commonly performed using a handheld engine that can reach rotational speeds of 18,000–35,000 rpm. Rapid planing of the skin is achieved through the combination of this rotational speed, the abrading attachment, and pressure applied by the operator. Because of the importance of the skill of the operator, patients should select doctors with significant experience with the procedure.

There are three types of abrading attachments in common use: diamond fraises, wire brushes, and serrated wheels. Diamond fraises are stainless steel wheels

Dermabrasion

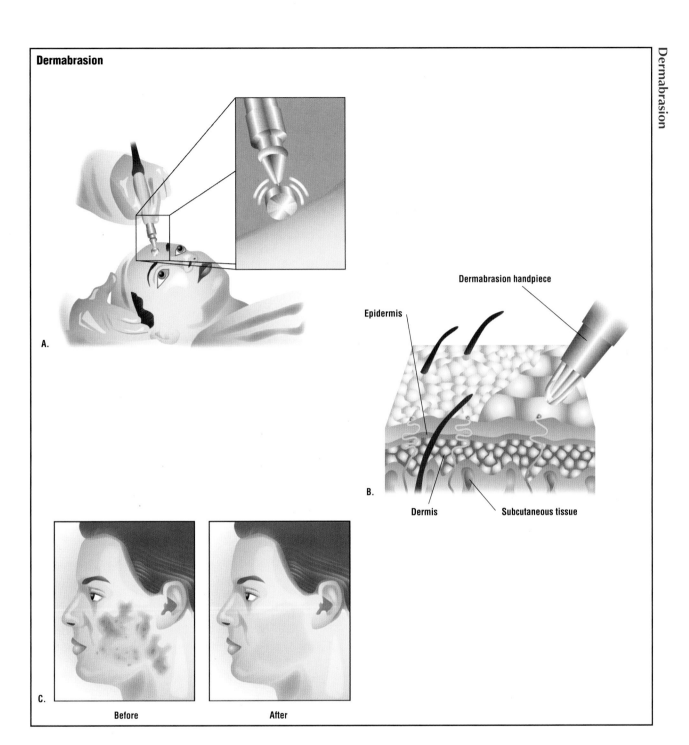

A.

Dermabrasion handpiece

Epidermis

B.

Dermis   Subcutaneous tissue

C.

Before   After

A doctor performs dermabrasion with a high-speed rotary wheel (A). The tool takes off the top layers of the skin (B) to improve the appearance of wrinkles or scars (C). *(Illustration by GGS Information Services. Cengage Learning, Gale.)*

that have diamond chips of varying coarseness bonded to its surface. Cylinder and pear-shaped diamond fraises are also used for work in various locations. The wire brush is a wheel with wires attached at various angles. In experienced hands, it is the most effective attachment for deep scars. The serrated wheel or diamond fraise is often used to soften the edges of skin removed with a wire brush.

Before the procedure begins, medication is often given to relax the patient and reduce pain. For small areas, local anesthetic nerve blocks are often used to

Chemical peel—A skin treatment that uses the application of chemicals, such as phenol or trichloroacetic acid (TCA), to remove the uppermost layer of skin.

Cryoanesthesia—The use of the numbing effects of cold as a surgical anesthetic. For dermabrasion, this involves the spraying of a cold-inducing chemical on the area being treated.

Epithelium—The cellular covering of the body. This covering is disturbed during dermabrasion and heals.

Gentian violet—An antibacterial, antifungal dye that is commonly applied to the skin during dermabrasion.

Keloid—An abnormal type of scarring that involves progressive enlargement, elevated edges, and irregular shapes because of excessive collagen formation during healing.

Laser skin resurfacing—The use of laser light to remove the uppermost layer of skin. Two types of lasers commonly used in this manner are CO_2 and erbium.

Punch grafting—A method of treating a deep scar involving excision of the damaged area, followed by the suturing in of similarly shaped punch of skin that is often taken from behind the ear.

Rosacea—A disease of the skin marked by constant flushing and acne-like lesions.

numb the area being treated. Alternatively, topical cryoanesthesia (numbing the skin using cold) can be used. This is done by spraying a cold-inducing agent on the skin. Sometimes the skin is pre-chilled with ice to increase the anesthetic effect.

During the procedure, patients lie on their backs on the surgical table, eyes covered with disposable eye patches. The area being treated is parted with Gentian violet, a stain that will help gauge how deep the treatment is going. A gloved and gowned assistant holds the skin taut while each section of the face is abraded using the handheld engine. The surgeon works in sections to avoid obvious lines of demarcation in the final results. If the entire face is to be dermabraded, laser is commonly used for the lower eyelids and lip as less than satisfactory results often occur in these areas.

Diagnosis/Preparation

Because there are several different skin-surfacing techniques now available, the initial meetings with the

This procedure should be performed by a dermatological or plastic surgeon with experience in dermabrasion. It is done in an outpatient suite. Hospitalization is not required.

dermatological or plastic surgeon must ensure that dermabrasion is the technique of choice for the particular skin abnormality and location that is being treated. Although controversial, some studies have reported abnormal scarring in patients previously treated with 13 cis-retinoic acid (Accutane); consequently, many surgeons will require a six-month break from the medication before performing dermabrasion. A second contraindication for dermabrasion is HIV or hepatitis infection, as small droplets of blood becomes aerosolized (distributed within the air) during the treatment, creating a risk for the doctor and other staff.

Finally, even if there is no patient history of cold sores, it is important that antiviral medicine is administered to anyone undergoing the procedure, as an outbreak after dermabrasion can be very severe and spread beyond the mouth to other areas of the face.

Aftercare

After the procedure, any treated areas are dressed for healing. For example, a dressing that is primarily water held on a mesh support, called Vigilon, can be used to cover the wound. It is changed daily for about five days, and then the wound is left open to the air. This kind of treatment speeds the restoration of the epithelium, the cellular covering of the body. Using this technique, healing occurs in 5–7 days.

Generally, the patient is given pain medication, **antibiotics**, and anti-swelling medication during recovery. Antiviral drugs are also continued. Patients should avoid the sun during the healing process.

Risks

The most common complication of the procedure is the formation of keloid, a type of abnormal scar that results from excessive collagen production. Because this type of scarring tends to be associated with darker skin types, patients with this kind of skin should approach dermabrasion with caution. Other potential complications include abnormal pigmentation of the

American Society of Plastic Surgeons. 444 E. Algonquin Rd. Arlington Heights, IL 60005. (800) 475-2784. http://www.plasticsurgery.org (accessed March 16, 2008).

Michelle Johnson, MS, JD
Rosalyn Carson-DeWitt, MD

Diabetes surgery *see* **Islet cell transplantation**

Dialysis, kidney *see* **Kidney dialysis**

Differential count *see* **White blood cell count and differential**

Dilatation and curettage

Definition

Dilatation and curettage (D & C) is a gynecological procedure in which the cervix is dilated (expanded) and the lining of the uterus (endometrium) is scraped away.

Purpose

D & C is used to diagnose and treat heavy or irregular bleeding from the uterus. Possible reasons for abnormal uterine bleeding include:

- Hormonal imbalance. Often women with abnormal bleeding are first treated with hormones in an attempt to normalize bleeding. D & C may be used to determine the cause of bleeding if hormone treatment is ineffective.
- Endometrial polyps. Polyps are benign growths that may protrude from the uterus by a stem or stalk, usually to the endometrium or cervix. D & C may be used to diagnose polyps or to remove them.
- Uterine fibroids. Also called leiomyomas, fibroids are benign growths in the smooth muscle of the uterus. Abnormal bleeding is often the only symptom of fibroids. D & C is often used to diagnose fibroids and may be used to scrape away small tumors; additional surgery may be needed to remove more extensive growths.
- Endometrial hyperplasia (EH). EH is a condition where the endometrium grows excessively, becoming too thick and causing abnormal bleeding. Tissue samples procured during D & C can be assessed for early signs of cancer.
- Cancer. D & C may be used to obtain tissue for microscopic evaluation to rule out cancer. Women over the age of 40 are at an increased risk of developing endometrial cancer.

---

treated skin, persistent redness of the skin, and a localized dilation of small groups of blood vessels called telangiectasia. Finally, the formation of milia, bumps that form due to obstruction of the sweat glands, although this can be treated after healing with retinoic acid.

Normal results

Normal results include significant improvement in the appearance of the skin's surface after healing of the skin. It should be emphasized, however, that many scars will not be completely removed and the change in appearance occurs due to a softening of the edges of the abnormality, not elimination. If a patient cannot tolerate a residual presence of the scar or other abnormality, the treatment should not be used.

Morbidity and mortality rates

The morbidity and mortality rate of this cosmetic procedure is extremely low.

Alternatives

A variety of other skin-resurfacing techniques are available and include chemical (phenol or trichloroacetic acid [TCA]) peels, and laser (CO_2 and erbium) resurfacing.

Resources

BOOKS

Habif, T. P. *Clinical Dermatology*. 4th ed. St. Louis: Mosby, 2004.

PERIODICALS

Roenigk, Henry H. "Dermabrasion: State of the Art 2002." *Journal of Cosmetic Dermatology* 1 (2002): 72–87.

ORGANIZATIONS

American Society for Aesthetic Plastic Surgery, 11081 Winners Circle, Los Alamitos, CA 90720. (800) 364-2147 or (562) 799-2356. http://www.surgery.org (accessed March 16, 2008).

Dilatation and curettage

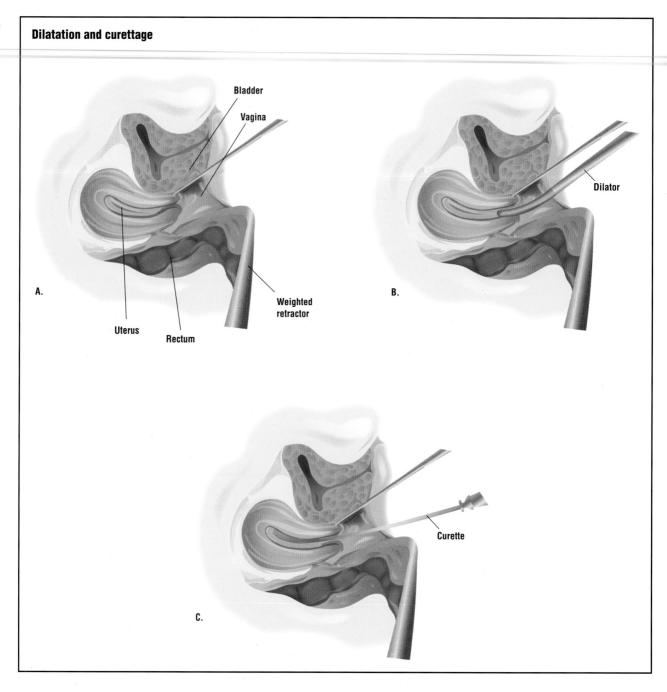

For a D&C, the patient lies on her back, and a weighted retractor is placed in the vagina (A). A dilator is used to open the cervix (B), and a curette is used to scrape the inside of the uterus (C). *(Illustration by GGS Information Services. Cengage Learning, Gale.)*

- Miscarriage, incomplete abortion, or childbirth. Abnormal bleeding may result if some of the products of pregnancy remain in the uterus after a miscarriage or induced abortion, or if parts of the placenta are not expelled naturally after childbirth. These retained products can be scraped out by D & C.

Description

D & C is usually performed under **general anesthesia**, although local or epidural anesthesia can also be used. **Local anesthesia** lessens risk and costs, but the woman will feel cramping during the procedure. The type of anesthesia used often depends on the reason for the D & C.

KEY TERMS

Endometrial polyps—Growths in the lining of the uterus (endometrium) that may cause bleeding and can develop into cancer.

Epidural anesthesia—A type of anesthesia that is injected into the epidural space of the spinal cord to numb the nerves leading to the lower half of the body.

Uterine fibroid—A non-cancerous tumor of the uterus that can range from the size of a pea to the size of a grapefruit. Small fibroids require no treatment, but those causing serious symptoms may need to be removed.

During the procedure, which takes only minutes to perform, the doctor inserts an instrument called a speculum to hold open the vaginal walls, and then stretches the opening of the uterus (the cervix) by inserting a series of tapering rods, each thicker than the previous one, or by using other specialized instruments. This process of opening the cervix is called dilation.

Once the cervix is dilated, the physician inserts a spoon-shaped surgical device called a curette into the uterus. The curette is used to scrape away the uterine lining. One or more small tissue samples from the lining of the uterus or the cervical canal are sent for analysis by microscope to check for abnormal cells.

Although simpler, less expensive techniques such as a vacuum aspiration are quickly replacing the D & C as a diagnostic method, it is still often used to diagnose and treat a number of conditions.

Diagnosis/Preparation

If general anesthesia will be used, the patient will be instructed to refrain from eating and drinking for at least eight hours before the procedure. The doctor may order blood and/or urine tests to scan for certain abnormalities. Because opening the cervix can be painful, sedatives may be given before the procedure begins. Deep breathing and other relaxation techniques may help ease cramping during cervical dilation.

Aftercare

A woman who has had a D & C performed in a hospital can usually go home the same day or the next day. Many women experience backache and mild cramps after the procedure, and may pass small blood clots for a day or so. Vaginal staining or bleeding may continue for several weeks.

Most women can resume normal activities almost immediately. Patients should avoid sexual intercourse, douching, and tampon use for at least two weeks to prevent infection while the cervix is closing and to allow the endometrium to heal completely.

Risks

The primary risk after the procedure is infection. A woman should report to her doctor if she experiences any of the following symptoms:

- fever
- heavy bleeding
- severe cramps
- foul-smelling vaginal discharge

D & C is a surgical operation that has certain risks associated with general anesthesia such as pulmonary aspiration and failed intubation. Rare complications include perforation of the uterus (which usually heals on its own) or puncture of the bowel or bladder (which requires further surgery to repair).

Extensive scarring of the uterus may occur after over-aggressive scraping during D & C, leading to a condition called Asherman's syndrome. The major symptoms of Asherman's syndrome are light or absent menstrual periods, infertility, and recurrent miscarriages. Scar tissue can be removed with surgery in most women, although approximately 20–30% of women will remain infertile after treatment.

Normal results

Removal of the uterine lining will normally cause no side effects, and may be beneficial if the lining has thickened so much that it causes heavy periods. The uterine lining soon grows again normally, as part of the menstrual cycle.

Morbidity and mortality rates

D & C has been associated with a 4–10% rate of postoperative complications.

Alternatives

There are a number of alternatives to D & C, depending on the reason for doing the procedure. Examples of procedures that allow doctors alternative ways of evaluating, sampling, or treating disorders of the inner lining of the uterus include:

WHO PERFORMS THE PROCEDURE AND WHERE IS IT PERFORMED?

D & C is generally performed by an obstetrician/gynecologist, a medical doctor who has completed specialized training in the areas of women's general health, pregnancy, labor and childbirth, prenatal testing, and genetics. Samples of the uterine lining may be sent to a pathologist for analysis. A pathologist is a medical doctor who has completed specialized training in the diagnosis of diseases from microscopic analysis of cells and tissues.

The health of the patient and the type of anesthesia used determines where a D & C is performed. The procedure is generally done in a hospital or an outpatient setting.

- Expectant management of spontaneous abortion. D & C is the most commonly used method of treatment for incomplete abortion; one study showed that more than 90% of women who visited hospital emergency rooms for incomplete spontaneous abortion were treated by D & C. Recent studies, however, have shown that expectant management (i.e., no active intervention) is a viable option for women who do not wish to undergo surgery and who are in otherwise good health. Up to 72% of women indicated that that expectant management of incomplete abortion was preferable to medical or surgical intervention.

- Endometrial biopsy. This procedure is similar to D & C in that a curette is used to obtain a sample of endometrial tissue. Little or no cervical dilation is necessary, however, because the curette used in endometrial biopsy is narrower. The cervix is numbed with a local anesthetic, but the patient will still experience cramping.

- Vacuum scraping. A thin plastic tube attached to a suction machine is passed through the cervix and scraped along the endometrium. Vacuum scraping has been shown to have similar success in diagnosing uterine cancer as D & C. Local anesthesia is also used for this procedure.

- Hysteroscopy. A thin telescope called a hysteroscope is inserted through the cervix and used to view the inside of the uterus after it has been expanded with a liquid or gas. The view afforded by the hysteroscope can help to diagnose abnormal growths, accumulation of scar tissue, or other conditions.

- Hysterectomy. A total hysterectomy permanently removes the uterus and cervix. This procedure is

QUESTIONS TO ASK THE DOCTOR

- Why is D & C recommended for my condition?
- Where will the procedure be performed?
- What alternative therapies are available to me?
- What are my options in terms of anesthesia during the procedure?
- What risks are involved with the procedure?

generally recommended only if a woman no longer desires to have children and no other forms of treatment have been successful. Most hysterectomies are done to treat uterine fibroids and endometriosis (a condition in which the endometrium grows outside of the uterus).

Resources

BOOKS

Gabbe, S. G., et al. *Obstetrics: Normal and Problem Pregnancies.* 5th ed. London: Churchill Livingstone, 2007.

Katz, V. L., et al. *Comprehensive Gynecology.* 5th ed. St. Louis: Mosby, 2007.

PERIODICALS

Geyman, John, Lynn Oliver, and Sean Sullivan. "Expectant, Medical, or Surgical Treatment of Spontaneous Abortion in First Trimester of Pregnancy?" *Journal of the American Board of Family Practice* 12, no. 1 (1999): 55–64.

Molnar, Alexandra, Lynn Oliver, and John Geyman. "Patient Preferences for Management of First-Trimester Incomplete Spontaneous Abortion." *Journal of the American Board of Family Practice* 13, no. 5 (2000): 333–7.

ORGANIZATIONS

American College of Obstetricians and Gynecologists. 409 12th St., SW, PO Box 96920, Washington, DC 20090-6920. http://www.acog.org (accessed March 16, 2008).

OTHER

"Asherman's Syndrome." *International Adhesions Society.* April 24, 2002 [cited February 24, 2003]. http://www.adhesions.org/asherman.htm (accessed March 16, 2008).

"Dilatation and Curettage." *eTenet.* 2001 [cited February 24, 2003]. http://www.etenet.com/ (accessed March 16, 2008).

"Dilatation and Curettage." *Patient Education Institute.* December 21, 2001 [cited February 24, 2003]. http://www.nlm.nih.gov/medlineplus/ency/article/002914.htm (accessed March 16, 2008).

"Dysfunctional Uterine Bleeding." WomenOne.org. 2001 [cited February 24, 2003. http://www.womenone.org/health04.htm (accessed March 16, 2008).

"Endometrial Hyperplasia." *American College of Obstetricians and Gynecologists.* 2001 [cited February 24, 2003]. http://www.medem.com/search/article_display.cfm?path =∖\TANQUERAY\M_ContentItem&mstr =/ M_ContentItem/ZZZ7Z2GWQMC.html&soc = ACOG&srch_typ = NAV_SERCH (accessed March 16, 2008).

"Hysterectomy." *American College of Obstetricians and Gynecologists.* 2001 [cited February 24, 2003]. http://www.medem.com/search/article_display.cfm?path =& setmn;\TANQUERAY\M_ContentItem&mstr =/M_ ContentItem/ZZZL67R927C.html&soc = ACOG&srch_ typ = NAV_SERCH.

"Hysteroscopy." American College of Obstetricians and Gynecologists. 2001 [cited February 24, 2003]. http:// www.medem.com/search/article_display.cfm?path = ∖\TANQUERAY\M_ContentItem&mstr =/ M_ContentItem/ZZZAXX8MA7C.html&soc = ACOG &srch_typ = NAV_SERCH (accessed March 16, 2008).

Williams, Carmine. "Dilation and Curettage." eMedicine. April 26, 2001 [cited February 24, 2003]. http://www. emedicine.com/aaem/topic156.htm (accessed March 16, 2008).

Carol A. Turkington
Stephanie Dionne Sherk
Rosalyn Carson-DeWitt, MD

Discharge from the hospital

Definition

Discharge from the hospital is the point at which the patient leaves the hospital and either returns home or is transferred to another facility such as a rehabilitation center or to a nursing home. Discharge involves the medical instructions that the patient will need to fully recover. Discharge planning is a service that considers the patient's needs after the hospital stay and may involve several different services such as visiting nursing care, physical therapy, and home blood drawing.

Description

Hospitalization is often a short-term event, so planning for discharge may begin shortly after admission. The physicians, nurses, and case managers involved in a patient's care are part of an assessment team that keeps in mind the patient's preadmission level of functioning, and whether the patient will be able to return home following the current hospital admission. Information that could affect the discharge plan should be noted in the patient's medical record so that it will be taken into account when discharge is being scheduled. The primary questions include:

- Can this patient return to his or her preadmission situation?
- Has there been a change in the patient's ability to care for him- or herself?
- Is the patient in need of services to be able to care for him- or herself?
- Which services will the patient need?
- Are there mental health needs that must be met?
- Does the patient agree with the discharge plan?

While a person has been in the hospital, physicians other than the primary-care physician have been in charge of the patient's care. Good discharge planning involves clear communication between the hospital physician(s) and the primary care physician. This may be done by telephone and/or in writing. The information to be conveyed includes:

- a summary of the hospital stay
- a list of test and surgeries performed, with results
- a list of test results still pending
- a list of tests needed after discharge, such as a repeat chest x ray
- a list of medications the patient is being discharged with, including the dosage and frequency
- a copy of the patient's discharge instructions
- when the patient should see the primary-care physician for a follow-up appointment
- the plan for outpatient treatment, such as home intravenous antibiotics or parenteral nutrition, to ensure that responsibility for this treatment has been clearly transferred and that the primary care physician accepts the treatment responsibility
- discharge instructions to the patient on activity level, diet, and wound care

Before leaving the hospital, the patient will receive discharge instructions that should include:

- an explanation of the care the patient received in the hospital
- a list of medications the patient will be taking (the dosage, times, and frequency)
- a list of potential side effects of any newly prescribed medications
- a prescription for any newly prescribed medications
- when to see the primary-care physician for a follow-up appointment
- home-care instructions, such as activity level, diet, restrictions on bathing, wound care, as well as when

KEY TERMS

Ombudsman—A patient representative who investigates patient complaints and problems related to hospital service or treatment. He or she may act as a mediator between the patient, the family, and the hospital.

Parenteral nutrition—The administration of liquid nutrition through an intravenous catheter placed in the patient's vein.

the patient can return to work or school, or resume driving

- signs of infection or worsening condition, such as pain, fever, bleeding, difficulty breathing, or vomiting
- an explanation of any services the patient will now be receiving, such as visiting nurse care, including contact information

The term discharge planning may be used to refer to the service provided to help patients arrange for services such as rehabilitation, physical therapy, occupational therapy, visiting nurses, or nursing **home care**. This service may be provided by a case manager or by the hospital's social service department. The patient may request this service, or the physician may make the request in the form of a referral to the department. The patient will need to be evaluated to see what services he or she requires, as well as what services he or she qualifies for (such as Meals on Wheels), or what services the patient's insurance will cover. The patient may be discharged to the home with a visit from a visiting nurse taking place later the same day to assess the patient's need for these services and to make arrangements for him or her in the home. A person may be discharged home only when certain equipment, such as a hospital-style bed and oxygen, has been delivered to the home. If a patient feels he or she is being discharged before he or she is ready, the patient can file a complaint with the hospital's ombudsman.

A follow-up from the hospital staff, either physician, nurse, or case manager, should take place within two weeks of discharge to review the results of any tests that were done in the hospital that came in after the patient was discharged, to remind the patient of the follow-up appointment with the physician, to see if the patient has any questions about any new medications that were added in the hospital, and to be sure that no problems arose after discharge that have not been addressed. Such follow-up calls help to ensure a successful recovery.

A patient may experience a complication or an adverse event, an injury that happens because of medical management, as a result of care received in the hospital. In the February 2003 issue of *The Annals of Internal Medicine*, researchers reported how often these adverse events arose, and how severe they were. Four hundred patients were interviewed by telephone a few weeks after discharge. Seventy-six patients had suffered an adverse event during the two-week period after discharge, such as a new or worsening symptom, medication-related problems, or the need for an unexpected visit to the doctor. Of that number, 23 were determined to have been caused by error, and 24 were found to have adverse events that could have been made less severe by better care. Of all the events, about 66% were drug related and 17% were related to procedures. Three percent of the patients studied suffered permanent disability.

Resources

BOOKS

Wachter, Robert M., Lee Goldman, and Harry Hollander, eds. *Hospital Medicine.* Baltimore: Lippincott Williams & Wilkins, 2000.

PERIODICALS

Forster, A. J., et al. "The Incidence and Severity of Adverse Events Affecting Patients after Discharge from the Hospital." *Annals of Internal Medicine,* 138 (February 2003): 161–167.

ORGANIZATIONS

The American Hospital Association. One North Franklin, Chicago, IL 60606.

National Center for Health Statistics. *National Hospital Discharge Survey,* Vital Health Stat. 153 (November 2002): 1–194.

National Institute on Aging. http://www.nih.gov/nia (accessed March 19, 2008).

Esther Csapo Rastegari, RN, BSN, EdM
Fran Hodgkins

Disk removal

Definition

Disk removal is one of the most common types of back surgery. Diskectomy (also called discectomy) is the removal of an intervertebral disk, the flexible plate that connects any two adjacent vertebrae in the spine. Intervertebral disks act as shock absorbers, protecting the brain and spinal cord from the impact produced by the body's movements.

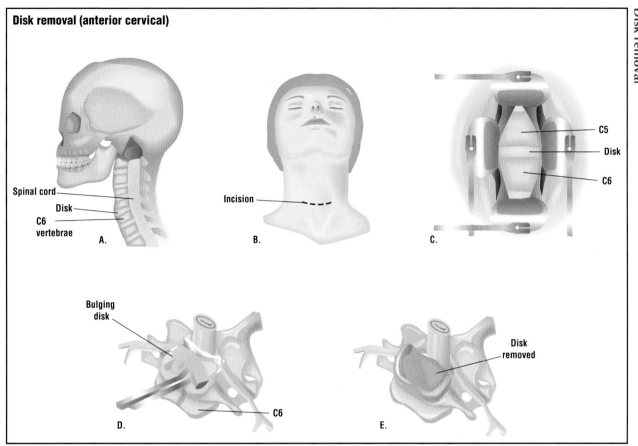

Disk removal (anterior cervical)

In the anterior cervical disk removal, and incision is made into the patient's neck (B). The cervical disk, which may be herniated, is visualized (C). It is removed completely (D and E). *(Illustration by GGS Information Services. Cengage Learning, Gale.)*

Purpose

Removing the invertebral disk is performed after completion of unsuccessful conservative treatment for back pain that has been present for at least six weeks. Surgery is also performed if there is pressure on the lumbosacral nerve roots that causes weakness, bowel dysfunction, or bladder dysfunction.

As a person ages, the disks between vertebrae degenerate and dry out, and tears form in the fibers holding them in place. Eventually, the disk can develop a blister-like bulge, compressing nerves in the spine and causing pain. This is called a "prolapsed" (or herniated) disk. If such a disk presses on a nerve root and causes muscle weakness, or problems with the bladder or bowel, immediate disk removal surgery may be needed.

The goal of the surgery is to relieve all pressure on nerve roots by removing the pulpy material from the disk, or the entire disk. If it is necessary to remove material from several nearby vertebrae, the spine may become unsteady. In this case, the surgeon will perform a **spinal fusion**, removing all disks between two or more vertebrae, and roughening the bones so that the vertebrae heal together. Bone strips taken from the patient's leg or hip may be used to help hold the vertebrae together. Spinal fusion decreases pain, but decreases spinal mobility.

Demographics

Approximately 150,000 Americans undergo disk removal each year in the United States.

Description

The surgery is performed under **general anesthesia**. The surgeon cuts an opening into the vertebral canal, and moves the dura and the bundle of nerves called the "cauda equina" (horse's tail) aside, which exposes the disk. If a portion of the disk has moved out from between the vertebrae and into the nerve canal, it is simply removed. If the disk itself has

Cauda equina—A bundle of nerve roots in the lower back (lumbar region) of the spinal canal that controls the leg muscles and functioning of the bladder, intestines, and genitals.

Computed tomography (CT) scan—A special type of x ray that produces detailed images of structures inside the body.

Diskectomy (or discectomy)—The surgical removal of a portion of an invertebral disk.

Dura—The strongest and outermost of three membranes that protect the brain, spinal cord, and nerves of the cauda equina.

Fusion—A union, joining together; e.g., bone fusion.

Herniated disk—A blister-like bulging or protrusion of the contents of the disk out through the fibers that normally hold them in place. Also called ruptured disk, slipped disk, or displaced disk.

Intervertebral disk—Cylindrical elastic-like gel pads that separate and join each pair of vertebrae in the spine.

Laminectomy—An operation in which the surgeon cuts through the covering of a vertebra to reach a herniated disk in order to remove it.

Magnetic resonance imaging (MRI)—A test that provides pictures of organs and structures inside the body by using a magnetic field and pulses of radio wave energy to detect tumors, infection, and other types of tissue disease or damage, or conditions affecting blood flow. The area of the body being studied is positioned inside a strong magnetic field.

Myelogram—The film produced by myelography; a graphic representation of the differential count of cells found in a stained representation of bone marrow.

Percutaneous—Denoting the passage of substances through unbroken skin; also refers to passage through the skin by needle puncture, including introduction of wires and catheters by the Seldinger technique.

Vertebra—The bones that make up the back bone (spine).

become fragmented and partially displaced, or is not fragmented but bulges extensively, the surgeon removes the damaged part of the disk and the part that lies in the space between the vertebrae.

There are minimally invasive surgical techniques for disk removal, including microdiskectomy. In this procedure, the surgeon uses a magnifying instrument or special microscope to view the disk. Magnification makes it possible to remove a herniated disk with a smaller incision, causing less damage to nearby tissue. Video-assisted arthroscopic microdiskectomy has exhibited good results with less use of narcotics and a shortened period of disability. Newer forms of diskectomy are still in the research stage, and are not yet widely available. These include laser diskectomy and automated percutaneous diskectomy.

Total disk replacement research in the United States is underway. Products under investigation include the ProDisc (made by Spine Solutions, Inc.), and the SB Charite III (made by Link Spine Group, Inc.). In these clinical studies, a significant number of patients who received artificial disk implants report a reduction in back and leg pain; 92.7% state they are satisfied or extremely satisfied with the procedure.

Diagnosis/Preparation

The physician will obtain x rays and neuroimaging studies, including a computed tomography (**CT**) **scan**, myelogram, and **magnetic resonance imaging** (**MRI**); and clinical exams to determine the precise location of the affected disk.

An hour before surgery, the patient is given an injection to dry up internal fluids and encourage drowsiness.

Aftercare

After the operation, the patient is lying flat and face down when he or she awakens. This position must be maintained for several days, except for occasional positional changes to avoid **bedsores**. There may be slight pain or stiffness in the back area.

Patients usually leave the hospital on the fourth or fifth day after surgery. They must:

- Avoid sitting for more than 15–20 minutes.

- Use a reclined chair.

- Avoid bending at the waist, twisting, or lifting heavy objects.

- Begin gentle walking (indoors or outdoors), and gradually increase exercise. Exercise should be continued for the next four weeks.
- Begin stationary biking or gentle swimming after two weeks.
- Sleep on a firm mattress.
- Slow down if they experience more than minor pain in the back or leg.
- Refrain from sitting in one place for an extended period of time (e.g., long car ride).

Patients should be able to resume normal activities in four to six weeks.

Risks

All surgery carries some risk due to heart and lung problems or the anesthesia itself, but this risk is generally very small. (The risk of **death** from general anesthesia for all types of surgery, for example, is only approximately one in 1,600 surgeries.)

The most common risk of the surgery is infection, which occurs in 1–2% of cases. Rarely, the surgery damages nerves in the lower back or major blood vessels in front of the disk. Occasionally, there may be some residual paralysis of a leg or bladder muscle after surgery, but this is the result of the disk problem that necessitated the surgery, not the operation itself.

Normal results

In properly evaluated patients, there is a very good chance that disk removal will be successful in easing pain. The surgery can relieve pain in 90% of cases; however, there are some people who do not achieve pain relief. This depends on a number of factors, including the length of time that they had the condition requiring surgery. Disk surgery has a "good to excellent" result in 87% of patients over age 60. The surgery can relieve both back and leg pain, especially the latter.

Alternatives

Prior to disk removal surgery, a patient usually undergoes treatment with medical or physical therapy.

Disk removal surgery may be indicated if these treatments are ineffective, or if emergency symptoms (i.e., bladder and bowel dysfunction) develop.

Resources

BOOKS

Beauchamp, M.D., Daniel R., Mark B. Evers, M.D., Kenneth L. Mattox, M.D., Courtney M. Townsend, and David C. Sabiston (Editors). *Sabiston Textbook of Surgery: The Biological Basis of Modern Surgical Practice,* 16th edition. London: W. B. Saunders Co., 2001.

Bogduk, Nikolai, Brian McGuirk, and Boriana Dirk Van Der Deliiska. *Medical Management of Acute and Chronic Low Back Pain.*Philadelphia, PA: Elsevier Health Sciences, 2002.

Cailliet, Rene.*Low Back Disorders: A Medial Enigma.*Philadelphia, PA: Lippincott Williams & Wilkins, 2003.

Lawrence, Peter F., Richard M. Bell, and Merril T. Dayton, eds. *Essentials of General Surgery,* 3rd edition. Philadelphia, PA: Lippincott, Williams & Wilkins, 2000.

Resnick, Daniel K., ed. *Surgical Management of Low Back Pain (Neurosurgical Topics).* 2nd edition. Rolling Meadows, IL: American Association of Neurological Surgeons, 2001.

Watkins, Robert G. *Surgical Approaches to the Spine,* 2nd edition. Berlin, Germany: Springer Verlag. 2003.

PERIODICALS

Alini, M., P.J. Roughley, J. Antoniou, T. Stoll, and M. Aebi. "A Biological Approach to Treating Disc Degeneration: Not for Today, But Maybe for Tomorrow." *European Spine Journal* 11, no. 2 (October 2002): S215-20.

Deyo, R., and J. Weinstein. "Low Back Pain." *New England Journal of Medicine* 344, no. 5 (2001): 363-70.

Oskouian, R.J., Jr., J.P. Johnson, and J.J. Regan. "Thoracoscopic Microdiscectomy." *Neurosurgery* 5, no. 1 (January 2002): 103-9.

Silber, J.S., D.G. Anderson, V.M. Hayes, and A.R. Vaccaro. "Advances in Surgical Management of Lumbar Degenerative Disease." *Orthopedics* 25, no.7 (July 2002): 767-71.

ORGANIZATIONS

National Institutes of Health. 9000 Rockville Pike, Bethesda, MD 20892. (301) 496-4000. Email: NIHInfo @OD.NIH.GOV. http://www.nih.gov/.

North American Spine Society. 22 Calendar Court, 2nd Floor, LaGrange, IL 60525. (877) Spine-Dr. E-mail: info@spine.org. http://www.spine.org.

OTHER

American Academy of Orthopaedic Surgery (AAOS) and American Association of Orthopaedic Surgery. *Low Back Surgery*. 2001. http://orthoinfo.aaos.org/booklet/ thr_report.cfm?thread_id = 10&topcategory = sp. [cited March 19, 2003].

Spine Health.com. *Total Disc Replacement*.2003. http:// www.spine-health.com/research/discupdate/artificial/ artificial04.html. [cited March 19, 2003].

Carol A. Turkington
Crystal H. Kaczkowski, MSc.

Diskectomy *see* **Disk removal**

Diuretics

Definition

Diuretics are drugs that help to reduce the amount of water in the body. They are sometimes called water pills.

Purpose

Diuretics are used to treat the buildup of excess fluid in the body. Medical conditions such as congestive heart failure, liver disease, kidney disease, and hormonal imbalances can cause fluid to accumulate and tissues to swell (edema). Certain medications can also cause water retention. When there is too much fluid in the body, blood pressure increases and the heart must work harder to pump. Therefore, diuretics are also often the first drug prescribed to treat high blood pressure (hypertension). They are the least expensive drug that effectively treats hypertension in many people.

When blood enters the kidney, water, waste products, and dissolved charged particles (ions) such as sodium (Na) and potassium (K) are filtered out of the blood and into special tubules in the kidneys. As they travel through these tubules, some water and particles are reabsorbed, and the rest are excreted as urine. In general, diuretics work by increasing the amount of ions and water that are excreted, thus increasing urine output and reducing the fluid load of the body. This, in turn, lowers blood pressure and reduces tissue swelling so that the heart does not have to work as hard.

Diuretics also may be used in surgery to reduce blood pressure and swelling. For example, mannitol, an osmotic diuretic, may be used to reduce swelling in the brain in some neurosurgical procedures.

Description

There are several classes of diuretics. Each class works in a slightly different way, although the end function of all diuretics is to eliminate excess water from the body. The different classes of diuretics include:

- Loop diuretics include bumetanide (Bumex), furosemide (Lasix), torsemide (Cemadex), and ethacrynic acid (Edecrin). They get their name from the loop-shaped part of the kidney tubules (the loop of Henle) where they have their effect.

- Thiazide and thiazide-like diuretics include such commonly used diuretics as hydrochlorothiazide (HydroDIURIL, Esidrix), chlorothiazide (Diuril), and chlorthalidone (Hygroton).

- Potassium-sparing diuretics help the body retain potassium while losing sodium and water. With many diuretics, potassium is lost from the body along with sodium. Too little potassium can cause serious health problems, because potassium plays a critical role in many metabolic functions. Examples of potassium-sparing diuretics are spironolactone (Aldactone), (amiloride (Midamor) and triamterene (Dyrenium).

- Osmotic diuretics keep water from being reabsorbed in the kidney. Mannitol, which is given by intravenous drip, is commonly used to reduce cerebral edema (swelling of the brain). Glycerol is also an osmotic diuretic. Osmotic diuretics are used under special circumstances and are not routinely given to control high blood pressure.

- Carbonic anhydrase inhibitors cause water loss through the kidneys by changing the acidity of urine, but their most common use is in treatment of glaucoma, an eye disease caused by increased pressure in the eye. Acetazolamide (Diamox), dichlorphenamide (Daranide), and methazolamide (Nepatazane) are often given by mouth, even though they primarily treat an eye condition.

In addition, some drugs contain combinations of two diuretics. The brands Dyazide and Maxzide, for example, contain the thiazide diuretic hydrochlorothiazide along with the potassium-sparing diuretic triamterene.

KEY TERMS

Lupus erythematosus—A chronic autoimmune disease that affects the skin, joints, and certain internal organs.

Pancreas—A gland located near the liver, the pancreas produces enzymes and fluids that help to breakdown food. It also produces the hormone insulin that the body must have to utilize sugar (glucose).

Potassium—A mineral found in whole grains, meat, legumes, and some fruits and vegetables. Potassium is important for many body processes, including proper functioning of nerves and muscles.

Triglyceride—A substance formed in the body from the breakdown of fat in the diet. Triglycerides are the main fatty materials in the blood. Triglyceride levels are important in the diagnosis and treatment of many diseases, including high blood pressure, diabetes, and heart disease.

Some nonprescription (over-the-counter, OTC) medicines and herbal remedies also function as diuretics. However, the drugs described here cannot be bought without a physician's prescription. They are available in tablet, capsule, liquid, and injectable forms.

Recommended dosage

The recommended dosage depends on the type of diuretic, the condition it treats, and the individual's size, age, and health. Patients should check with the physician who prescribed the drug or the pharmacist who filled the prescription for the correct dosage and then take the medicine exactly as directed.

Precautions

Seeing a physician regularly while taking a diuretic is important. The physician may order blood work and will do a **physical examination** to make sure the diuretic is working as it should without unwanted side effects.

For patients taking a class of diuretic that can cause large amounts of potassium to be excreted, physicians may recommend adding potassium-rich foods such as bananas to the diet, and they may suggest taking a daily potassium supplement. If the physician recommends any of these measures, the patient must make sure to closely follow the directions. The patient should not make other significant diet changes or take any dietary supplements without checking with the physician. People who are taking potassium-sparing diuretics should not add potassium to their diets, as too much potassium may be harmful.

Patients taking potassium-sparing diuretics should know the signs of too much potassium and should check with a physician as soon as possible if any of these symptoms occur, including:

- irregular heartbeat
- breathing problems
- numbness or tingling in the hands, feet, or lips
- confusion or nervousness
- unusual tiredness or weakness
- weak or heavy feeling in the legs

Patients taking diuretics that cause potassium loss should know the signs of too little potassium and should check with a physician as soon as possible if they have any of these symptoms, including:

- fast or irregular heartbeat
- weak pulse
- nausea or vomiting
- dry mouth
- excessive thirst
- muscle cramps or pain
- unusual tiredness or weakness
- mental or mood changes

People who become ill with gastrointestinal diseases while taking diuretics may lose too much water or potassium if they have severe vomiting and diarrhea.

Diuretics drugs make some people feel lightheaded, dizzy, or faint when they get up after sitting or lying down. Older people are especially likely to have this problem. Drinking alcohol, exercising, standing for long periods, or being outdoors in hot weather may make the problem worse. To lessen this problem, a person should get up gradually and hold onto something for support if possible. The patient should avoid or limit the amount of alcohol he or she drinks and be careful in hot weather or when exercising or standing for a long time.

People who take a diuretic should tell the healthcare professional before having surgical or dental procedures, medical tests, or emergency treatment.

Special conditions

People who have certain medical conditions or who are taking certain other drugs may encounter problems if they take diuretics. Before taking diuretic drugs, they should be sure to let the physician know about these conditions.

ALLERGIES. Anyone who has had unusual reactions to diuretics or **sulfonamides** (sulfa drugs) in the past should let the physician know. The physician should also be told about any allergies to foods, dyes, preservatives, or other substances.

PREGNANCY. Diuretics will not help the swelling of hands and feet that some women experience during pregnancy. Pregnant women should not use diuretics unless prescribed by their obstetrician or other physician. Although studies have not been done on pregnant women, studies of laboratory animals show that some diuretics can cause harmful effects when taken during pregnancy.

BREASTFEEDING. Some diuretics pass into breast milk, but no reports exist of problems in nursing babies whose mothers use this medicine. However, thiazide diuretics may decrease the flow of breast milk. Women who are breastfeeding and need to use a diuretic should check with the physician.

OTHER MEDICAL CONDITIONS. Side effects of some diuretics may be more likely in people who have had a recent heart attack or who have liver disease or severe kidney (renal) disease. Other types of diuretics may not work properly in people with liver disease or kidney disease. Diuretics may worsen certain medical conditions such as gout, kidney stones, pancreatitis, lupus erythematosus, and hearing problems. In addition, people with diabetes should be aware that a diuretic may increase blood sugar levels. People with heart or blood vessel disease should know that some diuretics increase cholesterol or triglyceride levels. The risk of an allergic reaction to certain diuretics is greater in people with bronchial asthma. Before using diuretics, people with any of these medical conditions should make their physicians aware of their medical history. Also, people who have trouble urinating or who have high blood levels of potassium may not be able to take diuretics and should discuss these conditions with their physician before using them.

Side effects

Some people feel unusually tired when they first start taking diuretics. This effect usually becomes less noticeable over time, as the body adjusts to the medicine. Other side effects, such as loss of appetite, nausea, vomiting, stomach cramps, diarrhea, and dizziness, usually lessen or go away as the body adjusts to the diuretic drug. These problems usually do not need

medical attention unless they continue or interfere with normal activities.

Some diuretics make the skin more sensitive to sunlight. Even brief exposure to sun can cause severe sunburn, itching, a rash, redness, or other changes in skin color. While being treated with this medicine, the person should avoid being in direct sunlight; wear a hat and tightly woven clothing that covers the arms and legs; use a sunscreen with a skin protection factor (SPF) of at least 15; protect the lips with a sun-block lipstick; and not use tanning beds, tanning booths, or sunlamps. People with fair skin may need to use a sunscreen with a higher SPF.

Because diuretics increase urine output, people who take this medicine may need to urinate more often, even during the night. Healthcare professionals can help patients schedule their doses to avoid interfering with their sleep or regular activities.

Interactions

Diuretics may interact with other drugs, herbs, or dietary supplements. When this occurs, the effects of one or both of the drugs become either more or less effective or the risk of side effects may increase. Anyone who takes a diuretic should inform the healthcare providers about all other prescription and over-the-counter drugs, herbs, and dietary supplements that he or she is taking in order to avoid harmful interactions.

Some common drugs that may interact with diuretics include:

- Angiotensin-converting enzyme (ACE) inhibitors such as benazepril (Lotensin), captopril (Capoten), and enalapril (Vasotec), which are used to treat high blood pressure. Taking these drugs with potassium-sparing diuretics may cause levels of potassium in the blood to be too high, increasing the chance of side effects.
- Cholesterol-lowering drugs such as cholestyramine (Questran) and colestipol (Colestid). Taking these drugs with combination diuretics such as Dyazide and Maxzide may keep the diuretic from working. The person should take the diuretic at least one hour before or four hours after the cholesterol-lowering drug.
- Cyclosporine (Sandimmune), a drug that suppresses the immune system. Taking this medicine with potassium-sparing diuretics may increase the chance of side effects by causing levels of potassium in the blood to be too high.
- Potassium supplements, other drugs or supplements containing potassium, or salt substitutes that contain

potassium. Taking these with potassium-sparing diuretics may lead to too much potassium in the blood, increasing the chance of side effects.

- Lithium, used to treat bipolar disorder (manic-depressive illness). Using this medicine with potassium-sparing diuretics may allow lithium to build up to poisonous levels in the body.

- Digitalis, also called digoxin (Lanoxin) or digitoxin. Using this medicine with combination diuretics such as triamterene-hydrocholorthiazide (Dyazide, Maxzide) increases the chance of irregular heartbeat.

The list above does not include every drug or herb that may interact with diuretics. The patient should check with a physician or pharmacist before combining diuretics with any other prescription or over-the-counter drugs, herbal medicines, or dietary supplements.

Resources

BOOKS

Rubin, Alan L. *High Blood Pressure for Dummies* 2nd ed. Indianapolis, IN: Wiley Pub., 2007.

ORGANIZATIONS

American Heart Association. 7272 Greenville Avenue, Dallas, TX 75231. (800) 242-8721. http://www.american heart.org (accessed March 19, 2008).

OTHER

Anaizi, Nasr "Diuretics." The Drug Monitor [cited January 3, 2008]. http://www.thedrugmonitor.com/diuretics.html (accessed March 19, 2008).
"Diuretics." *Mayo Clinic.* December 22, 2006 [cited January 3, 2008]. http://www.mayoclinic.com/health/diuretics/HI00030 (accessed March 19, 2008).
"Diuretics Key Factor in Preventing Heart Failure." American Heart Association. May 1, 2006 [cited January 3, 2008]. http://www.americanheart.org/presenter.jhtml? identifier = 3039311 (accessed March 19, 2008).

Nancy Ross-Flanigan
Sam Uretsky, PharmD
Tish Davidson, AM

Diverticulectomy *see* Meckel's diverticulectomy

Diverticulitis

Definition

Diverticulitis is a condition in which tiny outpouchings of the colon (large intestine) become inflamed and infected. These outpouchings are called

diverticuli; the term that describes the presence of many of these diverticuli is "diverticulosis." Together, these conditions are referred to as diverticular disease.

Demographics

People can have diverticulosis without having any symptoms, and not all people with diverticulosis go on to develop diverticulitis. About 10% of people over 40 have diverticulosis; of these, about 10-25% will eventually develop diverticulitis in one or more of the diverticular pouches.

Description

Although the cause of diverticular disease is not completely understood, a low-fiber diet is thought to be an important factor. People who live in industrialized countries where low-fiber diets are prevalent (the United States, Great Britain, Australia) have higher rates of diverticular disease than do individuals living in arts of the world where higher-fiber diets are common (such as Asia). Low-fiber diets often result in some degree of constipation, requiring straining during defecation. This straining causes increased pressure in the colon, which may result in the development of diverticuli. When a bit of stool blocks the diverticulum, bacteria within the pouch may have the opportunity to grow, resulting in the infection of diverticulitis.

While some people can have diverticulosis without any recognizable symptoms, other people have clear-cut discomfort related to the condition, including bloating, cramps, and constipation. Diverticulitis causes more severe symptoms, such as

- Severe abdominal pain and cramping
- Fever and chills
- Nausea and vomiting
- Bleeding
- Fistula formation (most commonly between the colon and the bladder)
- Intestinal obstruction

Severe complications of untreated diverticulitis can result in a walled off, pus-filled area of infection called an abscess. Perforation of the diverticular pouch, may also occur, resulting in leakage of intestinal contents into the abdomen, and peritonitis (a severe and life-threatening infection of the lining of the abdominal cavity.

Diagnosis/Preparations

Asymptomatic cases of diverticulosis are often diagnosed during medical exams (such as colonoscopy) done for screening or other purposes. Diverticular disease can also be diagnosed with **barium enema** or **CT scan**. If bleeding is suspected, a radionuclide angiogram may be ordered, in order to evaluate the extent of bleeding.

Treatment

Treatment of diverticulosis starts with increasing fiber in the diet. However, once diverticulitis sets in, dietary interventions are insufficient. Diverticulitis must be treated with hospitalization, intravenous **antibiotics** (such as ampicillin, piperacillin, ciprofloxacin, and cefoxitin), nasogastric tube and suction to remove accumulating gastric juices (in the case of intestinal obstruction), and bowel rest (taking nothing by mouth or staying on a liquid diet until the intestine has healed sufficiently).

In some cases, surgical intervention will be required. Surgery may utilize a traditional open incision (**laparotomy**) or may be achieved through minimally invasive, laparoscopic techniques (**laparoscopy**), using several tiny incisions, a lighted fiberoptic scope, and miniaturized surgical instruments. The section of the colon with the infected diverticuli will be removed (bowel resection). In uncomplicated cases of diverticulosis, the two remaining ends of intestine will be attached to each other, restoring an intact gastrointestinal tract.

When severe inflammation and infection are present, however, the remaining ends cannot be rejoined immediately.The remaining end of the colon closest to the rectum will be closed off temporarily. The end of the colon that is continuous with the small intestine will be brought to the surface of the abdomen and connected up with a temporary stoma (hole) through the abdomen. This allows stool to exit through this **colostomy**, into a special bag that can be put over the stoma to catch the feces. After a few months, a second operation will be performed to close the stoma and reattach the ends of the colon to each other.

Resources

BOOKS

Feldman, M., et al. *Sleisenger & Fordtran's Gastrointestinal and Liver Disease.* 8th ed. St. Louis: Mosby, 2005.

Khatri, V. P., and J. A. Asensio. *Operative Surgery Manual.* 1st ed. Philadelphia: Saunders, 2003.

Townsend, C. M., et al. *Sabiston Textbook of Surgery.* 17th ed. Philadelphia: Saunders, 2004.

Rosalyn Carson-DeWitt, MD

DNR order *see* **Do not resuscitate order (DNR)**

Do not resuscitate (DNR) order

Definition

A do not resuscitate (DNR) order is a kind of advanced medical directive allowed by a 1991 federal law. The law expanded the notion of patient autonomy to situations in which patients may not be able to make crucial medical decisions due to incapacitation. A DNR order instructs medical personnel not to perform life-saving **cardiopulmonary resuscitation** (CPR) or other procedures to restart the heart or breathing once it has ceased. By law, the DNR directive must be offered as an option to patients by health providers in and, in some states, outside a hospital setting. Once signed, the DNR directive must be placed in the patient's chart.

Purpose

With such advanced cardiopulmonary techniques as CPR, it is possible to keep almost any patient's heart and lungs functioning, independent of how terminal or hopeless his or her medical condition becomes. The DNR program is designed to help people in the final stages of a terminal illness or those who are suffering from intractable pain the option for deciding against life-saving measures that may only prolong their pain and inevitable **death**. The option of deciding against life-saving measures is considered to be a formal part of patient autonomy and is respected as an ethical subset of medical **informed consent**.

Description

DNR orders affect a small group of patients and are designed to avoid the suffering of a terminal illness or other serious conditions that are medically irreversible. The order actually authorizes medical treatment to be

KEY TERMS

Advanced medical directive—A legal document drafted by a patient, in advance, ordering specific medical procedures to be offered or withheld if they are incapacitated.

Cardiopulmonary resuscitation (CPR)—A set of medical procedures used in an emergency to restart the heart and lungs.

Medical agent—A designated representative for the patient who, in advance, is legally empowered to carry out their wishes with respect to medial care.

Medical surrogate—Another name for a medical agent or person legally designated to represent the patient with medical providers.

withheld. It is included with the medical orders in the medical chart, and with it, hospital and pre-hospital personnel are restricted from using CPR techniques and other measures to revive the patient.

Some states allow DNR orders only in hospital settings. Other states allow DNR orders to be honored by emergency responders working outside the hospital setting. Over half of the states in the United States have pre-hospital DNR orders. A physician must sign the pre-hospital DNR directives. The state's emergency medical service (EMS) department or state medical association administers the programs. In some states, the DNR may be called a pre-hospital medical care directive or a comfort care-only document.

A DNR order can be revoked at any time in any way that effectively communicates the patient's desire. It can come from the patient in the form of a letter or document. It can come from the patient telling an emergency provider to disregard the order. The revocation can be invoked by removing any bracelet or medallion that indicates DNR status. It can be communicated by the designated health agent or patient representative who has the power to express the patient's wishes to health providers. Some states maintain a registry for individuals with DNR orders. It is important to find out about a state's service for DNR and its particular legal forms and requirements. Many patients who die in a hospital have had a DNR order.

Preparation

Do not resuscitate orders are a part of advanced medical directives. Advanced directives are legal documents that place limits on medical treatment, guide medical providers on the wishes and options of the patient,

and help family members and providers make decisions in accordance with the patient's wishes. Advanced directives are prepared in advance and may include a **living will** that details the patient's wishes should he or she become incapacitated. A DNR order is a very specific order that medical treatment be withheld, especially CPR. Finally, a medical agent or a person with a durable medical **power of attorney** is usually appointed to carry out all wishes of the patient and to make sure that specific wishes, like DNR, are honored.

An advanced directive for withholding resuscitation can be prepared by requesting a form from the physician, by writing down that wish, by having a lawyer draft a living will, or by using computer software for legal documents. States differ in the respect of whether the documents must be cosigned or notarized. Crucial to the effort is that the physician be told of the wishes of the patient.

Normal results

DNR law varies from state to state, but the common features include:

- Formal documents that providers or responders can readily recognize in charts or on display in the home.
- DNR bracelets or medallions that the patient wears and providers are trained to recognize.
- DNR must be signed by a physician before responders or other providers may honor them.
- Once in effect, DNR orders include only certain life-preserving procedures, like CPR. Comfort treatment is not withheld, and the alleviation of pain is still pursued by providers.
- Physicians or other providers who are unwilling to carry out the order (for moral or professional reasons) are required to transfer the care of the patient to another provider who will carry out the DNR order.

Resources

PERIODICALS

Kish, S.K. "Advance Directives in Critically Ill Cancer Patients." In *Critical Care Nursing Clinics North America* 12 (September 1, 2000): 373–83.

Matousek, M. "Start the Conversation: The Modern Maturity Guide to End-of-Life Care" and "The Last Taboo." *Modern Maturity/AARP* (September–October 2000).

ORGANIZATIONS

Cancer Information Service. (800) 4-CANCER (800-422-6237). TTY: (800)332-8615. http://www.cancer.gov (accessed March 19, 2008).

Partnership for Caring. 1620 Eye St., NW, Suite 202, Washington, DC 20006. (202) 296-8071. Fax: (202) 296-8352. Toll-free hotline: (800) 989-9455 (option 3). http://www.partnershipforcaring.org/ (accessed March 19, 2008).

OTHER

"Advanced Directives and Do Not Resuscitate Orders." American Academy of Family Physicians. March 2002 [cited May 5, 2003]. http://familydoctor.org/handouts/003.html (accessed March 19, 2008).

"Choosing a Health Care Agent." *Healthwise* WebMD Health [cited May 5, 2003]. http://www.WebMD.com (accessed March 19, 2008).

"Death and Dying." *Health Topics* National Library of Medicine, NIH/MedlinePlus [cited May 5, 2003]. http://www.nlm.nih.gov/medlineplus/deathanddying.html (accessed March 19, 2008).

"Death and Dying." In *Merck Manual, Home Edition* [cited May 5, 2003]. http://www.merck.com/mmhe/index.html (accessed March 19, 2008).

Nancy McKenzie, PhD
Fran Hodgkins

Dopamine *see* **Adrenergic drugs**

Doppler echocardiography *see*
Echocardiography

Doxycycline *see* **Tetracyclines**

Dressings *see* **Bandages and dressings**

Drug-resistant organisms

Definition

Drug-resistant organisms include bacteria and other pathogens that are not affected by one or more pharmaceutical products. Stated differently, one or more drugs are no longer able to control or kill a particular bacterium or pathogen.

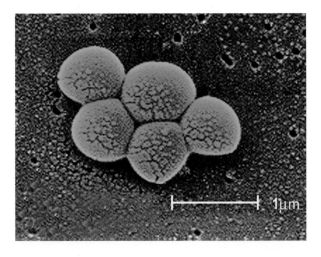

Methicillin-resistant staph bacteria. *(Scott Camazine / Alamy)*

Purpose

With the possible exception of being used as a biological weapon, there is no desired purpose for a drug-resistant organism.

Demographics

In the 1940s, penicillin resistance to *staphylococcus aureus* was first reported. Other strains of pathogens have become drug resistant since that time. The rate of drug resistance is increasing more rapidly than the number of new drugs that are being discovered.

Description

Drug-resistant organisms are pathogens that have become immune to the effects of one or more drugs that once controlled or eliminated them. One common mechanism for creating drug resistance is inadequate treatment. People discontinue use of a drug before all pathogens have been eliminated. Those that remain tend to be hardier and more difficult to kill. Over time, the remaining pathogens are likely to mutate and acquire immunity to a drug used to treat them.

Some pathogens have become resistant to more than one drug. Tuberculosis is an example of a pathogen that has become resistant to multiple drugs.

Examples of drug-resistant organisms include the following:

- MRSA—methicillin-resistant *Staphylococcus aureus*
- MRSE—methicillin-resistant *Staphylococcus epidermitis*
- VRE—vancomycin-resistant *enterococcus*
- PRSP—penicillin-resistant *Streptococcus pneumonia*
- TB—*mycobacterium tuberculosis*

Diagnosis/Preparation

Drug-resistant organisms are identified by isolation and drug susceptibility testing. These procedures are conducted in a clinical laboratory by a medical technologist or a clinical microbiologist.

Aftercare

Appropriate treatment after being exposed to a drug-resistant organism is to administer a different drug to which an organism or pathogen is sensitive.

The Centers for Disease Control and Prevention recommend that the following steps be taken after possible contact or exposure to a drug-resistant organism:

- Washing one's hands with soap and hot water
- Wearing disposable gloves if contact with body fluids contaminated with drug-resistant organisms is likely to occur; wash hands after removing the gloves
- Towels and bedding used by persons with a drug-resistant organism should be regularly changed
- Towels used by caregivers should be washed in hot water or discarded after use

Risks

Healthy persons have a low risk for contracting drug-resistant organisms. Centers for Disease Control and Prevention guidelines permit (but do not encourage) casual touching or brief hugging of persons with drug-resistant organisms. Washing hands with hot water and soap after casual contact with a person infected with drug-resistant organism is strongly encouraged.

The following risk factors increase the likelihood of becoming infected with a drug-resistant organism:

- Having a serious or severe illness such as diabetes mellitus
- Having chronic renal failure
- Experiencing open skin lesions or a dermatitis

- Having been recently catheterized or undergone renal dialysis
- Having been previously treated for a drug-resistant organism
- Being over age 65
- Taking a steroid or other drug that can suppress the immune system
- Being hospitalized for more than 10 days

Normal results

An alternate drug, if available, must be found when an organism becomes drug-resistant.

Morbidity and mortality rates

Alternative drugs may have unwanted side-effects.

Accurate morbidity and mortality data are not generally available.

Alternatives

Alternatives may or may not be available. They may have unwanted side-effects or be more expensive than th drug to which a pathogen has become resistant.

An alternate drug, if available, must be found when an organism becomes drug-resistant.

Resources

BOOKS

Fischbach, F. T. and M. B. Dunning. *A Manual of Laboratory and Diagnostic Tests.* 8th ed. Philadelphia: Lippincott Williams & Wilkins, 2008.

McGhee, M. *A Guide to Laboratory Investigations.* 5th ed. Oxford, UK: Radcliffe Publishing Ltd, 2008.

Price, C. P. *Evidence-Based Laboratory Medicine: Principles, Practice, and Outcomes.* 2nd ed. Washington, DC: AACC Press, 2007.

Scott, M.G., A. M. Gronowski, and C. S. Eby. *Tietz's Applied Laboratory Medicine.* 2nd ed. New York: Wiley-Liss, 2007.

Springhouse, A. M.. *Diagnostic Tests Made Incredibly Easy!* 2nd ed. Philadelphia: Lippincott Williams & Wilkins, 2008.

PERIODICALS

Izumeda, M., M. Nagai, A. Ohta, et al. "Epidemics of drug-resistant bacterial infections observed in infectious disease surveillance in Japan, 2001–2005." *Journal of Epidemiology* 17, Supplement (2007): S42–S47.

Kato, Y., M. Fukayama, T. Adachi, et al. "Multidrug-resistant typhoid fever outbreak in travelers returning from Bangladesh." *Emerging Infectious Disease* 13, no. 12 (2007): 1954–1955.

Koenig, R. "Drug-resistant tuberculosis. In South Africa, XDR TB and HIV prove a deadly combination." *Science* 319, no. 5865 (2008): 894–897.

Sjolund, M., J. Bonnedahl, J. Hernandez, et al. "Dissemination of multidrug-resistant bacteria into the Arctic." *Emerging Infectious Disease* 14, no. 1 (2008): 70–72.

ORGANIZATIONS

American Academy of Family Physicians. 11400 Tomahawk Creek Parkway, Leawood, KS 66211-2672. (913) 906-6000. E-mail: fp@aafp.org. http://www.aafp.org.

American Academy of Pediatrics. 141 Northwest Point Boulevard, Elk Grove Village, IL 60007-1098. (847) 434-4000, Fax: (847) 434-8000. E-mail: kidsdoc@aap.org. http://www.aap.org/default.htm.

American College of Physicians. 190 N. Independence Mall West, Philadelphia, PA 19106-1572. (800) 523-1546, x2600, or (215) 351-2600. http://www.acponline.org.

American Medical Association. 515 N. State Street, Chicago, IL 60610. (312) 464-5000. http://www.ama-assn.org.

OTHER

AIDS Treatment Data Network. "Information about drug resistance." 2008 [cited February 25, 2008]. http://www.atdn.org/simple/resistance.html.

Centers for Disease Control and Prevention. "Information about drug resistance." 2008 [cited February 22, 2008]. http://www.cdc.gov/drugresistance/.

National Institute of Allergy and Infectious Disease. "Information about drug resistance." 2008 [cited February 24, 2008]. http://www3.niaid.nih.gov/topics/antimicrobialresistance/.

World Health Organization. "Information about drug resistance." 2008 [cited February 24, 2008]. http://www.who.int/drugresistance/en/.

L. Fleming Fallon, Jr, MD, DrPH

Drugs used in labor *see* **Uterine stimulants**

Durable medical power of attorney *see* **Power of attorney**

Dying *see* **Death and dying**

Ear, nose, and throat surgery

Definition

Ear, nose, and throat surgery is the surgical treatment of diseases, injuries, or deformations of the ears, nose, throat, head, and neck areas.

Purpose

The purpose of surgery to the ears, nose, throat, head, and neck is to treat an abnormality, such as a defect or disease, in these anatomical areas. An anatomical deformity is a change that usually occurs during embryological development, leaving the affected person with the apparent defect. A disease in this area usually develops later in life, such as head and neck cancer. Additionally, the specialty known as otorhinolaryngology (ears [*oto*], nose [*rhino*], and throat [*laryn*], referring to the larynx or throat) also includes surgical intervention for diseases in the head and neck regions. Most ears, nose, and throat (ENT) surgeons in the United States are referred to as otolaryngologist and the specialty as otolaryngology. Ear surgery is usually performed to correct specific causes of hearing loss. Nose surgery can include different types of procedures necessary to treat sinus problems, like sinus surgery. Throat surgery can include complicated procedures such as cancer of the larynx resulting in a **laryngectomy**, or more simple procedures such as surgical removal of the adenoids, known as an **adenoidectomy**, or tonsils, known as a **tonsillectomy**. Head and neck surgery may be necessary to remove a tumor or reconstruct an area after disfigurement from trauma or injury.

Demographics

Ears, nose, and throat surgery comprises many different types of surgical procedures and spans over all age groups regardless of gender or ethnicity. Pediatric otolaryngology, a subspecialty, is the branch that treats ENT problems for infants and children.

Description

ENT surgery is the oldest surgical specialty in the United States, and it is one of the most elaborate fields of surgical specialty services, using advanced technology and a broad range of procedures that also includes major **reconstructive surgery** to correct deformity or injury. **Cosmetic surgery** can include surgical procedures to improve wrinkles in the face, contours of the nose and ears, chin augmentation, and **hair transplantation**.

Typically, ear surgery corrects defects causing hearing loss or impairment. Such procedures include **stapedectomy**, the removal of all or part of a bone in the middle ear called the stapes; **tympanoplasty**, or reconstruction of the ear drum; and **cochlear implants**, which is implantation of a device to stimulate nerve ends within the inner portion of the ear to enable hearing. Surgery of the ear also includes myringotomy, or insertion of ear tubes to drain fluid in persons with chronic ear infections.

Common surgical procedures of the throat include removal of tonsils (tonsillectomy) or adenoids (adenoidectomy). The tonsils, found on either side and in back of the throat, and adenoids, which are higher up the throat behind the nose, are masses of lymph tissue that play an active role in body defenses to fight infection. The tonsils and adenoids can get chronically infected, in which case surgical removal is usually indicated to relieve breathing problems and infection recurrence. Furthermore, chronic inflammation of the adenoids can cause repeated middle ear infections that can ultimately impair hearing.

Surgery of the nose can include procedures that treat sinus diseases. Advanced endoscopic surgery for sinus and nasal disorders can eliminate the need for external incisions and greater surgical precision. Other common surgical procedures include correction of a

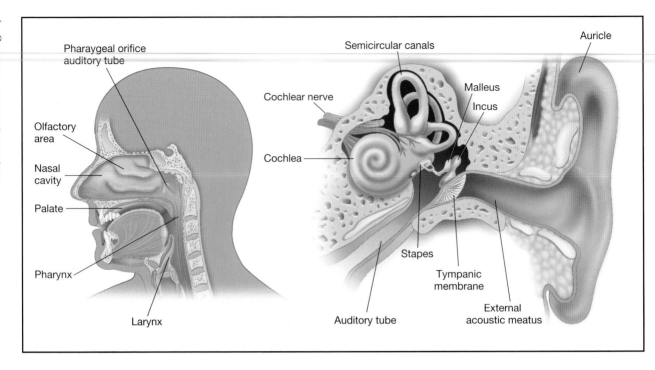

Pharaygeal orifice
auditory tube

Olfactory
area

Nasal
cavity

Palate

Pharynx

Larynx

Semicircular canals

Auricle

Cochlear nerve

Malleus

Incus

Cochlea

Stapes

Tympanic
membrane

Auditory tube

External
acoustic meatus

(Illustration by Electronic Illustrators Group.)

deviated nasal septum (**septoplasty**) and for chronic nasal obstruction (congestion).

Surgery of the neck region can commonly include **tracheotomy**, a surgical procedure in which an opening is made in the trachea or windpipe. Tracheotomy is indicated for a person who is unable to deliver enough oxygen to the lungs. ENT surgeons also perform complicated surgical procedures for the treatment of malignant head and neck cancers. In addition to **tumor removal**, when indicated, ENT surgeons may perform an operation called **radical neck dissection**, during which the ENT will remove cancer that has spread via lymphatic vessels to regional neck lymph nodes. Neck dissection is also useful since specimens can be removed for pathological examination, which can provide important information concerning metastasis, or spread, and can direct the treatment plan (i.e., radiation therapy and/or chemotherapy may be recommended for aggressive cancers). ENT surgeons also treat sleep-related disorders such as sleep apnea and excessive snoring; a procedure called laser-assisted uvula palatoplasty (LAUP) will remove tissue to allow for unobstructed airflow.

Other ENT procedures include surgical reconstruction of ear deformities (otoplasties), special surgery for diseases in the inner ear, and skull-based surgeries (neuro-otology). As well, ENT surgeons can surgically treat abnormalities near the eye, perform oral surgery for treatment of dental and jaw injury, and remove skin cancer within the head and neck region. ENT surgeons also perform special surgical techniques that can preserve nerve and blood vessel function (**microsurgery**) and reconstruction of bone and soft tissue.

Diagnosis/Preparation

A careful history and **physical examination** of the ears, nose, throat, head, and neck is a standard approach during initial consultation. Different instruments with light sources, like an otoscope for ear examinations, enable ENT surgeons to quickly visualize the ears, nose, and throat. Visualization of these areas can reveal the severity of the disease or deformity. The head and neck area is inspected and the neck and throat area is typically felt with the surgeon's hands, a technique known as palpation. Special technological advancements have enabled ENT surgeons to further visualize deep internal anatomical structures. Nasal endoscopy allows visualization of the upper airway to detect anatomical problems related to sinuses. Videostroboscopy can be used to visualize the vocal cords, and triple endoscopy (laryngoscopy, esophagoscopy, and **bronchoscopy**) can diagnose and stage head and neck cancers. Preparation before surgery is fairly standardized and includes blood work-up and instructions to have nothing to eat or drink after midnight of the night before the procedure.

Aftercare

The aftercare for ENT surgery depends on the procedure and state of the health of the patient. The aftercare for a patient who is 60 years old with head/neck cancer is more extensive than a tonsillectomy performed in a young adolescent or child. Generally, aftercare should be directed toward **wound care** and knowledge gained from the surgeon specifically detailing the expected length of average convalescence. Wound care, such as cleansing and dressing changes, and postoperative follow-up with the ENT surgeon is essential. Medications for pain may be prescribed. Patients stay in the hospital for eight to 10 hours for the effects of anesthesia to subside for same-day surgical procedures like a tonsillectomy, or they may be admitted for a few days for more complicated procedures, such as those related to cancer treatment. Aftercare and convalescence may take longer for complicated procedures such as advanced cancer, temporal-bone surgery for nerve disorders that can affect balance, or for tumors.

Risks

The risk of ENT surgery depends on the procedure and the health status of the patient. Some procedures do not have much risk, while complications for other procedures can carry considerable risk. For example, the risk of a complicated operation such as neck dissection could result in loss of ear sensation, since the nerve that provides the feeling of sensation is commonly severed during the procedure.

Normal results

There will be a cure or an improvement of the primary disease. Ear surgery should help individuals hear well. Throat surgery can help remove chronically inflamed tonsils, adenoids, polyps, or cancer. Nose surgery for deviated septums or nasal congestion will improve breathing problems and help a person breath more easily and effectively through the nose. Neck surgery can help remove diseased tissue and prevent

further spread of cancer. Surgery for sleep apnea will remove redundant tissue that blocks airways and obstructs normal airflow.

Morbidity and mortality rates

Outcome and disease progression vary for each disease state. There are no general statistics for all ENT procedures. Some procedures are generally correlated with excellent morbidity, such as over 90% success rates for all cases receiving tympanoplasty, and no mortality, while others may be associated with poor outcome and much illness, like advanced head/neck cancer.

Alternatives

Usually, surgery is indicated when benefit from surgery is a clear-cut primary intervention or when medical, or conservative treatment has failed to provide sustained symptomatic improvement. A person diagnosed with cancer may not have an alternative conservative treatment, depending on the stage of their cancer; however, a person with sinus problems may be treated conservatively with **antibiotics**, saline nasal spray wash, steroid nasal spray, and/or antihistamine spray before indication or necessity for surgery. There are many other services that the ENT surgeon uses to treat specific diseases, including audiology services for diagnostic and therapeutic purposes, like hearing aids, and services to treat disorders of speech and voice.

Resources

BOOKS

Corbridge, Rogan, and Nicholas Steventon. *Oxford Handbook of ENT and Head and Neck Surgery*. New York: Oxford University Press, 2006.

McPhee, Stephen, et al. "Ears, Nose, and Throat." In *Current Medical Diagnosis and Treatment,* 35th ed. Stamford, CT: Appleton & Lange, 1995.

Stamm, Aldo C. and Wolfgang Craf. *Micro-endoscopic Surgery of the Paranasal Sinuses and the Skull Base*. New York: Springer, 2000.

ORGANIZATIONS

American Academy of Otolaryngology-Head and Neck Surgery, One Prince Street, Alexandria, VA, 22314-3357, (703) 836-4444, http://www.entnet.org.

American Hearing Research Foundation, 8 S. Michigan Avenue, Suite 814, Chicago, IL, 60603, (312) 726-9670, http://www.american-hearing.org/.

American Speech-Language-Hearing Association, 2200 Research Boulevard, Rockville, MD, 20850-3289, (800) 638-8255, http://www.asha.org.

Laith Farid Gulli, M.D., M.S.
Robert Ramirez, B.S.
Laura Jean Cataldo, R.N., Ed.D.

Ear surgery *see* **Otoplasty**

Ear tubes *see* **Myringotomy and ear tubes**

Eardrum repair *see* **Tympanoplasty**

ECCE *see* **Extracapsular cataract extraction**

ECG *see* **Electrocardiography**

Echocardiography

Definition

Echocardiography is a noninvasive diagnostic test that uses **ultrasound** waves to produce an moving image of the heart.

Purpose

Echocardiography is one of the most widely used diagnostic tests for heart disease. Ultrasound waves generated by a device placed on the skin rebound or echo off the heart and are processed by a computer. The resulting image can show the size, shape, and movement of the heart's valves and chambers, as well as the flow of blood through the heart.

Echocardiography may reveal abnormalities such damage to the heart tissue from a heart attack or as a poorly functioning heart valve. Echocardiography is especially useful for assessing disorders of the heart valves. It not only allows doctors to evaluate the condition of the heart valves, but also can show abnormalities in the pattern of blood flow. For example, echocardiography can show the backward flow of blood through heart valves that remain partially open and should be fully closed.

By assessing the motion of the heart wall, echocardiography can help detect the presence and assess the severity of coronary artery disease, as well as help determine whether chest pain is related to heart disease. Additionally, echocardiography can help detect hypertrophic cardiomyopathy, a condition in which

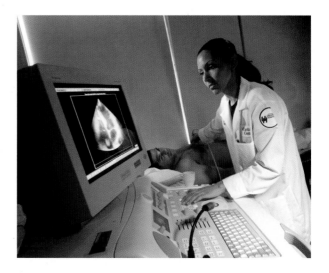

Echocardiography. *(Yoav Levy/Phototake. Reproduced by permission.)*

the walls of the heart thicken in an attempt to compensate for heart muscle weakness.

Echocardiography is also used to evaluate heart murmurs (abnormal heart sounds), determine the causes of congestive heart failure, assess enlarged hearts, hearts with septal defects (holes between pumping chambers), and to monitor the heart in patients with diseases that may affect heart function (e.g., lupus erythematosus, lung diseases). The biggest advantage to echocardiography is that it is noninvasive (it does not involve breaking the skin or entering body cavities), and it has no known risks or side effects. It also gives a more detailed picture of the heart than other imaging techniques. Echocardiography is often used in conjunction with other diagnostic tests for the heart such as **electrocardiography**.

Echocardiography is usually performed in the cardiology department at a hospital, but may also be performed in a cardiologist's office or an outpatient imaging center. Because the ultrasound scanners used to perform echocardiography are portable (handheld) or mobile, echocardiography can be performed in a hospital emergency department or at the bedside of patients who cannot be moved.

Description

Echocardiography creates an image of the heart using ultra-high-frequency sound waves—sound waves that are too high in frequency to be heard by the human ear. The technique is very similar to ultrasound scanning commonly used to visualize the fetus during pregnancy.

An echocardiography examination generally lasts 15–30 minutes. The patient lies bare-chested on an examination table. A special gel is spread over the chest to help the transducer make good contact and to slide smoothly over the skin. The transducer, also called a probe, is a small handheld device at the end of a flexible cable. The transducer is placed against the chest and directs ultrasound waves into the chest. Some of the waves get echoed (or reflected) back to the transducer. Since different tissues and blood reflect ultrasound waves differently, these returning sound waves can be translated into a meaningful image of the heart that is displayed on a monitor and recorded. The patient does not feel the sound waves, and the entire procedure is painless.

Occasionally, variations of the echocardiography test are used. For example, Doppler echocardiography employs a special transducer that allows technicians to measure and analyze the direction and speed of blood flow through blood vessels and heart valves. This makes it especially useful for detecting and evaluating backflow through the heart valves. By assessing the speed of blood

flow at different locations around an obstruction, it can also help to precisely locate the obstruction.

An **exercise** echocardiogram, or stress echo, is an echocardiogram performed during exercise, when the heart muscle must work harder to supply blood to the body. This allows doctors to detect heart problems that might not be evident when the body is at rest and needs less blood. For patients who are unable to exercise, certain drugs can be used to mimic the effects of exercise by dilating the blood vessels and making the heart beat faster.

A transesophageal is done when it is difficult to get a clear picture of the heart using standard **electrocardiogram** techniques (e.g., interference from internal scar tissue, obesity). A transducer is attached to an endoscope, a thin tube that is threaded down the throat after it has been numbed. This position allows a clearer picture of the heart.

During the examination, a trained sonographer takes measurements and, using the ultrasound scanner's computer, make calculations, including measuring blood flow speed. Most ultrasound scanners are equipped with videotape recorders or digital imaging/archiving devices to record the real-time examination, and with medical image printers to print out hard copies of still images. Information from the echocardiogram is then evaluated by a cardiologist.

Preparation

The patient removes any clothing and jewelry above the waist.

Aftercare

No special measures need to be taken following echocardiography. The procedure is painless.

Risks

There are no known complications associated with the use of echocardiography. There is a slight risk of having a heart attack during an exercise echocardiogram, due to the stress put on the heart during the test, mostly for patients with a history of heart attack or other risk factors.

Normal results

A normal echocardiogram shows a normal heart structure and the normal flow of blood through the heart chambers and heart valves. However, a normal echocardiogram does not rule out the possibility certain types of heart disease.

An echocardiogram may show a number of abnormalities in the structure and function of the heart, including:

- thickening of the wall of the heart muscle (especially the left ventricle)
- abnormal motion of the heart muscle
- blood leaking backward through the heart valves
- decreased blood flow through a heart valve due to narrowing of the valve (stenosis)

Resources

ORGANIZATIONS

American College of Cardiology. Heart House. 2400 N Street, NW | Washington, DC 20037. (202) 375-6000. http://www.acc.org (accessed March 19, 2008).

American Heart Association. 7272 Greenville Avenue, Dallas, TX 75231. (800) 242-8721. http://www.american heart.org (accessed March 19, 2008).

American Registry of Diagnostic Medical Sonographers.51 Monroe Street, Plaza One East, Rockville, MD 20850. (800) 541-9754. http://www.ardms.org (accessed March 19, 2008).

American Society of Echocardiography. 1500 Sunday Drive, Suite 102, Raleigh, NC 27607. (919) 861-5574. http://www.asecho.org (accessed March 19, 2008).

OTHER

"Echocardiogram." *Medline Plus* April 12, 2007 [cited January 4, 2008]. http://www.nlm.nih.gov/medlineplus/ency/article/003869.htm (accessed March 19, 2008).

"Echocardiogram: Sound Imaging of the Heart." *Mayo Clinic* July 14, 2006 [cited January 4, 2008]. http://www.mayoclinic.com/health/echocardiogram/HB00012 (accessed March 19, 2008).

Jennifer E. Sisk, MA
Lee Shratter, MD
Tish Davidson, AM

Ectopic pregnancy treatment *see* **Salpingostomy**

EECP *see* **Enhanced external counterpulsation**

EEG *see* **Electroencephalography**

EKG *see* **Electrocardiography**

Elective abortion *see* **Abortion, induced**

Elective surgery

Definition

An elective surgery is a planned, non-emergency surgical procedure. It may be either medically required (e.g., cataract surgery), or optional (e.g., breast augmentation or implant) surgery.

Purpose

Elective surgeries may extend life or improve the quality of life physically and/or psychologically. Cosmetic and reconstructive procedures, such as a facelift (rhytidectomy), tummy tuck (**abdominoplasty**), or **nose surgery** (**rhinoplasty**), may not be medically indicated, but they may benefit the patient in terms of raising self-esteem. Other procedures, such as cataract surgery, improve functional quality of life even though they are not medically necessary.

Some elective procedures are necessary to prolong life, such as an **angioplasty**. However, unlike **emergency surgery** (e.g., **appendectomy**), which must be performed immediately, a required elective procedure can be scheduled at the patient's and surgeon's convenience.

Demographics

According to the National Center for Health Statistics of the U.S. Centers for Disease Control and Prevention (CDC), in 2005 over 44 million inpatient surgical procedures were performed in the United States. Heart disease and delivery surgeries were the most frequently performed types of surgery. Statistically, women were more likely to have surgery, accounting for 59% of inpatient procedures. This data includes both emergency and elective procedures.

Description

There are hundreds of elective surgeries in modern medical practice, spanning all the systems of the body. Several major categories of common elective procedures include:

- Plastic surgery. Cosmetic or reconstructive surgery that improves appearance and, in some cases, physical function.
- Refractive surgery. Laser surgery for vision correction.
- Gynecological surgery. Either medically necessary or optional surgery (e.g., hysterectomy, tubal ligation).

- Exploratory or diagnostic surgery. Surgery to determine the origin and extent of a medical problem, or to biopsy tissue samples.
- Cardiovascular surgery. Nonemergency procedures to improve blood flow or heart function, such as angioplasty or the implantation of a pacemaker.
- Musculoskeletal system surgery. Orthopedic surgical procedures, such as hip replacement and ACL reconstruction.

Diagnosis/Preparation

In some cases, insurance companies may require a **second opinion** before approving payment on elective surgical procedures. Anyone considering an elective surgery should review their coverage requirements with their health insurance carrier before scheduling the procedure.

Diagnostic and/or radiological testing may be performed to confirm the diagnosis or assist the surgeon in planning the surgical procedure. Typically, a complete medical history, **physical examination**, and laboratory tests (e.g., **urinalysis**, **chest x ray**, blood work, and **electrocardiogram**) are administered as part of the preoperative evaluation.

Other preoperative preparations will depend on the surgery itself. If a general anesthetic is to be used, dietary restrictions may be placed on the patient prior to the operation. If blood loss is expected during the procedure,

advance banking of blood by the patient (known as autologous donation) may be recommended.

Aftercare

Recovery time and **postoperative care** will vary by the elective procedure performed. Patients should receive complete, written postoperative care instructions prior to returning home after surgery, and these instructions should be explained completely to them by the physician or nursing staff.

Risks

The risks for an elective surgery will vary by the type of procedure performed. In general, by their invasive nature most surgeries carry a risk of infection, hemorrhage, and circulatory problems such as shock or thrombosis (clotting within the circulatory system). The anesthesia used may also present certain risks for complications such as anaphylactic shock (an allergic reaction).

Normal results

Elective surgical results depend on the type of procedure performed. Optimal results for an elective procedure should be discussed with the patient's health care team prior to surgery. In some cases, the "normal" results from a surgery may only be temporary (i.e., follow-up surgery may be required at a later date), while other results are life long. For example, a facelift may eventually require a second procedure as a patient ages, whereas a **tubal ligation** offers permanent results.

Morbidity and mortality rates

Success, morbidity, and mortality rates also depend on the elective procedure itself. A physician and/or surgeon should be able to provide a patient with statistical information on success rates for a specific elective surgery.

Alternatives

The alternatives available for a particular surgery will depend on the purpose of the procedure. For example, other birth control options would be an alternative to any elective surgery for the purpose of sterilization (i.e., tubal ligation, **vasectomy**, **hysterectomy**). Other elective surgeries may not have a treatment alternative other than foregoing the surgery and living with the medical consequences. As part of **informed consent**, a patient's physician should review all possible treatment options, surgical and otherwise, before scheduling elective surgery.

Resources

BOOKS

Morrey, Bernard F., ed. *Joint Replacement Arthroplasty*, 3rd Edition. New York: Churchill Livingstone, 2003.

Thorne, Charles H., et al., eds. *Grabb and Smith's Plastic Surgery*, 6th Edition. Philadelphia: Wolters Kluwer Health/Lippincott Williams & Wilkins, 2007.

PERIODICALS

Wright, Charles J., G. Keith Chambers, and Yoel Robens-Paradise. "Evaluation of Indications for and Outcomes of Elective Surgery." *CMAJ* (September 2002): 167–72.

ORGANIZATIONS

American College of Surgeons. 633 N. St. Clair Drive, Chicago, IL 60611. 1-312-202-5001. Email: postmaster@facs.org. http://www.facs.org (accessed March 19, 2008).

Paula Ford-Martin
Robert Bockstiegel

Electrocardiogram

Definition

An electrocardiogram is a test that detects and records electrical activity of the heart. It is also called an EKG or ECG.

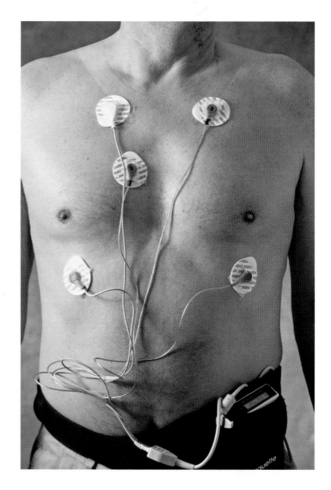

Electrocardiogram. *(blphoto / Alamy)*

Purpose

An electrocardiogram is used to detect and locate the source of heart irregularities.

Description

Electrical impulses are generated by specialized tissues in the heart called the sinoatrial node. These electrical impulses cause the muscles of the heart to contract generating heartbeats. The sinoatrial node is located in the right atrium. The electrical impulses travel from the right atrium to the left ventricle, casing the muscle to contract as they travel through the heart. As the heart contracts, it pumps blood out to the rest of the body. The electrical impulses can be detected by sensors. An electrocardiogram is a paper record of the electrical activity in the heart.

An electrocardiogram records how fast the heart beats. By recording many heartbeats in succession, the pattern and regularity of heartbeats can be observed. AN electrocardiogram records the strength and timing of the electrical impulses as they travel through each portion of the heart.

Many diseases of the heart cause changes in the pattern of electrical impulses that are generated. Recordings of these electrical impulses can help to diagnose many different heart problems. These include the following conditions.

• Interrupted or stopped heart beats (a heart attack)
• Changes in the flow of blood to the muscles of the heart
• Irregularities in heartbeats (either too fast or too slow)
• Changes in the force of pumping by the heart or the volume of blood pumped
• Changes in the thickness of heart muscles
• Changes in the size of any of the four chambers in the heart
• Evidence of birth defects in the heart
• Diseases affecting heart valves
• Changes in the speed of electrical impulses

Electrocardiogram recordings can assist in diagnosing a heart attack. Changes can be detected by comparing EKG tracings that are made at different times.

Preparation

An electrocardiogram requires minimal preparation. All drugs (prescription, over the counter, and herbal products) that have been used in the previous 24 to 48 hours should be disclosed. This is necessary as many such products can affect electrocardiograms.

Jewelry and clothing that contains metal should be removed.

Areas on the arms, legs, and chest where electrodes (small metal discs) are placed are cleaned. They may be shaved to provide a clean, smooth surface for attaching the electrode.

Disposable electrodes that require no preparation are most commonly used. These are attached to skin on the chest, arms and a leg. These are connected to the electrocardiogram recorder by wires.

Electrocardiograms only record electrical impulses generated by the body.

Precautions

Other than removing metal, no other precautions are needed prior to having an EKG test.

Side effects

The only known side effect of an electrocardiogram is slight pulling of skin when the electrodes are removed.

Interactions

Since an electrocardiogram only records and does not generate any electrical impulses, it does not interact with any bodily system or drugs.

Merck Manual. "Information about electrocardiography." 2008 [cited February 24, 2008]. http://www.merck.com/mmpe/sec05/ch047/ch047c.html.

National Library of Medicine. "Information about electrocardiography." 2008 [cited February 25, 2008]. http://www.ncbi.nlm.nih.gov/books/bv.fcgi?rid = cm.chapter.1019.

L. Fleming Fallon, Jr, MD, DrPH

KEY TERMS

Sinoatrial node—Specialized tissue in he right atrium that initiates electrical activity in the heart

Resources

BOOKS

Bickley, L. S., and P. G. Szilagyi. *Bates' Guide to Physical Examination and History Taking*. 9th ed. Philadelphia: Lippincott Williams and Wilkins, 2007.

Jarvis, C. *Physical Examination and Health Assessment*. 5th ed. Philadelphia: Saunders, 2007.

Seidel. H. M., J. Ball, J. Dains, and W. Bennedict. *Mosby's Physical Examination Handbook*. 6th ed. St. Louis: MOsby, 2006.

Swartz, M. H. *Textbook of Physical Diagnosis: History and Examination*. 5th ed. Philadelphia: Saunders, 2005.

PERIODICALS

Holmqvist, F., D. Husser, J. M. Tapanianen et al. "Interatrial conduction can be accurately determined using standard 12-lead electrocardiography: Validation of P-wave morphology using electroanatomic mapping in man." *Heart Rhythm* 5, no. 3 (2008): 413–418.

Nikus, K. C. "Electrocardiography." *Timely Topics I Medicine* 11, (2007): E29–E37.

Silverman, M. E. " Electrocardiographic-Clinical-Patho logic Sleuthing (by Dr. J. Willis Hurst)." *American Journal of Cardiology* 101, no. 4 (2008): 550–552.

Song, Z. Z. "Electrocardiography-synchronized multi-detector row CT of right ventricular function." *Radiology* 246, no. 3 (2008): 986–988.

ORGANIZATIONS

American Academy of Family Physicians. 11400 Tomahawk Creek Parkway, Leawood, KS 66211-2672. (913) 906-6000. E-mail: fp@aafp.org. http://www.aafp.org.

American Academy of Pediatrics. 141 Northwest Point Boulevard, Elk Grove Village, IL 60007-1098. (847) 434-4000; Fax: (847) 434-8000. E-mail: kidsdoc@aap.org. http://www.aap.org/default.htm.

American College of Physicians. 190 N Independence Mall West, Philadelphia, PA 19106-1572. (800) 523-1546, x2600, or (215) 351-2600. http://www.acponline.org.

American Medical Association. 515 N. State Street, Chicago, IL 60610. (312) 464-5000. http://www.ama-assn.org.

OTHER

American Heart Association. "Information about electrocardiography." 2008 [cited February 24, 2008]. http://www.americanheart.org/presenter.jhtml?identifier = 3004613.

Kid's Health. "Information about electrocardiography." 2008 [cited February 22, 2008]. http://www.kids health.org/parent/general/sick/ekg.html.

Electrocardiography

Definition

Electrocardiography is a commonly used, noninvasive procedure for recording electrical changes in the heart. The record, which is called an **electrocardiogram** (ECG or EKG), shows the series of waves that relate to the electrical impulses that occur during each beat of the heart. The results are printed on paper and/or displayed on a monitor to provide a visual representation of heart function. The waves in a normal record are named P, Q, R, S, and T, and follow in alphabetical order. The number of waves may vary, and other waves may be present.

Purpose

Electrocardiography is a starting point for detecting many cardiac problems, including angina pectoris, stable angina, ischemic heart disease, arrhythmias (irregular heartbeat), tachycardia (fast heartbeat), bradycardia (slow heartbeat), myocardial infarction (heart attack), and certain congenital heart conditions. It is used routinely in physical examinations and for monitoring a patient's condition during and after surgery, as well as in the intensive care setting. It is the basic measurement used in **exercise** tolerance tests (i.e., stress tests) and is also used to evaluate symptoms such as chest pain, shortness of breath, and palpitations.

Demographics

According to the U.S. Centers for Disease Control (CDC), nearly 23 million EKG procedures were performed in doctor's offices in the year 2000.

Men are more likely to experience heart attacks than women, although a woman's risk of heart attack rises after menopause. African-Americans, Hispanics, and Native Americans are all at greater risk for cardiovascular disease than Caucasians, in part because of the higher incidence of diabetes mellitus (a major risk factor for cardiovascular disease) in these populations.

KEY TERMS

Ambulatory monitoring—ECG recording over a prolonged period during which the patient can move around.

Arrhythmia or dysrhythmia—Abnormal rhythm in hearts that contract in an irregular way.

ECG or EKG—A record of the waves that relate to the electrical impulses produced at each beat of the heart.

Ectopic beat—Abnormal heart beat arising elsewhere than from the sinoatrial node.

Electrodes—Tiny wires in adhesive pads that are applied to the body for ECG measurement.

Fibrillation—Rapid, uncoordinated contractions of the upper or the lower chambers of the heart.

Lead—Name given the electrode when it is attached to the skin.

Reperfusion therapy—Restoration of blood flow to an organ or tissue; following a heart attack, quickly opening blocked arteries to reperfuse the heart muscles to minimize damage.

Description

The patient disrobes from the waist up, and electrodes (tiny wires in adhesive pads) are applied to specific sites on the arms, legs, and chest. When attached, these electrodes are called leads; three to 12 leads may be employed for the procedure.

Muscle movement may interfere with the recording, which lasts for several beats of the heart. In cases where rhythm disturbances are suspected to be infrequent, the patient may wear a small Holter monitor in order to record continuously over a 24-hour period. This is known as ambulatory monitoring.

Special training is required for interpretation of the electrocardiogram. To summarize in the simplest manner the features used in interpretations, the P wave of the electrocardiogram is associated with the contraction of the atria—the two chambers of the heart that receive blood from the veins. The QRS series of waves, or QRS complex, is associated with ventricular contraction, with the T wave coming after the contraction. The ventricles are the two chambers of the heart that receive blood from the atria and that send the blood into the arteries. Finally, the P-Q or P-R interval gives a value for the time taken for the electrical impulse to travel from the atria to the ventricle (normally less than 0.2 seconds).

Diagnosis/Preparation

Patients are asked not to eat for several hours before a **stress test**. Before the leads are attached, the skin is cleaned to obtain good electrical contact at the electrode positions and, occasionally, shaving the chest may be necessary.

Heart problems are diagnosed by the pattern of electrical waves produced during the EKG, and an abnormal rhythm can be called dysrhythmia. The cause of dysrhythmia is ectopic beats. Ectopic beats are premature heartbeats that arise from a site other than the sinus node—commonly from the atria, atrio-ventricular node, or the ventricle. When these dysrhythmias are only occasional, they may produce no symptoms or simply a feeling that the heart is turning over or "flip-flopping." These occasional dysrhythmias are common in healthy people, but they also can be an indication of heart disease.

The varied sources of dysrhythmias provide a wide range of alterations in the form of the electrocardiogram. Ectopic beats display an abnormal QRS complex. This can indicate disease associated with insufficient blood supply to the heart muscle (myocardial ischemia). Multiple ectopic sites lead to rapid and uncoordinated contractions of the atria or ventricles. This condition is known as fibrillation. When the atrial impulse fails to reach the ventricle, a condition known as heart block results.

Aftercare

To avoid skin irritation from the salty gel used to obtain good electrical contact, the skin should be thoroughly cleaned after removal of the electrodes.

Risks

The EKG is a noninvasive procedure that is virtually risk-free for the patient. There is a slight risk of heart attack for individuals undergoing a stress test EKG, but patients are carefully screened for their suitability for this test before it is prescribed.

Risk factors for heart disease include obesity, hypertension (high blood pressure), high triglycerides and total blood cholesterol, low HDL ("good") cholesterol, tobacco smoking, and increased age. People who have diabetes mellitus (either type 1 or type 2) are also at increased risk for cardiovascular disease.

Normal results

When the heart is operating normally, each part contracts in a specific order. Contraction of the muscle is triggered by an electrical impulse. These electrical impulses travel through specialized cells that form a conduction system. Following this pathway ensures that contractions will occur in a coordinated manner.

When the presence of all waves is observed in the electrocardiogram, and these waves follow the order defined alphabetically, the heart is said to show a normal sinus rhythm, and impulses may be assumed to be following the regular conduction pathway.

In the normal heart, electrical impulses—at a rate of 60–100 times per minute—originate in the sinus node. The sinus node is located in the first chamber of the heart, known as the right atrium, where blood reenters the heart after circulating through the body. After traveling down to the junction between the upper and lower chambers, the signal stimulates the atrioventricular node. From here, after a delay, it passes by specialized routes through the lower chambers or ventricles. In many disease states, the passage of the electrical impulse can be interrupted in a variety of ways, causing the heart to perform less efficiently.

The heart is described as showing arrhythmia or dysrhythmia when time intervals between waves, or the order or the number of waves do not fit the normal pattern described above. Other features that may be altered include the direction of wave deflection and wave widths.

Morbidity and mortality rates

According to the American Heart Association, cardiovascular disease is the number one cause of **death** in the United States. It is also the leading cause of death among people with diabetes.

Alternatives

Electrocardiography is the gold standard for detecting heart conditions involving irregularities in electrical conduction and rhythm. Other tests that may be used in conjunction with an EKG include an echocardiogram (a sonogram of the heart's pumping action) and a stress test—an EKG that is done in conjunction with treadmill or other supervised exercise to observe the heart's function under stress—may also be performed.

Resources

BOOKS

Beasley, Brenda. *Understanding EKGs: A Practical Approach,* 2nd ed. Upper Saddle River, NJ: Prentice Hall, 2002.

PERIODICALS

Fergusun, J. D., et al. "The Prehospital 12-Lead Electrocardiogram: Impact on Management of the Out-of-Hospital Acute Coronary Syndrome Patient." *American Journal of Emergency Medicine* 21, no. 2 (March 2003): 136–42.

Kadish, Alan, et al. "ACC/AHA Clinical Competence Statement on Electrocardiography and Ambulatory Electrocardiography." *Journal of The American College of Cardiology* 38, no. 7 (2001). http://www.acc.org/clinical/competence/ECG/pdfs/ECG_pdf.pdf.

ORGANIZATIONS

The American College of Cardiology. Heart House, 9111 Old Georgetown Road, Bethesda, MD 20814-1699. (800) 253- 4636. http://www.acc.org.

American Heart Association. 7272 Greenville Ave., Dallas, TX 75231. (800) 242-8721. http://www.americanheart.org.

Maggie Boleyn, R.N., B.S.N.
Paula Ford-Martin

Electroencephalography

Definition

Electroencephalography, or EEG, is a neurological test that involves attaching electrodes to the head of a person to measure and record electrical activity in the brain over time.

Purpose

The EEG, also known as a brain wave test, is a key tool in the diagnosis and management of epilepsy and other seizure disorders. It is also used to assist in the diagnosis of brain damage and diseases such as strokes, tumors, encephalitis, mental retardation, and sleep disorders. An EEG may also be used to monitor brain activity during surgery to assess the effects of anesthesia. It is also used to determine brain status and brain **death**.

Demographics

The number of EEG tests performed each year can only be estimated. It is not a reportable event and is used in the diagnostic workup for a number of disorders. The number of EEG tests per year is estimated to be in the range of 10–25 million.

Description

Before an EEG begins, a nurse or technologist attaches approximately 16–21 electrodes to a person's scalp using an electrically conductive, washable paste. The electrodes are placed on the head in a standard pattern based on head circumference measurements. Depending on the purpose for the EEG, implantable, or invasive, electrodes are occasionally used. Implantable electrodes include sphenoidal electrodes, which are fine wires inserted under the zygomatic arch, or cheekbone. Depth electrodes, or subdural strip electrodes, are surgically implanted into the brain and are used to localize a seizure focus in preparation for epilepsy surgery. Once in place, even implantable electrodes do not cause pain. The electrodes are used to measure the electrical activity in various regions of the brain over the course of the test period.

For the test, a person lies on a bed, padded table, or comfortable chair and is asked to relax and remain still while measurements are being taken. An EEG usually takes no more than one hour, although long-term monitoring is often used for diagnosis of seizure disorders. During the test procedure, a person may be asked to breathe slowly or quickly. Visual stimuli such as flashing lights or a patterned board may be used to stimulate certain types of brain activity. Throughout the procedure, the electroencephalography unit makes a continuous graphic record of the person's brain activity, or brain waves, on a long strip of recording paper or computer screen. This graphic record is called an electroencephalogram. If the display is computerized, the test may be called a digital EEG, or dEEG.

The sleep EEG uses the same equipment and procedures as a regular EEG. Persons undergoing a sleep EEG are encouraged to fall asleep completely rather than just relax. They are typically provided a bed and a quiet room conducive to sleep. A sleep EEG lasts up to three hours, or up to eight or nine hours if it is a night's sleep.

In an ambulatory EEG, individuals are hooked up to a portable cassette recorder. They then go about normal activities and take normal rest and sleep for a period of up to 24 hours. During this period, individuals and their family members record any symptoms or abnormal behaviors, which can later be correlated with the EEG to see if they represent seizures.

An extension of the EEG technique, called quantitative EEG (qEEG), involves manipulating the EEG signals with a computer using the fast Fourier transform algorithm. The result is then best displayed using a colored gray scale transposed onto a schematic map of the head to form a topographic image. The brain map produced in this technique is a vivid illustration of electrical activity in the brain. This technique also has the ability to compare the similarity of the signals between different electrodes, a measurement known as spectral coherence. Studies have shown the value of this measurement in diagnosis of Alzheimer's disease and mild closed-head injuries. The technique can also identify areas of the brain having abnormally slow activity when the data are both mapped and compared to known normal values. The result is then known as a statistical or significance probability map (SPM). This allows differentiation between early dementia (increased slowing) or otherwise uncomplicated depression (no slowing).

Diagnosis/Preparation

An EEG is generally performed as one test in a series of neurological evaluations. Rarely does the EEG form the sole basis for a particular diagnosis.

Full instructions should be given to individuals receiving an EEG when they schedule their test. Typically, individuals taking medications that affect the central nervous system, such as anticonvulsants, stimulants, or antidepressants, are told to discontinue their prescription for a short time prior to the test (usually one to two days). However, such requests should be cleared with the treating physician. EEG test candidates may be asked to avoid food and beverages that contain caffeine, a central nervous system stimulant. They may also be asked to arrive for the test with clean hair that is free styling products to make attachment of the electrodes easier.

Individuals undergoing a sleep EEG may be asked to remain awake the night before their test. They may be given a sedative prior to the test to induce sleep.

Aftercare

If an individual has suspended regular medication for the test, the EEG nurse or technician should advise as to when to begin taking it again.

Risks

Being off certain medications for one to two days may trigger seizures. Certain procedures used during EEG may trigger seizures in persons with epilepsy. Those procedures include flashing lights and deep breathing. If the EEG is being used as a diagnostic for epilepsy (i.e., to determine the type of seizures an individual is experiencing) this may be a desired effect, although the person needs to be monitored closely so that the seizure can be aborted if necessary. This type of test is known as an ictal EEG.

Normal results

In reading and interpreting brain wave patterns, a neurologist or other physician will evaluate the type of brain waves and the symmetry, location, and consistency of brain wave patterns. Brain wave response to certain stimuli presented during the EEG test (such as flashing lights or noise) will also be evaluated.

The four basic types of brain waves are alpha, beta, theta, and delta, with the type distinguished by frequency. Alpha waves fall between 8 and 13 Hertz (Hz), beta are above 13 Hz, theta between 4 and 7 Hz, and delta are less than 4 Hz. Alpha waves are usually the dominant rhythm seen in the posterior region of the brain in older children and adults, when awake and relaxed. Beta waves are normal in sleep, particularly for infants and young children. Theta waves are normally found during drowsiness and sleep and are normal in wakefulness in children, while delta waves are the most prominent feature of the sleeping EEG. Spikes and sharp waves are generally abnormal; however, they are common in the EEG of normal newborns.

Different types of brain waves are seen as abnormal only in the context of the location of the waves, a person's age, and one's conscious state. In general, disease typically increases slow activity, such as theta or delta waves, but decreases fast activity, such as alpha and beta waves.

Not all decreases in wave activity are abnormal. The normal alpha waves seen in the posterior region of the brain are suppressed merely if a person is tense. Sometimes the addition of a wave is abnormal. For example, alpha rhythms seen in a newborn can signify seizure activity. Finally, the area where the rhythm is seen can be telling. The alpha coma is characterized by alpha rhythms produced diffusely, or, in other words, by all regions of the brain.

Some abnormal beta rhythms include frontal beta waves that are induced by sedative drugs. Marked asymmetry in beta rhythms suggests a structural lesion on the side lacking the beta waves. Beta waves are also commonly measured over skull lesions, such as fractures or burr holes, in activity known as a breach rhythm.

Usually seen only during sleep in adults, the presence of theta waves in the temporal region of awake, older adults has been tentatively correlated with vascular disease. Another rhythm normal in sleep, delta rhythms, may be recorded in the awake state over localized regions of cerebral damage. Intermittent delta rhythms are also an indication of damage of the relays between the deep gray matter and the cortex of

WHO PERFORMS THE PROCEDURE AND WHERE IS IT PERFORMED?

Electroencephalography is often administered by specially trained technicians who are supervised by a neurologist or other physician with specialized training in administering and interpreting the test. Because of the equipment involved, an EEG is usually administered in a hospital setting. It may be conducted in a professional office.

QUESTIONS TO ASK THE DOCTOR

- How many EEG procedures has the technician performed?
- What preparations are being made to treat an induced seizure?
- Is the supervising physician appropriately certified to interpret an EEG?

the brain. In adults, this intermittent activity is found in the frontal region whereas in children, it is in the occipital region.

The EEG readings of persons with epilepsy or other seizure disorders display bursts, or spikes, of electrical activity. In focal epilepsy, spikes are restricted to one hemisphere of the brain. If spikes are generalized to both hemispheres of the brain, multifocal epilepsy may be present. The EEG can be used to localize the region of the brain where the abnormal electrical activity is occurring. This is most easily accomplished using a recording method, or montage, called an average reference montage. With this type of recording, the signal from each electrode is compared to the average signal from all the electrodes. The negative amplitude (upward movement, by convention) of the spike is observed for the different channels, or inputs, from the various electrodes. The negative deflection will be greatest as recorded by the electrode that is closest in location to the origin of the abnormal activity. The spike will be present but of reduced amplitude as the electrodes move farther away from the site producing the spike. Electrodes distant from the site will not record the spike occurrence.

A final variety of abnormal result is the presence of slower-than-normal wave activity, which can either be a slow background rhythm or slow waves superimposed on a normal background. A posterior dominant rhythm of 7 Hz or less in an adult is abnormal and consistent with encephalopathy (brain disease). In contrast, localized theta or delta rhythms found in conjunction with normal background rhythms suggest a structural lesion.

Morbidity and mortality rates

There are few adverse conditions associated with an EEG test. Persons with seizure disorders may induce seizures during the test in reaction to flashing lights or by deep breathing. Mortality from an EEG has not been reported.

Alternatives

There are no equivalent tests that provide the same information as an EEG.

Resources

BOOKS

Chin, W. C., and T. C. Head. *Essentials of Clinical Neurophysiology,* 3rd ed. London: Butterworth-Heinemann, 2002.

Daube, J. R. *Clinical Neurophysiology,* 2nd ed. New York: Oxford University Press, 2002.

Ebersole, J. S., and T. A. Pedley. *Current Practice of Clinical Electroencephalography,* 3rd ed. Philadelphia: Lippincott Williams & Wilkins, 2002.

Rowan, A. J., and E. Tolunsky. *Primer of EEG.* London: Butterworth-Heinemann, 2003.

PERIODICALS

De Clercq, W., P. Lemmerling, S. Van Huffel, and W. Van Paesschen. "Anticipation of epileptic seizures from standard EEG recordings." *Lancet* 361, no. 9361 (2003): 971–972.

ORGANIZATIONS

American Association of Neuromuscular and Electrodiagnostic Medicine (AANEM). 421 First Avenue SW, Suite 300 East, Rochester, MN 55902. (507) 288–0100. Fax: (507) 288–1225. Email: aanem@aanem.org. http://www.aanem.org/index.cfm.

American Board of Registration for Electroencephalographic Technologists. P.O. Box 916633, Longwood, FL 32791-6633.

American Board of Registration of Electroencephalographic and Evoked Potential Technologists, Inchttp://www.abret.org.

American Society of Electroneurodiagnostic Technologists Inc, 204 W. 7th Carroll, IA 51401. (712) 792–2978. http://www.aset.org/.

Epilepsy Foundation. 4351 Garden City Drive, Landover, MD 20785-7223. (800) 332–1000 or (301) 459–3700. http://www.efa.org.

OTHER

Dowshen, Steven, M.D. "EEG (Electroencephalography)." Kid's Health For Parents. September 2007. http://kids health.org/parent/system/medical/eeg.html [Accessed April 11, 2008].

National Society for Epilepsy. "Epilepsy Information: Electroencephalography." October 2006. http://www.epilepsynse.org.uk/pages/info/leaflets/eeg.cfm [Accessed April 11, 2008].

L. Fleming Fallon, Jr., MD, DrPH
Laura Jean Cataldo, RN, EdD

Electrolyte tests

Definition

Electrolytes are positively and negatively charged molecules, called ions, that are found within the body's cells and extracellular fluids, including blood plasma. A test for electrolytes includes the measurement of sodium, potassium, chloride, and bicarbonate. These ions are measured to assess renal (kidney), endocrine (glandular), and acid-base function, and are components of both renal function and comprehensive metabolic biochemistry profiles. Other important electrolytes routinely measured in serum or plasma include calcium and phosphorus. These are measured together because they are both affected by bone and parathyroid diseases, and often move in opposing directions. Magnesium is another electrolyte that is routinely measured. Like calcium, it will cause tetany (uncontrolled muscle contractions) when levels are too low in the extracellular fluids.

Purpose

Tests that measure the concentration of electrolytes are needed for both the diagnosis and management of renal, endocrine, acid-base, water balance, and many other conditions. Their importance lies in part with the serious consequences that follow from the relatively small changes that diseases or abnormal conditions may cause. In short, diagnosis and management of a patient with an electrolyte disturbance is best served by measuring all four electrolytes.

Description

Sodium levels are directly related to the water concentration in blood plasma. Since water will often follow sodium, loss of sodium leads to dehydration, and retention of sodium leads to edema (swelling, water retention). Conditions that promote increased sodium, called hypernatremia, do so without promoting an equivalent gain in water. Such conditions include diabetes insipidus (water loss by the kidneys), Cushing's disease, and hyperaldosteronism (increased sodium reabsorption).

Many other conditions, such as congestive heart failure, cirrhosis of the liver, and renal disease result in renal retention of sodium, but an equivalent amount of water is retained as well. This results in a condition called total body sodium excess, which causes hypertension and edema, but not an elevated serum sodium concentration. Low serum sodium, called hyponatremia, may result from Addison's disease, excessive diuretic therapy, the syndrome of inappropriate secretion of antidiuretic hormone (SIADH), burns, diarrhea, vomiting, and cystic fibrosis. In fact, the diagnosis of cystic fibrosis is made by demonstrating an elevated chloride concentration (greater than 60 mmol/L) in sweat.

Potassium is the electrolyte used as a hallmark sign of renal failure. Like sodium, potassium is freely filtered by the kidney. In renal failure, the combination of decreased filtration and decreased secretion combine to cause increased plasma potassium. Hyperkalemia is the most significant and life-threatening complication of renal failure. Hyperkalemia is also commonly caused by hemolytic anemia (release from hemolysed red blood cells), diabetes insipidus, Addison's disease, and digitalis toxicity. Frequent causes of low serum potassium include alkalosis, diarrhea and vomiting, excessive use of thiazide **diuretics**, Cushing's disease, intravenous fluid administration, and SIADH.

The reference range for potassium is 3.6-5.0 mmol/L (or mEq/L). Potassium is often a STAT (needed immediately) test because values below 3.0 mmol/L (or mEq/L) are associated with arrhythmia (irregular heartbeat), tachycardia (rapid heartbeat), and cardiac arrest, and values above 6.0 mmol/L (or mEq/L) are associated with bradycardia (slow heartbeat) and heart failure. Abnormal potassium cannot be treated without reference to bicarbonate, which is a measure of the buffering capacity of the plasma. Sodium bicarbonate and dissolved carbon dioxide act together to resist changes in blood pH. For example, an increased plasma bicarbonate indicates a condition called metabolic alkalosis, which results in blood pH that is too high. This may cause hydrogen ions to shift from the cells into the extracellular fluid in exchange for potassium. As potassium moves into the cells, the plasma concentration falls. The low plasma potassium, called hypokalemia, should not be treated by administration of potassium, but by identifying and eliminating the cause of the alkalosis. Administration of potassium would result in hyperkalemia (too much potassium) when the acid-base disturbance is corrected.

Sodium measurements are very useful in differentiating the cause of an abnormal potassium result. Conditions such as the overuse of diuretics (drugs that promote lower blood pressure) often result in low levels of both sodium and potassium. On the other hand, Cushing's disease (adrenocortical over-activity) and Addison's disease (adrenocortical under-activity) drive the sodium and potassium in opposing directions. Chloride levels will follow sodium levels except in the case of acid-base imbalances, in which chloride may move in the opposing direction of bicarbonate.

Calcium and phosphorus are measured together because they are both likely to be abnormal in bone and parathyroid disease states. Parathyroid hormone causes resorption of these minerals from bone. However, it promotes intestinal absorption and renal reabsorption of calcium, and renal excretion of phosphorus. In hyperparathyroidism, serum calcium will be increased and phosphorus will be decreased. In hypoparathyroidism and renal disease, serum calcium will be low but phosphorus will be high. In vitamin D dependent rickets (VDDR), both calcium and phosphorus will be low; however, calcium is normal while phosphorus is low in vitamin D resistant rickets (VDRR).

Differential diagnosis of an abnormal serum calcium is aided by the measurement of ionized calcium (i.e., calcium not bound by protein). Only the ionized calcium is physiologically active, and the level of ionized calcium is regulated by parathyroid hormone (PTH) via negative feedback (high ionized calcium inhibits secretion of PTH). While hypoparathyroidism, VDDR, renal failure, hypoalbuminemia, hypovitaminosis D, and other conditions may cause low total calcium, only hypoparathyroidism (and alkalosis) will result in low ionized calcium. Conversely, while hyperparathyroidism, malignancies (those that secrete parathyroid hormone-related protein), multiple myeloma, antacids, hyperproteinemia, dehydration, and hypervitaminosis D cause an elevated total calcium, only hyperparathyroidism, malignancy, and acidosis cause an elevated ionized calcium.

Serum magnesium levels may be increased by hemolytic anemia, renal failure, Addison's disease, hyperparathyroidism, and magnesium-based antacids. Chronic alcoholism is the most common cause of a low serum magnesium owing to poor nutrition. Serum magnesium is also decreased in

KEY TERMS

Arrhythmia—Abnormal rhythm of the heartbeat.

Bradycardia—Slow heart beat, usually under 60 beats per minute.

Hyperkalemia—An abnormally high concentration of potassium in the blood.

Hypocalcemia—An abnormally small concentration of calcium in the blood.

Hypokalemia—An abnormally small concentration of potassium in the blood.

Tachycardia—Rapid heart beat, generally over 100 beats per minute.

Tetany—Inappropriately sustained muscle spasms.

diarrhea, hypoparathyroidism, pancreatitis, Cushing's disease, and with excessive diuretic use. Low magnesium can be caused by a number of **antibiotics** and other drugs and by administration of intravenous solutions. Magnesium is needed for secretion of parathyroid hormone, and therefore, a low serum magnesium can induce hypocalcemia (too little calcium). Magnesium deficiency is very common in regions where the water supply does not contain sufficient magnesium salts. Magnesium acts as a calcium channel blocker, and when cellular magnesium is low, high intracellular calcium results. This leads to hypertension, tachycardia, and tetany.

Measurement of electrolytes

Electrolytes are measured by a process known as potentiometry. This method measures the voltage that develops between the inner and outer surfaces of an ion selective electrode. The electrode (membrane) is made of a material that is selectively permeable to the ion being measured. This potential is measured by comparing it to the potential of a reference electrode. Since the potential of the reference electrode is held constant, the difference in voltage between the two electrodes is attributed to the concentration of ion in the sample.

Precautions

Electrolyte tests are performed on whole blood, plasma, or serum, usually collected from a vein or capillary.

Special procedures are followed when collecting a sweat sample for electrolyte analysis. This procedure, called pilocarpine iontophoresis, uses electric current applied to the arm of the patient (usually an infant) in order to convey the pilocarpine to the sweat glands where it will stimulate sweating. Care must be taken to ensure that the collection device (macroduct tubing or gauze) does not become contaminated and that the patient's parent or guardian understands the need for the electrical equipment employed.

Preparation

Usually no special preparation is necessary by the patient. Samples for calcium and phosphorus and for magnesium should be collected following an eight-hour fast.

Aftercare

Discomfort or bruising may occur at the puncture site, or the person may feel dizzy or faint. Pressure to the puncture site until the bleeding stops reduces bruising. Applying warm packs to the puncture site relieves discomfort.

Risks

Minor temporary discomfort may occur with any blood test, but there are no complications specific to electrolyte testing.

Normal results

Electrolyte concentrations are similar whether measured in serum or plasma. Values are expressed as mmol/L for sodium, potassium, chloride, and bicarbonate. Magnesium results are often reported as milliequivalents per liter (meq/L) or in mg/dL. Total calcium is usually reported in mg/dL and ionized calcium in mmol/L. Since severe electrolyte disturbances can be associated with life-threatening consequences such as heart failure, shock, coma, or tetany, alert values are used to warn physicians of impending crisis. Typical reference ranges and alert values are cited below:

- serum or plasma sodium: 135–145 mmol/L; alert levels: less than 120 mmol/L and greater than 160 mmol/L
- serum potassium: 3.6–5.4 mmol/L (plasma, 3.6–5.0 mmol/L); alert levels: less than 3.0 mmol/L and greater than 6.0 mmol/L
- serum or plasma chloride: 98–108 mmol/L
- sweat chloride: 4–60 mmol/L
- serum or plasma bicarbonate: 18–24 mmol/L (as total carbon dioxide, 22–26 mmol/L); alert levels: less than 10 mmol/L and greater than 40 mmol/L
- serum calcium: 8.5–10.5 mg/dL (2.0–2.5 mmol/L); alert levels: less than 6.0 mg/dL and greater than 13.0 mg/dL
- ionized calcium: 1.0–1.3 mmol/L
- serum inorganic phosphorus: 2.3–4.7 mg/dL (children, 4.0–7.0 mg/dL); alert level: less than 1.0 mg/dL
- serum magnesium: 1.8–3.0 mg/dL (1.2–2.0 meq/L or 0.5–1.0 mmol/L)
- ionized magnesium: 0.53–0.67 mmol/L
- osmolality (calculated) 280–300 mosm/Kg

Resources

BOOKS

Tierney, Lawrence M., Stephen J. McPhee, and Maxine A. Papadakis. *Current Medical Diagnosis and Treatment 2008.* 47th ed. New York: Lange Medical Books/ McGraw-Hill, 2007.
Wallach, Jacques. *Interpretation of Diagnostic Tests.* 8th ed. Philadelphia, PA: Lippincott Williams & Wilkins, 2006.

OTHER

"Electrolytes." Lab Tests Online. April, 11 2005. http:// www.labtestsonline.org/understanding/analytes/ electrolytes/test.html [Accessed April 11, 2008].
"Electrolytes." MedLine Plus. August 14, 2007. http:// www.nlm.nih.gov/medlineplus/ency/article/ 002350.htm [Accessed April 11, 2008].
Stöppler, Melissa Conrad, MD, and William C. Shiel, Jr, MD, FACP, FACR. "Electrolytes." MedicineNet. January 1, 2006. http://www.medicinenet.com/ electrolytes/article.htm [Accessed April 11, 2008].

Erika J. Norris
Mark A. Best, MD
Laura Jean Cataldo, RN, EdD

Electrophysiology study of the heart

Definition

An electrophysiology study (EPS) of the heart is a test performed to analyze the electrical activity of the heart. The test uses cardiac catheters and sophisticated computers to generate **electrocardiogram** (EKG) tracings and electrical measurements with exquisite precision from within the heart chambers.

Purpose

Heart disease is the leading killer in the United States, accounting for more than 50% of all annual deaths. The normal function of the heart depends on its electrical activity, and the effect of this activity on each of its cells. When a heart is diseased, impaired electrical activity is often the factor that leads to sudden **death**, thus the need for EPS tests.

An EPS can be performed solely for diagnostic purposes or to pinpoint the exact location of electrical signals (cardiac mapping) in conjunction with a therapeutic procedure called catheter ablation (tissue removal). A cardiologist may recommend an EPS when the standard EKG, Holter monitor, event recorder, **stress test**, echocardiogram, or angiogram cannot provide enough information to evaluate an abnormal heart rhythm (arrhythmia).

An EPS offers more detailed information about the heart's electrical activity than many other non-invasive tests because electrodes are placed directly *on* heart tissue. This placement allows the electrophysiologist to determine the specific location of an arrhythmia and, often, to correct it during the same procedure. This corrective treatment is considered a permanent cure; in many cases, the patient may not need to take heart medications.

EPS may be helpful in assessing:

- certain tachycardias (fast heartbeats) or bradycardias (slow heartbeats) of unknown cause
- patients who have been resuscitated after experiencing sudden cardiac arrest
- various symptoms of unknown cause, such as chest pain, shortness of breath, fatigue, or syncope (dizziness/fainting)
- response to anti-arrhythmic therapy

Precautions

Pregnant patients should not undergo EPS because the study requires exposure to radiation, which may harm the growing baby. Patients who have coronary artery disease may need to be treated prior to EPS. EPS is contraindicated in patients with an acute myocardial infarction, as the infarct may be extended with rapid pacing. The test is also contraindicated for patients who are uncooperative.

Description

The rhythmic pumping action of the heart, which is essentially a muscle, is the result of electrical impulses traveling throughout the walls of the four heart chambers. These impulses originate in the sinoatrial (SA) node (specialized cells situated in the right atrium, or top right chamber of the heart). Normally, the SA node, acting like a spark plug, spontaneously generates the impulses, which travel through specific

---

KEY TERMS

Ablation—Removal or destruction of tissue, such as by burning or cutting.

Angiogram—X ray of a blood vessel after special x-ray dye has been injected into it.

Bradycardia—Relatively slow heart action, usually considered as a rate under 60 beats per minute.

Cardiac catheter—Long, thin, flexible tube, which is threaded into the heart through a blood vessel.

Cardiologist—Doctor who specializes in diagnosing and treating heart diseases.

Echocardiogram—Ultrasound image of the heart.

Electrocardiogram—Tracing of the electrical activity of the heart.

Electrode—A medium, such as platinum wires, for conducting an electrical current.

Electrophysiology—Study of how electrical signals in the body relate to physiologic function.

Event recorder—A small machine, worn by a patient usually for several days or weeks, that is activated by the patient to record his or her EKG when a symptom is detected.

Fibrillation—Rapid, random contraction (quivering).

Holter monitor—A small machine worn by a patient usually for 24 hours, that continuously records the patient's EKG during usual daily activity.

Stress test—Recording a patient's EKG during exercise.

Supraventricular tachycardia (SVT)—A fast heartbeat that originates above the ventricles.

Tachycardia—Fast heartbeat.

Thrombophlebitis—Venous inflammation with the formation of thrombus (a clot in the cardiovascular system).

---

pathways throughout the atria to the atrioventricular (AV) node. The AV node is a relay station sending the impulses to more specialized muscle fibers throughout the ventricles (the lower chambers of the heart). If these pathways become damaged or blocked or if extra (abnormal) pathways exist, the heart's rhythm may be altered (too slow, too fast, or irregular), which can seriously affect the heart's pumping ability.

To undergo EPS, the patient is placed on a table in the EPS lab and connected to various monitors. Sterile technique is maintained. A minimum of two catheters are inserted into the right femoral (thigh) vein in the groin area. Depending on the type of arrhythmia, the number of catheters used and their route to the heart may vary. For certain tachycardias, two additional catheters may be inserted in the left groin and one in the internal jugular (neck) vein or in the subclavian (below the clavicle) vein. The catheters are about 0.08 in (2 mm) in diameter, about the size of a spaghetti noodle. The catheters used in catheter ablation are slightly larger.

With the help of fluoroscopy (x rays on a television screen), all catheters are guided to several specific locations in the heart. Typically, four to 10 electrodes are located on the end of the catheters, which have the ability to send electrical signals to stimulate the heart (called pacing) and to receive electrical signals from the heart, but not at the same time (just as a walkie-talkie cannot send and receive messages at the same time).

First, the electrodes are positioned to receive signals from inside the heart chambers, which allows the doctor to measure how fast the electrical impulses travel in the patient's heart at that time. These measurements are called the patient's baseline measurements. Next, the electrodes are positioned to pace. That is, the EPS team tries to induce (sometimes in combination with various heart drugs) the arrhythmia that the patient has previously experienced so the team can observe it in a controlled environment, compare it to the patient's clinical or spontaneous arrhythmia, and decide how to treat it.

Once the arrhythmia is induced and the team determines that it can be treated with catheter ablation, cardiac mapping is performed to locate the precise origin and route of the abnormal pathway. When this is accomplished, the ablating electrode catheter is positioned directly against the abnormal pathway, and high radio-frequency energy is delivered through the electrode to destroy (burn) the tissue in this area.

Pediatric patients present challenges for EPS. In 2001, an analysis of 45 children who underwent EPS was conducted. The researchers concluded that success rates and the prevention of complications in children may be increased by using **ultrasound** guidance for access to the internal jugular vein for coronary sinus cannulation (insertion of a tube for the transport of fluid) during EPS. Access was successfully obtained in all 45 of the patients without major complications using this technique.

Diagnosis/Preparation

The following preparations are made for an EPS:

- Blood tests usually are ordered one week prior to the test.
- The patient may be advised to stop taking certain medications, especially cardiac medications, that may interfere with the test results.
- The patient fasts for six to eight hours prior to the procedure. Fluids may be permitted until three hours before the test.
- The patient undergoes conscious sedation (awake but relaxed) during the test.
- A local anesthetic is injected at the site of catheter insertion.
- Peripheral pulses are marked with a pen prior to catheterization. This permits rapid assessment of pulses after the procedure.

Aftercare

The patient needs to rest flat in bed for several hours after the procedure to allow healing at the catheter insertion sites. The patient often returns home either the same day or the next day. Someone should drive the patient home. To minimize bleeding and pain, the patient is advised to keep the extremity in which the catheter was placed immobilized and straight for several hours after the test.

Risks

EPS and catheter ablation are considered low-risk procedures. There is a risk of bleeding and/or infection at the site of catheter insertion. Blood clot formation may occur and is minimized with anticoagulant medications administered during the procedure. Vascular injuries causing hemorrhage or thrombophlebitis are possible. Cardiac perforations are also possible. If the right internal jugular vein is accessed, the potential for puncturing the lung with the catheter exists and could lead to a collapsed lung.

Because ventricular tachycardia or fibrillation (lethal arrhythmias) may be induced in the patient, the EPS lab personnel must be prepared to defibrillate the patient as necessary.

Patients should notify their health care provider if they develop any of these symptoms:

• numbness or tingling in the extremities
• heavy bleeding
• change in color and/or temperature of extremities
• loss of function in extremities

Normal results

Normal EPS results show that the heart initiates and conducts electrical impulses within normal limits.

Abnormal results include confirmation of arrhythmias, such as:

• supraventricular tachycardias
• ventricular arrhythmias
• accessory pathways
• bradycardias

Resources

BOOKS

Grubb, Blair P., and Brian Olshansky. *Syncope: Mechanisms and Management.* 2nd ed. Malden, MA: Blackwell Publishing, 2005.

Hummel, J. D., S. J. Kalbfleisch, and J. M. Dillon. *Pocket Guide for Electrophysiology.* Philadelphia: W. B. Saunders Co., 1999.

Josephson, M. E. *Clinical Cardiac Electrophysiology: Techniques and Interpretations.* Philadelphia: Lippincott Williams & Wilkins Publishers, 2008.

Pagana, Kathleen D., and Timothy J. Pagana. *Diagnostic Testing and Nursing Implications* 5th ed. St. Louis: Mosby, 1999.

Singer, Igor. *Interventional Electrophysiology* 2nd ed. Baltimore, MD: Lippincott Williams & Wilkins, 2001.

PERIODICALS

Asirvatham, S. J., C. J. Bruce, and P. A. Friedman. "Advances in imaging for cardiac electrophysiology." *Coronary Artery Disease* 14 (February 2003): 3–13.

Kocic, I. "Sudden cardiac death: from molecular biology and cellular electrophysiology to therapy." *Current Opinions in Investigative Drugs* 3 (July 2002): 1045–1050.

Liberman, L., A. J. Hordof, D. T. Hsu, and R. H. Pass. "Ultrasound-Assisted Cannulation of the Right Internal Jugular Vein during Electrophysiologic Studies in Children." *Journal of Interventional Cardiology and Electrophysiology* 5, no. 2 (June 2001): 177–179.

ORGANIZATIONS

American Association of Critical-Care Nurses. 101 Columbia, Aliso Viejo, CA 92656-4109. (800) 899–2226. www.aacn.org/.

The American College of Cardiology Heart House, 9111 Old Georgetown Road, Bethesda, MD 20814-1699. (800) 253–4636 www.acc.org.

American Heart Association. 7272 Greenville Ave., Dallas TX 75231-4596. (800) 242–1793. www.amhrt.org.

Cardiac Arrhythmia Research and Education Foundation (C.A.R.E.). 2082 Michelson Dr. #301, Irvine, CA 92612. (800) 404–9500. www.longqt.com/.

Cardiac Electrophysiology Society. http://www.cardiaceps.org/.

Maggie Boleyn, RN, BSN
Monique Laberge, PhD
Laura Jean Cataldo, RN, EdD

Electrosurgery *see* **Curettage and electrosurgery**

Emergency airway puncture *see* **Cricothyroidotomy**

Emergency surgery

Definition

Emergency surgery is nonelective surgery performed when the patient's life or well-being is in direct jeopardy. Largely performed by surgeons specializing in emergency medicine, this surgery can be conducted for many reasons but occurs most often in urgent or critical cases in response to trauma, mass casualties, cardiac events, poison episodes, brain injuries, and pediatric medicine.

Purpose

Most surgery is elective and is performed after a diagnosis based on a history and **physical examination** of the patient, with differential test results and the development of strategies for management of the condition. With emergency surgery, the **surgical team** as well as the surgeon may have less information about the patient than would ordinarily be required and must work under time-dependent conditions to save a patient's life, help avoid critical injury or systemic deterioration of the patient, or alleviate severe pain. Because of the unique conditions for urgent acute surgery, operations are usually performed by a surgical team specially trained for management of a critical or life-threatening event.

Acute surgical emergencies include:

- invasive resuscitation for acute respiratory failure, pulmonary embolism, and pulmonary obstructions
- injuries resulting from blasts, explosions, or the release of dangerous chemicals, as in terrorist attacks, industrial accidents, pipeline leaks, or aviation accidents
- injuries resulting from buildings collapsing as a result of earthquakes, tornadoes, or hurricanes
- blunt or penetrating injuries to the head, chest, or abdomen, largely from automobile accidents and gunshot wounds
- injuries resulting in the loss or amputation of body parts (teeth, fingers, ears, toes, etc.) from human or animal bites, knife wounds, industrial accidents, etc.
- burns
- cardiac events, including heart attacks, cardiac shock, and cardiac arrhythmia
- aneurysms
- brain injuries and other neurological conditions
- complications of pregnancy
- abdominal disorders, including perforated ulcer, appendicitis, and peritonitis

Description

Emergency surgery can take place in any hospital or battlefield setting. However, trauma centers or trauma sections of hospitals handle most emergency surgeries. Forty-one states have ACS-verified trauma centers as of 2008, some states with better systems than others. There is an additional ACS-verified trauma center in Landstuhl, Germany.

One major difficulty remaining in the early 2000s is that trauma centers are unevenly distributed across the United States. A study published in the *Journal of the American Medical Association* reported in 2005 that 26.7% and 27.7% of the population of the United States had access to level I or II trauma centers by helicopter only within time periods of 45 and 60 minutes, respectively; and 1.9% and 3.1% of Americans had access only by helicopter to level I or II centers from trauma centers or base helipads outside their home states within those time periods. Most of these people live in rural areas. By contrast, 69.2% of people in the United States living in large cities can get to a level I or level II trauma center within 45 minutes, and 84.1% can reach a trauma center within 60 minutes.

Trauma centers in the United States are classified by the American College of Surgeons (ACS) as levels I, II, III, and IV, respectively. A level I trauma center, the most advanced of the trauma center system, is equipped to get the patient to surgery beginning with trained first responders. The system relies on available operating rooms, readily available laboratory personnel, anesthesiologists, x-ray and blood bank access, intensive care nurses, and ward nurses—all trained to take the patient to the **operating room** within 60 minutes of the incident. If patients are in surgery within an hour, they have a 25% chance of survival. Level I trauma centers also carry on research and maintain programs on trauma prevention.

Level II trauma centers work in collaboration with level I centers. They provide 24-hour availability of all essential specialties, personnel, and equipment but are not required to have research or residency programs. Level III centers do not have the full range of specialists, but have resources for emergency resuscitation, surgery, and intensive care of most trauma patients; they also have transfer agreements with level I and level II centers for the care of severely injured patients. Level IV centers stabilize and treat patients in remote areas where no other emergency care is available.

Diagnosis/Preparation

Emergency surgery follows a path from resuscitation and stabilization of the patient with a patient management team, to preparation of the patient for surgery, to postoperative and recovery procedures—all designed to deal quickly with the life-threatening situation. There is often little time or possibility for extensive diagnosis or the gathering of a patient history. Decisions are made quickly about surgery, often without family members present. The possibility of emergency surgery due to trauma, injury, emergency medical conditions, and cardiac events make it wise for all patients to have a **living will** detailing their medical care wishes and to carry it with them at all times.

Emergency surgery related to situations in which there are mass casualties, as in aviation disasters, railroad collisions, factory explosions, terrorist attacks, or such natural disasters as earthquakes, is often performed on site rather than in a trauma center, as there

KEY TERMS

Aneurysm—A bulge in the wall of a blood vessel caused by the weakening of the vessel wall. Aneurysms can be fatal if the affected blood vessel bursts.

Arrhythmia—An abnormal heart rhythm.

Embolism—The obstruction of a blood vessel by an air bubble or foreign particle.

First responder—A term used to describe the first medically trained responder to arrive on scene of an emergency, accident, natural or human-made disaster, or similar event. First responders may be police officers, fire fighters, emergency medical services personnel, or bystanders with some training in first aid.

Peritonitis—Inflammation of the layer of tissue that lines the inside of the abdominal cavity.

Trauma centers—Specialized hospital facilities that are equipped to deal with emergency life-threatening conditions.

Triage—Prioritizing the needs of patients according to the urgency of their need for care and their likelihood of survival.

may not be time to transport survivors to a hospital. In these situations, first responders typically carry out triage, which is the sorting out and giving medical assistance to patients in order to maximize the number of survivors. In most cases, triage involves focusing efforts on those whose survival depends on receiving prompt care rather than on those who will survive without immediate treatment and those who are past help. In mass casualty situations, survivors may need to be treated for burns, decontaminated from dangerous chemicals, or taken outside the immediate danger zone before surgical interventions can be carried out.

Normal results

Mortality rates are high for emergency surgeries. For instance, the rupture of an abdominal aneurysm results in **death** in about 50% of cases due to kidney failure from shock or disrupted blood supply. An untreated aneurysm is always fatal. Certain gastrointestinal disorders require emergency surgery, including bleeding in the digestive tract, obstructions, appendicitis, and peritonitis (inflammation of the lining of the abdomen). Pediatric emergency surgery includes birth defects of the heart. One in 120 infants is born with a heart defect requiring surgery to unblock the flow of blood or to treat a malformed aortic valve. Heart attacks are very effectively treated with emergency surgery depending upon the part of the heart affected, on whether there is arterial blockage, and on the patient's overall health. Arrhythmias can develop as well as stroke. The first 48 hours are the most crucial with cardiac events and whether there is immediate medical and surgical attention. Many cardiac surgeries result in bypass procedures, with a higher death rate associated with bypass surgery done on an emergency basis. Women have emergency heart bypass operations more often than men, probably due to lack of earlier cardiac care.

Resources

BOOKS

Marx, John A., ed. *Rosen's Emergency Medicine: Concepts and Clinical Practice*, 6th ed. Philadelphia: Mosby/Elsevier, 2006.

Peitzman, Andrew B., ed. *The Trauma Manual: Trauma and Acute Care Surgery*, 3rd ed. Philadelphia: Lippincott Williams and Wilkins, 2007.

Wyatt, Jonathan P. *Oxford Handbook of Emergency Medicine*, 3rd ed. New York: Oxford University Press, 2006.

PERIODICALS

Branas, Charles C., Ellen J. MacKenzie, Justin C. Williams, et al. "Access to Trauma Centers in the United States." *Journal of the American Medical Association* 293 (June 1, 2005): 2626–2633.

Cancio, L. C. "Airplane Crash in Guam, August 6, 1997: The Aeromedical Evacuation Response." *Journal of Burn Care and Research* 27 (September–October 2006): 642–648.

Judy, M. B. "Planning for the Utilization of Air Medical Resources for Large-Scale Incidents." *Emergency Medical Services* 36 (February 2007): 42–43.

Moore, E. E., M. M. Knudson, C. W. Schwab, et al. "Military-Civilian Collaboration in Trauma Care and the Senior Visiting Surgeon Program." *New England Journal of Medicine* 357 (December 27, 2007): 2723–2727.

Vella, M., M. R. Masood, and W. S. Hendry. "Surgery for Ulcerative Colitis." *Surgeon* 5 (December 2007): 356–362.

ORGANIZATIONS

American College of Emergency Physicians (ACEP). 1125 Executive Circle, Irving, TX 75038-2522. (800) 798-1822 or (972) 550-0911.http://www.acep.org (accessed March 19, 2008).

American College of Surgeons (ACS). 633 North St. Clair Street, Chicago, IL 60611. (800) 621-4111. http://www.facs.org/ (accessed March 19, 2008).

OTHER

DeNoon, D. "Trauma Centers: Life-or-Death Difference." *WebMD Medical News* October 23, 2002 [cited June 17, 2003]. http://www.webmd.com (accessed March 19, 2008).

Smith, I. M. "U.S. Trauma Centers." *Virtual Hospital* April 2003 [cited June 17, 2003]. http://www.vh.org/adult/

patient/internalmedicine/aba30/2003/traumacenter.
html (accessed March 19, 2008).

Stevens, Everett. "EMS and Terrorism." *eMedicine*, March 10,
2005. http://www.emedicine.com/emerg/topic712.htm
[cited January 10, 2008] (accessed March 19, 2008).

Nancy McKenzie, PhD
Rebecca Frey, PhD

Endarterectomy, carotid *see* **Carotid
endarterectomy**

Endarterectomy, peripheral *see* **Peripheral
endarterectomy**

Endocardial resection *see* **Myocardial
resection**

Endolymphatic shunt

Definition

An endolymphatic shunt is a surgical procedure in which a very small silicone tube is placed in the membranous labyrinth of the inner ear to drain excess fluid.

Purpose

An endolymphatic shunt is placed as part of the treatment of Ménière's disease, a disorder of the inner ear whose causes are still unknown. Ménière's disease is characterized by the following symptoms:

- a rise in the level of endolymphatic fluid in the labyrinth of the inner ear
- hearing loss that comes and goes

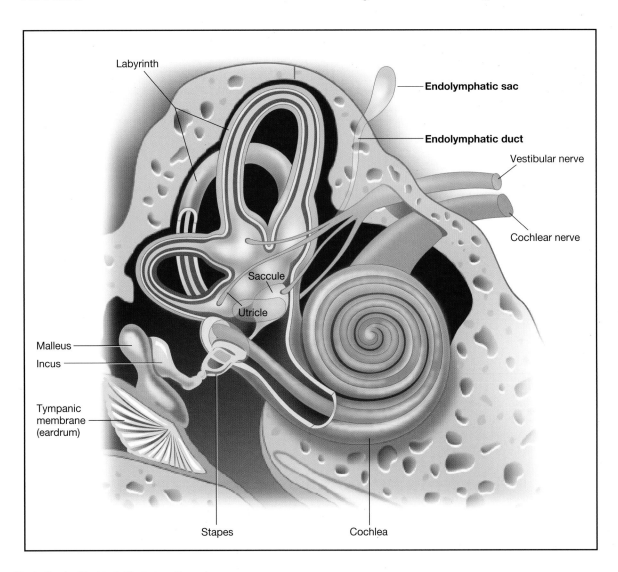

Labyrinth

Endolymphatic sac

Endolymphatic duct

Vestibular nerve

Cochlear nerve

Saccule

Utricle

Malleus

Incus

Tympanic
membrane
(eardrum)

Stapes

Cochlea

(Illustration by Electronic Illustrators Group.)

- a sensation that the environment or oneself is revolving or spinning (vertigo)
- ringing, buzzing, or hissing noises in the ears (tinnitus)
- a feeling that the ears are blocked or plugged

Endolymphatic shunt surgery is one of the surgical procedures available to treat Ménière's disease, which is also known as endolymphatic hydrops. The surgery is based on the theory that the disorder causes the inner ear to become overloaded with fluid and that draining this fluid will relieve the symptoms. The fluid is drained by opening the endolymphatic sac, a pouch located next to the mastoid bone at the end of the endolymphatic duct. The endolymphatic duct is a canal that leads to the inner ear.

Demographics

According to the National Institute on Deafness and Other Communication Disorders (NIDCD), there were an estimated three to five million cases of Ménière's disease in the United States in 1998, with nearly 100,000 new cases diagnosed annually. In most cases only one ear is affected, but as many as 15–40% of patients are affected in both ears. The onset of Ménière's disease occurs most often in adults between the ages of 20 and 50. Men and women are affected in equal numbers.

Description

An endolymphatic shunt is placed with the patient under **general anesthesia**. The operation takes about two hours to perform. The patient is usually positioned lying on the back with the head turned to one side and the affected ear lying uppermost. The head is immobilized and supported with a pad or brace. The operation itself begins with opening the mastoid bone and identifying the endolymphatic sac. To find the sac, the surgeon removes the bony cover of the sigmoid sinus, which is an S-shaped cavity behind the mastoid bone. The surgeon leaves intact a small rectangle of thin bone called Bill's Island (named for Dr. William House). The sigmoid sinus is then collapsed with gentle pressure. The surgeon exposes the endolymphatic sac and makes an incision in it in order to insert the shunt.

Diagnosis/Preparation

The diagnosis of Ménière's disease is based on the patient's medical history, a **physical examination**, and the results of hearing tests, balance tests, an electronystagmogram, and imaging studies. An MRI or CT scan is performed to rule out a tumor as the cause of the patient's symptoms. A hearing test (audiogram) identifies the hearing loss that is typical of Ménière's disease. Balance function tests are administered to assess the patient's vertigo.

KEY TERMS

Bony labyrinth—A series of cavities contained in a capsule inside the temporal bone of the skull. The endolymph-filled membranous labyrinth is suspended in a fluid inside the bony labyrinth.

Electronystagmogram—A test that involves the graphic recording of eye movements.

Endolymph—The watery fluid contained in the membranous labyrinth of the inner ear.

Endolymphatic sac—The pouch at the end of the endolymphatic duct that connects to the membranous labyrinth of the inner ear.

Mastoid—A large bony process at the base of the skull behind the ear. It contains air spaces that connect with the cavity of the middle ear.

Membranous labyrinth—A complex arrangement of communicating membranous canals and sacs, filled with endolymph and suspended within the cavity of the bony labyrinth.

Ménière's disease—Also known as idiopathic endolymphatic hydrops, Ménière's disease is a disorder of the inner ear. It is named for Prosper Ménière (1799–1862), a French physician.

Shunt—A channel through which blood or another body fluid is diverted from its normal path by surgical reconstruction or the insertion of a synthetic tube.

Sigmoid sinus—An S-shaped cavity on the inner side of the skull behind the mastoid process.

Tinnitus—A sensation of ringing, buzzing, roaring, or clicking noises in the ear.

Vertigo—An illusory feeling that either one's self or the environment is revolving. It is usually caused either by diseases of the inner ear or disturbances of the central nervous system.

The patient is prepared for surgery by having the hair removed and the skin shaved over an area of at least 1.5 in (3.8 cm) around the site of the incision. A mild solution of soap and water is commonly used to cleanse the outer ear and surrounding skin.

Aftercare

The operated ear is covered with a Glassock dressing, which is a special dressing applied to keep pressure on the site to reduce swelling. There is usually some tenderness and discomfort in the operated ear and the throat (from the breathing tube inserted during

An endolymphatic shunt is performed in a hospital or ambulatory surgery center on an outpatient basis. It is done by an otolaryngologist, who is a surgeon specializing in disorders of the ear, nose, and throat.

- What are the alternatives to an endolymphatic shunt procedure?
- Will I regain my hearing if I have this surgery?
- Can I expect improvement in any of the other symptoms of Ménière's disease?
- How long will it take to recover from the surgery?
- How many endolymphatic shunts do you perform each year?

surgery), which can be controlled by such analgesic medications as meperidine (Demerol) or oxycodone (Percocet).

Risks

There are few risks associated with endolymphatic shunt surgery. The operation is considered the first-line surgical treatment for Ménière's disease precisely because it is very safe. The chance of hearing loss from the procedure is about 0.5%.

Normal results

Endolymphatic shunt surgery relieves the vertigo associated with Ménière's disease, with restoration of hearing dependent on the severity of the disease. The patient's ear may protrude slightly shortly after surgery but usually returns to its original position within two to three weeks after the operation. Numbness around the ear is a common complication that may last for several months.

Morbidity and mortality rates

Endolymphatic shunt surgery is considered a low-morbidity procedure. It has been reported to achieve complete or substantial control of vertigo in 81% of patients, with significant improvement in hearing in about 20%. Overall, there is a 60% chance of curing the vertigo, a 20% chance that the attacks will remain at the same level of severity, and a 20% chance that the attacks will get worse. The patient's vertigo usually improves even if hearing does not improve.

Alternatives

Nonsurgical alternatives

There are several nonsurgical treatments recommended for patients with Ménière's disease:

- Vestibular suppressants. These are drugs designed to control vertigo attacks; they include mechzine (Antivert), diazepam (Valium), and dimenhydrinate (Dramamine).

- Diuretics. Medications that increase the body's output of urine can also help reduce the frequency of vertigo attacks in some patients by lowering the amount of fluid in the body.

- Dietary changes. Although the benefits of a low salt diet have not been confirmed by formal scientific research, many patients with Ménière's disease have noted that their symptoms improve when they restrict their salt intake.

- Steroids. Prednisone and other steroids have been used to treat patients in the early stages of Ménière's disease. Their use in this disorder, however, is still considered experimental as of 2003.

Surgical

Surgical alternatives to the placement of an endolymphatic shunt include:

- Selective vestibular neurectomy. In this procedure, the surgeon cuts the vestibular nerve, which relays balance, position and movement signals from the inner ear to the brain. Vestibular neurectomy prevents the transmission of faulty information from the affected ear and eliminates attacks of vertigo in many patients.

- Labyrinthectomy. In this procedure, the membranous labyrinth of the inner ear is removed. Labyrinthectomy is more successful than other surgeries in eliminating vertigo, but the patient suffers complete and permanent loss of hearing in the operated ear.

Resources

BOOKS

Graham, M. D. *Treatment Options for Ménière's Disease: Endolymphatic Sac Surgery: Do It or Don't Do It and Why?* San Diego: Singular Publishing, 1998.

Haybach, P. J., and J. Underwood. *Ménière's Disease: What You Need to Know.* Portland, OR: Vestibular Disorders Association, 1998.

"Ménière's Disease." Section 7, Chapter 85 in *The Merck Manual of Diagnosis and Therapy*, edited by Mark H. Beers, MD, and Robert Berkow, MD. Whitehouse Station, NJ: Merck Research Laboratories, 1999.

PERIODICALS

Brookler, K. H. "A Patient with Endolymphatic Hydrops Refractory to Shunt Surgery." *Ear Nose Throat Journal* 79 (July 2000): 493.

Goksu, N., Y. A. Bayazit, A. Abdulhalik, and Y. K. Kemaloglu. "Vestibular Neurectomy with Simultaneous Endolymphatic Subarachnoid Shunt." *European Archives of Otorhinolaryngology* 259 (May 2002): 243-246.

Mason, T. P. "What is Ménière's Disease, and How is it Treated?" *Health News* 9 (April 2003): 12.

Ostrowski, V. B., and J. M. Kartush. " Endolymphatic Sac-Vein Decompression for Intractable Ménière's Disease: Long Term Treatment Results." *Otolaryngology Head and Neck Surgery* 128 (April 2003): 550-559.

Welling, D. B., and H. N. Nagaraja. "Endolymphatic Mastoid Shunt: a Reevaluation of Efficacy." *Otolaryngology Head and Neck Surgery* 122 (March 2000): 340-345.

ORGANIZATIONS

American Academy of Otolaryngology—Head and Neck Surgery. One Prince Street, Alexandria, VA 22314. (703) 806-4444. www.entnet.org.

National Institute on Deafness and Other Communication Disorders (NIDCD). 31 Center Drive, MSC 2320, Bethesda, MD 20892-2320. (800) 241-1044. www.nidcd.nih.gov/.

Vestibular Disorders Association (VEDA). PO Box 4467, Portland, OR 97208-4467. (800) 837-8428. www.vestibular.org.

OTHER

"Ménière's Disease—Surgical Therapy." UPennHealth. www.uphs.upenn.edu/balance/patient%20education%20brochures/Meniere's-Surgical%20Treatment.htm.

Monique Laberge, Ph.D.

Endometriosis surgery *see* **Laparoscopy for endometriosis**

Endoscopic retrograde cholangiopancreatography

Definition

Endoscopic retrograde cholangiopancreatography (ERCP) is an imaging technique used to diagnose diseases of the pancreas, liver, gallbladder, and bile ducts. It combines endoscopy and x-ray imaging.

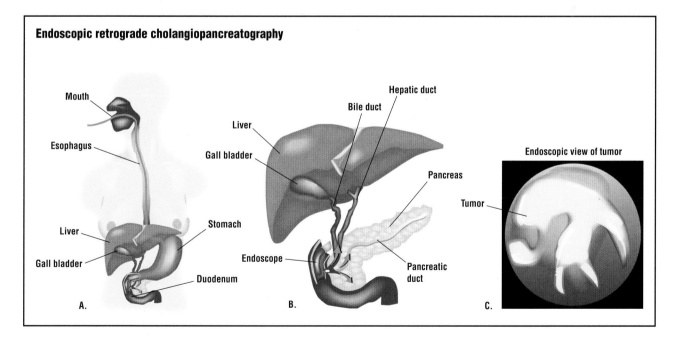

Endoscopic retrograde cholangiopancreatography

In endoscopic retrograde cholangiopancreatography, an endoscope is introduced into the patient's mouth and fed through the esophagus, stomach, and duodenum (small intestine) (A). A dye is released into the ducts (B). A series of x rays is taken, and a tumor may be visible with the endoscope (C). *(Illustration by GGS Information Services. Cengage Learning, Gale.)*

Purpose

ERCP is used in the management of diseases that affect the gastrointestinal tract, specifically the pancreas, liver, gall bladder, and bile ducts. The pancreas is an organ that secretes pancreatic juice into the upper part of the intestine. Pancreatic juice is composed of specialized proteins that help to digest fats, proteins, and carbohydrates. Bile is a substance that helps to digest fats; it is produced by the liver, secreted through the bile ducts, and stored in the gallbladder. Bile is released into the small intestine after a person has eaten a meal containing fat.

A doctor may recommend ERCP if a patient is experiencing abdominal pain of unknown origin, weight loss, or jaundice. These may be symptoms of biliary disease. For instance, gallstones that form in the gallbladder or bile ducts may become stuck there, causing cramping or dull pain in the upper right area of the abdomen, fever, and/or jaundice. Other causes of biliary obstruction include tumors, injury from gallbladder surgery, or inflammation. The bile ducts may also become narrowed (called a biliary stricture) as a result of cancer, blunt trauma to the abdomen, pancreatitis (inflammation of the pancreas), or primary biliary cirrhosis (PBC). PBC may be caused by a condition called primary sclerosing cholangitis, an inflammation of the bile ducts that may cause pain, jaundice, itching, or other symptoms. These symptoms may also be experienced by a patient with cholangitis, or with infection of the bile ducts caused by bacteria or parasites.

ERCP can also be used to diagnose a number of pancreatic disorders. Pancreatitis is an inflammation of the pancreas, caused by chronic alcohol abuse, injury, obstruction of the pancreatic ducts (e.g., by gallstones), or other factors. The condition may be either acute (having a severe but short course) or chronic (persistent). Symptoms of pancreatitis include abdominal pain, weight loss, nausea, and vomiting. ERCP may be used to diagnose cancer of the pancreas; pancreatic pseudocysts (collections of pancreatic fluid); or strictures of the pancreatic ducts. Certain congenital disorders may also be identified by ERCP, such as pancreas divisum, a condition in which parts of the pancreas fail to fuse together during fetal development.

Demographics

Diseases of the pancreas and biliary tract affect millions of Americans each year. According to the National Health and Nutrition Survey, gallbladder disease affects approximately 6.3 million men and 14.2 million women in the United States between the

ages of 24 and 74. Approximately one million new cases of gallstones are diagnosed each year. The incidence of gallstones is higher among women; adults over the age of 40; and people who are overweight. Primary sclerosing cholangitis occurs at a rate of two to seven cases per 100,000 persons. The rate of gallbladder cancer is approximately 2.5 out of 100,000 persons. In addition, approximately 87,000 cases of pancreatitis and 30,000 cases of pancreatic cancer are diagnosed each year in the United States.

Description

ERCP is performed with the patient given either a sedative or **general anesthesia**. The physician then sprays the back of the patient's throat with a local anesthetic. The endoscope (a thin, hollow tube attached to a viewing screen) is then inserted into the mouth. It is threaded down the esophagus, through the stomach, and into the duodenum (upper part of the small intestine) until it reaches the spot where the bile and pancreatic ducts empty into the duodenum. At this point a small tube called a cannula is inserted through the endoscope and used to inject a contrast dye into the ducts. The term "retrograde" in the name of the procedure refers to the backward direction of the dye as it is injected through the ducts. A series of x rays are then taken as the dye moves through the ducts.

If the x rays show that a problem exists, ERCP may be used as a therapeutic tool. Special instruments can be inserted into the endoscope to remove gallstones, take samples of tissue for further examination (e.g., in the case of suspected cancer), or place a special tube called a stent into a duct to relieve an obstruction.

Diagnosis/Preparation

ERCP is generally not performed unless other less invasive diagnostic tests have first been used to determine the cause of a patient's symptoms. Such tests include:

- complete medical history and physical examination
- blood tests (certain diseases can be diagnosed by abnormal levels of blood components)
- ultrasound imaging (a procedure that uses high-frequency sound waves to visualize structures in the human body)
- computed tomography (CT) scan (an imaging device that uses x rays to produce two-dimensional cross-sections on a viewing screen)

Before undergoing ERCP, the patient will be instructed to refrain from eating or drinking for at least six hours to ensure that the stomach and upper part of the intestine are empty. Arrangements should be made for someone to take the patient home after the procedure, as he or she will not be able to drive. The physician should also be given a complete list of all prescription, over-the-counter, and alternative medications or preparations that the patient is taking. The patient should also notify the doctor if he or she is allergic to iodine because the contrast dye contains it.

Aftercare

After the procedure, the patient will remain at the hospital or outpatient facility until the effects of the sedative wear off and no signs of any complications have appeared. A longer stay may be warranted if the patient experiences complications or if other procedures were performed.

Risks

Complications that have been reported with ERCP include pancreatitis; cholangitis (inflammation of the bile ducts); cholecystitis (inflammation of the gallbladder); injury to the duodenum; pain; bleeding;

WHO PERFORMS THE PROCEDURE AND WHERE IS IT PERFORMED?

ERCP is usually performed in the x-ray department of a hospital or outpatient facility by a gastroenterologist, a medical doctor who has completed specialized training in the diagnosis and treatment of diseases of the digestive system. An anesthesiologist administers the anesthetic, and a radiologist may be consulted in interpreting the images obtained by the dye injection.

infection; and formation of blood clots. Factors that increase the risk of complications include liver damage, bleeding disorders, a history of post-ERCP complications, and a less experienced endoscopist.

Normal results

Following ERCP, the patient's biliary and pancreatic ducts should be free of stones and show no strictures, obstructions, or evidence of infection or inflammation.

Morbidity and mortality rates

The overall complication rate associated with ERCP is approximately 11%. Pancreatitis may occur in up to 7% of patients. Cholangitis and cholecystitis occur in less than 1% of patients. Infection, injury, bleeding, and blot clot formation also occur in less than 1%. The mortality rate for ERCP is approximately 0.1%.

Alternatives

Although less invasive techniques exist (such as computed tomography and ultrasonography) to help to diagnose gastrointestinal diseases, these imaging studies are often not precise enough to allow for definite diagnosis of certain conditions. Percutaneous transhepatic cholangiography (PTCA) is an alternative to ERCP that involves the insertion of a long, flexible needle through the skin to the bile ducts; contrast dye is then injected into the ducts so that they may be visualized by x ray. PTCA may be recommended if ERCP fails or cannot be performed. Magnetic resonance cholangiopancreatography (MRCP) is an imaging technology that allows for noninvasive examination of the biliary and pancreatic ducts. Its disadvantage, however, is that unlike ERCP, it cannot be used for therapeutic procedures as well as imaging.

Bethesda, MD: NDDIC, 2002. [cited April 7, 2003]. http://www.niddk.nih.gov/health/digest/pubs/diagtest/ercp.htm.

Stephanie Dionne Sherk

Endoscopic sclerotherapy *see* **Sclerotherapy for esophageal varices**

QUESTIONS TO ASK THE DOCTOR

- Why is ERCP recommended in my case?
- What diagnostic tests will be performed prior to ERCP?
- How long will the procedure take?
- When will I find out the results?
- Will you treat the problem if one is found during the procedure?

Resources

BOOKS

Feldman, Mark, et al. *Sleisenger & Fordtran's Gastrointestinal and Liver Disease*, 7th ed. Philadelphia: Elsevier Science, 2002.

PERIODICALS

Ahmed, Aijaz, and Emmet B. Keeffe. "Gallstones and Biliary Tract Disease." *WebMD Scientific American Medicine* February 28, 2003 [cited April 7, 2003]. http://www.medscape.com/viewarticle/449563_1.

Aronson, Naomi, Carole Flamm, Rhonda L. Bohn, et al. "Evidence-Based Assessment: Patient, Procedure, or Operator Factors Associated with ERCP Complications." *Gastrointestinal Endoscopy* 56, no. 6 (December 2002)(6 Suppl): S294-S302.

Freeman, Martin L. "Adverse Outcomes of ERCP." *Gastrointestinal Endoscopy* 56, no. 6 (December 2002) (6 Suppl): S273-S282.

Vandervoort, Jo, et al. "Risk Factors for Complications After Performance of ERCP." *Gastrointestinal Endoscopy* 56, no. 5 (November 2002): 652-656.

Yakshe, Paul. "Biliary Disease." *eMedicine*, March 29, 2002 [cited April 7, 2003]. http://www.emedicine.com/MED/topic225.htm.

Yakshe, Paul. "Pancreatitis, Chronic." *eMedicine*, January 8, 2003 [cited April 7, 2003]. http://www.emedicine.com/med/topic1721.htm.

ORGANIZATIONS

American College of Gastroenterology. 4900 B South 31st St., Arlington, VA 22206. (703) 820-7400. http://www.acg.gi.org.

American Gastroenterological Association. 7910 Woodmont Ave., 7th Floor, Bethesda, MD 20814. (301) 654-2055. http://www.gastro.org.

American Society for Gastrointestinal Endoscopy. 1520 Kensington Rd., Suite 202, Oak Brook, IL 60523. (630) 573-0600. http://www.asge.org.

OTHER

National Digestive Diseases Information Clearinghouse. *Endoscopic Retrograde Cholangiopancreatography*.

Endoscopic sinus surgery

Definition

Functional endoscopic sinus surgery (FESS) is a minimally invasive surgical procedure that opens up sinus air cells and sinus ostia (openings) with an endoscope.

The use of FESS as a sinus surgical method has now become widely accepted, and the term "functional" is meant to distinguish this type of endoscopic surgery from nonendoscopic, more conventional sinus surgery procedures.

Purpose

The purpose of FESS is to restore normal drainage of the sinuses. This function requires ventilation through the ostia (mouth-like opening) and is facilitated by a mucociliary transport process that maintains a constant flow of mucus out of the sinuses. All sinuses need ventilation to prevent infection and inflammation, a condition known as sinusitis. In healthy individuals, sinus ventilation occurs through the ostia into the nose. The sinuses open into the middle meatus (curved passage in each nasal cavity) under the middle turbinate (thin, bony process that is the lower portion of the ethmoid bone in each nasal cavity), which together are known as the osteomeatal complex, the key area of the nose. The hair-like cilia direct the flow of mucus toward the ostia.

Sinusitis develops when there is a problem in the area where the maxillary and frontal sinuses meet near the nose or, occasionally, a dental infection. When sinusitis occurs, the cilia work less efficiently, preventing the flow of mucus. The mucous membranes of the sinuses become engorged, resulting in ostia closure. Poor ventilation and accumulation of mucus then produce the conditions required for bacterial infection.

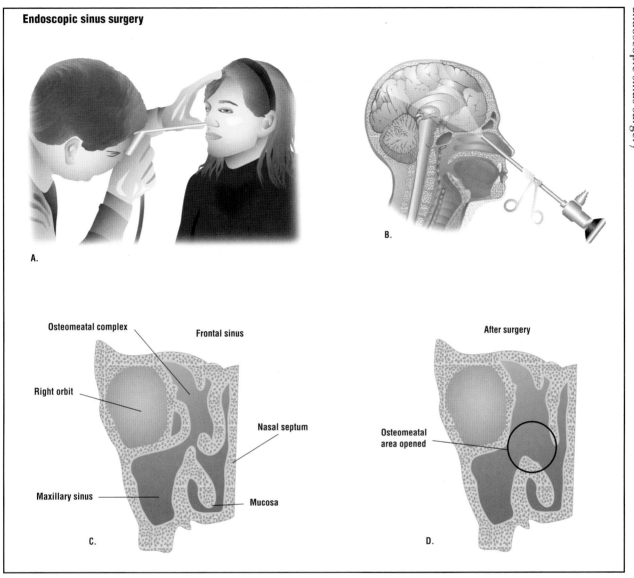

Endoscopic sinus surgery

During endoscopic sinus surgery, a doctor uses an endoscope to view the inner cavities of the nose (A and B). Using special instruments, the sinuses are opened to alleviate problems with sinusitis (C and D). *(Illustration by GGS Information Services. Cengage Learning, Gale.)*

Demographics

Sinusitis is a very common condition, affecting 31 million Americans each year; 30% of the U.S. population have sinusitis at some point in their lives. The average adult has three to four upper respiratory infections a year; 1% of these infections are complicated by sinusitis, accounting for 16 million visits to the doctor each year.

Description

After inducing adequate vasoconstriction with cocaine or ephedrine, the surgeon locates the middle turbinate, the most important landmark for the FESS procedure. On the side of the nose at the level of the middle turbinate lies the uncinate process, which the surgeon removes. The surgeon opens the back ethmoid air cells, to allow better ventilation, but leaves the bone covered with the mucous membrane. Following this step, the ostium located near the jaw is checked for obstruction and, if necessary, opened with a middle meatal antrostomy. This surgical procedure often greatly improves the function of the osteomeatal complex and provides better ventilation of the sinuses.

FESS offers several advantages:

KEY TERMS

Antrostomy—The operation of opening an antrum for drainage.

Antrum—The cavity of a sinus.

Caldwell-Luc procedure—A surgical procedure in which the surgeon enters the maxillary sinus by making an opening under the upper lip above the teeth.

Cilia—Short hairlike processes that are capable of a lashing movement.

CT scan—A sectional imaging of the body constructed by computed tomography.

Endoscope—An instrument for visualizing the interior of a hollow organ.

Ethmoid sinuses—Paired labyrinth of air cells between the nose and eyes.

Maxillary sinuses—Sinuses located in the cheek under the eye next to the ethmoid sinus.

Meatus—A general term for an opening or passageway in the body.

Middle meatus—A curved passage in each nasal cavity located below the middle nasal concha and extending along the entire superior border of the inferior nasal concha.

Middle turbinate—The lower of two thin bony processes on the ethmoid bone on the lateral wall of each nasal fossa that separates the superior and middle meatus of the nose.

Mucociliary—Involving cilia of the mucous membranes of the respiratory system.

Mucous membrane—A membrane rich in mucous glands that lines body passages and cavities communicating directly or indirectly with the exterior of the body (as for example, the alimentary, respiratory, and genitourinary tracts). Mucous membranes functions in protection, support, nutrient absorption, and secretion of mucus, enzymes, and salts.

Mucus—A viscous, slippery secretion that is produced by mucous membranes which it moistens and protects.

Nasal concha—Any of three thin bony plates on the lateral wall of the nasal fossa on each side with or without their covering of mucous membrane.

Ostia—A mouth-like opening in a bodily part.

Polyp—A projecting mass of swollen and hypertrophied or tumorous tissue.

Sinus—A cavity in a bone of the skull that usually communicates with the nostrils and contains air.

Sinusitis—Inflammation of a sinus.

Stenosis—Narrowing of a duct or canal.

Turbinate—Relating to a nasal concha.

Uncinate process—A downwardly and backwardly directed process of each lateral mass of the ethmoid bone that joins with the inferior nasal conchae.

Vasoconstriction—Narrowing of blood vessels, especially as a result of vasomotor action.

- It is a minimally invasive procedure.
- It does not disturb healthy tissue.
- It is performed in less time with better results.
- It minimizes bleeding and scarring.

Diagnosis/Preparation

As with many diseases, the history of a patient with sinusitis represents a key part of the preoperative evaluation. Before considering FESS, the ear, nose and throat (ENT) specialist will proceed with a thorough diagnostic examination. The development of such diagnostic tools as the fiberoptic endoscope and CT scanning has greatly improved the treatment of sinus disease. The fiberoptic endoscope is used to examine the nose and all its recesses thoroughly. The specific features that the physician must examine and evaluate are the middle turbinate and the middle

meatus, any anatomic obstruction, and the presence of pus and nasal polyps.

CT scanning can also be used to identify the diseased areas, a process that is required for planning the surgery. It shows the extent of the affected sinuses, as well as any abnormalities that may make a patient more susceptible to sinusitis.

FESS is usually performed under **local anesthesia** with intravenous sedation on an outpatient basis with patients going home one to two hours after surgery. It usually does not cause facial swelling or bruising, and does not generally require nasal packing.

Aftercare

FESS usually does not cause severe postoperative sinus pain. After the procedure, it is important to keep the nose as free from crust build-up as possible. To

WHO PERFORMS THE PROCEDURE AND WHERE IS IT PERFORMED?

This procedure is usually performed on an outpatient basis by an ear, nose, and throat (ENT) specialist, such as an otolaryngologist or an ophthalmic surgeon. ENT physicians are graduates of a school of medicine and typically undergo an otolaryngology residency with further specialization in sinus disease and endoscopic sinus surgery.

QUESTIONS TO ASK THE DOCTOR

- Why is sinus surgery required?
- What are the risks involved?
- How many endoscopic sinus surgeries do you perform in a year?
- How much time will I need to recover from the procedure?
- Is the procedure painful?
- What are the alternatives?

achieve this, the surgeon may perform a lengthy cleaning two to three times per week, or the patient may perform a simple nasal douching several times a day. Normal function usually reappears after one or two months. In patients with severe sinusitis or polyps, a short course of systemic steroids combined with **antibiotics** may quicken recovery.

Risks

The most serious risk associated with FESS is blindness resulting from damage to the optic nerve. However, the chances of this complication occurring are extremely low. Cerebrospinal fluid leak represents the most common major complication of FESS, but it occurs in only about 0.2% of cases in the Unites States. The leak is usually recognized at the time of surgery and can easily be repaired. Other less serious and rare complications include orbital hematoma and nasolacrimal duct stenosis. All of these complications are also associated with conventional sinus surgery and not only with FESS.

Normal results

The FESS procedure is considered successful if the patient's sinusitis is resolved. Nasal obstruction and facial pain are usually relieved. The outcome has been compared with that of the Caldwell-Luc procedure and, although both methods are considered effective, there is a strong patient preference for FESS. The extent of the disease before surgery dictates the outcome, with the best results obtained in patients with limited nasal sinusitis.

Morbidity and mortality rates

According to the American Academy of Family Physicians (AAFP), FESS usually has a good outcome, with most studies reporting an 80–90% rate of success. Good results have also been obtained in patients who have had previous sinus surgery.

Alternatives

- Image-guided endoscopic surgery. This method uses image guidance techniques that feature a three-dimensional mapping system combining CT scanning and real-time data acquisition concerning the location of the surgical instruments during the procedure. It allows surgeons to navigate more precisely in the affected area. The surgeon can monitor the exact location of such vital organs as the brain and eyes as well as positively identifying the affected areas.
- Caldwell-Luc procedure. This procedure is improves drainage in the maxillary sinus region located below the eye. The surgeon reaches the region through the upper jaw above one of the second molars. He or she creates a passage to connect the maxillary sinus to the nose in order to improve drainage.

Resources

BOOKS

Bhatt, N. J. *The Frontal Sinus: Advanced Surgical Techniques*. Independence, KY: Singular Publishing Group, 2002.

Marks, S. C. and W. A. Loechel. *Nasal and Sinus Surgery*. Philadelphia: W. B. Saunders Co., 2000.

PERIODICALS

Engelke, W., W. Schwarzwaller, A. Behnsen, and H. G. Jacobs. "Subantroscopic laterobasal sinus floor augmentation (SALSA): an up-to-5-year clinical study." *International Journal of Oral and Maxillofacial Implants* 18 (January-February 2003): 135–143.

Graham, S. M., and K. D. Carter. "Major complications of endoscopic sinus surgery: a comment." *British Journal of Ophthalmology* 87 (March 2003): 374–377.

Larsen, A. S., C. Buchwald, and S. Vesterhauge. "Sinus barotrauma—late diagnosis and treatment with computer-aided endoscopic surgery." *Aviation & Space Environmental Medicine* 74 (February 2003): 180–183.

Ramadan, H. H. "Relation of age to outcome after endoscopic sinus surgery in children." *Archives of Otolaryngology & Head and Neck Surgery* 129 (February 2003): 175–177.

Wormald, P. J. "Salvage frontal sinus surgery: the endoscopic modified Lothrop procedure." *Laryngoscope* 113 (February 2003): 276–283.

ORGANIZATIONS

American Academy of Otolaryngology-Head and Neck Surgery. One Prince St., Alexandria, VA 22314-3357. (703) 836-4444. http://www.entnet.org/.

Association for Research in Otolaryngology. 19 Mantua Rd., Mt. Royal, NJ 08061. (856) 423-0041. (301) 733-3640. http://www.aro.org/index.html.

North American Society for Head and Neck Pathology. Department of Pathology, H179, P.O. Box 850, Milton S. Hershey Medical Center, Penn State University School of Medicine, Hershey, PA 17033. (717) 531-8246. http://www.headandneckpathology.com/.

OTHER

"Factsheet: Sinus Surgery." American Academy of Otolaryngology—Head and Neck Surgery. http://www.entnet.org/HealthInformation/SinusSurgery.cfm [Accessed April 11, 2008].

Monique Laberge, PhD
Laura Jean Cataldo, RN, EdD

Endoscopic ultrasound

Definition

Endoscopic ultrasound is an imaging test which combines an endoscopic examination with an ultrasound examination. A very thin flexible tube is passed through the mouth, into the throat, and then on through either the bronchi into the lungs or through the esophagus into the stomach. Alternatively, the tube can be passed through the anus and into the lower gastrointestinal tract. A tiny ultrasound transducer is built into this tube, allowing close examination of areas of either the upper or lower gastrointestinal tract, or the respiratory tract. Endoscopic ultrasound can be used to diagnose conditions, to stage cancer, and to access biopsy samples.

Purpose

Endoscopic ultrasound can be used to evaluate a number of conditions, including:

- Cancer of the esophagus, stomach, pancreas or rectum
- Lung cancer

- Gallstones in the bile duct
- Pancreatitis
- Pancreatic cysts
- Dysfunctional anal sphincter
- Incontinence
- Barrett's esophagus
- Rectal fistulas

Precautions

Patients who are taking blood thinners, aspirin, or nonsteroidal anti-inflammatory medications may need to discontinue their use in advance of the test, to avoid increasing the risk of bleeding.

Description

After the patient is adequately sedated, he or she will be placed in the appropriate position, depending on what type of examination is being performed. For upper gastrointestinal or respiratory exams, the throat will be sprayed with a local anesthetic which will prevent the gag reflex from interfering with introduction of the endoscope. Air may be introduced into the gastrointestinal tract, in order to expand the area for more easy visualization of the structures.

The endoscope will be passed either through the mouth into the trachea and then through the bronchial tree into the lungs, or through the mouth into the esophagus and on into the stomach. From the stomach, the endoscope can be passed further into the small intestine, where it can be used to access the pancreas as well. Alternatively, the endoscope can be introduced through the rectum into the large intestine for examination of the bowel.

The progression of the endoscope past the various structures will be visible to the examiner on a television monitor. A separate ultrasound monitor allows the examiner to view ultrasound images during the course of the examination. Fine needle biopsy can be performed through the endocscope in order to obtain biopsy samples.

Preparations

Patients will need to stop eating and drinking for at least six hours prior to the exam. For examinations involving the gastrointestinal tract, enemas and/or laxatives may be used to empty the GI tract of feces. An intravenous line will be placed in order to provide the patient with fluids and sedation during the exam. Sedation will make the passage of the endoscopy tube less traumatic and uncomfortable. The patient will be attached to a variety of monitors to keep track of

Barrett's esophagus—A condition in which the esophageal tissue closest to the stomach contains highly abnormal cells that have a great likelihood of converting to frank cancer.

Endoscope—A narrow, flexible tube with a fiber optic light on it, used to pass into the body for a variety of medical examinations.

Fine needle biopsy—Use of a very thin type of needle to withdraw cells from an organ, a tumor, or other body tissue, in order to examine those cells for abnormalities (such as malignancy)in a pathology laboratory.

Fistula—An abnormal opening occurring between two organs or an abnormal opening leading to the outside of the body.

Pancreatitis—Inflammation of the pancreas.

Transducer—The instrument that sends sound waves into organs of the body, in order to produce ultrasound images.

blood pressure, heart rate, and blood oxygen level throughout the procedure.

Aftercare

After the test, patients will rest until the sedative wears off. Once their gag reflex has returned, they can begin drinking fluids. After some hours, they can progress to a light diet. Most people can resume their normal diet and activity level within 24 hours of this type of test.

Risks

In general, endoscopic ultrasound examinations that are performed without final needle aspiration are relatively low risk. Only about one in 2,000 patients undergoing this procedure develop any kind of complication from it. Possible problems include reaction to the sedatives (such as nausea, vomiting, hives, or skin rash), or swelling or infection of the area where the intravenous line was placed. The most serious complication involves inadvertent perforation (puncture) of the intestinal wall, requiring surgical repair. This is an extremely rare complication.

There is a slightly higher rate of complication when endoscopic ultrasound is performed in conjunction with a fine needle aspiration. Complication rates for this procedure are about 0.5-1.0%. In this case,

there is some chance of bleeding if the needle accidentally passes through the intestinal wall. This may require that the patient be hospitalized for observation, or, even more rarely, for a blood transfusion. Infection can also occur following fine needle aspiration. When the procedure involves the pancreas, there is a risk of pancreatic inflammation or pancreatitis, requiring some days of hospitalization and treatment.

Normal results

Normal results mean that there are no structural abnormalities visualized during the course of the examination. If biopsies are performed, a normal examination would mean that only normal tissue was identified upon pathological examination.

Abnormal results

Abnormal results range from the discovery and identification of tumors, cysts, or gallstones, to the demonstration of cancerous tissue upon examination of biopsy material in the pathology laboratory.

Resources

BOOKS

Feldman, M, et al. *Sleisenger & Fordtran's Gastrointestinal and Liver Disease,* 8th ed. St. Louis: Mosby, 2005.

Goldman, L., D. Ausiello, eds. *Cecil Textbook of Internal Medicine,* 23rd ed. Philadelphia: Saunders, 2008.

Grainger, R. G., et al. *Grainger & Allison's Diagnostic Radiology: A Textbook of Medical Imaging,* 4th ed. Philadelphia: Saunders, 2001.

Mettler, F. A. *Essentials of Radiology,* 2nd ed. Philadelphia: Saunders, 2005.

Townsend, C. M., et al. *Sabiston Textbook of Surgery,* 17th ed. Philadelphia: Saunders, 2004.

Rosalyn Carson-DeWitt, MD

Endotracheal intubation

Definition

Endotracheal intubation is the placement of a tube into the trachea (windpipe) in order to maintain an open airway in patients who are unconscious or unable to breathe on their own. Oxygen, anesthetics, or other gaseous medications can be delivered through the tube.

Endotracheal intubation

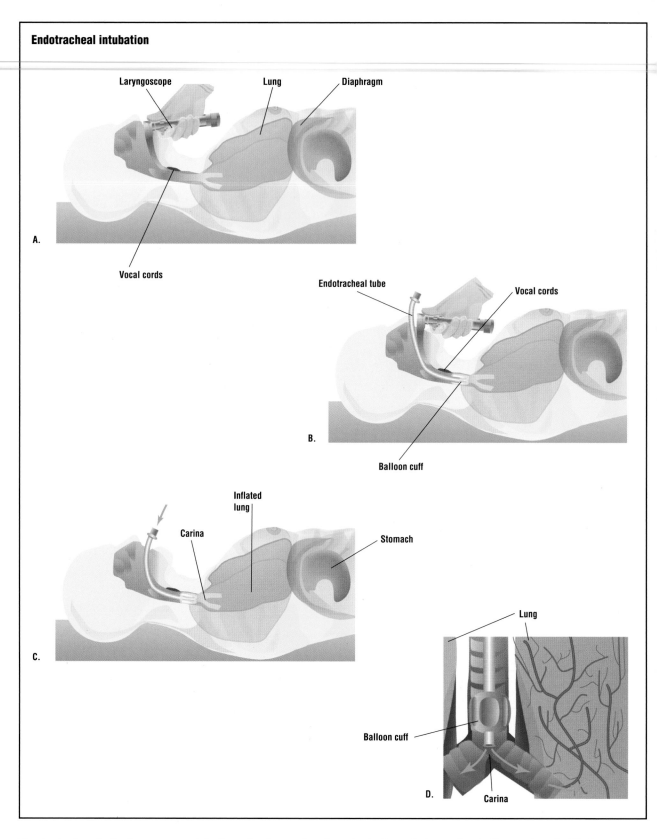

The doctor inserts the laryngoscope into the patient's mouth, advancing to through the trachea to the vocal cords (A). An endotracheal tube is inserted into the airway (B). The balloon cuff is inflated, and the laryngoscope is removed (C). *(Illustration by GGS Information Services. Cengage Learning, Gale.)*

Purpose

Specifically, endotracheal intubation is used for the following conditions:

- respiratory arrest
- respiratory failure
- airway obstruction
- need for prolonged ventilatory support
- Class III or IV hemorrhage with poor perfusion
- severe flail chest or pulmonary contusion
- multiple trauma, head injury and abnormal mental status
- inhalation injury with erythema/edema of the vocal cords
- protection from aspiration

Description

To begin the procedure, an anesthesiologist opens the patient's mouth by separating the lips and pulling on the upper jaw with the index finger. Holding a laryngoscope in the left hand, he or she inserts it into the mouth of the patient with the blade directed to the right tonsil. Once the right tonsil is reached, the laryngoscope is swept to the midline keeping the tongue on the left to bring the epiglottis into view. The laryngoscope blade is then advanced until it reaches the angle between the base of the tongue and the epiglottis. Next, the laryngoscope is lifted upwards towards the chest and away from the nose to bring the vocal cords into view. Often an assistant has to press on the trachea to provide a direct view of the larynx. The anesthesiologist then takes the endotracheal tube, made of flexible plastic, in the right hand and starts inserting it through the mouth opening. The tube is inserted through the cords to the point that the cuff rests just below the cords. Finally, the cuff is inflated to provide a minimal leak when the bag is squeezed. Using a **stethoscope**, the anesthesiologist listens for breathing sounds to ensure correct placement of the tube.

Preparation

For endotracheal intubation, the patient is placed on the operating table lying on the back with a pillow under the head. The anesthesiologist wears gloves, a gown, and goggles. **General anesthesia** is administered to the patient before starting intubation.

Risks

The anesthesiologist should evaluate and follow the patient for potential complications that may

KEY TERMS

Anesthesia—The loss of feeling or sensation. Anesthesia is administered during surgery by an anesthesiologist.

Edema—The presence of abnormally large amounts of fluid in the intercellular tissue spaces of the body.

Emphysema—A pathological accumulation of air in tissues or organs, especially in the lungs.

Endotracheal—Located inside the trachea.

Epiglottis—A cartilaginous lidlike appendage that closes the glottis while food or drink is passing through the pharynx.

Glottis—The vocal part of the larynx, consisting of the vocal cords and the opening between them.

Laryngoscope—An instrument used to examine the larynx.

Larynx—The voice box.

Pharynx—The cavity at the back of the mouth.

Pneumothorax—A collapse of the lung due to an abrupt change in the intrapleural pressure within the chest cavity.

Trachea—The windpipe; a tough, fibrocartilaginous tube passing from the larynx to the bronchi before the lungs.

Stethoscope—A rubber Y-shaped device used to listen to sounds produced by the human body.

include edema, bleeding, tracheal and esophageal perforation, pneumothorax (collapsed lung), and aspiration. The patient should be advised of the potential signs and symptoms associated with life-threatening complications of airway problems. These signs and symptoms include, but are not limited to, sore throat, pain or swelling of the face and neck, chest pain, subcutaneous emphysema, and difficulty swallowing.

Normal results

The endotracheal tube inserted during the procedure maintains an open passage through the upper airway and allows air to pass freely to and from the lungs in order to ventilate them.

Alternatives

Alternatives to endotracheal intubation include:

- Esophageal tracheal combitube (ETC). The ETC is a double-lumen tube, combining the function of an esophageal obturator airway and a conventional endotracheal airway. The esophageal lumen has an open upper end, perforations at the pharyngeal level, and a closed distal end. The tracheal lumen has open ends. The lumens are separated by a wall and each is linked via a short tube with a connector. An oropharyngeal balloon serves to seal the oral and nasal cavities after insertion. At the lower end, a second cuff serves to seal either the trachea or esophagus.

- Laryngeal mask airway (LMA). The LMA consists of an inflatable silicone ring attached diagonally to a flexible tube. The ring forms an oval cushion that fills the space around and behind the larynx. It achieves a low pressure seal between the tube and the trachea without insertion into the larynx.

- Tracheostomy. A tracheostomy is a surgically created opening in the neck that allows direct access to the trachea. It is kept open with a tracheostomy tube. A tracheostomy is performed when it is not possible to intubate the patient.

Resources

BOOKS

Finucane, B. T., and A. H. Santora. *Principles of Airway Management.* New York: Springer Verlag, 2003.

Roberts, J. T. *Fundamentals of Tracheal Intubation.* New York: Grune & Stratton, 1983.

Stewart, C. E. *Advanced Airway Management.* St. Louis: Quality Medical Publishing, 2002.

PERIODICALS

Bochicchio, G. V., et al. "Endotracheal intubation in the field does not improve outcome in trauma patients who present without an acutely lethal traumatic brain injury." *Journal of Trauma Injury, Infections and Critical Care* 54 (February 2003): 307–311.

Erhan, E., et al. "Tracheal intubation without muscle relaxants: Remifentanil or alfentanil in combination with propofol." *European Journal of Anaesthesiology* 20 (January 2003): 37–43.

Udobi, K. F., E. Childs, and K. Touijer. "Acute respiratory distress syndrome." *American Family Physician* 67 (January 2003): 315–322.

Van de Leur, J. P., J. H. Zwaveling, B. G. Loef, and C. P. Van der Schans. "Endotracheal suctioning versus minimally invasive airway suctioning in intubated patients: A prospective randomized controlled trial." *Intensive Care Medicine* 186 (February 8, 2003).

ORGANIZATIONS

American Society of Anesthesiologists. 520 N. Northwest Highway, Park Ridge, IL 60068-2573. (847) 825-5586. http://www.asahq.org/.

OTHER

"Endotracheal intubation." Health_encyclopedia. http://www.austin360.com/search/healthfd/shared/health/adam/ency/article/003449.html.

"Endotracheal intubation." PennHealth. http://www.pennhealth.com/ency/article/003449.htm.

"Intubation." Discovery_Health. http://health.discovery.com/diseasesandcond/encyclopedia/1219.html.

Monique Laberge, Ph.D.

Endovascular stent surgery

Definition

Endovascular stent surgery is a minimally invasive surgical procedure that uses advanced technology and instrumentation to treat disorders of the circulatory system such as blockage or damage to blood vessels caused by the buildup of plaque (fatty deposits, calcium deposits, and scar tissue) in the arteries, a condition called atherosclerosis (hardening of the arteries). The surgeon may recommend the placement of an endovascular stent, a small wire-mesh tube that surgeons call a scaffold, in an affected artery. The procedure may be done in conjunction with cleaning or repairing the artery. The twofold procedure opens, enlarges, and supports artery walls for a long-lasting improvement in blood flow and a decrease in the risk

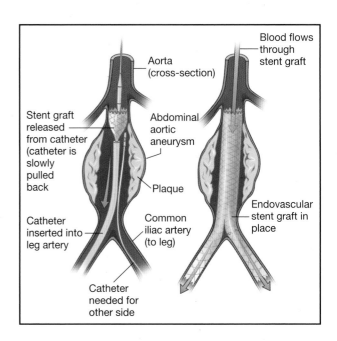

(Illustration by Electronic Illustrators Group.)

of heart attack or stroke. In endovascular stent surgery (*endo*, within, and *vascular,* blood vessel), all of the work done by the surgeon is within the blood vessels themselves. Nearly all of the medium-sized and large blood vessels in the body's vascular system can be accessed from within the vessels. This fact contributes to a rapid increase in the performance of endovascular stent surgery.

Purpose

The purpose of endovascular stent surgery is to improve or restore the flow of blood and oxygen throughout the body, a process called coronary revascularization. Endovascular stent surgery is used most often to correct the narrowing in medium-sized and large arteries blocked by plaque. Stents have been used in coronary arteries, the carotid arteries in the neck, and renal (kidney) or biliary (gallbladder) arteries. They are rarely used for smaller arteries in the legs, for example, or other smaller vessels in the body.

Endovascular stenting is also the newest treatment for emergency vascular events, such as abdominal or thoracic (related to chest and lung area) aortic aneurysms. Aortic aneurysms are life-threatening bulges in the walls of the aorta, the largest artery in the body, usually the result of progressive atherosclerosis.

Demographics

Candidates for endovascular stent surgery are patients with atheroslerosis who are at high risk for heart attack and stroke. Heart disease and stroke are the leading causes of **death** and disability in the United States for both men and women. People at greatest risk have high blood pressure and high cholesterol, and sometimes diabetes. Typically these people may also smoke, be overweight, and have close relatives with heart disease or coronary artery disease or who have had a stroke. More than 700,000 people per year have stent surgeries to clear obstructions in the coronary arteries. Abdominal aortic aneurysms are the 13th leading cause of death in the United States, occurring primarily in people over age 67. More than 190,000 aortic aneurysms are diagnosed each year; of these, 45,000 people have surgery. Although the use of stent grafting is increasing, most aneurysms are treated with conventional open surgery procedures.

Description

The conditions most often treated by endovascular stent surgery are: coronary artery disease; narrowing (stenosis) of the carotid artery in the neck, a risk factor for stroke; and aortic aneurysm.

- Coronary artery disease is a circulatory disorder resulting from plaque blockages in the arteries of the heart. The heart is a muscle that requires a constant flow of blood and oxygen through its blood vessels so that it can perform the critical function of supplying the whole body with blood. When fatty deposits form in the heart's two main arteries, the arteries become narrowed and the flow of blood and oxygen is blocked. Blockages can cause pain in the chest (angina) and eventually, when the blood vessels are occluded (closed up), a heart attack.

- The carotid arteries in the neck carry blood and oxygen to the brain. When these major arteries are blocked by plaque, the narrowing can interrupt the flow of blood to the brain and cause a disabling stroke. A carotid endarterectomy is a surgical procedure performed on people with significant stenosis (50 to 70% narrowing); in this procedure, a surgeon removes the fatty deposits to correct the narrowing and allow blood and oxygen to flow freely to the brain. Although an effective surgical measure, it is a surgery that presents high risks to patients who are already greatly compromised. Endovascular stent surgery is a less invasive procedure, with fewer risks, and is sometimes the surgeon's choice to prevent stroke in certain high-risk patients.

- An aortic aneurysm, which is a life-threatening bulging of the aorta, can occur anywhere along this major artery, either in the abdomen (abdominal aortic aneurysm or AAA) or in the chest area (thoracic aneurysm). When the aorta is blocked by significant amounts of plaque, pressure may cause it to bulge like a balloon directly above or below the blockage, causing a weakening of the vessel wall. The aorta may eventually rupture, causing massive bleeding and death. Sometimes the aneurysm is diagnosed when the victim complains of pain, but there may also be no obvious symptoms. Sometimes the vessel ruptures, causing massive internal bleeding and eventual loss of consciousness, requiring emergency surgery. Endovascular stent surgery is the least invasive method of surgical intervention to repair an aneurysm.

Coronary artery disease and carotid stenosis can be treated in three ways: medically, which is the use of therapeutic drugs in combination with changes in diet and **exercise**; by such open surgery as the highly invasive coronary artery bypass surgery (CABG); or by such minimally invasive procedures as stent implantation, balloon **angioplasty**, and atherectomy or endarterectomy (the cutting of plaque from the inside of vessel walls). Sometimes combinations of these methods are used. The goal of all these procedures is to improve the flow of blood and oxygen throughout the

KEY TERMS

Aorta—The largest artery in the body, which passes through the abdomen and chest, supplying blood to the stomach and legs.

Aneurysm—A life-threatening enlargement or bulge in an artery caused by a weakening of the artery wall above or below an area of blockage.

Balloon angioplasty—X-ray-guided insertion of a balloon catheter into a blocked blood vessel to remove plaque and open the vessel for better blood flow.

Endovascular—Within the walls of a blood vessel.

Graft—Replacement of a diseased or damaged part of the body with a compatible substitute that can be artificial (metal or other substance) or taken from the body itself, such as a piece of skin, healthy tissue, or bone.

Revascularization—Restoring the body's blood flow after an interruption or blockage has disrupted normal circulation.

Rupture—The bursting of a blood vessel or organ that has suffered enlargement, bulging, and weakening from unusual pressure.

Stent—A specially designed wire-mesh device that is placed inside a blood vessel to open or support it.

Thoracic—Pertaining to the chest cavity, including the lungs and the area around the lungs.

Vascular—Pertaining to the blood vessels of the body that make up the circulatory system; veins and arteries.

body, reduce symptoms, and reduce the risk of heart attack or stroke.

Endovascular stent surgery was introduced in the 1980s to treat occlusive (blocking) coronary artery disease, without using open surgery. More recently, endovascular stent grafting, a variation of the procedure, is also being used to repair life-threatening aortic aneurysms, which formerly could be treated only with open surgery. Because the incision for endovascular procedures is just large enough to allow passage of a small tube (catheter) into a blood vessel, the procedure does not disturb the patient's body processes as much as conventional **vascular surgery**. This advance in technique helps reduce the patient's stay in the hospital and makes recovery faster. At the same time, it satisfies a common goal of surgeons to use less

invasive methods that offer patients the best result with the fewest risks.

An endovascular stent is a tiny wire mesh tube that can look like a cage or a coiled spring, depending on the manufacturer's design. The implantation of stents is performed through a tiny incision, using a catheter to deliver it to the site of treatment in a vessel. The stent provides a mechanical way to hold a blood vessel open and improve blood flow over the long term. Stents are sometimes implanted through the same incision after balloon angioplasty has been performed. The balloon angioplasty is another catheter-guided procedure that uses a balloon device to stretch the waxy plaque formation and open the vessel walls. Before stents were used, some patients undergoing angioplasty (in 5–10% of angioplasty procedures) suffered acute closure, which is the complete closing down of the treated artery either during or after the procedure. Stents reduce the likelihood of this medical emergency and the need for immediate cardiac surgery to correct it. Stents are implanted both to treat new blockages and to treat the repeat build-up of plaque after prior surgical treatment, a process called restenosis. Endovascular stent implantation has been shown to reduce the likelihood of restenosis. Some stents can deliver anti-plaque drugs to the area of blockage. These are called drug-eluting stents; they are aimed at preventing restenosis and eliminating the need for further surgery.

Endovascular stent surgery is performed in a **cardiac catheterization** laboratory equipped with a fluoroscope, a special x-ray machine and an x-ray monitor that looks like a regular television screen. The patient will be placed on an x-ray table and covered with a sterile sheet. An area on the inside of the upper leg will be washed and treated with an antibacterial solution to prepare for the insertion of a catheter. The patient is given **local anesthesia** to numb the insertion site and will usually remain awake during the procedure. To implant stents in arteries, the stent is threaded through an incision in the groin up into the affected blood vessel on a catheter with a deflated balloon at its tip and inside the stent. The surgeon views the entire procedure with a fluoroscope. The surgeon guides the balloon catheter to the blocked area and inflates the balloon, causing the stent to expand and press against the vessel walls. The balloon is then deflated and taken out of the vessel. The entire procedure takes from an hour to 90 minutes to complete. The stent remains in the vessel permanently to hold the vessel walls open and allow blood to pass freely as in a normally functioning healthy artery. Cells and tissue will begin to grow over the stent until its inner surface is covered. It then becomes a permanent part of the functioning artery.

Stent surgery for emergency treatment of aortic aneurysm is called endovascular stent grafting or endovascular repair. Candidates for this treatment have either aortic aneurysms or other abnormal conditions of the aorta, such as an **arteriovenous fistula** (abnormal communication between an artery and a vein), or other kinds of aortic blockage. Formerly these conditions were treated by highly invasive surgical procedures, with incisions that reached from the breastbone to the navel, to access the aorta, open it, and insert and attach a slender fabric-covered tube called a graft. During the less invasive endovascular stent surgery, a collapsed metal stent-graft (also called an endograft) is threaded through an artery beginning from a small incision in the groin and ending in the aorta. Threading is done through a tube-like delivery system lying in the vessel, which allows catheters and stents to move up and down during the procedure. A stent graft is similar to the stents used in coronary artery procedures, but it has a ring of tiny hooks and barbs at each end that allow it to connect to the inner wall of the artery, replacing and repairing (grafting) the weakened area. The surgeon guides the stent graft into the aneurysm by using fluoroscopic x-ray imaging. When the stent graft is in place, its outer sheath is withdrawn and the stent graft is expanded. It will anchor itself to the inside of the artery wall with the hooks and barbs on each end. Some stent-graft systems also use balloons to push the hooks into the vessel wall. Because the procedure is minimally invasive, patients recover quickly and are usually able to eat the same day, walk on the second day, and go home in two to three days after the surgery.

Diagnosis/Preparation

Often the first test done to diagnose coronary artery disease is an **electrocardiogram**, to show the heart's rhythm. A **stress test**, or exercise electrocardiogram, may be performed as well, though the test can be too strenuous for some patients. Cardiac catheterization is considered the most definitive test. It requires the injection of a special dye into the coronary arteries at the same time a catheter is threaded up into the heart's arteries and x rays are displayed on a monitor to show any narrowing or blockage. To diagnose clogged arteries in other areas of the body, imaging techniques, such as computed tomography (CT) or **magnetic resonance imaging** (MRI) may be used to visualize the presence and extent of narrowing in the blood vessels. Diagnostic procedures for aneurysm may include these same imaging tests; but often,

because of the emergency nature of aneurysm, there is little time to conduct extensive testing beyond immediate confirmation of the presence of the aneurysm.

For up to 12 hours before a stent procedure or combined angioplasty and stent surgery, the patient will have to avoid eating or drinking. An intravenous line will be inserted so that medications (anticoagulants to prevent clot formation and radioactive dye for x rays) can be administered during the surgery. The patient's groin area will be shaved and cleaned with an antiseptic to prepare for the incision. About an hour before the procedure, the patient may be given a mild sedative to ensure that he or she will relax sufficiently for the procedure.

Aftercare

After stent surgery, the patient will spend several hours in the **recovery room** to be monitored for **vital signs** (temperature, heart rate, and breathing) and heart sounds. Pressure will be applied to the catheter insertion site in the groin to prevent bleeding; a weight may be applied to the leg to restrict movement. For the first 24 hours, the patient will have to lie flat and limit activities. Drinking fluids will be especially important to help flush out the dye that was used for x rays during the procedure. Stent recipients are usually placed on **aspirin** therapy or anti-clotting (anticoagulant) medication immediately after surgery. They will remain on it indefinitely to prevent clots from occurring in the stent. There are no other postoperative precautions, although dietary and lifestyle changes may be recommended to reduce such risk factors as high cholesterol and smoking that could lead to new blockages from ongoing buildup of plaque in the body's blood vessels. Patients are advised not to have magnetic resonance imaging (MRI) procedures after the surgery because of the effect of magnetism on the metal stents. Stents are not affected by metal detectors.

Risks

The greatest risk with stent implantation is the formation of clots within the stent. Aspirin and oral anti-clotting medications are usually given after stent placement to minimize this risk, which has been reported to occur in about 1–1.5% of patients undergoing endovascular stent surgeries. There has been no evidence of long-term complications from stent implantation, according to the American Heart Association.

A variety of complications can occur with stent grafting for emergency aneurysm repair. Movement of the stent within the vessel can occur in up to 10% of cases, requiring repeat surgery. Clots can occur in the vessel and migrate to other areas of the body, causing heart attack or stroke. About 2% of patients will require an additional open surgical procedures to correct the aneurysm or complications that occur after emergency endovascular repair.

Normal results

People undergoing endovascular stent surgeries usually recover within a week or so, compared to months of recovery from conventional open surgery. They can quickly resume normal activities with a reduction of symptoms and little chance of repeat stenosis, depending upon their general health. The American Heart Association reports that 70–90% of procedures for coronary artery disease are endovascular stenting procedures. Stents have been shown to reduce the risk of restenosis after angioplasty or other catheter-based procedures have been performed.

Morbidity and mortality rates

Deaths have not been reported either during or immediately following endovascular stent surgeries that are linked to the surgical procedure. Stent procedures have been shown to increase survival (by reducing restenosis) among people with coronary artery disease.

The mortality rate for surgically treated abdominal aortic aneurysm is about 5% and increases to 50% for aneurysms that rupture. Thoracic aneurysms also have a mortality rate of about 5%, rising to 67% if ruptured. Stent grafting has been shown overall to have lower rates of morbidity and mortality than conventional open procedures.

Prevention

Preventive measures are the same as those taken to prevent heart attack and stroke. Any adult can reduce the likelihood of plaque formation by making dietary and lifestyle changes, such as:

- Eating a healthy diet rich in fruits, vegetables, and whole grains, with limited meat and dairy. Especially avoid trans-fatty-acids found in chemical- or heat-extracted oils such as margarine, some vegetable oils, and butter substitutes.
- Keeping blood pressure down by reducing the use of table salt and avoiding salty foods, such as chips, processed meats, pickles and sauerkraut, as well as prepared and packaged foods.
- Losing weight, if necessary, which helps to reduce blood pressure. Excess weight strains the whole circulatory system.

- Engaging in moderate exercise several times a week. Exercise that works up a sweat and increases heart rate is recommended. A brisk walk for 20 minutes, three days a week is thought to be sufficient for people who are less physically active.
- Controlling cholesterol through diet and certain medications.
- Having a heart examination at least once a year with an electrocardiogram. The patient should also consult the doctor about taking aspirin for clot prevention.
- Quitting smoking. Smoking encourages the build-up of plaque. Nicotine raises blood pressure and carbon monoxide in smoke reduces the amount of oxygen circulating in the blood. Strong links have been made between smoking and heart attack or stroke.
- Keeping alcohol use moderate. Moderate alcohol use, one or two drinks a day, has been shown to help increase the levels of "good" cholesterol, improve circulation, and reduce the risk of clots forming in the blood.

Alternatives

Stent implantation helps to clear blocked arteries. There are no mechanical alternatives; however, there are alternative ways to reduce plaque formation. Nutritional supplements and alternative therapies that have been recommended to help reduce risks and promote good vascular health include:

- Vitamins B_6 and B_{12} help to lower homocysteine, an amino acid that is believed to contribute to atherosclerosis. B_6 is also a mild diuretic and helps to balance fluids in the body.
- Folic acid helps lower homocysteine levels and increases the oxygen-carrying capacity of red blood cells.
- Antioxidant vitamins C and E work together to promote healthy blood vessels and improve circulation.
- Angelica, an herb that contains coumadin, a recognized anticoagulant, may help to prevent blood clot formation.

- Garlic has been shown in studies to reduce cholesterol and help prevent atherosclerosis.
- Essential fatty acids help reduce blood pressure and cholesterol, and maintain elasticity of blood vessels.
- Chelation therapy can be used to break up plaque and improve circulation.
- Citrin is an herbal extract that inhibits the synthesis of dangerous fats in the body.
- Certain herbs have been shown to improve circulation and help prevent plaque formation, including cayenne, chickweed, ginkgo biloba, and hawthorn berries.
- A vegetarian diet, with plenty of whole grains (brown rice, oats, spelt, whole wheat) showed a reversal of coronary artery disease in a U.S. study called the Lifestyle Heart Trial.

Resources

BOOKS

Heart and Stroke Facts, and Stent Procedure. American Heart Association, 2002.

ORGANIZATIONS

American Heart Association. 7320 Greenville Ave. Dallas, TX 75231. (214) 373-6300. http://www.americanheart.org.

OTHER

"Performing Endovascular Surgery: New Minimally Invasive Approach to Treating Vascular Disease." Patient Care. Department of Surgery, State University of New York, Stony Brook. http://galactica.informatics.sunysb.edu/surgery/endovasc-3.html [Accessed April 11, 2008].

L. Lee Culvert
Laura Jean Cataldo, RN, EdD

Enhanced external counterpulsation

Definition

Enhanced external counterpulsation (EECP) is a noninvasive procedure in which a set of inflatable cuffs (much like blood pressure cuffs) mechanically compress the blood vessels in the patient's lower limbs to increase blood flow in the coronary arteries of the heart. The blood pressure cuffs (also called stockings) are wrapped around the patient's calves, lower thighs, and upper thighs. Computer technology, **electrocardiography**, and blood pressure monitors enable the pressure cuffs to be inflated and deflated in time with the patient's heartbeat and blood pressure.

Purpose

EECP is performed to restore blood flow to the heart and to relieve chest pain (angina pectoris) and ischemia. The goals of the procedure are to relieve the symptoms of coronary artery disease, enable the patient to resume a normal lifestyle, and lower the risk of a heart attack or other heart problems. EECP may encourage blood vessels to open small channels (called collateral blood vessels) to eventually bypass blocked vessels and improve blood flow to the heart.

Demographics

The concept of counterpulsation is not new; it was first introduced in 1953 at Harvard, and refined in the late 1950s. Early models of EECP, however, used non-sequenced pulsation; that is, compression of the patient's blood vessels was performed simultaneously along the full length of the body. In the 1970s, researchers in China reported on a sequential compression system in which four sets of pressure cuffs were applied to the patient's legs, buttocks, and arms. Favorable reports about the effectiveness of sequential compression encouraged a research team at SUNY Stony Brook to develop the three-cuff EECP model in use in the early 2000s. The computerized technology currently available with EECP makes it a relatively new procedure compared to the systems used in the 1960s and early 1970s. As of 2008, it is available in about 200 centers across the United States.

EECP is used to treat patients with chronic stable angina, coronary artery disease, or high blood pressure. The Food and Drug Administration (FDA) approved EECP for the treatment of congestive heart failure (CHF) in the early 2000s. Researchers at the Ohio Heart and Vascular Center reported in 2006 that

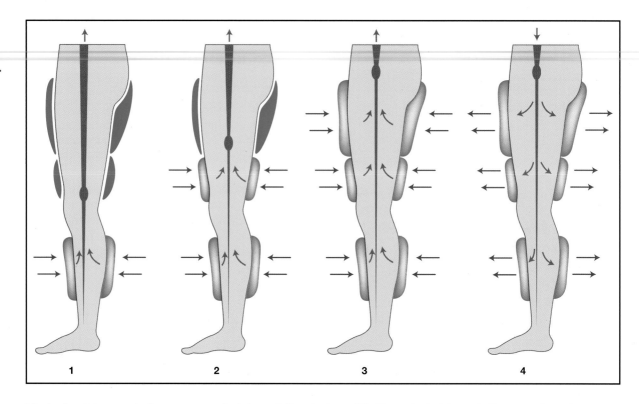

The horizontal arrows indicate pressure (in 1 through 3) and release (4). *(Illustration by Electronic Illustrators Group.)*

EECP improves **exercise** duration as well as quality of life in patients with CHF. The treatment may be appropriate for patients who are not eligible for such nonsurgical interventional procedures as balloon **angioplasty**, stent placement, rotablation, atherectomy, or brachytherapy. It may also be used for patients who do not qualify for such surgical treatments as **coronary artery bypass graft surgery**.

EECP is not the first-line treatment for angina. Rather, it is reserved for patients who have not achieved good results from medication or interventional management of their symptoms. To be eligible for EECP, a patient must have coronary artery disease that includes at least one heart vessel with at least 70% obstruction. In addition, the patient must have evidence of either an infarction or significant ischemia on a **stress test** with nuclear or echocardiographic imaging.

EECP may benefit patients with such other medical conditions as erectile dysfunction, kidney disease, eye disease, diabetic neuropathy, restless legs syndrome, and other circulatory disorders. More research is needed to evaluate the outcomes of EECP for these patients.

Many insurance providers and **Medicare** have approved EECP treatment for reimbursement. Medicare pays about $5,500 for the full series of 35 treatments.

Contraindications

EECP is not recommended for patients who have certain types of valve disease, uncontrolled arrhythmias (irregular heart rhythms), severe hypertension, uncontrolled congestive heart failure, significant blockages or blood clots in the leg arteries, or those who have had a recent **cardiac catheterization**, angioplasty, or bypass surgery. It should also not be given to pregnant women.

Description

While the patient lies on a bed, the leg cuffs are deflated and inflated with each heartbeat. A computer synchronizes the compression of the cuffs with the heartbeat. The **electrocardiogram** indicates when each heartbeat begins, triggering the cuffs to be mechanically deflated. As each heartbeat ends, the cuffs are mechanically inflated in sequential order, starting with the cuffs on the calves and working upward to the cuffs on the lower and then the upper thighs. The pressure produced by the inflation of the cuffs when the heart is at rest pushes the blood in the legs upward toward the heart. The deflating action that occurs just when the heart begins to beat reduces the work of the heart as it pumps blood to other parts of the body. Inflation is controlled by a pressure monitor that

Angina—Also called angina pectoris; chest pain or discomfort that occurs when diseased blood vessels restrict blood flow to the heart.

Aorta—The main artery that carries blood from the heart to the rest of the body; the largest artery in the body.

Artery—A vessel that carries oxygen-rich blood to the body.

Atherectomy—A nonsurgical technique for treating diseased arteries with a rotating device that cuts or shaves away obstructing material inside the artery.

Atria (singular, atrium)—The right and left upper chambers of the heart.

Balloon angioplasty—A nonsurgical technique for treating diseased arteries by temporarily inflating a tiny balloon inside an artery.

Beta blocker—An antihypertensive drug that limits the activity of epinephrine, a hormone that increases blood pressure.

Brachytherapy—The use of radiation during angioplasty to prevent the artery from narrowing again (a process called restenosis).

Calcium channel blocker—A drug that lowers blood pressure by regulating calcium-related electrical activity in the heart.

Cardiac catheterization—An invasive procedure used to create x rays of the coronary arteries, heart chambers and valves.

Collateral vessel—A side branch or network of side branches of a large blood vessel.

Coronary artery disease—Also called atherosclerosis, it is a buildup of fatty matter and debris in the coronary artery wall that causes narrowing of the artery.

Echocardiogram—An imaging procedure used to create a picture of the heart's movement, valves and chambers.

Electrocardiogram (ECG, EKG)—A test that records the electrical activity of the heart, using small electrode patches attached to the skin on the chest.

Infarction—An area of dead tissue caused by obstruction of the blood supply to that tissue.

Ischemia—Decreased blood flow to an organ, usually caused by constriction or obstruction of an artery.

Rotablation—A nonsurgical technique for treating diseased arteries in which a special catheter with a diamond-coated tip is guided to the point of narrowing in the artery. The catheter tip spins at high speed and grinds away the blockage or plaque on the artery walls.

Stent—A device made of expandable metal mesh that is placed (by using a balloon catheter) at the site of a narrowing artery. The stent remains in place to keep the artery open.

Stress test—A test that determines how the heart responds to stress.

Vein—A blood vessel that returns oxygen-depleted blood from various parts of the body to the heart.

Ventricles—The lower pumping chambers of the heart that propel blood to the lungs and the rest of the body.

---

inflates the cuffs to about 300 mm Hg. When timed correctly, the procedure increases the cardiac output.

EECP treatments are performed on an outpatient basis and generally last one to two hours. Treatments must be repeated about five times a week for up to seven weeks to achieve improved circulation. This 35-hour regimen is generally followed because it was used in the first multicenter study of EECP in 1999.

Diagnosis/Preparation

Preparation

The patient is usually instructed to wear tight-fitting seamless cycling pants or athletic tights to prevent chafing, one of the main adverse side effects.

Before the procedure, the patient's weight, blood pressure, pulse, and breathing rate are measured and recorded. The patient's legs are examined for areas of redness and signs of potential vascular problems.

The patient is asked to record his or her symptoms during the course of treatment to determine whether and how symptoms improve over time. The patient should record the severity and duration of troublesome symptoms, the time the symptoms occurred, and any activities that may have triggered the symptoms. This patient record is reviewed before each treatment session.

PATIENT EDUCATION. The healthcare team will ensure that the patient understands the potential benefits and risks of the procedure. Informative and instructional handouts are usually provided to explain the procedure. Because the procedure requires multiple outpatient visits (generally 35 visits over a seven-week period), the patient must be able to meet the treatment schedule.

INFORMED CONSENT. Informed consent is an educational process between healthcare providers and patients. Before any procedure is performed, the patient is asked to sign a consent form. Before signing the form, the patient should understand the nature and purpose of the diagnostic procedure or treatment; the risks and benefits of the procedure; and alternatives, including the option of not proceeding with the test or treatment. During the discussion about the procedure, the healthcare providers are available to answer all of the patient's questions.

SMOKING CESSATION. Patients who will undergo any procedure to treat cardiovascular disease are encouraged to stop smoking and using any tobacco products before the procedure, and to make a commitment to be a nonsmoker after the procedure. There are several **smoking cessation** programs available in the community. The patient should ask a healthcare provider for more information if he or she needs help quitting smoking.

Aftercare

Discomfort

Patients report little or no discomfort during the procedure. Some people may feel tired after the first few treatments, but this loss of energy improves over time.

Lifestyle changes

To manage heart disease, the patient needs to make several lifestyle changes before and after the procedure, including:

- Quitting smoking. Smoking causes damage to blood vessels, increases the patient's blood pressure and heart rate, and decreases the amount of oxygen available in the blood.
- Managing weight. Maintaining a healthy weight, by watching portion sizes and exercising, is important. Being overweight increases the work of the heart.
- Participating in an exercise program. The cardiac rehabilitation exercise program is usually tailored for the patient, who will be supervised by professionals.
- Making dietary changes. Patients should eat a lot of fruits, vegetables, grains, and nonfat or low-fat dairy products, and reduce fats to less than 30% of all calories. Alcoholic beverages should be limited or avoided.

WHO PERFORMS THE PROCEDURE AND WHERE IS IT PERFORMED?

EECP is performed by healthcare providers trained in the procedure. Interventional cardiologists, registered nurses, and other healthcare professionals may perform the procedure. Currently, EECP credentialing is being investigated by the International EECP Therapists Association (IETA). EECP is generally performed in an outpatient clinic or hospital.

- Taking medications as prescribed. Aspirin and other heart medications may be prescribed, and the patient may need to take these medications for life.
- Following up with healthcare providers. The patient should visit the physician regularly for follow-up visits to control risk factors.

Risks

EECP is a relatively safe and effective treatment, and few adverse side effects have been reported. The main adverse side effect is chafing (skin irritation from the compression of the cuffs). To reduce or prevent this side effect, patients are instructed to wear tight-fitting cycling pants or athletic tights. Leg pain is another adverse side effect.

Normal results

The benefits of EECP are comparable to the results of angioplasty and coronary artery bypass graft surgery: 70–80% of patients experience significant improvement after EECP treatment for as long as five years. The largest research study on EECP indicates that after receiving treatment, patients used less medication, had fewer angina attacks with less severe symptoms, and increased their capacity to exercise without experiencing symptoms. EECP improves the patient's sense of well-being and overall quality of life, and in some cases, prolongs the patient's life. Benefits five years after EECP treatment are comparable to surgical outcomes.

The effects of EECP treatment last from three to five years and sometimes longer.

EECP does not prevent coronary artery disease from recurring; therefore, lifestyle changes are strongly recommended and medications are prescribed to reduce the risk of recurrent disease.

QUESTIONS TO ASK THE DOCTOR

- Why do you recommend this procedure?
- Who will perform the procedure? How many years of experience does this doctor have? How many other EECP procedures has this doctor performed?
- May I take my medications the day of the procedure?
- May I eat or drink the day of the surgery? If not, how long before the surgery should I stop eating or drinking?
- How long do the treatments last?
- What should I do if I experience chest discomfort or other symptoms similar to those I felt before the procedure?
- What types of symptoms should I report to my doctor?
- Will I be able to perform my normal activities during the course of treatment?
- When will I find out if the procedure was successful?
- Will I have any pain or discomfort after the procedure?
- What lifestyle changes (including diet, weight management, exercise, and activity changes) are recommended to improve my heart health?
- How often do I need to see my doctor for follow-up visits after the procedure?

Morbidity and mortality rates

Morbidity and mortality have not been reported with this procedure.

Alternatives

All patients with coronary artery disease can help improve their condition by making lifestyle changes such as quitting smoking, losing weight if they are overweight, eating healthful foods, reducing blood cholesterol, exercising regularly, and controlling diabetes and high blood pressure.

All patients with coronary artery disease should be prescribed medications to treat their condition. Such antiplatelet medications as **aspirin** or clopidogrel (Plavix) are usually recommended. Other medications used to treat angina may include beta blockers, nitrates, and angiotensin-converting enzyme (ACE) inhibitors. Medications may also be prescribed to lower lipoprotein levels, since elevated lipoprotein levels have been associated with an increased risk of cardiovascular problems.

Treatment with vitamin E is not recommended because it does not lower the rate of cardiovascular events in people with coronary artery disease. Although such antioxidants as vitamin C, beta-carotene, and probucol show promising results, they are not recommended for routine use. Treatment with folic acid and vitamins B_6 and B_{12} lowers homocysteine levels (reducing the risk for cardiovascular problems), but more studies are needed to determine if lowered homocysteine levels correlate with a reduced rate of cardiovascular problems in treated patients.

Such nonsurgical interventional procedures as balloon angioplasty, stent placement, rotablation, atherectomy, or brachytherapy can be performed to open a blocked artery.

Coronary artery bypass graft surgery is a surgical procedure in which one or more blocked coronary arteries are bypassed by a blood vessel graft to restore normal blood flow to the heart. These grafts usually come from the patient's own arteries and veins located in the leg, arm, or chest.

Resources

BOOKS

Elefteriades, John A., and Lawrence S. Cohen. *Your Heart: An Owner's Guide: Answers to Your Questions about Heart Disease*. Amherst, NY: Prometheus Books, 2007.

McGoon, Michael D., ed., and Bernard J. Gersh. *Mayo Clinic Heart Book: The Ultimate Guide to Heart Health*, 2nd ed. New York: William Morrow and Co., Inc., 2000.

Topol, Eric J., ed. *Textbook of Cardiovascular Medicine*, 3rd ed. Philadelphia: Lippincott Williams and Wilkins, 2007.

Trout, Darrell, and Ellen Welch. "Enhanced External Counterpulsation (EECP)." In *Surviving with Heart: Taking Charge of Your Heart Care*, Golden, CO: Fulcrum Publishing, 2002.

PERIODICALS

Abbottsmith, C. W., E. S. Chung, T. Varricchione, et al. "Enhanced External Counterpulsation Improves Exercise Duration and Peak Oxygen Consumption in Older Patients with Heart Failure: A Subgroup Analysis of the PEECH Trial." *Congestive Heart Failure* 12 (November–December 2006): 307–311.

Arora, R. R., et al. "The Multicenter Study of Enhanced External Counterpulsation (MUST-EECP): Effect of EECP on Exercise-Induced Myocardial Ischemia and Anginal Episodes." *The Journal of the American College of Cardiology* 33, no.7 (1999): 1833–1840.

Feldman, A. M., M. A. Silver, G. S. Francis, et al. "Enhanced External Counterpulsation Improves Exercise Tolerance in Patients with Chronic Heart Failure." *Journal of the American College of Cardiology* 48 (September 19, 2006): 1198–1205.

Feldman, A. M., M. A. Silver, G. S. Francis, et al. "Treating Heart Failure with Enhanced External Counterpulsation (EECP): Design of the Prospective Evaluation of EECP in Heart Failure (PEECH) Trial." *Journal of Cardiac Failure* 11 (April 2005): 240–245.

Lawson, W. E., J. C. Hui, E. D. Kennard, et al. "Effect of Enhanced External Counterpulsation on Medically Refractory Angina Patients with Erectile Dysfunction." *International Journal of Clinical Practice* 61 (May 2007): 757–762.

Machanda, A., and O. Soran. "Enhanced External Counterpulsation and Future Directions: Step beyond Medical Management for Patients with Angina and Heart Failure." *Journal of the American College of Cardiology* 50 (October 16, 2007): 1523–1531.

Urano, H., et al. "Enhanced External Counterpulsation Improves Exercise Tolerance, Reduces Exercise-Induced Myocardial Ischemia and Improves Left Ventricular Diastolic Filling in Patients with Coronary Artery Disease." *Journal of the American College of Cardiology* 37, no. 1 (2001): 93–99.

ORGANIZATIONS

American College of Cardiology. Heart House, 2400 N Street, NW, Washington, DC 20037. (202) 375-6000. http://www.acc.org (accessed March 19, 2008).

American Heart Association. 7272 Greenville Ave., Dallas, TX 75231. (800) 242-8721 or (214) 373-6300. http://www.americanheart.org (accessed March 19, 2008).

Cleveland Clinic Heart and Vascular Institute, The Cleveland Clinic Foundation. 9500 Euclid Avenue, F25, Cleveland, Ohio, 44195. (216) 445-9288. http://www.clevelandclinic.org/heartcenter (accessed March 19, 2008).

International EECP Therapists Association. P.O. Box 650005, Vero Beach, FL 32965-0005. (800) 376-3321, ext. 140. http://www.ietaonline.com (accessed March 19, 2008).

National Heart, Lung and Blood Institute (NHLBI). NHLBI Health Information Center, P.O. Box 30105, Bethesda, MD 20824-0105. http://www.nhlbi.nih.gov (accessed March 19, 2008).

Texas Heart Institute. Heart Information Service. P.O. Box 20345, Houston, TX 77225-0345. (832) 355-1000. http://www.texasheartinstitute.org/ (accessed March 19, 2008).

OTHER

Heart Information Network. http://www.heartinfo.org (accessed March 19, 2008).

Angela M. Costello
Rebecca Frey, PhD

Enucleation, eye

Definition

Enucleation is the surgical removal of the eyeball that leaves the eye muscles and remaining orbital contents intact.

Purpose

Enucleation is performed to remove large-sized eye tumors or as a result of traumatic injury when the eye cannot be preserved. In the case of tumors, the amount of radiation required to destroy a tumor of the eye may be too intense for the eye to bear. Within months to years, many patients who are treated with radiation for large ocular melanomas lose vision, develop glaucoma, and eventually have to undergo enucleation.

The two types of eye tumors that may require enucleation are:

- Intraocular eye melanoma. This is a rare form of cancer in which malignant cells are found in the part of the eye called the uvea, which contains cells called melanocytes that house pigments. When the melanocytes become cancerous, the cancer is called a melanoma. If the tumor reaches the iris and begins to grow, or if there are symptoms, enucleation may be indicated.
- Retinoblastoma. Retinoblastoma is a malignant tumor of the retina. The retina is the thin layer of tissue that lines the back of the eye; it senses light and forms images. If the cancer occurs in one eye, treatment may consist of enucleation for large tumors when there is no expectation that useful vision can be preserved. If there is cancer in both eyes, treatment may involve enucleation of the eye with the larger tumor, and radiation therapy to the other eye.

Demographics

Data from the U.S. National Center for Health Statistics estimate that nearly 2.4 million eye injuries occur in the United States annually. This report calculated that nearly one million Americans have permanent significant visual impairment due to injury, with more than 75% of these individuals being blind in one eye. Eye injury is a leading cause of monocular blindness in the United States, and is second only to cataract as the most common cause of visual impairment. While no segment of the population escapes the risk of eye injury, the victims are more likely to be young. The majority of all eye injuries occur in persons under thirty years of age. Trauma is considered the most

Enucleation, eye

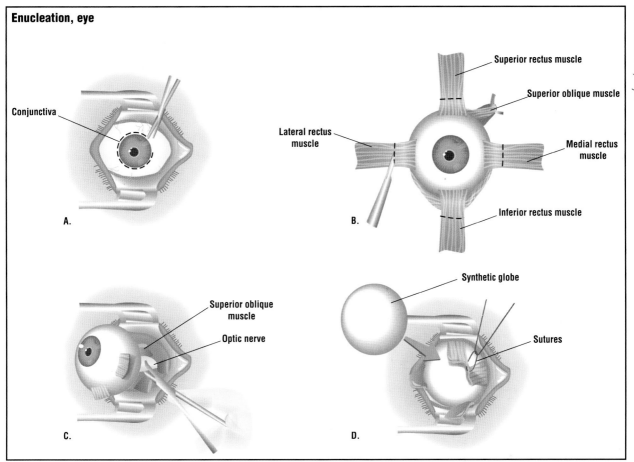

Conjunctiva

A.

Superior rectus muscle

Superior oblique muscle

Lateral rectus muscle

Medial rectus muscle

B.

Inferior rectus muscle

Superior oblique muscle

Optic nerve

C.

Synthetic globe

Sutures

D.

The conjunctiva (outer covering of eye) is removed with blunt scissors (A). The four rectus muscles are removed from their attachments to the eyeball (B). The optic nerve is severed (C), and the eyeball is removed. A synthetic globe replaces the eyeball in the socket, and the rectus muscles are sutured around it (D). (Illustration by GGS Information Services. Cengage Learning, Gale.)

common cause of enucleation in children over three years of age.

For the year 2000, Texas demographics for cancer of the eye and orbit were fewer than five per 100,000. According to the National Institutes of Health (NIH), there are about 2,200 cases of eye cancer diagnosed in the United States each year.

Description

Following anesthesia, the surgeon measures the dimensions of the eye globe, length of the optic nerve, and horizontal dimensions of the cornea. The surgeon then illuminates the globe of the eye before opening it. A dissecting microscope is used to detect major features and possible minute lesions. The eye is opened with a sharp razor blade by holding the globe with the left hand, cornea down against the cutting block, and holding the blade between the thumb and middle finger of the right hand. Enucleation proceeds with a sawing motion from back to front. The plane of

section begins adjacent to the optic nerve and ends at the periphery of the cornea. The plane of section is dependent on whether a lesion has been detected. If not, the globe is cut along a horizontal plane, using as surface landmarks the superior and inferior oblique insertions and the long postciliary vein. If a lesion has been found, the plane of section is modified so that the lesion is included in the slab.

Diagnosis/Preparation

Enucleation may be performed under general or **local anesthesia**. In either case, the injection is given in the retrobulbar space. An antibiotic and an anti-inflammatory medication such as dexamethasone are also given intravenously.

Aftercare

Because the eye is surrounded by bones, it is much easier for patients to tolerate enucleation than the loss of a lung or kidney. When surgery is performed under

KEY TERMS

Cornea—The transparent structure forming the anterior part of the fibrous tunic of the eye. It consists of five layers.

Glaucoma—A group of eye diseases characterized by an increase in intraocular pressure that causes changes in the optic disk and defects in the field of vision.

Intraocular melanoma—A rare form of cancer in which malignant cells are found in the part of the eye called the uvea.

Iris—The contractile eye membrane perforated by the pupil, and forming the colored portion of the eye.

Melanocytes—Color-containing cells in the uvea.

Melanoma—A malignant tumor arising from the melanocytic system of the skin and other organs.

Optic nerve—The nerve carrying impulses for the sense of sight.

Orbit—The cavity or socket of the skull in which the eye and its appendages are situated.

Retina—Thin nerve tissue that lines the back of the eye that senses light and forms images.

Retinoblastoma—Malignant (cancerous) tumor of the retina.

general anesthesia, patients do not feel or see anything until they regain consciousness. Additional local anesthesia is often given at the end of the surgery so that the patient will have the least pain possible when waking up in the **recovery room**. Most patients have a headache for 24–36 hours after surgery that is relieved with two regular headache medication pills, such as Tylenol, every four hours. A firm pressure dressing is maintained for four to six days; oral **antibiotics** are given for one week; and steroids, such as prednisone, adjusted according to patient status, are given three times daily for four days. The socket is evaluated after removal of the pressure dressing. If the edema has disappeared, the sutures are removed. **Topical antibiotics** are applied four times daily for four weeks.

Risks

Enucleation surgery is very safe. Only rarely do patients experience major complications, whicht may include bleeding, infection, scarring, persistent

Eye enucleation is usually performed by an ophthalmic surgeon or an ophthalmologist in a hospital setting. Young and healthy patients may undergo the surgery on an outpatient basis but most stay in the hospital for at least one night after surgery. Ophthalmic surgeons are members of the American College of Eye Surgeons, and are certified by the American Board of Eye Surgery after submitting to an extensive written application. Before ABES certification, they must be certified by the American Board of Ophthalmology (ABO). This certification indicates successful completion of an approved residency program and acquisition of sufficient knowledge in the areas of medical and surgical ophthalmology.

swelling, pain, wound separation, and the need for additional surgery. Complications may also occur with the orbital implants routinely used with patients who have undergone enucleation. Among these is the risk of infection.

Normal results

Within two to six weeks of enucleation surgery, patients are sent for a temporary ocular prosthesis (plastic eye). Besides the swelling and the black eye, patient features look normal. After a final prosthetic fitting, 90% of patients are usually quite happy with the way they look; 80% say others cannot even tell that they have only one eye.

Morbidity and mortality rates

In a study performed by the National Eye Institute on melanoma patients at five-year follow-up, 82% of the patients who underwent enucleation remained alive. At a 10-year follow-up, 31% remained alive. As of 2003, the study was ongoing and would follow all patients for up to 15 years.

Alternatives

There are no alternatives to enucleation because it is a procedure of last resort performed when other treatments have failed.

QUESTIONS TO ASK THE DOCTOR

- Why is enucleation required?
- Will there be pain after surgery?
- How many enucleation surgeries do you perform in a year?
- How much time will I need to recover from the operation?
- When can I get a prosthesis?

Resources

BOOKS

Linberg, J. W. *Oculoplastic and Orbital Emergencies.* New York: McGraw-Hill Professional, 1992.

Shields, J. A. and C. L. Shields. *Atlas of Orbital Tumors.* Philadelphia: Lippincott Williams & Wilkins Publishers, 1999.

Tasman, W., et al. *The Wills Eye Hospital Atlas of Clinical Ophthalmology.* Philadelphia: Lippincott Williams & Wilkins Publishers, 2001.

Vafidis, G. et al. *Perioperative Care of the Eye Patient.* Annapolis Junction, MD: BMJ Books, 2000.

PERIODICALS

Adenis, J. P., P. Y. Robert, and M. P. Boncoeur-Martel. "Abnormalities of orbital volume." *European Journal of Ophthalmology* 12 (September-October 2002): 345–350.

Burroughs, J. R., C. N. Soparkar, J. R. Patrinely, et al. "Monitored anesthesia care for enucleations and eviscerations." *Ophthalmology* 110 (February 2003): 311–313.

Chantada, G., A. Fandino, S. Casak, et al. "Treatment of overt extraocular retinoblastoma." *Medical Pediatric Oncology* 40 (March 2003): 158–161.

Gragoudas, E., W. Li, M. Goitein, et al. "Evidence-based estimates of outcome in patients irradiated for intraocular melanoma." *Archives of Ophthalmology* 120 (December 2002): 1665–1671.

Jordan, D. R., S. R. Klapper, and S. M. Gilberg. "The use of vicryl mesh in 200 porous orbital implants: a technique with few exposures." *Ophthalmologic and Plastic Reconstruction Surgery* 19 (January 2003): 53–61.

ORGANIZATIONS

American Academy of Ophthalmology. P.O. Box 7424, San Francisco, CA 94120-7424. (415) 561-8500. http://www.aao.org/index.html.

American College of Eye Surgeons. 2665 Oak Ridge Court, Suite A, Fort Myers, FL 33901. (239) 275-8881. http://www.aces-abes.org/.

National Cancer Institute. Suite 3036A, 6116 Executive Boulevard, MSC8322, Bethesda, MD 20892-8322.(800) 422-6237. <http://cancer.gov/>.

OTHER

Finger, Paul T., MD, FACS. "Enucleation." Eye Cancer Network. [cited May 5, 2003]. http://www.eyecancer.com/Enucleation/enuc.html.

Monique Laberge, Ph.D.

Enzyme immmunoassay *see* **Immunoassay tests**

Epidural therapy

Definition

An epidural is a local (regional) anesthetic delivered through a catheter (small tube) into a vacant space outside the spinal cord, called the epidural space.

The drugs commonly used in epidural anesthesia are bupivicaine (Marcaine, Sensorcaine), chloroprocaine (Nesacaine), and lidocaine (Xylocaine). The solutions of anesthetic should be preservative free.

Purpose

The anesthetic agents that are infused through the small catheter block spinal nerve roots in the epidural space and the sympathetic nerve fibers adjacent to them. Epidural anesthesia can block most of the pain of labor and birth for vaginal and surgical deliveries. Epidural analgesia is also used after cesarean sections to help control postoperative pain. More than 50% of women giving birth at hospitals use epidural anesthesia.

Description

Epidural anesthesia, because it virtually blocks all pain of labor and birth, is particularly helpful to women with underlying medical problems such as pregnancy-induced hypertension, heart disease, and pulmonary disease. Epidural anesthesia for labor is usually initiated at the woman's request, provided that the labor is progressing well, or if the mother feels severe pain during early labor.

Precautions

The primary problem associated with receiving epidural anesthesia is low blood pressure, otherwise known as hypotension, because of the blocking of sympathetic fibers in the epidural space. The decreased peripheral resistance that results in the circulatory system causes dilation of peripheral blood vessels. Fluid collects in the peripheral vasculature (vessels), simulating a condition that the body interprets as low fluid volume. A simple measure that prevents most hypotension is the infusion of 500–1000 cc of fluid intravenously into the patient prior to the procedure. Ringer's lactate is preferable to a solution containing dextrose because the elevated maternal glucose that accompanies the rapid infusion of solutions containing dextrose can result in hyperglycemia in the newborn with rebound hypoglycemia.

It is important not to place a woman flat on her back after she has an epidural because the supine position can bring on hypotension. If a woman's blood pressure does drop, then the proper treatment is to turn her on her side, administer oxygen, increase the flow of intravenous fluids, and possibly administer ephedrine if the hypotension is severe. Very rarely, convulsions can result from severe reactions. Seizure activity would be treated with short-acting **barbiturates** or diazepam (Valium).

Diagnosis/Preparation

To prepare for the administration of epidural anesthesia, the woman should have the procedure explained fully and sign required consent forms. An intravenous line is inserted, if not already in place. She is positioned on her side or in a sitting position and connected to a blood pressure monitoring device. The nurse/assistant has the following equipment available: oxygen, epidural insertion equipment, fetal monitor, and additional intravenous fluid.

The health-care provider cleans the area with an antiseptic solution, injects a local anesthetic to create a small wheal at the L 3–4 area (between the third and fourth lumbar vertebrae), and inserts a needle into the epidural space. Once it is ascertained that the needle is in the correct place, a polyethylene catheter is threaded through the needle. The needle is removed and a test dose of the anesthetic agent is administered. The catheter is taped in place along the patient's back with the end over her shoulder for easy retrieval when further doses are required.

If the patient responds well to the test dose, a complete dose is administered. Pain relief should come up to the level of the umbilicus. The epidural anesthesia lasts approximately 40 minutes to two hours, or longer as required. If necessary, additional doses of anesthetic, or top-up, are injected through the catheter or by continuous infusion on a special pump.

Epidural anesthesia can be given in labor in a "segmented" manner. In this instance, the laboring woman receives a small dose of anesthesia so that the perineal muscles do not fully relax. The baby's head is more apt to undergo internal rotation when the perineal muscles are not too loose, thus facilitating delivery. At the time of delivery, an additional dose can be administered for perineal relief.

Women who have cesarean deliveries may have additional medication injected into the epidural space to control intra-operative pain. Medications generally used are narcotics such as fentanyl or morphine (Duramorph). Side effects include severe itching, nausea, and vomiting. Treatment of these side effects with the appropriate medication can be helpful. Despite these problems, epidural analgesia is an effective method to relieve pain after cesarean delivery, allowing the woman to move easily and speed recovery.

Local anesthetics are generally safe when administered by the epidural route. There is a low frequency of allergic reaction to the drug. Most often the drug causes a mild skin reaction, but in more severe cases can cause breathing difficulty and an asthma-like reaction. A burning sensation at the site of injection may occur, sometimes with swelling and skin irritation. Other adverse reactions may occur if the epidural anesthetic is not properly administered.

Aftercare

It is important to carefully monitor **vital signs** after the administration of epidural anesthesia. Hypotension can result in fetal **death** and can also have grave consequences for the mother. The nurse should monitor the patient constantly and use a continuous blood pressure machine to obtain regular blood pressure readings for 20–30 minutes after each administration of anesthesia. The systolic blood pressure should not fall below 100 mm Hg or be 20 mm Hg less than a baseline systolic blood pressure for a hypertensive patient.

It is important to remind the woman to empty her bladder at least every two hours. With epidural anesthesia, there is loss of sensation of the need to void.

Sometimes, an overfull bladder can block the descent of the baby's head. A catheter can be inserted into the bladder to drain the urine. The nurse needs to closely monitor intake and output and assess the bladder for signs of distension.

Risks

Side effects and complications are rare, but sometimes the patient will experience a "spinal headache" due to leakage of cerebrospinal fluid (CSF).

When a woman receives epidural anesthesia for labor pains, at times the labor can be prolonged because of excessive relaxation of the muscles. Also, the baby's head may not rotate—especially if it is in the occiput-posterior position (the back of the head is facing toward the woman's back). The woman may not have the sensation that results in the desire to push during contractions when she is fully dilated. These complications may result in an increased incidence of births with the use of vacuum extraction, forceps, or even cesarean deliveries. Administering a Pitocin (oxytocin) drip intravenously can counter this problem. Pitocin is a medication that causes the uterus to contract. Allowing the epidural to wear off in the second stage of labor when the woman is pushing may avoid this problem, but the return of the labor pains may be overwhelming to the woman.

Occasionally, slow absorption of the medication from the epidural space into the circulation can result in toxic reactions evident by decreased level of consciousness, slurred speech, loss of coordination, drowsiness, nervousness, and anxiety. The health-care provider should look out for these signs, and also report any elevation in temperature before a top-up dose is administered.

Nomral results

Epidural anesthesia is a safe and effective method of giving pain relief to women during labor and delivery. It also can be used for cesarean births. It is believed that very little of the anesthetic is absorbed throughout the body (systemically), therefore epidural anesthesia is ideal because it does not pass the medication into the fetal circulation.

Resources

BOOKS

Pillitteri, Adele. *Maternal & Child Health Nursing*, 4th edition. Philadelphia: Lippincott, 2002.

ORGANIZATIONS

American Association of Nurse Anesthetists (AANA). 222 S. Prospect Avenue, Park Ridge, IL 60068. (847) 692-7050. http://www.aana.com.

OTHER

Anesthesia Options for Labor and Delivery: What Every Expectant Mother Should Know. AANA, 2001. http://www.aana.com/patients/options.asp.
Epidural Anesthesia. American Pregnancy Association, 2007. http://www.americanpregnancy.org/labornbirth/epidural.html

Nadine M. Jacobson, RN
Samuel D. Uretsky, PharmD
Renee Laux, M.S.

Epilepsy surgery *see* **Anterior temporal lobectomy; Corpus callosotomy; Hemispherectomy**

Epinephrine *see* **Adrenergic drugs**

Episiotomy

Definition

An episiotomy is a surgical incision made in the perineum, the area between the vagina and anus. Episiotomies are done during the second stage of labor to expand the opening of the vagina to prevent tearing of the area during the delivery of the baby.

Purpose

An episiotomy is usually done during the birthing process in order to deliver a baby without tearing the perineum and surrounding tissue. Reasons for an episiotomy might include:

- evidence of maternal or fetal distress (i.e., no time to allow perineum to stretch);
- the baby is premature or in a breech position, and his/her head could be damaged by a tight perineum;
- the baby is too large to be delivered without causing extensive tearing;
- delivery is being assisted by forceps;
- the mother is too tired or unable to push; or
- there is existing trauma to the perineum.

Some experts believe that an episiotomy speeds up the birthing process, making it easier for the baby to be delivered. Speed can be important if there is any sign of distress that may harm the mother or baby.

Episiotomy

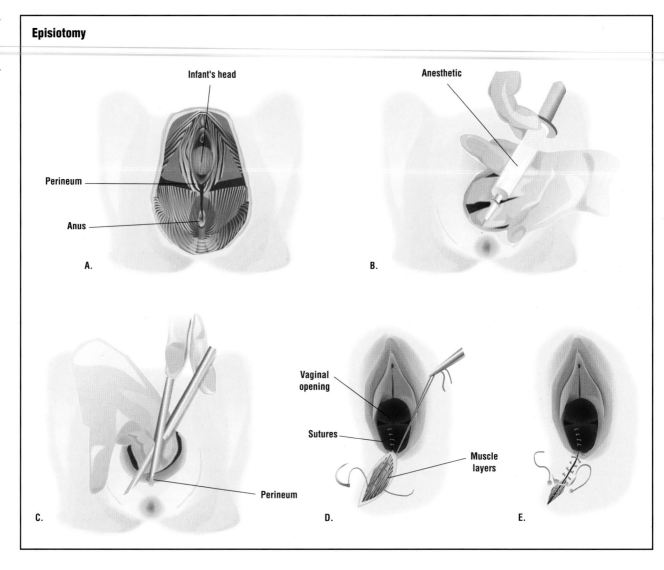

During childbirth, the area called the perineum is often cut to facilitate delivery (A). First, a local anesthetic may be given (B). The perineum is cut on an angle with scissors (C). After delivery, the layers of muscle and skin are repaired (D and E). *(Illustration by GGS Information Services. Cengage Learning, Gale.)*

Because tissues in this area may tear during the delivery, another reason for performing an episiotomy is that a clean incision is easier to repair than a jagged tear and may heal faster. Although episiotomies are sometimes described as protecting the pelvic muscles and possibly preventing future problems with urinary incontinence, it is not clear that the procedure actually helps.

Demographics

About 33% of all American women undergo episiotomy during labor and delivery. While this represents a dramatic drop from the 1983 rate of 69.4%, there are many experts who still believe that this represents too high a number. Episiotomy rates were higher among white women (32.1%) than African American women (11.2%). Similar differences have been reported in other obstetric procedures (e.g., **cesarean section** and epidural use).

Episiotomy rates differ according to care provider—patients of midwives have lower rates than patients of medical doctors. One study comparing perineal outcomes for women being cared for by midwives or medical doctors found the episiotomy rate among midwives at 25% and 40% among medical doctors. Younger doctors are also less likely to perform an episiotomy than older doctors; one study found the rate of episiotomies performed by residents to be 17%, while the rate among doctors in private practice was 66%.

Description

An episiotomy is a surgical incision, usually made with sterile scissors, in the perineum as the baby's head is being delivered. This procedure may be used if the tissue around the vaginal opening begins to tear or does not seem to be stretching enough to allow the baby to be delivered.

In most cases, the physician makes a midline incision along a straight line from the lowest edge of the vaginal opening toward the anus. In other cases, the episiotomy is performed by making a diagonal incision across the midline between the vagina and anus (called a mediolateral incision). This method is used much less often, may be more painful, and may require more healing time than the midline incision. After the baby is delivered through the extended vaginal opening, the incision is closed with **stitches**. A local anesthetic may be applied or injected to numb the area before it is sewn up (sutured).

Episiotomies are classified according to the depth of the incision:

- A first-degree episiotomy cuts through skin only (vaginal/perineal).
- A second-degree episiotomy involves skin and muscle and extends midway between the vagina and the anus.
- A third-degree episiotomy cuts through skin, muscle, and the rectal sphincter.
- A fourth-degree episiotomy extends through the rectum and cuts through skin, muscle, the rectal sphincter, and anal wall.

Diagnosis/Preparation

Although there are some reasons for anticipating an episiotomy before labor has begun (e.g., breech presentation of the baby), the decision to perform an episiotomy is generally not made until the second stage of labor, when delivery of the baby is imminent.

Aftercare

The area of the episiotomy may be uncomfortable or even painful for several days. Several practices can relieve some of the pain. Cold packs can be applied to the perineal area to reduce swelling and discomfort. Use of a sitz bath can ease the discomfort. This unit circulates warm water over the area. A squirt bottle with water can be used to clean the area after urination or defecation rather than wiping with tissue. Also, the area should be patted dry rather than wiped. Cleansing pads soaked in witch hazel (such as the brand Tucks) are very effective for soothing and cleaning the perineum.

Risks

Several side effects of episiotomy have been reported, including infection (in 0.3% of cases), increased pain, increased bleeding, prolonged healing time, and increased discomfort once sexual intercourse is resumed. There is also the risk that the incision will be deeper or longer than is necessary to permit the birth of the infant. An incision that is too long or deep may extend into the rectum, causing more bleeding and an increased risk of infection. Additional tearing or tissue damage may occur beyond the episiotomy itself.

Normal results

In a normal and well-managed delivery, an episiotomy may be avoided altogether. If an episiotomy is considered necessary, a simple midline incision will be made to extend the vaginal opening without additional tearing or extensive trauma to the perineal area. Although there may be some pain associated with the healing of the incision, relief can usually be provided with mild pain relievers and supportive measures, such as the application of cold packs.

Morbidity and mortality rates

Studies have found that the rates of urinary/fecal incontinence, postpartum perineal pain, and sexual dysfunction are generally the same between women who have had an episiotomy and those who had a spontaneous tear of the perineum. There does appear to be a higher risk of more extensive perineal trauma when an episiotomy is performed (20.9% experienced third- or fourth-degree lacerations) than when it is not (3.1% experienced major perineal damage).

Alternatives

It may be possible to avoid the need for an episiotomy. Pregnant women may want to talk with their care providers about the use of episiotomy during the delivery. Kegel exercises are often recommended during the pregnancy to help strengthen the pelvic floor muscles. Prenatal perineal massage may help to stretch and relax the tissue around the vaginal opening. During the delivery process, warm compresses can be applied to the area along with the use of perineal massage. Coaching and support are also important during the delivery process. Slowed, spontaneous pushing during the second stage of labor (when the mother gets the urge to push) may allow the tissues to stretch rather than tear. Also, an upright birthing position (rather than one where the mother is lying down) may decrease the need for an episiotomy.

Resources

BOOKS

Gabbe, S. G., et al. *Obstetrics: Normal and Problem Pregnancies,* 5th ed. London: Churchill Livingstone, 2007.

Katz V. L., et al. *Comprehensive Gynecology,* 5th ed. St. Louis: Mosby, 2007.

PERIODICALS

Goldberg, J., D. Holtz, T. Hyslop, and J. E. Tolosa. "Has the Use of Routine Episiotomy Decreased? Examination of Episiotomy Rates From 1983 to 2000." *Obstetrics and Gynecology* 99 (March 2002): 395–400.

Roberts, Joyce E. "The 'Push' for Evidence: Management of the Second Stage." *Journal of Midwifery and Women's Health* 47, no. 1 (January 2002): 2–15.

Yokoe, D. S., C. L. Christiansen, R. Johnson, et al. "Epidemiology of and Surveillance for Postpartum Infections." *Emerging Infectious Diseases* 7, no. 5 (September–October 2001): 837–841.

OTHER

"Episiotomy FAQ." Perinatal Education Associates, Inc. 2002. http://www.birthsource.com/scripts/article.asp?articleid = 80 (March 30, 2008).

Marcus, Adam. "Episiotomy Rates Dropping in U.S." Lifeclinic Health Management Systems. May 7, 2002. http://www.lifeclinic.com/healthnews/article_view.asp?story = 507067 (March 30, 2008).

ORGANIZATIONS

American College of Nurse-Midwives, 8403 Colesville Road, Suite 1550, Silver Spring, MD, 20910, (240) 485-1800, http://www.midwife.org.

American College of Obstetricians and Gynecologists, 409 12th St., SW, P.O. Box 96920, Washington, DC, 20090-6920, (202) 638-5577, http://www.acog.org.

Midwives Alliance of North America, 611 Pennsylvania Avenue, SE, #1700, Washington, DC, 20003-4303, (888) 923-MANA, http://www.mana.org.

Altha Roberts Edgren
Stephanie Dionne Sherk
Rosalyn Carson-DeWitt, MD

EPS *see* **Electrophysiology study of the heart**

ERCP *see* **Endoscopic retrograde cholangiopancreatography**

Erythromycins

Definition

Erythromycins are a group of medicines that kill bacteria or prevent their growth.

Purpose

Erythromycins are **antibiotics**, a type of medicine used to treat infections caused by microorganisms. Physicians prescribe these drugs for many types of infections caused by bacteria, including strep throat, sinus infections, pneumonia, ear infections, tonsillitis, bronchitis, gonorrhea, pelvic inflammatory disease (PID), and urinary tract infections. Some medicines in this group are also used to treat Legionnaires' disease and ulcers caused by bacteria. These drugs will not work for colds, flu, and other infections caused by viruses.

Drugs in the erythromycin group may be used to eliminate areas of infection, such as abscesses, prior to surgery. For this purpose, they have been used in dentistry, eye surgery, and intestinal surgery. In some cases, erythromycin has been used to treat brain abscesses.

Description

The drugs described here include erythromycins (Erythrocin, Ery-C, E-Mycin, and other brands) and medicines that are chemically related to erythromycins such as azithromycin (Zithromax) and clarithromycin (Biaxin). They are available only with a physician's prescription and are sold in capsule, tablet (regular and chewable), liquid, and injectable forms.

Recommended dosage

The recommended dosage depends on the type of erythromycin, the strength of the medicine, and the medical problem for which it is being taken. The person should check with the physician who prescribed the drug or the pharmacist who filled the prescription for the correct dosage.

The patient must always take erythromycins exactly as directed. The patient should never take larger, smaller, more frequent, or less frequent doses. To make sure the infection clears up completely, it is very important to take the medicine for as long as it has been prescribed. Patients must not stop taking the drug just because symptoms begin to improve. This is important with all types of infections, but it is especially important in streptococcal infections, which can lead to serious heart problems if they are not cleared up completely.

Erythromycins work best when they are at constant levels in the blood. To help keep levels constant, the medicine should be taken in doses spaced evenly through the day and night. The patient must not miss any doses. Some of these medicines are most effective when taken with a full glass of water on an empty

KEY TERMS

Abscess—A collection of pus, appearing in a localized infection, and associated with tissue destruction and frequently with swelling.

Bronchitis—Inflammation of the air passages of the lungs.

Gonorrhea—A sexually transmitted disease (STD) that causes infection in the genital organs and may cause disease in other parts of the body.

Inflammation—Pain, redness, swelling, and heat that usually develop in response to injury or illness.

Legionnaires' disease—A lung disease caused by a bacterium.

Microorganism—An organism that is too small to be seen with the naked eye.

Pelvic inflammatory disease (PID)—Inflammation of the female reproductive tract, caused by any of several microorganisms. Symptoms include severe abdominal pain, high fever, and vaginal discharge. Severe cases can result in sterility.

Pneumonia—A disease in which the lungs become inflamed. It may be caused by bacteria, viruses, or other organisms, or by physical or chemical irritants.

Sinus—Any of several air-filled cavities in the bones of the skull.

Strep throat—A sore throat caused by infection with *Streptococcus* bacteria. Symptoms include sore throat, chills, fever, and swollen lymph nodes in the neck.

Tonsillitis—Inflammation of a tonsil, a small mass of tissue in the throat.

Urinary tract—The passage through which urine flows from the kidneys out of the body.

stomach, but they may be taken with food if stomach upset is a problem. Others work equally well when taken with or without food. Patients should check package directions or ask the physician or pharmacist for instructions on how to take the medicine.

Precautions

There are warnings and cautions that apply to erythromycin and its related drugs when they are taken by mouth over a period of several days. These warnings may not apply when erythromycin is given intravenously (by vein), or as a single dose prior to or immediately after surgery.

Symptoms should begin to improve within a few days of beginning to take this medicine. If they do not, or if they get worse, the patient should check with the physician who prescribed the medicine.

Erythromycins may cause mild diarrhea, which usually goes away during treatment; however, severe diarrhea could be a sign of a very serious side effect. Anyone who develops severe diarrhea while taking erythromycin or related drugs should stop taking the medicine and call a physician immediately.

Special conditions

Taking erythromycins may cause problems for people with certain medical conditions or people who are taking certain other medicines. Before taking these drugs, the patient should tell the physician about any of these conditions.

ALLERGIES. Anyone who has had unusual reactions to erythromycins, azithromycin, or clarithromycin in the past should let the physician know before taking the drugs again. The physician should also be told about any allergies to foods, dyes, preservatives, or other substances.

PREGNANCY. Some medicines in this group may cause problems in pregnant women and have the potential to cause birth defects. Women who are pregnant or who may become pregnant should check with their physicians before taking these drugs.

BREAST-FEEDING. Erythromycins pass into breast milk. Mothers who are breast-feeding and who need to take this medicine should check with their physicians.

OTHER MEDICAL CONDITIONS. Before using erythromycins, people with any of these medical problems should make sure their physicians are aware of their condition:

- heart disease;
- liver disease; or
- hearing loss.

USE OF CERTAIN MEDICINES. Taking erythromycins with certain other drugs may affect the way the drugs work or may increase the chance of side effects.

Side effects

The most common side effects are mild diarrhea, nausea, vomiting, and stomach or abdominal cramps. These problems usually go away as the body adjusts to the drug and do not require medical treatment. Less common side effects, such as sore mouth or tongue and vaginal itching and discharge, also may occur. They do not need medical attention unless they persist or are bothersome.

More serious side effects are not common, but may occur. If any of the following side effects occur, the patient is advised to check with a physician immediately:

- severe stomach pain, nausea, vomiting, or diarrhea;
- fever;
- skin rash, redness, or itching; or
- unusual tiredness or weakness.

Although rare, very serious reactions to azithromycin (Zithromax) are possible, including extreme swelling of the lips, face, and neck; and anaphylaxis (a violent allergic reaction). Anyone who develops these symptoms after taking azithromycin should stop taking the medicine and get immediate medical help.

Other rare side effects may occur with erythromycins and related drugs. Anyone who has unusual symptoms after taking these medicines should get in touch with the physician.

Interactions

Erythromycins may interact with many other medicines. When an interaction occurs, the effects of one or both of the drugs may change or the risk of side effects may be greater. Anyone who takes erythromycins should let the physician know all other medicines he or she is taking. Drugs that may interact with erythromycins include:

- acetaminophen (Tylenol);
- medicine for overactive thyroid;
- male hormones (androgens);
- female hormones (estrogens);
- other antibiotics;
- blood thinners;
- disulfiram (Antabuse), used to treat alcohol abuse
- anti-seizure medicines such as valproic acid (Depakote, Depakene);
- caffeine;
- the antihistamine astemizole (Hismanal); and
- antiviral drugs such as zidovudine (Retrovir).

The list above does not include every drug that may interact with erythromycins. A physician or pharmacist should be consulted before combining erythromycins with any other prescription or nonprescription (over-the-counter) medicine.

Resources

BOOKS

AHFS: Drug Information. Washington, DC: American Society of Healthsystems Pharmaceuticals, 2008.

Brody, T. M., J. Larner, and K. P. Minneman. *Human Pharmacology Molecular to Clinical,* 2nd ed. St. Louis: Mosby, 1998.

Karch, A. M. *2008 Lippincott's Nursing Drug Guide.* Springhouse, PA: Lippincott Williams & Wilkins, 2007.

Sweetman, Sean C., ed. *Martindale: The Complete Drug Reference,* 35th ed. London: The Pharmaceutical Press, 2007.

PERIODICALS

"Steps to keep antibiotics working effectively." *Tufts University Health & Nutrition Letter.* Medford, MA: Tufts University, May 2003.

OTHER

'Erythromycin.' MedicineNet.com. December 31, 1997. http://www.medicinenet.com/erythromycin/article.htm (February 2008).

"Erythromycin." Medline Plus. April 1, 2003. http://www.nlm.nih.gov/medlineplus/druginfo/medmaster/a682381.html (February 2008).

Nancy Ross-Flanigan
Sam Uretsky, Pharm.D.
Laura Jean Cataldo, R.N., Ed.D.

Esophageal atresia repair

Definition

Esophageal atresia repair, also known as tracheoesophageal fistula or TEF repair, is a surgical procedure performed to correct congenital defects of the

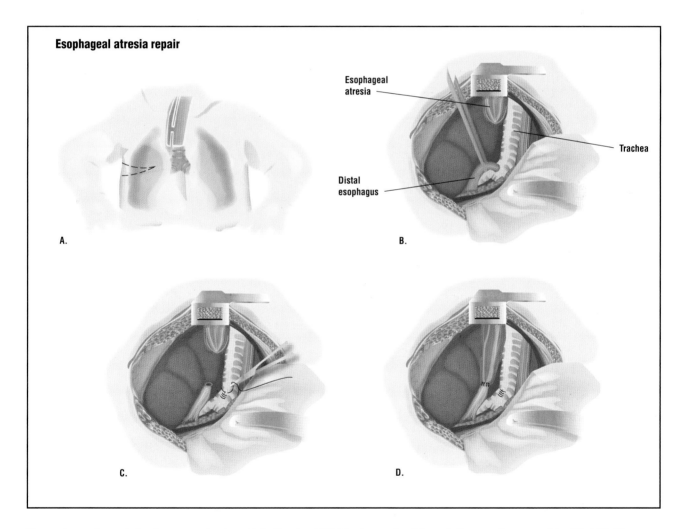

Esophageal atresia repair

A.

B.

Esophageal atresia

Distal esophagus

Trachea

C.

D.

To repair esophageal atresia, an opening is cut into the chest (A). The two parts of the existing esophagus are identified (B). The lower esophagus is detached from the trachea (C) and connected to the upper part of the esophagus (D). The wound in the trachea is closed, and the chest incision is repaired. *(Illustration by GGS Information Services. Cengage Learning, Gale.)*

esophagus (the muscular tube that connects the mouth to the stomach) and the trachea (the windpipe that carries air into the lungs). Esophageal atresia (EA) and tracheoesophageal fistula (TEF) are commonly found together (EA/TEF), but may also occur separately. As of 2003, there is no known cause for these congenital defects.

Purpose

In children born with EA, the esophagus has not developed as a continuous passage into the stomach but ends in a blind pouch. In the majority of cases (86%) it is also abnormally connected to the trachea by a small channel called a fistula. EA/TEF repair is performed to correct these defects, ensuring the survival of affected infants and their proper breathing and digestion.

Demographics

EA/TEF is reported to occur in about one in 4,500 births. It occurs equally among male and female infants and has been associated with prematurity. There are no other notable associations.

Description

The human esophagus and trachea are normally formed as two separate but parallel passageways early in fetal development. The esophagus leads from the throat to the stomach and digestive tract, and the trachea leads from the larynx to the lungs and respiratory system. Esophageal atresia occurs when the esophagus is incompletely formed; most typically, its upper portion ends in a pouch, failing to connect with the lower portion that leads to the stomach. Esophageal atresia with tracheoesophageal fistula, commonly known as EA/TEF, occurs when the membrane that divides the trachea from the esophagus (tracheoesophageal septum) is incompletely formed, leaving a fistula between the two normally separate organs. The combined defect is found in 86% of children who need esophageal atresia repair. Isolated esophageal atresia, or esophageal atresia without TEF, is a much less common congenital defect thought to occur later in fetal development and requiring a more complicated operation. The presence of TEF without EA occurs also, but with fewer noticeable symptoms in the infant, making it more difficult to diagnose. It may not be diagnosed until months or even years later when digestive disturbances occur. Surgery is required to correct all of these congenital defects.

KEY TERMS

Anastomosis—The connection of separate parts of a body organ or an organ system.

Anomaly (anomalies)—Abnormal development of a body organ or a defect in part of an organ system.

Aspiration—To take into the lungs by breathing.

Atresia—Absence of a normal opening.

Congenital—Present at birth.

Dysmotility—A lack of normal muscle movement (motility), especially in the esophagus, stomach, or intestines.

Dysplasia—The abnormal form or abnormal development of a body organ or organ system.

Esophagus—The upper portion of the digestive system, a tube leading from the mouth to the stomach.

Fistula—An abnormal tube-like passage between body organs or from a body organ to the body surface.

Trachea—The medical term for the windpipe.

A classification system is commonly used to describe five types of esophageal atresia, with and without TEF:

- Type A: Esophageal atresia (7.7% of cases). EA alone is a condition in which both segments of the esophagus, upper and lower, end in blind pouches with neither segment attached to the trachea.

- Type B: Esophageal atresia with upper tracheoesophageal fistula (0.8%). This is a rare type of EA/TEF, in which the upper segment of the esophagus forms a channel to the trachea (TEF) and the lower segment of the esophagus ends in a blind pouch (EA).

- Type C: Esophageal atresia with lower tracheoesophageal fistula (86.5%). This is the most common type of EA/TEF, in which the upper portion of the esophagus ends in a blind pouch and the lower segment of the esophagus is attached to the trachea by a fistula.

- Type D: Esophageal atresia with tracheoesophageal fistula (0.7%). Type D is the rarest form of EA/TEF, in which both segments of the esophagus are attached to the trachea.

- Type E: Tracheoesophageal fistula (4.2%). TEF alone is a condition in which a fistula is present between the esophagus and the trachea, while the esophagus has a normal connection to the stomach.

The incomplete esophagus in EA/TEF will not allow swallowed saliva, food, or liquids to pass into the stomach for normal digestion and nutrition. Because of the defect, normal eating or drinking can be dangerous because food and fluids have a direct route through the fistula into the lungs. Swallowed material in the dead-end esophagus as well as stomach fluids may be aspirated into the lungs through the fistula, compromising the child's breathing and potentially causing pneumonia or infection. The impossibility of normal eating, breathing, and digestion creates a life-threatening condition that requires immediate surgery.

The first signs of EA/TEF in a newborn infant may be tiny white frothy bubbles of mucus in the infant's mouth and sometimes in the nose as well. These bubbles reappear when they are suctioned away. Although the infant can swallow normally, the parents can often hear a rattling sound in the chest along with coughing and choking, especially when the baby is trying to nurse. Depending on the severity of the defect, some infants may develop a bluish complexion (cyanosis), caused by a lack of sufficient oxygen in the circulatory system. The infant's abdomen may be distended (swollen and firm) because the abnormally formed trachea will allow air to build up in the stomach and fill the space surrounding the abdominal organs. Saliva and stomach fluids may be aspirated into the lungs through the abnormal opening in the infant's trachea. Aspiration can lead to infection or even asphyxiation (impaired breathing or loss of consciousness due to lack of oxygen).

Other congenital defects are found in at least 50% of infants with EA/TEF. Typically more than one type of malformation will be found. These may include:

- heart defects (about 25% of affected infants)
- gastrointestinal (digestive) anomalies, including malformed anus (rectum) or twisting of the small intestine (about 16%)
- urinary tract and kidney defects (10%)
- musculoskeletal (muscle and bone) defects, especially of the ribs and limbs

The multiple anomalies that can occur with EA/TEF have been described by an acronym, VATER or VACTRRL. This acronym stands for vertebral defect, anorectal malformation, cardiac defect, tracheoesophageal fistula, renal anomaly, radial dysplasia, and limb defects. About 10% of children with EA have what is called the VATER syndrome. More infants with Type A esophageal atresia have multiple anomalies than those with Type B, the combined EA/TEF.

Healthy infants who have no complications, such as heart or lung problems or other types of intestinal malformations, can usually have esophageal surgery within the first 24 hours of life. The operation will be delayed for low birth weight infants or those with complicated malformations, usually until their nutritional status can be improved and other problems resolved sufficiently to reduce the risks of surgery. H-type TEF, which has fewer symptoms and is typically diagnosed when the child is at least four months old, is also easier to repair when the child's size and weight have increased. The esophagus can be dilated periodically during the growth period and a stomach tube used to decompress the stomach until the surgical repair is performed. All infants with some type of esophageal atresia will require surgery; many will have the repair performed in separate stages over a period of years. The procedures used to treat the five types of EA/TEF defects are similar.

Surgery is conducted while the infant is under **general anesthesia**, unconscious and free of pain. The surgeon makes an incision in the right chest wall between the ribs. If the gap between the two portions of the esophagus is short, the surgeon may join both ends of the esophagus together. This is called an anastomosis. If the upper portion of the esophagus is short and a long gap exists between the upper and lower portions, **reconstructive surgery** cannot be performed and the infant will have to be fed in another way to allow several months of growth. In this case, a **gastrostomy** (stomach tube) may be surgically placed directly into the stomach for feeding. In the most typical EA/TEF repair, the fistula will first be closed off, creating a separate airway. Then the blind esophageal pouch will be opened and connected to the other portion of the esophagus, creating a normal pathway directly into the stomach.

Diagnosis/Preparation

Diagnosis

A tentative diagnosis of EA/TEF may be made before the child is born. One of the first signs of esophageal atresia may be seen during the mother's prenatal **ultrasound** examination. Polyhydramnios, which is an excessive amount of amniotic fluid surrounding the fetus, is not always diagnostic but offers a warning sign. Fluid is normally exchanged between the fetus and the amniotic fluid through swallowing, urination, and discharges from the nose and mouth. In EA/TEF, the fetus may drool excessively because of a collection of fluid in the abnormal esophageal pouch, thus increasing the amount of amniotic fluid.

A newborn infant suspected of EA/TEF will be given an x-ray examination. The imaging study may reveal a dilated esophageal pouch that is larger than expected because it has collected a pool of amniotic fluid. During fetal development, the enlarged esophagus may also have pressed on and narrowed the trachea, a condition that may contribute to fistula development. Air in the stomach may confirm the presence of a fistula while gas in the large intestine will rule out duodenal atresia. The physician will also perform a comprehensive **physical examination**, looking for other congenital anomalies that are known to accompany EA/TEF. Chest x-rays may be taken to look for skeletal and cardiac abnormalities. Abdominal X-rays may be taken as well to look for intestinal obstruction and abnormalities. An echocardiogram (ECG) may be performed to evaluate heart function and an ultrasound of the kidneys performed to evaluate kidney function. A nasogastric (NG) tube may be placed in the infant; it may help to confirm a diagnosis of EA/TEF if it stops short of the usual distance (17 cm or about 6.7 in) to the stomach.

Preparation

When an infant is suspected of having EA/TEF, he or she will be transferred from the regular nursery to the neonatal (newborn) or pediatric intensive care department of the medical facility. Corrective surgery must be scheduled immediately to help ensure survival and promote proper swallowing, digestion, nutrition, and breathing. In patients with pneumonia or other lung problems, the doctor may clean out the baby's stomach and esophageal pouch with a suction tube to prevent the baby's stomach contents from being drawn through the fistula and into the trachea. A tube will be placed through the baby's mouth to continuously suction the esophageal pouch during surgery. The baby will be given fluids intravenously during surgery. **Oxygen therapy** will be administered if needed. An airway will be placed in the trachea if the baby has lung problems. **Antibiotics** may be given to treat or to prevent infection in the lungs, especially if the stomach contents have been drawn into the lungs. Preoperative blood and urine tests will also be performed.

Aftercare

Immediately after surgery, the patient will be cared for in the neonatal ICU with monitoring of breathing, **body temperature**, and heart and kidney function. Oxygen may be administered, and a mechanical respirator may also be necessary. Pain medication will be given if needed. Blood and urine tests may be performed to evaluate the infant's overall condition. Scans may be performed to evaluate esophageal functioning. The infant will be fed intravenously or will have a gastrostomy tube placed directly into the

EA/TEF repair is performed in a hospital operating room by a pediatric or general surgeon.

stomach until oral feedings can be swallowed and digested. Secretions may be suctioned from the throat and a nasogastric tube may be placed in the infant's nose to clear the stomach as needed. Hospitalization may be required for two weeks or longer, depending on the presence of complications or other underlying conditions. An x-ray procedure known as esophagography is usually performed at two months, six months, and one year of age to monitor the digestive function as the child grows. Long-term follow-up of patients who have had EA/TEF repair is essential.

Risks

There is some risk of postoperative breathing difficulties or respiratory complications, particularly infection or pneumonia due to aspiration of stomach contents. Pretreatment with antibiotics helps to prevent infection to some degree. Other risks of esophageal atresia repair include those that may occur with any surgery: reactions to anesthesia or medications; bleeding or clot formation; narrowing of the repaired organs; nerve injury; fluid imbalances; and collapsed lung (pneumothorax).

Complications that can occur in infants who have had EA/TEF repair include the following:

- Esophageal dysmotility. Dysmotility refers to weakness of the muscular walls of the esophagus. Some degree of dysmotility is expected to occur in all infants undergoing esophageal repair. This complication requires special precautions when the child is eating or drinking.

- About 50% of patients will develop gastroesophageal reflux disease (GERD) later in childhood or adult life. GERD is a condition in which the acid contents of the stomach flow back into the esophagus. The condition requires medical or surgical treatment.

- Recurrence of TEF. Recurrence is treated with repeat surgery.

- Swallowing difficulties (dysphagia). Dysphagia can cause food or pills to become stuck in the esophagus at the site of the surgical repair. Medications should be taken with water to prevent ulcers from developing.

- Breathing difficulties and choking. These complications are related to the slow passage of food, food stuck in the esophagus, or aspiration of food into the trachea.
- Chronic cough. The cough is characteristic of TEF repair; it is caused by weakness in the trachea and does not indicate a cold or illness.
- Increased susceptibility to colds, respiratory infections, and pneumonia. Precautions should be taken to avoid contact with other sick children. Parents and caregivers can seek advice about strengthening the child's immune system through appropriate nutrition and supplements.

Normal results

EA/TEF can usually be corrected with surgery, allowing the child to eat, breathe, and digest food in a normal fashion. Although almost 100% of children who have corrective surgery for EA/TEF survive the procedure, they may continue to have complications, some of which can be chronic. Ongoing medical care and additional surgery may be necessary.

Morbidity and mortality rates

The postoperative mortality rate in healthy infants is essentially zero. Prior to the development of a more advanced EA/TEF repair technique in 1939, the condition was often fatal. Pre- and postoperative neonatal care has also significantly improved the surgical outcome. Infants with multiple anomalies or cardiac or pulmonary problems are more subject to complications than otherwise healthy infants.

Alternatives

Esophageal atresia and tracheoesophageal fistula are congenital defects for which there are no recommended alternatives. These defects are commonly corrected surgically. There are no known measures to prevent these congenital defects.

Resources

BOOKS

Allan, W., MD, et al. *Pediatric Gastrointestinal Disease: Pathophysiology, Diagnosis, Management*, 3rd ed. Boston, MA: B.C. Decker, 2000.

ORGANIZATIONS

American Academy of Family Physicians. PO Box 11210, Shawnee Mission, KS 66207. (800) 274-2237. www.aafp.org.

EA/TEF Child and Family Support Connection. 111 West Jackson Blvd., Suite 1145, Chicago, IL 60604. (312) 987-9085. www.eatef.org.

OTHER

Allesandro, M. P., MD. *Esophageal Atresia and Tracheoesophageal Fistula (EA/TEF)*. Gastrointestinal Diseases, Virtual Children's Hospital Library. www.vh.org/pediatric/provider/radiology/PAP/GIDiseases/EATEF.html.

TEF/VATER International. *What is esophageal atresia?* www.tefvater.org.

L. Lee Culvert

Esophageal function tests

Definition

The esophagus is the muscular tube through which food passes on its way from the mouth to the stomach. The main function of the esophagus is to propel food into the stomach. To ensure that food does not move backward—a condition known as reflux—sphincters (constricting ring-shaped muscles) at either end of the esophagus close when the food is not passing through them in a forward direction. Esophageal function tests are used to determine whether the sphincters are working properly.

Purpose

The esophagus has two sets of sphincters at its upper and lower ends. Each of these muscular rings must contract in an exact sequence for swallowing to proceed normally. The upper esophageal sphincter normally stops the contents of the stomach from moving backward into the pharynx and larynx (voice box). The lower esophageal sphincter guards against stomach acid moving upward into the esophagus. The lower sphincter should be tightly closed except to allow food and fluids to enter the stomach.

The three major symptoms occurring with abnormal esophageal function are difficulty with swallowing (dysphagia); heartburn; and chest pain. Doctors perform a variety of tests to evaluate these symptoms. Endoscopy, which is not a test of esophageal function, is often used to determine if the lining of the esophagus has any ulcers, tumors, or areas of narrowing (strictures); however, many times endoscopy only shows the doctor if there is an injury to the esophageal lining; it does not always provide information about the cause of the problem. Tests that measure the functioning of the esophagus are sometimes needed in addition to endoscopy. There are three basic types of tests used to assess esophageal function:

- Manometry. Manometry is used to study the way the muscles of the esophagus contract, and is most useful for investigating dysphagia.
- Esophageal pH monitoring. This test measures changes in the acidity of the esophagus, and is valuable for evaluating patients with heartburn or gastroesophageal reflux disease (GERD).
- X-ray studies. This type of imaging study is used to investigate dysphagia, either by using a fluoroscope to follow the progress of a barium mixture during the process of swallowing, or by using radioactive scanning techniques.

Description

Manometry

This study is designed to measure the pressure changes produced by contraction of the muscular portions of the esophagus. An abnormality in the function of any one of the segments of the esophagus can cause difficulty in swallowing (dysphagia). A manometric examination is most useful in evaluating patients when an endoscopy yields normal results.

During manometry, the patient swallows a thin tube carrying a device that senses changes in pressures in the esophagus. Readings are taken at rest and during the process of swallowing. Medications are sometimes given during the study to aid in the diagnosis. The results are then transmitted to recording equipment. Manometry is most useful in

KEY TERMS

Achalasia—Failure to relax. The term is often applied to sphincter muscles.

Barium—A metallic element used in its sulfate form as a contrast medium for X-ray studies of the digestive tract.

Bolus—A mass of food ready to be swallowed, or a preparation of medicine to be given by mouth or IV all at once rather than gradually.

Cathartic—A medication or other agent that causes the bowels to empty.

Craniopharyngeal achalasia—A swallowing disorder of the throat.

Diffuse esophageal spasm (DES)—An uncommon condition characterized by abnormal simultaneous contractions of the esophagus.

Dysphagia—Difficulty or discomfort in swallowing.

Esophagus—The muscular passageway between the throat and the stomach.

Heartburn—A sensation of warmth or burning behind the breastbone, rising upward toward the neck. It is often caused by stomach acid flowing upward from the stomach into the esophagus.

Hiatal hernia—A condition in which part of the stomach pushes up through the same opening in the diaphragm that the esophagus passes through.

Motility—Ability to move freely or spontaneously. Esophageal motility refers to the ability of the muscle fibers in the tissue of the esophagus to contract in order to push food or other material toward the stomach.

Peristalsis—The wavelike contraction of the muscle fibers in the esophagus and other parts of the digestive tract that pushes food through the system.

Sphincter—A circular band of muscle fibers that constricts or closes a passageway in the body. The esophagus has sphincters at its upper and lower ends.

identifying diseases that produce disturbances of motility or contractions of the esophagus. In 2003, a solution containing five drops of peppermint oil in 10 mL (milliliters) of water was found to improve the manometric features of diffuse esophageal spasm (DES). The peppermint oil solution eliminated simultaneous esophageal contractions in all patients in the study.

Esophageal pH monitoring

This procedure measures the esophagus' exposure to acid reflux from the stomach. The test is ideal for evaluating recurrent heartburn or gastroesophageal reflux disease (GERD). Excessive acid reflux may produce ulcers, or strictures resulting from healed ulcers, in addition to the symptom of heartburn.

Normally, acid from the stomach washes backward into the esophagus in small amounts for short periods of time. The lower esophageal sphincter usually prevents excessive reflux in patients without disease. Spontaneous contractions that increase esophageal emptying and production of saliva also act to prevent damage to the esophagus.

Researchers have shown that in the esophagus, the presence of acid is damaging only if it lasts over long periods of time. Therefore, esophageal **pH monitoring** has been designed to monitor the level of acidity over a 24-hour period, usually in the patient's home. In this way, patients are able to maintain their daily routine, document their symptoms, and correlate symptoms with specific activities. During this period, a thin tube with a pH monitor remains in the esophagus to record changes in acidity. After the study, a computer is used to compare the changes with symptoms reported by the patient.

In addition to esophageal pH monitoring, the doctor may perform a Bernstein test (also known as the acid perfusion test) and an acid clearing test. In the Bernstein test, a small quantity of hydrochloric acid (HCl) is directed into the patient's esophagus. If the patient feels pain from the acid, the test is positive for reflux esophagitis. If there is no discomfort, another explanation must be sought for the patient's symptoms. In the acid clearing test, HCl is also directed into the esophagus. This test measures the patient's ability to quickly swallow the acid. If the patient has to swallow more than 10 times to move the acid down the esophagus, he or she has a problem with esophageal motility.

Monitoring of pH levels is usually performed before surgery to confirm the diagnosis and to judge the effects of drug therapy. In 2003, studies showed that integrated esophageal and gastric acidity provided better quantitative measures of esophageal dysfunction in GERD than conventional measurements of pH. This finding may suggest better ways to evaluate the effectiveness of different treatments for GERD.

X-ray tests

X-ray tests of esophageal function fall into two categories: (1) tests performed with barium and a fluoroscope; and (2) those performed with radioactive materials. Studies performed with fluoroscopy are especially useful in identifying structural abnormalities of the esophagus. Sometimes the patient is given a sandwich or marshmallow coated with barium in order to identify the site of an obstruction. Fluoroscopy can diagnose or provide important information about a number of disorders involving esophageal function, including cricopharyngeal achalasia (a swallowing disorder of the throat); decreased or reverse peristalsis; and **hiatal hernia**.

During fluoroscopy, the radiologist can observe the passage of material through the esophagus in real time, and also make video recordings. These observations are particularly useful when the swallowing symptoms appear to occur mostly in the upper region of the esophagus. The most common cause of difficulty swallowing is a previous stroke, although other diseases of the neuromuscular system (like myasthenia gravis) can produce similar symptoms.

Scans using low-dose radioactive materials are useful because they may demonstrate that food passes more slowly than usual through the esophagus. They can also measure the speed of the bolus' passage. These studies involve swallowing food coated with radioactive material, followed by a nuclear medicine scan. Scans are often used when other methods have failed to make a diagnosis, or if it is necessary to determine the degree of the abnormality.

Preparation

Patients should not eat or drink anything after midnight before an esophageal function test. Many medications affect the esophagus; doses may need to be adjusted or even discontinued prior to testing. Patients must inform their physician of any and all medications they take, including over-the-counter medications and herbal preparations. They must also tell the doctor about any known allergies.

Aftercare

No special care is needed after most esophageal function tests. Patients can usually return to their normal daily activities following almost all of these tests.

Risks

Exposure to x rays, especially in the first three months of a woman's pregnancy, can be harmful to the fetus. Barium swallows may also cause impaction (hardening) of fecal matter. Additionally, although the tubes passed through the esophagus during some of the esophageal function tests are small, and most patients adjust to them quite well, some patients may gag and aspirate (breathe into the lungs rather than passing through the esophagus) some gastric juices.

Normal results

Normal findings include:

- lower esophageal sphincter pressure, 10–20 mm Hg (millimeters of mercury);
- normal peristaltic waves;
- normal size, shape, position, patency, and filling of the esophagus;
- negative acid reflux;
- acid clearing in fewer than 10 swallows; and
- negative Bernstein test.

Manometry is used to diagnose abnormalities related to contraction or relaxation of the various muscular regions of the esophagus. These studies cannot distinguish whether injury to either the muscle or nerves of the esophagus is producing the abnormal results—only the final effect on esophageal muscle is identified. The results of this test should be interpreted in light of the patient's entire medical history. For example, there are many diseases that affect the relaxation of the lower esophageal sphincter; one such condition is called achalasia, and is a frequent finding in individuals with Down's syndrome. Achalasia is a type of esophageal motility disorder characterized by the lack of muscular contractions in the lower portion of the esophagus, In addition, there is failure of the valve at the bottom of the esophagus to open and let food into the stomach. This condition results in difficulty eating solid foods and in drinking fluids and may become more advanced over time, causing regurgitation and spasm of the chest wall muscles.

Abnormal results of pH tests can confirm symptoms of heartburn or indicate a cause of chest pain (or rarely, swallowing difficulties). The patient's doctor may want to prescribe or change medications based on these results, or even repeat the test using different doses of medication. As noted above, these studies should be done before surgical treatment of GERD.

X-ray tests can serve to document an abnormality in the esophagus. If the results are negative, other studies may be needed.

Resources

BOOKS

Castell, June A., and R. Matthew Gideon. "Esophageal Manometry," in Donald O. Castell and Joel E. Richter, eds., *The Esophagus,* 4th ed. Philadelphia, PA: Lippincott Williams & Wilkins, 2003.

Pagana, Kathleen D., and Timothy J. Pagana. *Diagnostic Testing and Nursing Implications*, 5th ed. St. Louis, MO: Mosby, 1999.

Smout, Andre. "Ambulatory Monitoring of Esophageal pH and Pressure," in Donald O. Castell and Joel E. Richter, eds., *The Esophagus,* 4th ed. Philadelphia, PA: Lippincott Williams & Wilkins, 2003.

PERIODICALS

Gardner, J. D., S. Rodriguez-Stanley, and M. Robinson. "Integrated Acidity and the Pathophysiology of Gastroesophageal Reflux Disease." *American Journal of Gastroenterology* 96, no. 5 (May 2001): 1363–1370.

Mujica, V. R., R. S. Mudipalli, and S. S. C. Rao. "Pathophysiology of Chest Pain in Patients with Nutcracker Esophagus." *American Journal of Gastroenterology* 96, no. 5 (May 2001): 1371–1377.

Pimentel, M., G. G. Bonorris, E. J. Chow, and H. C. Lin. "Peppermint Oil Improves the Manometric Findings in Diffuse Esophageal Spasm." *Journal of Clinical Gastroenterology* 33, no.1 (July 2001): 27–31.

Zarate, N., F. Mearin, A. Hidalgo, and J. R. Malagelada. "Prospective Evaluation of Esophageal Motor Dysfunction in Down's Syndrome." *American Journal of Gastroenterology* 96, no. 6 (June 2001): 1718–1724.

OTHER

Ferguson, Mark. "Achalasia and Esophageal Motility Disorders." January 26, 2000. Society of Thoracic Surgeons. http://www.sts.org/doc/4120 (March 30, 2008).

ORGANIZATIONS

American Society for Gastrointestinal Endoscopy, 1520 Kensington Road, Suite 202, Oak Brook, IL, 60523, (630) 573-0600, http://www.asge.org.

Society for Gastroenterology Nurses and Associates, 401 North Michigan Avenue, Chicago, IL, 60611-4267, (800) 245-7462, http://www.sgna.org.

Maggie Boleyn, R.N., B.S.N.
Lee Shratter, M.D.
Laura Jean Cataldo, R.N., Ed.D.

Esophageal radiography *see* **Upper GI exam**

Esophageal resection

Definition

An esophageal resection is the surgical removal of the esophagus, nearby lymph nodes, and sometimes a portion of the stomach. The esophagus is a hollow muscular tube that passes through the chest from the mouth to the stomach—a "foodpipe" that carries food and liquids to the stomach for digestion and nutrition. Removal of the esophagus requires reconnecting the remaining part of the esophagus to the stomach to allow swallowing and the continuing passage of food. Part of the stomach or intestine may be used to

KEY TERMS

Achalasia—Failure to relax. The term is often applied to sphincter muscles.

Adenocarcinoma—A type of cancer that develops in the esophagus near the opening into the stomach.

Anastomosis—A surgically created joining or opening between two organs or body spaces that are normally separate.

Barrett's esophagus—A potentially precancerous change in the type of cells that line the esophagus, caused by acid reflux disease.

Carcinoma—The common medical term for cancer.

Dysphagia—Difficulty and pain in swallowing.

Dysplasia—The presence of precancerous cells in body tissue.

Endoscopic ultrasound—An imaging procedure that uses high-frequency sound waves to visualize the esophagus via a lighted telescopic instrument (endoscope) and a monitor.

Esophagus—The upper portion of the digestive system, a tube that carries food and liquids from the mouth to the stomach.

Gastroesophageal reflux disease (GERD)—A condition of excess stomach acidity in which stomach acid and partially digested food flow back into the esophagus during or after eating.

Malignancy—The presence of tumor-causing cancer cells in organ tissue.

Metastasis (plural, metastases)—The spread of cancer cells from a cancerous growth or tumor into other organs of the body.

Resection—The surgical cutting and removing of a body organ, portion of an organ, or other body part.

Sphincter—A circular band of muscle fibers that constricts or closes a passageway in the body. The esophagus has sphincters at its upper and lower ends.

Squamous cell carcinoma—A type of cancer that develops in the cells in the top layer of tissue.

Thoracotomy—An open surgical procedure performed through an incision in the chest.

Thorascopy—Examination of the chest through a tiny incision using a thin, lighted tube-like instrument (thorascope).

---

make this connection. Several surgical techniques and approaches (ways to enter the body) are used, depending on how much or which part of the esophagus needs to be removed; whether or not part of the stomach will be removed; the patient's overall condition; and the surgeon's preference.

There are two basic esophageal resection surgeries. Esophagectomy is the surgical removal of the esophagus or a cancerous (malignant) portion of the esophagus and nearby lymph nodes. **Esophagogastrectomy** is the surgical removal of the lower esophagus and the upper part of the stomach that connects to the esophagus, performed when cancer has been found in both organs. Lymph nodes in the surrounding area are also removed.

An esophageal resection may be performed in combination with pre- and postoperative radiation and chemotherapy (chemoradiation).

Purpose

An esophagectomy is most often performed to treat early-stage cancer of the esophagus before the cancer has spread (metastasized) to the stomach or other organs. Esophagectomy is also a treatment for esophageal dysplasia (Barrett's esophagus), which is a precancerous condition of the cells in the lining of the esophagus. Lymph nodes are removed to be tested for the presence of cancer cells, which helps to determine if the cancer is spreading. Esophagectomy is also recommended when irreversible damage has occurred as a result of traumatic injury to the esophagus; swallowing of caustic (cell-damaging) agents; chronic inflammation; and complex motility (muscle movement) disorders that interfere with the passage of food to the stomach.

An esophagogastrectomy is performed when cancer of the esophagus has been shown to be spreading to nearby lymph nodes and to the stomach, creating new tumors. When cancer invades other tissues in this way, it is said to be metastatic. The goal of esophagogastrectomy is to relieve difficult or painful swallowing (dysphagia) in patients with advanced esophageal cancer, and to prevent or slow the spread of metastases to more distant organs such as the liver or the brain.

Demographics

The candidates for esophageal resection parallel those at high risk for esophageal cancer. Esophageal cancer is found among middle-aged and older adults, with the average age at diagnosis between 55 and 60. Esophageal cancer and esophageal dysplasia occur far more often in men than in women. One type of esophageal cancer (squamous cell carcinoma) occurs more frequently in African Americans; another type (adenocarcinoma) is more common in Caucasian males. Caucasian and Hispanic men with a history of gastroesophageal reflux disease (GERD) are also at increased risk, because GERD has been shown to cause changes in the cells of the esophagus that may lead to cancer. Higher risks are also associated with smoking (45%), alcohol abuse (20%), and lung disorders (23%).

Description

Esophageal cancer is diagnosed in about 13,000 people annually in the United States; it is responsible for approximately 1.5–5% of cancer deaths each year. Although it is not as prevalent as breast and colon cancer, its rate of occurrence is increasing. This rise is thought to be related to an increase in gastroesophageal reflux disease, or GERD.

The esophagus has a muscular opening, or sphincter, at the entrance to the stomach, which usually keeps acid from passing upward. In people with GERD, the esophageal sphincter allows partially digested food and excess stomach acid to flow back into the esophagus. This occurrence is known as regurgitation. Regurgitation continually exposes the lining of the esophagus to large amounts of acid, causing repetitive damage to the cells of the esophageal lining. The result is Barrett's esophagus, a condition in which the normal cells (squamous cells) of the esophageal lining are replaced by the glandular type of cells that normally line the stomach. Glandular cells are more resistant to acid damage but at the same time, they can more readily develop into cancer cells. Studies at New York's Memorial Sloan-Kettering Hospital have shown that only 30% of people diagnosed with Barrett's esophagus will later be diagnosed with cancer; the other 70% will not develop dysplasia, the precancerous condition. Effective medical treatment of acid reflux is thought to be a factor in the low incidence of cancer in people with Barrett's esophagus. Other types of cancer can also occur in the esophagus, including melanoma, sarcoma, and lymphoma.

The risk factors for esophageal cancer include:

- Use of tobacco. The highest risk for esophageal cancer is the combination of smoking and heavy alcohol use.

- Abuse of alcohol.

- Barrett's esophagus as a result of long-term acid reflux disease.

- A low-fiber diet; that is, a diet that is low in fruits and vegetables, and whole grains that retain their outer bran layer. Other dietary risk factors include vitamin and mineral deficiencies, such as low levels of zinc and riboflavin.

- Accidental swallowing of cleaning liquids or other caustic substances in childhood.

- Achalasia. Achalasia is an impaired functioning of the sphincter muscle between the esophagus and the stomach.

- Esophageal webs. These are bands of abnormal tissue in the esophagus that make it difficult to swallow.

- A rare inherited disease called tylosis, in which excess layers of skin grow on the hands and the soles of the feet. People with this condition are almost certain to develop esophageal cancer.

Cancer of the esophagus begins in the inner layers of the tissue that lines the passageway and grows outward. Cancer of the top layer of the esophageal lining is called squamous cell carcinoma; it can occur anywhere along the esophagus, but appears most often in the middle and upper portions. It can spread extensively within the esophagus, requiring the surgical removal of large parts of the esophagus. Adenocarcinoma is the type of cancer that develops in the lower end of the esophagus near the stomach. Both types of cancer may develop in people with Barrett's esophagus. Prior to 1985, squamous cell carcinoma was the most common type of esophageal cancer, but adenocarcinoma of the esophagus and the upper part of the stomach is increasing more rapidly than any other type of cancer in the United States. Up to 83% of patients undergoing esophagectomy have been shown to have adenocarcinoma. This development may be related to such changes in risk factors as decreased smoking and alcohol use as well as increased reflux disease. People at high risk for esophageal cancer should be examined and tested regularly for changes in cell types.

Esophageal cancer is classified in six stages determined by laboratory examination of tissue cells from the esophagus, nearby lymph nodes, and stomach. The six stages are:

- Stage 0. This is the earliest stage of esophageal cancer, in which cancer cells are present only in the innermost lining of the esophagus.

- Stage I. The cancer has spread to deeper layers of cells but has not spread into nearby lymph nodes or organs.

- Stage IIA. The cancer has invaded the muscular layer of the esophageal walls, sometimes as far as the outer wall.
- Stage IIB. The cancer has invaded the lymph nodes near the esophagus and has probably spread into deeper layers of tissue.
- Stage III. Cancer is present in the tissues or lymph nodes near the esophagus, especially in the trachea (windpipe) or stomach.
- Stage IV. The cancer has spread to more distant organs, such as the liver or brain.

Unfortunately, the symptoms of esophageal cancer usually don't appear until the disease has progressed beyond the early stages and is already metastatic. Without early diagnostic screening, patients may wait to consult a doctor only when there is little opportunity for cure. The symptoms of esophageal cancer may include difficulty swallowing or painful swallowing; unexplained weight loss; hiccups; pressure or burning in the chest; hoarseness; lung disorders; or pneumonia.

The decision to perform an esophageal resection will be made when staging tests have confirmed the presence of cancer and its stage. Two-thirds of people who undergo endoscopy, a close examination of the inside lining of the esophagus, and biopsies (testing esophageal tissue cells) will already have cancer, which can progress rapidly. Some will be treated with surgery and others with medical therapy, depending on the stage of the cancer, the patient's general health status, and the degree of risk. Removing the esophagus or the affected portion is the most common treatment for esophageal cancer; it can cure the disease if the cancer is in the early stages and the patient is healthy enough to undergo the stressful surgery. Esophagectomy will be recommended if early-stage cancer or a precancerous condition has been confirmed through extensive diagnostic testing and staging. Esophagectomy is not an option if the cancer has already spread to the stomach. In this case an esophagogastrectomy will usually be performed to remove the cancerous part of the esophagus and the upper part of the stomach.

Esophagectomy

An esophagectomy takes about six hours to perform. The patient will be given **general anesthesia**, keeping him or her unconscious and free of pain during surgery. One of several approaches or incisional strategies will be used, chosen by the surgeon to gain adequate access to the upper abdomen and remove the esophagus or the tumor and the nearby lymph nodes. The four common incisional approaches are:

transthoracic, which involves a chest incision; Ivor-Lewis, a side entry through the fifth rib; three-hole esophagectomy, which uses small incisions in the chest and abdomen to accommodate the use of instruments; and transhiatal, which involves a mid-abdominal incision. The approach chosen depends on the extent of the cancer, the location of the tumor or obstruction, and the overall condition of the patient.

In a minimum-access laparoscopic and thorascopic procedure, the surgeon makes several small incisions on the chest and abdomen through which he or she can insert thin telescopic instruments with light sources. The abdomen will be inflated with gas to enlarge the abdominal cavity and give the surgeon a better view of the procedure. First, the camera-tipped laparoscope will be inserted through one small incision, allowing images of the organs in the abdominal area to be displayed on a video monitor in the **operating room**. If the surgeon is going to use a portion of the stomach to replace the resected esophagus, he or she will first locate the fundus, or upper portion of the stomach. The fundus will be manipulated, stapled off, and removed laparoscopically, to be sutured in place (gastroplasty) as a replacement esophagus.

Next, the surgeon will pass thorascopic instruments into the chest through another incision. The esophagus or cancerous portion of the esophagus will be visualized, manipulated, cut and removed. Lymph nodes in the area will also be removed. Then the surgeon will either pull up a portion of the stomach and connect it to the remaining portion of the esophagus (anastomosis), or use a piece of the stomach or intestine, usually the colon, to reconstruct the esophagus. Either procedure will allow the patient to swallow and pass food and liquid to the stomach after recovery. As discussed above, other approaches may be used to gain access to the affected portion of the esophagus.

There are several variations of an esophagectomy, including:

- Standard open esophagectomy. This technique requires larger incisions to be made in the chest (thoracotomy) and in the abdomen so that the surgeon can dissect the esophagus or cancerous portion and remove it along with the nearby lymph nodes. The esophagus can then be reconnected to the stomach using a portion of either the stomach or the colon.
- Laparoscopic esophagectomy. This is a less invasive technique performed through several small incisions on the chest and abdomen with the camera-tipped laparoscope and a video monitor to guide removal of the esophagus or tumor along with nearby lymph glands.

• Vagal-sparing esophagectomy. This procedure preserves the branches of the vagus nerve that supply the stomach, with only minimal alteration of the size of the stomach and the nerves that control acid production and digestive functions.

Esophagogastrectomy

An esophagogastrectomy is also major surgery performed with the patient under general anesthesia. The surgeon will choose the incisional approach that allows the best possible access for resecting the lower portion of the esophagus and the upper portion of the stomach. The surgeon's decision will depend on the extent of the cancer, the amount of the esophagus that must be removed, and the patient's overall health status. An esophagogastrectomy can be performed as an open procedure through large incisions, or as a laparoscopic procedure through small incisions.

In a minimum-access laparoscopic procedure, several small incisions are made in the patient's abdomen. A laparoscope will be inserted through one small incision, allowing images of the abdominal organs to be displayed on a video monitor. As in an esophagectomy, gas may be used to inflate the abdominal cavity for better viewing and space for the surgeon to maneuver. The cancerous upper portion of the stomach will first be stapled off and resected. The cancerous portion of the esophagus will then be cut and removed along with nearby lymph nodes. Finally, a portion of the stomach will be pulled upward and connected to the remaining portion of the esophagus (anastomosis); or, if most of the esophagus has been removed, a piece of the colon will be used to construct a new esophagus. Sometimes the surgeon must make an incision in the neck in order to gain access to and resect the upper portion of the esophagus, followed by making an anastomosis between the esophagus and a portion of the stomach.

Diagnosis/Preparation

Diagnosis

The diagnosis of esophageal cancer begins with a careful history and a review of symptoms, and involves a number of different diagnostic examinations. An esophagoscopy may be performed in the doctor's office, allowing the doctor to examine the inside of the esophagus with a lighted telescopic tube (esophagoscope). A barium swallow is another common screening test, performed in the radiology (x-ray) department of the hospital or in a private radiology office. In a barium swallow, the patient drinks a small amount of radiopaque (visible on x ray) barium that will highlight any raised areas on the wall of the esophagus when chest x rays are taken. The x-ray studies will reveal irregular patches that may be early cancer or larger irregular areas that may narrow the esophagus and could represent a more advanced stage of cancer. If either of these conditions is present, the doctors will want to confirm the diagnosis of esophageal cancer; determine how far it has invaded the walls of the esophagus; and whether it has spread to nearby lymph nodes or organs. This staging process is essential in order to determine the best treatment for the patient.

One staging technique is a diagnostic procedure called **endoscopic ultrasound**. The doctor will thread an endoscope, which is a tiny lighted tube with a small **ultrasound** probe at its tip, into the patient's mouth and down into the esophagus. This procedure allows the inside of the esophagus to be viewed on a monitor to show how far a tumor has invaded the walls of the esophagus. At the same time, the doctor can perform biopsies of esophageal tissue by cutting and removing small pieces for microscopic examination of the cells for cancer staging. Staging tests may also include computed tomography (**CT scans**); thorascopic and laparoscopic examinations of the chest and abdomen; and **positron emission tomography (PET)**.

Preparation

The patient will be admitted to the hospital on the day of the operation or the day before, and will be taken to a preoperative nursing unit. The surgeon and anesthesiologist will visit the patient to describe the resection procedure and answer any questions that the patient may have. The standard preoperative blood and urine tests will be performed. Intravenous lines (IV) will be inserted in the patient's vein for the administration of fluids and pain medications during and after the surgery. Sedatives may be given before the patient is taken to the operating room.

Aftercare

Immediately after surgery the patient will be taken to a recovery area where the pulse, **body temperature**, and heart, lung, and kidney function will be monitored. Several hours later, the patient will be transferred to a concentrated care area. Surgical wound **dressings** will be kept clean and dry. Pain medication will be given as needed. A chest tube inserted during surgery will be checked for drainage and removed when the drainage stops. A nasogastric (nose to stomach) tube, also placed during surgery, will be used to drain stomach secretions. Nurses will check it regularly and rinse it out. It will eventually be removed by the surgeon. Until the patient is able to swallow soft foods, he or she will be fed intravenously or through a feeding tube that was placed in the small intestine during surgery. Patients will be encouraged to cough and to breathe deeply after surgery to fully expand the lungs and help prevent infection and collapse of the lungs. Walking and movement will also be encouraged to promote a quicker recovery.

About 10–14 days after the surgery, the patient will be given another barium swallow so that the doctor can examine the esophagus for any areas of leaking fluid. If none are seen, the nasogastric tube can be removed. The patient can then begin to sip clear liquids, followed gradually by small amounts of soft foods. Patients being treated for esophageal cancer may begin chemotherapy (cytotoxic or cell-killing medications), radiation therapy, or both, before or soon after **discharge from the hospital**. Patients typically remain in the hospital as long as two weeks after surgery if no complications have occurred.

When the patient goes home, any remaining **bandages** must be kept clean and dry. Frequent walking and gentle **exercise** are encouraged. Because laparoscopic and thorascopic surgery is less invasive and uses only small incisions, there is less trauma to the body and activity can be resumed more quickly than with open procedures that require larger incisions. The patient should report any fever or chills, persistent pain, or incision drainage to the surgeon. The patient's diet will typically be restricted for a while to soft foods and small portions; a normal diet can be resumed in about a month, but with smaller quantities. Patients are advised not to drive if they are still taking prescribed narcotic pain medications. Daily care and assistance at home is recommended during the recuperation period. Regular medical care and periodic diagnostic testing, such as endoscopic ultrasound, is essential to monitor the condition of the esophagus and to detect recurrence of the cancer or the development of new tumors.

Risks

One of the primary risks associated with esophageal resection surgeries is leakage at the site of the anastomosis, where a new feeding tube was sutured (stitched) to the remaining esophagus. As many as 9% of all patients have been reported to develop leaks, most occurring when a portion of the stomach rather than the colon was used to construct the new section of the esophagus.

Other risks include:

- formation of blood clots that can travel to the heart, lungs, or brain
- nerve injury, which can cause defective emptying of the stomach

- infection
- breathing difficulties and pneumonia
- adverse reactions to anesthesia
- narrowing of the remaining esophagus (strictures), which may cause swallowing problems
- increased acid reflux and heartburn as a result of injury to or removal of the esophageal sphincter

Normal results

Esophageal resection, especially esophagectomy, can be curative if cancer has not spread beyond the esophagus. About 75% of patients undergoing esophagectomy will be found to have metastatic disease that has already spread to other organs. Esophagectomy will reduce symptoms in most patients, especially swallowing difficulties, which will improve the patient's nutritional status as well. Patients whose esophagectomy is preceded and followed by a combination of chemotherapy and radiation treatments have longer periods of survival.

The typical result of an esophagogastrectomy is palliation, which is the relief of symptoms without a cure. Because esophagogastrecomy is always performed when metastases have already been found elsewhere in the body, the procedure may relieve pain and difficulty in swallowing, and may delay the spread of the cancer to the liver and brain. Cure of the disease, however, is not an expectation.

Patients having less invasive laparoscopic and thorascopic resection procedures will experience less pain and fewer complications than patients undergoing open procedures.

Morbidity and mortality rates

Because 75% of all esophagectomy patients and 100% of all esophagogastrectomy patients will have metastatic disease, morbidity and mortality rates for these procedures are high. Thirty-day mortality for esophagectomy ranges from 6–12%; it is 10% or higher for esophagogastrectomy. Survival of early-stage cancer patients after esophagectomy ranges from 17 to 34 months if surgery alone is the treatment.

The mortality rate for early-stage cancer patients having esophagectomy alone is higher than when surgery is combined with pre- and postoperative chemoradiation. The three-year survival rate for early-stage cancer patients who received pre- and post-esophagectomy chemoradiation is about 63%. Better staging techniques, more careful selection of patients, and improved surgical techniques are also believed to be responsible for the increase in postoperative survival rates. Recurrence of cancer in esophagectomy patients has been shown to be about 43%. A higher percentage of patients undergoing esophageal resections survive beyond the 30-day postoperative period in hospitals where the surgeons perform these procedures on a regular basis.

Alternatives

People with Barrett's esophagus can be treated with medicine and dietary changes to reduce acid reflux disease. These nonsurgical approaches are effective in relieving heartburn, calming inflamed tissues, and preventing further cell changes.

Fundoplication, or anti-reflux surgery, can strengthen the barrier to acid regurgitation when the lower esophageal sphincter does not work properly, curing GERD and reducing the exposure of the esophagus to excessive amounts of acid.

Photodynamic therapy (PDT) is the injection of a cytotoxic (cell killing) drug in conjunction with laser treatments, delivering benefits comparable to more established treatments. Endoscopic laser treatments that deliver short, powerful laser beams to the tumor through an endoscope can improve swallowing difficulties; however, multiple treatments are required and the benefits are neither long-lasting nor shown to prevent cancer.

Resources

BOOKS

American Cancer Society. *The American Cancer Society's Complementary and Alternative Cancer Methods Handbook*. Atlanta, GA: American Cancer Society, 2002.

Harpham, Wendy S., MD. *Diagnosis Cancer: Your Guide Through the First Few Months*. New York: W. W. Norton, Inc., 1998.

Heitmiller, R. F., et al. "Esophagus," in Martin D. Abeloff, ed., *Clinical Oncology*, 2nd ed. New York: Churchill Livingstone, 2000.

ORGANIZATIONS

American Cancer Society. 1599 Clifton Road NE, Atlanta, GA 30329. (800)ACS-2345. www.cancer.org.

American Gastroenterological Association. 4930 Del Ray Avenue, Bethesda, MD 20814. (301) 654-2055. www.gastro.org.

OTHER

Ferguson, Mark, MD. *Esophageal Cancer*. Society of Thoracic Surgeons. www.sts.org/doc4121.

National Cancer Institute (NCI). *General Information About Esophageal Cancer*. Bethesda, MD: NCI, 2003.

L. Lee Culvert

Esophagogastrectomy

Definition

Esophagogastrectomy is a surgical procedure in which a section of diseased esophagus is removed, along with part of the stomach and neighboring lymph nodes. The remaining piece of the esophagus is then reattached to the remaining stomach.

Purpose

Esophagogastrectomy is performed to treat cancer of the esophagus. There are two types of esophageal cancer: squamous cell and adenocarcinoma. Squamous cell cancer of the esophagus used to be the most common type, but now is only responsible for fewer than 50% of cases of esophageal cancer. Squamous cell cancer occurs when the cells of the esophageal lining convert into malignant cells. This type of esophageal cancer is more common in white patients. Adenocarcinoma of the esophagus often follows a condition called Barrett's esophagus, in which the lower cells of the esophagus convert into cells resembling the glandular cells of the stomach. Over time, these abnormal Barrett's cells have the potential of converting into truly malignant cells. Adenocarcinoma of the esophagus is the more common type of esophageal cancer in African-American patients.

Men are three to four times more likely to develop esophageal cancer than are women, and African-Americans are about 50% more likely to develop the condition. According to the American Cancer Society, about 16,470 new cases of esophageal cancer will be diagnosed in the United States in 2008, and the disease will be responsible for about 14,280 deaths. The disease is much more common in other countries, such as Iran, northern China, India, and southern Africa, where rates are between ten and 100 times as high as they are in the United States. Still, esophageal cancer rates among white men in Western countries are increasing steadily, at a rate of about 2% per year; the rate has held steady among white women. Among patients diagnosed at all stages of esophageal cancer, five-year survival rates are about 18% in white patients and 11% in African-American patients.

Precautions

Patients who are taking blood thinners, aspirin, or nonsteroidal anti-inflammatory medications may need to discontinue their use in advance of the test, to avoid increasing the risk of bleeding.

Description

Patients undergoing esophagogastrectomy require general anesthesia. This will be administered in the form of intravenous medications as well as anesthetic gasses that are inhaled. The patient will be intubated for the duration of the surgery, and a ventilator will breathe for them.

Esophagogastrectomy can be achived through a traditional upper abdominal incision, or through multiple very small laparoscopic incision. Traditional open abdominal esophagogastrectomy exposes the entire upper abdomen in order to allow careful visual inspection of all the structures and lymph nodes surrounding the stomach an esophagus. Laparoscopic esophagogastrectomy involves the introduction of a scope through one of the keyhole incisions, and the use of other tiny incisions for introducing the miniature

surgical instruments necessary for the operation. The exact technique utilized in the surgery will depend on where in the esophagus the cancerous segment is located, and how much of the stomach is involved. Surgical preference is to be able to preserve part of the esophagus, in order to allow it to be reconnected to the remaining stomach. In some cases, however, so much esophagus must be removed that there is not enough left to reattach to the stomach. When this occurs, a piece of intestine can be removed and used to connect the throat to the stomach. Requiring this step considerably increases the complexity and risks of the operation.

Preparations

Patients will need to stop eating and drinking for about 12-16 hours prior to their operation. The evening before the operation, a series of enemas and/or laxatives are used to empty the GI tract of feces. An intravenous line will be placed in order to provide the patient with fluids, general anesthesia agents, sedatives, and pain medicines during the operation. A urinary catheter will be placed in the patient's bladder. The patient will be attached to a variety of monitors to keep track of blood pressure, heart rate, and blood oxygen level throughout the procedure.

Aftercare

Esophagogastrectomy is major surgery, and often requires that the patient remain hospitalized for recuperation for as much as two weeks after the operation. Over this time, the patient's diet will slowly be reinstated, progressing gradually from liquids to soft foods to solids. Because esophageal cancer often causes symptoms of dysphagia (difficulty swallowing), a therapist specializing in re-teaching swallowing may be needed to help design a rehabilitative program.

Risks

Esophagogastrectomy carries a number of significant risks, including the general risks accompanying major surgery, such as blood clots, bleeding, heart attack, and infection. Specific complications that can occur with esophagogastrectomy include:

- Leakage of the new esophageal-stomach connection
- Slow stomach emptying due to surgical effects on the nerves controlling this function, sometimes resulting in chronic nausea and vomiting
- Severe heartburn if the lower part of the esophagus and upper part of the stomach are weakened by the surgery, allowing stomach contents to reflux back up into the esophagus
- Strictures or narrowing of the esophagus due to scarring from the surgery

The risk of fatal complications from esophagogastrectomy may range from about three to about seventeen percent. In general, studies have shown that hospital and surgeon experience with esophagogastrectomy reduces the risk of morbidity and mortality for patients.

Normal results

Normal results occur when the cancerous tissue is completely removed, and a patent, functional connection is created between the remaining esophageal and stomach tissue.

Abnormal results

Abnormal results range from remaining malignant tissue, to those complications detailed above, such as a leaky esophageal-stomach connection, chronic nausea secondary to nerve damage and slow stomach emptying, dysphagia due to strictures, etc.

Resources

BOOKS

Abeloff, M. D., et al. *Clinical Oncology,* 3rd ed. Philadelphia: Elsevier, 2004.

Goldman, L., D. Ausiello, eds. *Cecil Textbook of Internal Medicine,* 23rd ed. Philadelphia: Saunders, 2008.

Khatri, VP and JA Asensio. *Operative Surgery Manual,* 1st ed. Philadelphia: Saunders, 2003.

Rosalyn Carson-DeWitt, MD

▌Esophagogastroduodenoscopy

Definition

An esophagogastroduodenoscopy (EGD), which is also known as an upper endoscopy or upper gastrointestinal endoscopy, is a diagnostic procedure that is performed to view the esophagus, stomach, and duodenum (part of the small intestine). In an EGD, the doctor uses an endoscope, a flexible, tube-like, telescopic instrument with a tiny camera mounted at its tip, to examine images of the upper digestive tract displayed on a monitor in the examination room. Small instruments may also be passed through the tube to treat certain disorders or to perform biopsies (remove small samples of tissue).

Purpose

An EGD is performed to evaluate, and sometimes to treat, such symptoms relating to the upper gastrointestinal tract as:

- pain in the chest or upper abdomen
- nausea or vomiting
- gastroesophageal reflux disease (GERD)
- difficulty swallowing (dysphagia)
- bleeding from the upper intestinal tract and related anemias

In addition, an EGD may be performed to confirm abnormalities indicated by such other diagnostic procedures as an upper gastrointestinal (upper GI) x-ray series or a CT scan. It may be used to treat certain conditions, such as an area of narrowing (stricture) or bleeding in the upper gastrointestinal tract.

Description

Upper endoscopy is considered to be more accurate than x-ray studies for detecting inflammation, ulcers, or tumors. It is used to diagnose early-stage cancer and can frequently help determine whether a growth is benign or malignant. The doctor can obtain biopsies of inflamed or suspicious tissue for examination in the laboratory by a pathologist or cytologist. Cell scrapings can also be taken by introducing a small brush through the endoscope; this technique is especially helpful in diagnosing cancer or an infection.

Besides its function as an examining tool, an endoscope has channels that permit the passage of instruments. This feature gives the physician an opportunity to treat on the spot many conditions that may be seen in the esophagus, stomach, or duodenum. These treatments may include:

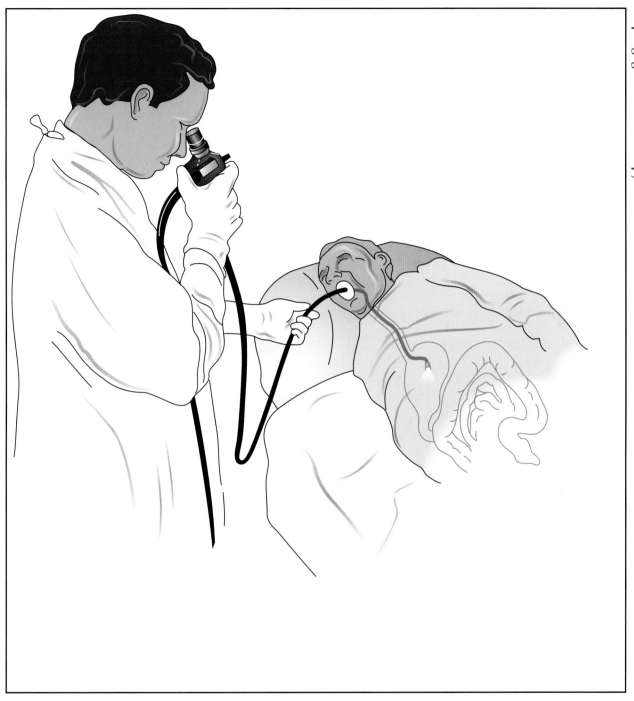

Esophagogastroduoenoscopy (EGD) is performed to evaluate or treat symptoms relating to the upper gastrointestinal tract. By inserting an endoscope into the mouth and guiding it through the gastrointestinal tract, the esophagus, stomach and duodenum can be examined and abnormalities treated. *(Illustration by Electronic Illustrators Group. Cengage Learning, Gale.)*

- removal of polyps and other noncancerous (benign) tissue growths

- stretching narrowed areas (strictures) in the esophagus

- stopping bleeding from ulcers or blood vessels

- removing foreign objects that have been swallowed, such as coins, pins, buttons, small nails, and similar items

KEY TERMS

Cytologist (cytology)—A medical technologist who specializes in preparing and examining biopsy specimens and cell specimens for changes that may indicate precancerous conditions or a specific stage of cancer.

Diverticulum (plural, diverticula)—A blind tubular sac or pouch created when the mucous tissue lining the esophagus or colon herniates through its muscular wall.

Duodenum—The first portion of the small intestine below the stomach.

Endoscope—A tube-like telescopic tool used to view areas of the body that cannot be directly observed, such as the esophagus, stomach, or colon, and to allow treatment of these areas.

Endoscopist—A physician or other medical professional highly trained in the use of the endoscope and related diagnostic and therapeutic procedures.

Esophagus— The hollow muscular tube that passes from the mouth to the stomach, carrying food and liquids to the stomach to be digested and absorbed.

Gastroenterologist—A physician who specializes in digestive disorders and diseases of the organs of the digestive tract, including the esophagus, stomach, and intestines.

Gastroesophageal reflux disease (GERD)—A condition of excess stomach acidity in which stomach acid and partially digested food flow back into the esophagus during or after meals.

Pathologist (pathology)—A doctor who specializes in the anatomic (structural) and pathologic (disease-causing) chemical changes in the body and the related results of diagnostic testing.

Stricture—An abnormal narrowing of the esophagus or other duct or canal in the body.

Some of the diseases and conditions that are investigated, identified, or treated using EGD include:

- abdominal pain
- achalasia, a defect in the muscular opening between the esophagus and the stomach
- Barrett's esophagus, a precancerous condition of the cells lining the esophagus
- Crohn's disease and inflammatory disease of the small intestine
- esophageal cancer

- gastroesophageal reflux disease (GERD), a condition caused by excess stomach acid
- hiatal hernia
- irritable bowel syndrome
- rectal bleeding
- stomach cancer
- stomach ulcers
- swallowing problems

An EGD procedure is usually performed by a gastroenterologist, who is a physician specializing in the diagnosis and treatment of disorders of the digestive tract. GI (gastrointestinal) assistants, **operating room** nurses, or technicians may be involved in the collection of samples and care of the patient. Patients will be asked to either gargle using a local anesthetic or will have an anesthetic sprayed into their mouths onto the back of the throat to numb the gag reflex. Then the endoscopist will guide the endoscope through the mouth into the upper gastrointestinal tract while the patient is lying on his or her left side. The lens or camera at the end of the instrument allows the endoscopist to examine each portion of the upper gastrointestinal tract by observing images on a monitor. Photographs are usually taken for reference. During the procedure, air is pumped in through the instrument to expand the structure that is being studied and allow better viewing. Biopsies and other procedures will be performed as needed. The patient's breathing will not be disturbed and there will be little if any discomfort. Many patients fall asleep during all or part of the procedure.

Some patients should not have an EGD. This examination is contraindicated in patients who have:

- severe upper gastrointestinal (UGI) bleeding
- history of such bleeding disorders as platelet dysfunction or hemophilia
- esophageal diverticula, which are small pouches in the esophagus that can trap food or pills and become infected
- suspected perforation (puncture or rupture) of the esophagus or stomach
- recent surgery of the upper gastrointestinal tract (throat, esophagus, stomach, pyloric valve, duodenum)

An EGD is also contraindicated for those patients who are unable to cooperate fully with the procedure or whose overall condition includes a severe underlying illness that increases the risk of complications.

Diagnosis/Preparation

Certain medications (such as **aspirin** and the anti-inflammatory drugs called NSAIDs) should be discontinued at least seven days before an EGD to reduce the risk of bleeding. Patients will be asked not to eat or drink anything for at least six to 12 hours before the procedure to ensure that the upper intestinal tract will be empty. Before the procedure, patients may be given a sedative and/or pain medication, usually by intravenous injection.

Aftercare

After the procedure, the patient will be observed in the endoscopy suite or in a separate recovery area for an hour, or until the sedative or pain medication has worn off. Someone should be available to take the patient home and stay with them for a while. Eating and drinking should be avoided until the local anesthetic has worn off in the throat and the gag reflex has returned, which may take two to four hours. To test if the gag reflex has returned, a spoon can be placed on the back of the tongue for a few seconds with light pressure to see if the patient gags. Hoarseness and a mild sore throat are normal after the procedure; the patient can drink cool fluids or gargle to relieve the soreness.

The patient may experience some bloating, belching, and flatulence after an EGD because air is introduced into the digestive tract during the procedure. To prevent any injury to the esophagus from taking medications by mouth, patients should drink at least 4 or more ounces of liquid with any pill, and remain sitting upright for 30 minutes after taking pills that are likely to cause injury. The doctor should be notified if the patient develops a fever; difficult or painful swallowing (dysphagia); breathing difficulties; or pain in the throat, chest, or abdomen.

Risks

Endoscopy is considered a safe procedure when performed by a gastroenterologist or other medical professional with special training and experience in endoscopy. The overall complication rate of EGD performance is less than 2%; many of these complications are minor, such as inflammation of the vein through which medication is given. Serious complications can and do occur, however, with almost half being related to the heart or lungs. Bleeding or perforations are also reported, especially when tumors or strictures have been treated or biopsied. Infections have been reported, though rarely; careful attention to cleaning the instrument should prevent this complication. Perforation, which is the puncture of an organ, is very rare and can be surgically repaired if it occurs during an EGD.

Normal results

The results of the procedure or probable findings are often available to the patient prior to discharge from the endoscopy suite or the recovery area. The results of tissue biopsies or cell tests (cytology) will take from 72–96 hours. Normal results will show that the esophagus, stomach and duodenum are free of strictures, ulcers or erosions, diverticula, tumors, or bleeding. Abnormal results include the presence of any of these problems, as well as esophageal infections, fissures, or tears. An increasingly common finding is medication-induced esophageal injury, caused by tablets and capsules that have lodged in the esophagus. These injuries are thought to be associated with damage to the esophageal tissue from gastrointestinal reflux disease (GERD) and the related exposure of the esophagus to large amounts of stomach acid.

Resources

BOOKS

Edmundowicz, Steven. "Endoscopy." In *The Esophagus*, 3rd ed., edited by Donald O. Castell and Joel E. Richter. Philadelphia, PA: Lippincott, 1999.

Pagana, Kathleen D., and Timothy J. Pagana. *Diagnostic Testing and Nursing Implications*, 5th ed. St. Louis, MO: Mosby, 1999.

ORGANIZATIONS

American Society for Gastrointestinal Endoscopy (ASGE). 13 Elm Street, Manchester, MA 01944-1314. (978) 526-8330. www.asge.org.

Society for Gastroenterology Nurses and Associates (SGNA). 401 North Michigan Avenue, Chicago, IL 60611-4267. (800) 245-7462. www.sgna.org.

Maggie Boleyn, RN, BSN
L. Lee Culvert

Essential surgery

Definition

Essential surgery is an operative procedure that is considered to be vitally necessary for treating a disease or injury. Postponing or deciding against an essential procedure may result in a patient's **death** or permanent impairment.

Description

Essential surgery may be performed on either an elective or emergency basis. **Elective surgery** is defined as surgery that can be scheduled in advance and is not considered an emergency. Some elective surgeries, however, may be considered essential. For example, an aortic aneurysm is a weak spot in the wall of the aorta, a major blood vessel. If an aortic aneurysm is found during a **physical examination** or imaging procedure, an aneurysmectomy (surgical repair of an aneurysm) may be scheduled as an elective procedure. In most cases, complications can be avoided if the aneurysm is repaired in a timely manner. If no repair is performed, however, the aneurysm may grow larger and eventually burst; this serious medical emergency is most often fatal.

In other cases, essential surgery arises out of a medical emergency, giving the patient and physician less time to prepare for surgery or seek alternatives. An example of such an emergency is appendicitis, or an infection of the appendix (a pouch-shaped organ in the abdomen). If left untreated, appendicitis may result in a ruptured appendix, which is a life-threatening condition. An **appendectomy** (surgical removal of the appendix) is usually considered essential in treating appendicitis and avoiding rupture. Another example is trauma surgery, or surgery to repair serious injuries to the body.

A surgical procedure may be optional under some circumstances, and essential under others. An example is surgery for Crohn's disease, or chronic inflammation of the intestines. This condition is associated with such symptoms as abdominal pain, fatigue, fever, loss of appetite, and weight loss. Patients who are not able to manage their symptoms with medication may choose surgical treatment (such as the removal of a segment of bowel) as a means of improving their quality of life. Without surgery, a patient's condition would not necessarily deteriorate. In contrast, the presence of severe bleeding, a bowel obstruction, or a hole in the intestinal wall—all potential complications of Crohn's disease— would be considered a medical emergency. Surgery subsequently becomes necessary to prevent permanent damage or to save the patient's life.

Whether a surgical procedure is essential is important in determining whether it will be covered by health insurance. If a procedure is not considered "medically necessary" (i.e., is considered elective), most insurance companies will not pay for the procedure, or will

KEY TERMS

Aorta—The largest artery in the body; carries oxygenated blood from the heart to the extremities and major organs.

Appendix—A pouch-shaped organ that is attached to the upper part of the large intestine.

Cosmetic surgery—Surgery that is intended to improve a patient's appearance or correct disfigurement. It is also called aesthetic surgery.

Elective surgery—Surgery that would be beneficial to the patient but is not urgent, and is therefore a matter of choice.

provide only minimal coverage. A common example of an elective procedure that is not usually covered by insurance is **cosmetic surgery**. In some cases, however, an elective procedure is covered by health insurance because it is considered essential in improving the patient's quality of life. An example is **breast reconstruction** following **mastectomy** (surgical removal of the breast). While breast reconstruction is an elective procedure according to most definitions (i.e., it is not medically necessary nor considered an emergency), it is considered essential in restoring a woman's self-image following the removal of a breast for the treatment of cancer. A 1998 federal law (the Women's Health and Cancer Rights Act) states that insurance companies are required to cover breast reconstruction in patients who are covered for mastectomy.

Resources

BOOKS

Khatri, V. P., and J. A. Asensio. *Operative Surgery Manual* 1st ed. Philadelphia: Saunders, 2003.

Townsend, C. M., et al. *Sabiston Textbook of Surgery* 17th ed. Philadelphia: Saunders, 2004.

ORGANIZATIONS

American College of Surgeons. 633 N. Saint Clair St., Chicago, IL 60611-3211. (312) 202-5000. http://www.facs.org (accessed March 20, 2008).

American Society of Plastic Surgeons (ASPS). 444 East Algonquin Road, Arlington Heights, IL 60005. (847) 228-9900. http://www.plasticsurgery.org (accessed March 20, 2008).

OTHER

Centers for Medicare and Medicaid Services. *The Women's Health and Cancer Rights Act*, January 20, 2003 [cited May 18, 2003]. http://www.cms.hhs.gov/ (accessed March 20, 2008).

Crohn's and Colitis Foundation of America. http://www. ccfa.org/ (accessed March 20, 2008).

O'Connor, Robert. "Aneurysms, Abdominal." *eMedicine*, February 11, 2002 [cited May 18, 2003]. http://www. emedicine.com/emerg/topic27.htm (accessed March 20, 2008).

Stephanie Dionne Sherk
Rosalyn Carson-DeWitt, MD

Excessive sweating surgery *see*
Sympathectomy

Excimer laser photoreflective keratectomy
see Photorefractive keratectomy (PRK)

Exenteration

Definition

Exenteration is a major operation during which all the contents of a body cavity are removed. Pelvic exenteration refers to the removal of the pelvic organs and adjacent structures; orbital exenteration refers to the removal of the entire eyeball, orbital soft tissues, and some or all of the eyelids.

Purpose

The pelvis is the basin-shaped cavity that contains the bladder, rectum, and reproductive organs. The internal reproductive organs include the ovaries, fallopian tubes, uterus, and cervix for women, and the prostate and various ducts and glands for men. Pelvic exenteration is performed to surgically remove cancer that involves these organs and that has not responded well to other types of treatment. Pelvic exenteration is also indicated when cancer returns after an earlier treatment. In women, the operation is performed mostly for advanced and invasive cases of endometrial, ovarian, vaginal, and cervical cancer; for aggressive prostate cancer in men; and rectal cancer in either sex.

Orbital exenteration is performed to remove the eye and surrounding tissues when cancer of the orbital contents cannot be controlled by simple removal or irradiation. It is often the only course of treatment for advanced cancers of the eyelid, eyeball, optic nerve, or retina.

Exenteration is a major operation for both patient and surgeon; it is technically very challenging because it involves elaborate **reconstructive surgery**. Although it is a radical surgical procedure, exenteration often provides the only opportunity available for patients to eliminate the cancer and to prevent it from recurring.

Demographics

No data are available regarding the demographic nature of patients undergoing exenteration, given the numerous conditions that may warrant it. Cancer affects individuals of any age, sex, race, or ethnicity, although incidence may differ among these groups by cancer type.

Description

Both pelvic and orbital exenterations are considered to be major surgery and are performed under **general anesthesia**. The exact surgical procedure performed depends on the type of exenteration.

Pelvic exenteration

Pelvic exenterations start with an incision in the lower abdomen. Blood vessels are clamped and the organs specified by the procedure are removed. The site of incision is then stitched up. There are three types of pelvic exenteration: anterior, posterior, and total.

ANTERIOR EXENTERATION. This operation is called anterior exenteration because it removes organs toward the front of the pelvic cavity. It usually involves the removal of the female reproductive organs, bladder, and urethra. (In males, an operation that removes the bladder and prostate is called a cystoprostatectomy.) Patients selected for this operation have cancers in areas that allow the rectum to be spared.

A new method for excreting urine must be created. One common approach, called an ileal conduit, diverts the ureters to a pouch made of small intestine, which is then connected to the abdominal wall. Urine exits the body through a small opening called a stoma, and collects in a small bag attached to the body. Vaginal reconstruction may also be performed during the exenteration, or in a later procedure.

POSTERIOR EXENTERATION. Posterior exenteration removes organs that are located in the back part of the pelvic cavity. These include the reproductive organs, plus the lower part of the bowel; the bladder and urethra are kept intact. A patient who has undergone posterior exenteration will require a **colostomy**, a procedure that connects the colon to the abdominal wall; waste exits the body through a stoma and is collected in a small bag.

Exenteration

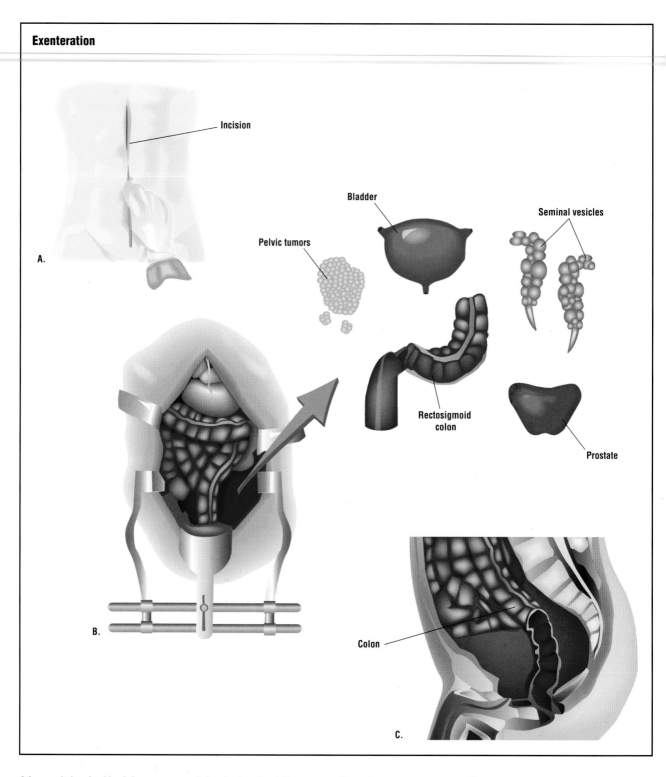

A large abdominal incision exposes abdominal and pelvic contents for pelvic exenteration (A). Contents of the lower abdominal cavity, including the rectosigmoid colon, prostate and seminal vesicles (if male), bladder, and any pelvic tumors are removed (B). *(Illustration by GGS Information Services. Cengage Learning, Gale.)*

TOTAL PELVIC EXENTERATION. This operation removes the bladder, urethra, rectum, anus, and supporting muscles and ligaments, together with the reproductive organs. Total pelvic exenteration is performed when there is no opportunity to perform a less extensive operation, because of the location and size of the cancer. A urinary stoma and a colostomy stoma will be created to collect waste.

Orbital exenteration

This operation removes the eyeball and surrounding tissues of the orbit. (Since the eye is surrounded by bone, orbital exenteration is often easier to tolerate than pelvic exenteration.) Orbital exenteration with partial preservation of eyelids and conjunctiva can sometimes be achieved. After the surgical site has healed, patients can be fitted with a temporary ocular prosthesis (plastic eye), although many patients prefer to wear an eye patch. Later, facial prostheses can be attached to the facial skeleton.

Diagnosis/Preparation

The evaluation of patients before pelvic exenteration includes a thorough physical exam with rectal and pelvic examination. Endorectal **ultrasound** and imaging studies such as computed tomography scans (**CT scans**) and **magnetic resonance imaging** (MRI) are routinely used to obtain pictures of the abdominal and pelvic areas and evaluate the spread of the cancer.

Ocular ultrasound examination, CT scan, and **angiography** evaluation (used to image blood vessels) are usually performed to prepare for orbital exenteration.

Some patients begin treatment with chemotherapy and/or radiation before the procedure. Surgery is typically performed approximately six weeks later.

In the case of pelvic exenteration, the patient will be given a bowel prep to cleanse the colon and prepare it for surgery. This procedure is required to lower the level of intestinal bacteria, thus helping to prevent **post-surgical infections**. **Antibiotics** are also typically given to help decrease bacteria levels in the bowel.

Aftercare

Pelvic exenteration

After a pelvic exenteration, a drainage tube is inserted at the site of the incision. There usually is some bleeding, discharge, and considerable tenderness and pain for a few days. At least a three- to five-day hospital stay is usually required. Side effects depend on the type of pelvic exenteration performed, but often include urination difficulty, especially if adjustment to a catheter is required; and a very painful lower abdomen.

Stitches are usually removed from the skin on the third day, or before the patient is sent home. A prescription for pain medication is usually given as well as instructions for follow-up care.

Ocular exenteration

After ocular exenteration, most patients have a headache for several days, which goes away with over-the-counter pain medications. An eye ointment is also prescribed that contains antibiotics and steroids to help the healing process.

Risks

As with any operation, there is a risk of complications due to anesthesia, wound infection, or injury to adjacent organs or structures.

In the case of pelvic exenteration, the following complications are also possible:

- hemorrhage that may require a blood transfusion
- injury to the bowel
- urinary tract infection
- urinary retention requiring permanent use of a catheter
- bowel obstruction

After removal of the reproductive organs, women will no longer have monthly periods nor will they be able to become pregnant. For men, surgery involving the prostate and the nerves around the rectum may also result in the inability to produce sperm or to have an erection.

WHO PERFORMS THE PROCEDURE AND WHERE IS IT PERFORMED?

As exenteration is considered to be major surgery, the procedure is performed under the strict conditions that a hospital operating room affords. A team of physicians, nurses, and other health care workers are involved in the procedure. Pelvic exenteration may be performed by a gynecologist, gynecologic oncologist, urologist, and/or plastic surgeon. Orbital exenteration may be performed by an ophthalmologist and/or oculoplastic surgeon.

In the case of orbital exenteration, the following complications have been known to occur:

- growth of an orbital cyst (rare)
- chronic throbbing orbital pain
- sinusitis (nasal stuffiness)
- ear problems
- reoccurrence of malignancy

Normal results

During and after recovery from exenteration, it is normal for a patient to undergo a period of psychological adjustment to the major change in lifestyle (e.g., learning to care for a urostomy or colostomy) or appearance (e.g., following orbital exenteration). It is important that all aspects of the procedure be discussed with the patient before undergoing surgery, and that any psychosocial distress that the patient experiences after exenteration be addressed.

Morbidity and mortality rates

There is a 30–44% chance of complications during pelvic exenteration, and the operative mortality rate ranges from 3–5%. About one-third of patients will experience postoperative complications such as bowel obstruction, fistula formation, inflammation or failure of the kidneys, narrowing of the ureters, or pulmonary embolism (a blood clot that travels to the lungs). The five-year survival rate after pelvic exenteration ranges from 23% to 61%. For patients who undergo pelvic or orbital exenteration, short- and long-term morbidity and mortality rates depend on the particular condition that required the procedure.

Alternatives

Exenteration is generally pursued only if no other less invasive options are available to the patient.

QUESTIONS TO ASK THE DOCTOR

- Why is exenteration recommended in my case?
- What organs or other structures will be removed?
- In the case of pelvic exenteration, what methods of urinary/fecal diversion will be performed?
- In the case of orbital exenteration, what are my options in terms of cosmetic prostheses?
- What non-surgical options are available to me?
- How long after surgery may I resume normal activity?

Alternatives, however, include chemotherapy, radiation therapy, and more conservative surgery.

Resources

BOOKS

Yanoff, Myron, and Jay Duker. *Ophthamology,* 1st ed. London: Mosby International Ltd., 1999.

PERIODICALS

Clarke, A., N. Rumsey, J. R. O. Collin, and M. Wyn-Williams. "Psychosocial Distress Associated with Disfiguring Eye Conditions." *Eye* 17, no. 1 (January 2003): 35–40.

Ramamoorthy, Sonia L., and James W. Fleshman. "Surgical Treatment of Rectal Cancer." *Hematology/Oncology Clinics of North America* 16, no. 4 (August 2002): 927.

Sevin, B. U., and O. R. Koechlie. "Pelvic Exenteration." *Surgical Clinics of North America,* 81, no. 4 (August 1, 2001): 771–9.

Turns, D. "Psychosocial Issues: Pelvic Exenterative Surgery." *Journal of Surgical Oncology* 76 (March 2001): 224–36.

ORGANIZATIONS

American Academy of Ophthalmology. P.O. Box 7424, San Francisco, CA 94120-7424. (415) 561-8500. http://www.aao.org.

American Cancer Society. 1599 Clifton Road NE, Atlanta, GA 30329. (800) ACS-2345. http://www.cancer.org.

American College of Obstetricians and Gynecologists. 409 12th St., SW, P.O. Box 96920, Washington, DC 20090-6920. http://www.acog.org.

OTHER

Juretzka, Margrit M. "Pelvic Exenteration." *eMedicine,* February 2, 2006. http://www.emedicine.com/med/topic3332.htm (accessed June 12, 2008).

Monique Laberge, PhD
Stephanie Dionne Sherk

Exercise

Definition

The Surgeon General of the United States defines exercise as physical activity that involves planned, structured, and repetitive bodily movements in order to improve or maintain physical fitness. As an element of health, exercise involves both strength training of the muscles and cardiovascular fitness, with stretching activities for flexibility. Most research on physical activity for fitness stresses the intensity and regularity of exercise as key elements. Typical exercise activities include fast walking, running, cycling, swimming, or aerobics classes. The latest Centers for Disease Control and Prevention (CDC) report, in conjunction with the American Council on Sports Medicine, recommends that all adults perform 30 or more minutes a day of moderate-intensity activity for five to seven days per week. The National Institutes of Health Consensus Development Conference Statement on Physical Activity and Cardiovascular Health identifies inactivity as a major public health problem in the United States. They have recommended exercise regimens five to seven days a week for people who are already active, and such leisure activities as gardening, walking, using stairs instead of an elevator, cleaning house, and recreational pursuits, etc., for people who are largely sedentary.

Purpose

One important purpose of exercise is speeding recovery from surgery. Nowhere is being fit as important as when a person is facing surgery or recovering from surgery. Regular exercise leads to important health advantages, including weight loss; greater cardiovascular efficiency; lower cholesterol levels; increased musculoskeletal strength and flexibility; increased bone density; and better functioning of the metabolic, endocrine, and immune systems. These effects diminish with lack of exercise within two weeks if physical activity is substantially reduced; the fitness effects disappear altogether within two to eight months if physical activity is not resumed.

With regard to **preparing for surgery**, the effects of regular exercise on all body systems create optimal responses both to the surgical procedures itself and during the postoperative recovery period.

Demographics

Most adults in North America would benefit from increasing their level of physical activity. The majority of adults in the United States (65%) are overweight, and two-thirds of those with weight problems are likely also to have diabetes, heart disease, high blood pressure, or other obesity-related conditions. A sedentary lifestyle and unhealthy eating patterns are responsible for at least 300,000 deaths each year from chronic diseases. It is estimated that two-thirds of people over 65 have at least one chronic condition, with 36 million Americans suffering from some form of arthritis. More than 300,000 total joint replacement procedures are performed each year due to osteoarthritis. Lack of physical activity contributes substantially to conditions like osteoarthritis, low back pain, and osteoporosis.

Obesity reached epidemic proportions among adults in the United States in the years between 1987 and 2008. Over 45 million adults are obese; in addition, the percentage of young people who are overweight has more than doubled in the last 20 years. Despite the benefits of physical activity, more than 60% of American adults do not get enough physical activity to provide health benefits. More than 25% are not active in their leisure time. Insufficient activity increases with age; it is also more common in women than men and among those with lower levels of economic stability and educational achievement. On the other hand, the CDC reported in 2007 that more adult Americans are getting more regular exercise than was the case in the recent past; the rate of women exercising at least 30 minutes per day increased by 8.6% from 2001 to 2005, and the rate for men increased by 3.5%.

The direct consequences of obesity include:

- Heart disease and stroke, the leading causes of death and disability in the United States.

- Type 2 diabetes (also known as NIDDM, or non-insulin-dependent diabetes mellitus).

- Cancer. Obesity increases the risk of cancer of the uterus, gallbladder, cervix, ovary, breast, and colon in women; it increases the risk of cancer of the colon, rectum, and prostate in men.

- Osteoarthritis. Obesity adds to daily "wear and tear" on joints, primarily the knees, as well as the hips and lower back.

- Gallbladder disease. The risk of gallbladder disease and gallstones increases as a person's weight increases.

- Stress incontinence in women, especially those over 65 years old.

- Gastroesophageal reflux disease (GERD).

KEY TERMS

Aerobic exercise—Any type of exercise that is intended to increase the body's oxygen consumption and improve the functioning of the cardiovascular and respiratory systems.

Body mass index (BMI)—A measurement that has replaced weight as the preferred determinant of obesity. The BMI can be calculated (in English units) as 703.1 times a person's weight in pounds divided by the square of the person's height in inches.

Obesity—Excessive weight gain due to accumulation of fat in the body, sometimes defined as a BMI of 30 or higher, or body weight greater than 30% above one's desirable weight on standard height-weight tables.

Physical activity—Any activity that involves moving the body and results in the burning of calories.

Physical fitness—The combination of muscle strength and cardiovascular health usually attributed to regular exercise and good nutrition.

Sedentary—Characterized by inactivity and lack of exercise. A sedentary lifestyle is a major risk factor for becoming overweight or obese.

Diagnosis/Preparation

More than 30 million Americans undergo surgery each year. Each patient's **surgical risk**, complications, and outcomes will depend on how fit they are; how well their cardiovascular and pulmonary systems withstand the stress of anesthesia; how quickly their bones and muscles recover after surgical procedures; and how well their metabolic and immune systems respond to surgery and the risk of infection. The general physical status of the patient is the most important factor in preparing for surgery. This status is determined by the physician, including his or her evaluation of the specific procedures to be performed. On the other hand, however, the patient's lifestyle may affect management of the surgery both before and after the actual procedures. A healthful diet, regular exercise, and quitting smoking are highly recommended before surgery. Each of these factors has an important role to play in optimal functioning of the circulatory and pulmonary systems. Smoking should cease two weeks before surgery to be beneficial.

Aftercare

After surgery, it is important to return to daily activities when the physician gives permission to do so. Most doctors encourage their patients to be as active as possible as soon as possible. While aftercare is individualized, and physicians may place certain limitations on physical activity for specific patients, walking as soon as the patient is able to walk is generally recommended. The patient should be as active as possible within the limits set by the physician for postoperative recovery, with the goal of returning to his or her normal daily activities and exercise routines. The patient should ask the physician for explicit guidelines about returning to an established exercise program or other physical or recreational activities.

Risks

The benefits of exercise before and after surgery, and continuing as a daily life activity cannot be overemphasized. There are risks, however, for people who begin an exercise program without having had one in the past. Patients should always have a **physical examination** before taking up an exercise program for the first time or after a long period of inactivity. It is also a good idea to look for a form of exercise that one finds personally appealing or interesting; studies have found that people are more likely to stick with an exercise program when they enjoy the sport or activity, whether it is an individual form of exercise (walking, running, cycling, yoga, tai chi, swimming) or one that involves a team or an exercise partner (dancing, martial arts, fencing, golf, tennis, volleyball, softball, etc.). One reason that walking is often recommended as a form of exercise is that it can be combined with a number of activities that many people enjoy, such as nature walks, bird watching, visiting an art or science museum, socializing with a friend, or exercising a pet dog. For some people, participation in a team sport is also a good way to make friends, as well as to commit to an exercise program.

Too much exercise can be as harmful to the body as too little; overuse of certain muscles and joints can lead to such health problems as tennis elbow and shin splints. Many exercise programs now recommend days of rest as well as regularly scheduled periods of exercise, as inadequate rest increases the risk of stroke and circulatory disorders. In particular, pregnant women should not exercise two days in a row.

Such high-intensity exercise regimens as high-impact aerobics and jogging are not recommended as often as they once were for helping patients attain a specific fitness level as measured by resting heart rate and muscle mass. Running in particular is hard on the knees and ankle joints; in addition, runners are frequently injured by falls. Walking, swimming, and gardening can all contribute to aerobic fitness. Strength training with resistance exercises for the arms and legs using weights or bands is now an important aspect of physical fitness. These exercises can be done at a moderate rate, with the number of repetitions increased over time. Stretching is very important to both kinds of exercise activities; yoga is often recommended for stretching, bending, and improving overall flexibility.

People who have specific health problems can still find ways to exercise that will not make their injuries or disorders worse. The American Council on Exercise (ACE) offers articles on exercising for the elderly and for adults with such problems as bad knees, shoulder injuries, asthma, chronic pain, arthritis, and flat feet.

Morbidity and mortality rates

Without exercise and a healthful diet, people burn fewer calories than they take in, resulting in increasing weight gain. While the formula is familiar, the outcomes are surprising. According to studies based on a newer index for obesity—the body mass index (BMI)—people who are overweight or obese have dramatically shorter life spans. This correlation was confirmed by a study published in the *Journal of the American Medical Association* in 2007. In fact, some studies are showing that individuals who are fat in middle age are as likely to lose years of life as those who smoke. Researchers have found obesity and overweight combined are the second leading cause of preventable **death** in the United States, behind tobacco use. Correlating the BMI—calculated from a person's weight in kilograms divided by height in meters squared—and the mortality of different cohorts of subjects in large longitudinal studies, researchers have found that the lowest mortality rates from all causes were found among those having a BMI between 23.5 and 24.9 for men and 22.0–23.4 for women. The strongest association between obesity and death from all causes are found among individuals with the highest BMI—people with a BMI of 40 +. Clinical obesity is defined as a BMI of 30 or above. Morbid obesity is defined as a BMI of 40 or above.

With respect to health care, people who are obese have higher rates of complications in the hospital. Researchers in New York studied a group of patients who were in the **intensive care unit** (ICU) for a variety of causes, and found that those who were morbidly obese were far more likely to die of their illness than those who were closer to their desirable weight (23.3% vs. 6.1%). Patients who were morbidly obese had higher rates of transfers to **nursing homes** from the ICU, rather than being discharged to their homes—over 16% for the obese patients compared to 3% for patients who were less overweight.

Resources

BOOKS

Corbin, Charles C., and Ruth Lindsey. *Fitness for Life*, 5th ed. Champaign, IL: Human Kinetics, 2007.

Murphy, Wendy. *Weight and Health*. Minneapolis, MN: Twenty-First Century Books, 2008.

Prentice, William. *Get Fit, Stay Fit*, 4th ed. Boston: McGraw-Hill Higher Education, 2007.

Sheen, Barbara. *Keeping Fit*. Chicago: Heinemann Library, 2008.

PERIODICALS

Bolliger, C. T. "Evaluation of Operability Before Lung Resection." *Current Opinion in Pulmonary Medicine* 9 (July 2003): 321–326.

Centers for Disease Control and Prevention (CDC). "Prevalence of Regular Physical Activity among Adults—United States, 2001 and 2005." *MMWR: Morbidity and Mortality Weekly Report* 56 (November 23, 2007): 1209–1212.

Cummings, S., E. S. Parham, and G. W. Strain. "Position of the American Dietetic Association: Weight Management." *Journal of the American Dietetic Association* 102 (August 2002): 1145–1155.

Morey, M. C., and C. W. Zhu. "Improved Fitness Narrows the Symptom-Reporting Gap Between Older Men and Women." *Journal of Women's Health (Larchmont)* 12 (May 2003): 381–390.

Pollock, M. L., et al. "Resistance Exercise in Individuals With and Without Cardiovascular Disease: American Heart Association Advisory." *Circulation* 101 (February 22, 2000): 828–833.

Sui, X., M. J. LaMonte, J. N. Laditka, et al. "Cardiorespiratory Fitness and Adiposity as Mortality Predictors in Older Adults." *Journal of the American Medical Association* 298 (December 5, 2007): 2507–2516.

Wallace, J. "Exercise in Hypertension: A Clinical Review." *Journal of Sports Medicine* 33 (2003): 585–598.

ORGANIZATIONS

American College of Sports Medicine (ACSM). P.O. Box 1440, Indianapolis, IN 46206-1440. (317) 637-9200. http://www.acsm.org/AM/Template.cfm?Section=Home (accessed March 20, 2008).

American Council on Exercise (ACE). 4851 Paramount Drive, San Diego, CA 92123. (888) 825-3636. http://www.acefitness.org/default.aspx (accessed March 20, 2008).

Shape Up America! c/o WebFront Solutions Corporation, 15757 Crabbs Branch Way, Rockville, MD 20855. (301) 258-0540. http://www.shapeup.org (accessed March 20, 2008).

Weight-control Information Network (WIN). 1 WIN Way, Bethesda, MD 20892-3665. (202) 828-1025 or (877) 946-4627.

OTHER

Agency for Health Care Practice and Research. http://www.ahcpr.gov/ (accessed March 22, 2008).

American Association of Orthopaedic Surgeons. http://www.aaos.org/ (accessed March 22, 2008).

National Center for Chronic Disease Prevention and Health Promotion, Centers for Disease Control and Prevention. *Nutrition and Physical Activity.* http://www.cdc.gov/nccdphp/dnpa/physical/index.htm (accessed March 22, 2008).

National Institutes of Health, National Institute of Diabetes & Digestive & Kidney Diseases (NIDDK). *Active At Any Size.* Bethesda, MD: NIDDK, 2007. NIH Publication No. 04-4352.

National Institutes of Health, National Institute of Diabetes & Digestive & Kidney Diseases (NIDDK). *Walking: A Step in the Right Direction.* Bethesda, MD: NIDDK, 2007. NIH Publication No. 07-4155.

National Institutes of Health, National Institute of Diabetes & Digestive & Kidney Diseases (NIDDK). *Weight Loss for Life.* Bethesda, MD: NIDDK, 2006. NIH Publication No. 94-3700.

Nancy McKenzie, PhD
Rebecca Frey, PhD

Exercise electrocardiogram *see* **Stress test**

Exercise stress test *see* **Stress test**

Exploratory laparotomy *see* **Laparotomy, exploratory**

Extracapsular cataract extraction

Definition

Extracapsular cataract extraction (ECCE) is a category of eye surgery in which the lens of the eye is removed while the elastic capsule that covers the lens is left partially intact to allow implantation of an intraocular lens (IOL). This approach is contrasted with intracapsular cataract extraction (ICCE), an older procedure in which the surgeon removed the complete lens within its capsule and left the eye aphakic (without a lens). The patient's vision was corrected after intracapsular extraction by extremely thick eyeglasses or by contact lenses.

There are two major types of ECCE: manual expression, in which the lens is removed through an incision made in the cornea or the sclera of the eye; and phacoemulsification, in which the lens is broken into fragments inside the capsule by **ultrasound** energy and removed by aspiration.

Purpose

Historical background

The purpose of ECCE is to restore clear vision by removing a clouded or discolored lens and replacing it with an IOL. Cataract operations are among the oldest recorded surgical procedures; there are references to cataract surgery in the *Code of Hammurabi* in 1750 B.C., and in the treatises written around 600 B.C. by Susruta, a famous surgeon from India. In the ancient world, lenses damaged by cataracts were dislocated rather than removed in the strict sense; the surgeon used a lance to push the clouded lens backward into the vitreous body of the eye. This operation, known as couching, was standard practice until the mid-eighteenth century. Couching is still performed by some traditional healers in Africa and parts of Asia.

The first extracapsular extraction of a cataract was performed by a French surgeon named Jacques Daviel in 1753. Daviel removed the lens through a fairly long incision in the cornea of the eye. In 1865, the German ophthalmologist Albrecht von Graefe refined the operation by removing the lens through a much smaller linear incision in the sclera of the eye. After von Graefe, however, intracapsular extraction gradually became the favored method of cataract removal even though it left the patient without a lens inside the eye. The two inventions that made extracapsular extraction preferable again were the operating microscope and the intraocular lens. The first eye surgery performed with an operating microscope was done in Portland, Oregon, in 1948; in the same year, a British ophthalmologist named Harold Ridley implanted the first IOL in the eye of a cataract patient. Between 1948 and the 1980s, manual expression was the standard form of ECCE. Although phacoemulsification was first introduced in 1967, it was not widely accepted at first because it requires special techniques that take time for the surgeon to learn, as well as expensive specialized equipment. As of 2007, phacoemulsification is now performed more often in the United States and Europe than "standard" ECCE. The manual expression technique, however, is still widely used in developing countries with large numbers of patients with eye disorders and limited hospital budgets.

Lens and cataract formation

The lens, which is sometimes called the crystalline lens because it is transparent, is located immediately behind the iris. In humans, the lens is about 0.35 in (9 mm) long and 0.15 in (4 mm) wide. It consists of protein fibers and water, with the fibers arranged in a

Acuity—Sharpness or clarity of vision.

Aphakic—Without a lens. An older form of cataract surgery known as intracapsular extraction left patients' eyes aphakic.

Aspiration—Removal by suction.

Brunescent—Developing a brownish or amber color over time; nuclear cataracts are sometimes called brunescent.

Capsulorrhexis—The creation of a continuous circular tear in the front portion of the lens capsule during cataract surgery to allow for removal of the lens nucleus.

Capsulotomy—A procedure that is sometimes needed after ECCE to open a lens capsule that has become cloudy.

Cataract—A cloudy or opaque area on or in the lens of the eye.

Cornea—The transparent front portion of the exterior cover of the eye.

Couching—The oldest form of cataract surgery, in which the lens is dislocated and pushed backward into the vitreous body with a lance.

Endophthalmitis—An infection on the inside of the eye that may result in vision loss.

Hyphema—Bleeding inside the anterior chamber of the eye.

Keratometer—A device that measures the curvature of the cornea. It is used to determine the correct power for an IOL prior to cataract surgery.

Lens capsule—A clear elastic membrane-like structure that covers the lens of the eye.

Macula—A small yellowish depression on the retina of the eye slightly below the optic disk that is the central point of sharpest vision. Its primary function is the absorption of shorter wavelengths of light.

Ophthalmology—The branch of medicine that deals with the diagnosis and treatment of eye disorders.

Phacoemulsification—A method of extracapsular cataract extraction in which the lens is broken apart by ultrasound energy and the fragments removed by suction.

Sclera—The tough white fibrous membrane that forms the outermost covering of the eyeball.

Uvea—The middle of the three coats of tissue surrounding the eye, comprising the choroid, iris, and ciliary body. The uvea is pigmented and well supplied with blood vessels.

Uveitis—Inflammation of any part of the uvea.

Vitreous body—The transparent gel that fills the inner portion of the eyeball between the lens and the retina. It is also called the vitreous humor or crystalline humor.

---

pattern that allows light to pass through the lens. There are three layers of cells in the lens: a central nucleus, which becomes denser and harder as a person ages; a cortex surrounding the nucleus, which contains cells that are metabolically active and continue to grow and divide; and a layer of cells between the cortex and the lens capsule known as the subcapsular epithelium.

Although a few people are born with cataracts or develop them in childhood, most cataracts are the result of the aging process. Between 5 and 10 million people around the world each year develop cataracts severe enough to impair their vision. As people grow older, the protein fibers in the lens become denser, start to clump together, and form cloudy or opaque areas in the lens. Cataracts vary considerably in their speed of progression; they may develop in a few months or over a period of many years. Some people have cataracts that stop growing at an early stage of development and do not interfere with their vision. Although most people develop cataracts in both eyes, they do not usually progress at the same rate, so that the person has much better vision in one eye than in the other.

Ophthalmologists classify cataracts according to their location in the lens. It is possible for a person to have more than one type of cataract, including:

- Nuclear cataracts. Nuclear cataracts grow slowly over many years but can become very large and hard, which complicates their removal. They are sometimes called brunescent cataracts because they are characterized by deposits of brown pigment that give the lens an amber color. Nuclear cataracts are most commonly associated with age and with smoking as risk factors.

- Cortical cataracts. Cataracts in the cortex of the lens develop more rapidly than nuclear cataracts but remain softer and are easier to remove. They are thought to be caused by an increase in the water content of the lens. Risk factors for cortical cataracts include female sex and African or Caribbean heritage.

- Posterior subcapsular (PSC) cataracts. This type of cataract, which develops between the back of the lens and the lens capsule, is the softest and most rapidly growing type. PSC cataracts tend to scatter light at night and thus interfere with nighttime driving. Risk factors for PSC cataracts include diabetes, high blood pressure, and a history of treatment with steroid medications.

Demographics

Cataract extraction is one of the most frequently performed surgical procedures in industrialized countries. It is estimated that 300,000–400,000 cases of visually disabling cataracts occur each year in the United States alone, and that between 1 and 1.5 million cataract extractions are performed annually in the United States. This frequency reflects the importance of cataracts as a major public health problem. The World Health Organization (WHO) estimated in 1997 that cataracts were responsible for 50% of cases of blindness around the world, or 19 million people. By the year 2020, that figure is expected to rise to 50 million. More recent publications estimate that 1.2% of the general population of Africa is blind, with cataracts responsible for 36% of these cases of blindness.

About one person in every 50 in the general American population will eventually have to have a cataract removed. However, it is difficult to compare the rates of cataract formation among various subgroups because present published studies use a number of different grading systems for defining and detecting cataracts. In addition, the elderly are often underrepresented in general population studies even though age is the greatest single risk factor for cataract development. Three recent research projects carried out in the United States, Australia, and England, respectively, reported that 50% of people over the age of 60 have some degree of cataract formation, with the figure rising to 100% for those over 80. As of 2007, little conclusive information is available regarding the incidence of cataracts in different racial and ethnic groups in the United States.

A variety of risk factors in addition to age have been associated with cataracts, but their precise significance is debated among researchers, including:

- Genetic factors. Twin studies show that the identical twin of a patient with a nuclear cataract has a 48% chance of developing one.

- Sex. Women are slightly more likely than men to develop cataracts. One American study found that 53.3% of women over 60 had nuclear cataracts compared to 49.7% of the men; 25.9% of the women had cortical cataracts versus 21.1% of the men.

- Exposure to ultraviolet radiation. Cortical cataracts are more likely to develop in people with frequent exposure to sunlight; however, nuclear cataracts are not related to sun exposure.

- Exposure to infrared light waves. Occupations as different as military surveillance, weather forecasting, spectroscopy, thermal efficiency analysis, and astronomy expose workers to infrared radiation.

- Smoking. People who smoke more than 25 cigarettes per day are three times as likely as nonsmokers to develop nuclear or PSC cataracts. Smoking does not appear to be related to cortical cataracts.

- Alcohol consumption. Heavy drinking has been reported to increase the risk of developing all three types of cataracts.

- Diabetes. Patients with diabetes are at increased risk of developing all three types of cataracts.

- Use of steroid medications. PSC cataracts are known to be induced by steroids, even though they represent less than 10% of all cataracts.

- Socioeconomic status (SES). People with college or professional-school education have lower rates of cataract formation than people who did not finish high school, even attempting to correct for environmental and nutritional factors. There is, however, no obvious biochemical or medical explanation for this correlation, and some researchers treat it with caution.

- Chronic dehydration, diarrhea, and malnutrition. Studies carried out in India indicate that severe malnutrition or repeated episodes of diarrhea in childhood carry a three- to fourfold increase in risk of developing cataracts in later life. It is not yet known, however, whether this statistic would hold true for people in other countries.

Description

Conventional extracapsular cataract extraction

Although phacoemulsification has become the preferred method of extracapsular extraction for most cataracts in the United States since the 1990s, conventional or standard ECCE is considered less risky for patients with very hard cataracts or weak epithelial tissue in the cornea. The ultrasound vibrations that are used in phacoemulsification tend to stress the cornea.

A conventional extracapsular cataract extraction takes less than an hour to perform. After the area around the eye has been cleansed with antiseptic, sterile drapes are used to cover most of the patient's face. The patient is given either a local anesthetic to numb the tissues around the eye or a topical anesthetic to numb the eye itself. An eyelid holder is used to hold the eye open during the procedure. If the patient is very nervous, the doctor may administer a sedative intravenously.

The surgeon makes an incision in the cornea at the point where the sclera and cornea meet. Although the typical length of a standard ECCE incision was 0.39–0.47 in (10–12 mm) in the 1970s, the development of foldable acrylic IOLs has allowed many surgeons to work with incisions that are only 0.19–0.23 in (5–6 mm) long. This variation is sometimes referred to as small-incision ECCE. After the incision is made, the surgeon makes a circular tear in the front of the lens capsule; this technique is known as capsulorrhexis. The surgeon then carefully opens the lens capsule and removes the hard nucleus of the lens by applying pressure with special instruments. After the nucleus has been expressed, the surgeon uses suction to remove the softer cortex of the lens. A special viscoelastic material is injected into the empty lens capsule to help it keep its shape while the surgeon inserts the IOL. After the intraocular lens has been placed in the correct position, the viscoelastic substance is removed and the incision is closed with two or three **stitches** using a very fine monofilament suture. A newer technique uses a laser rather than stitches to close the incision, and appears to give equally good results.

Phacoemulsification

In phacoemulsification, the surgeon uses an ultrasound probe inserted through the incision to break up the nucleus of the lens into smaller pieces. The newer technique offers the advantages of a smaller incision than standard ECCE, fewer or no stitches to close the incision, and a shorter recovery time for the patient. Its disadvantages are the need for specialized equipment and a steep learning curve for the surgeon. One study found that surgeons needed to perform about 150 cataract extractions using phacoemulsification before their complication rates fell to a baseline level. As of 2007, there is a need for more residency programs in eye surgery that give residents sufficient practice in this technique of cataract extraction.

Diagnosis/Preparation

Diagnosis

The diagnosis of cataract is usually made when the patient begins to notice changes in his or her vision and consults an eye specialist. In contrast to certain types of glaucoma, there is no pain associated with the development of cataracts. The specific changes in the patient's vision depend on the type and location of the cataract. Nuclear cataracts typically produce symptoms known as myopic shift (in nearsighted patients) and second sight (in farsighted patients). What these terms mean is that the nearsighted person becomes more nearsighted while the farsighted person's near vision improves to the point that there is less need for reading glasses. Cortical and posterior subcapsular cataracts typically reduce visual acuity; in addition, the patient may also complain of increased glare in bright daylight or glare from the headlights of oncoming cars at night.

Because visual disturbances may indicate glaucoma as well as cataracts, particularly in older adults, the examiner will first check the intraocular pressure (IOP) and the anterior chamber of the patient's eye. The examiner will also look closely at the patient's medical history and general present physical condition for indications of diabetes or other systemic disorders that affect cataract development. The next step in the diagnostic examination is a test of the patient's visual acuity for both near and far distances, commonly known as the Snellen test. If the patient has mentioned glare, the Snellen test will be conducted in a brightly lit room.

The examiner will then check the patient's eyes with a slit lamp in order to evaluate the location and size of the cataract. After the patient's eyes have been dilated with eye drops, the slit lamp can also be used to check the other structures of the eye for any indications of metabolic disorders or previous eye injury. Lastly, the examiner will use an ophthalmoscope to evaluate the condition of the optic nerve and retina at the back of the eye. The ophthalmoscope can also be used to detect the presence of very small cataracts.

Imaging studies of the eye (ultrasound, MRI, or **CT scan**) may be ordered if the doctor cannot see the back of the eye because of the size and density of the cataract.

Preparation

ECCE is almost always elective surgery—emergency removal of a cataract is performed only when the cataract is causing glaucoma or the eye is severely injured or infected. After the surgery has been scheduled, the patient will need to have special testing known as keratometry if an IOL is to be implanted.

The testing, which is painless, is done to determine the strength of the IOL needed. The ophthalmologist measures the length of the patient's eyeball with ultrasound and the curvature of the cornea with a device called a keratometer. The measurements obtained by the keratometer are entered into a computer that calculates the correct power for the IOL.

The IOL is a substitute for the lens in the patient's eye, not for corrective lenses. If the patient was wearing eyeglasses or contact lenses before the cataract developed, he or she will continue to need them after the IOL is implanted. The lens prescription should be checked after surgery, however, as it is likely to need adjustment.

Aftercare

Patients can use their eyes after ECCE, although they should have a friend or relative drive them home after the procedure. The ophthalmologist will place some medications—usually steroids and antibiotics—in the operated eye before the patient leaves the office. Patients can go to work the next day, although the operated eye will take between three weeks and three months to heal completely. At the end of this period, they should have their regular eyeglasses checked to see if their lens prescription should be changed. Patients can carry out their normal activities within one to two days after surgery, with the exception of heavy lifting, severe chronic coughing, or extreme bending. Most ophthalmologists recommend that patients wear their eyeglasses during the day and tape an eye shield over the operated eye at night. They should wear sunglasses on bright days and avoid rubbing or bumping the operated eye. In addition, the ophthalmologist will prescribe eye drops for one to two weeks to prevent infection, manage pain, and reduce swelling. It is important for patients to use these eye drops exactly as directed.

Patients recovering from cataract surgery will be scheduled for frequent checkups in the first few weeks following ECCE. In most cases, the ophthalmologist will check the patient's eye the day after surgery and about once a week for the next several weeks.

About 25% of patients who have had a cataract removed by either extracapsular method will eventually develop clouding in the lens capsule that was left in place to hold the new IOL. This clouding, which is known as posterior capsular opacification (PCO), is not a new cataract but may still interfere with vision. It is thought to be caused by the growth of epithelial cells left behind after the lens was removed. PCO is treated by capsulotomy, which is a procedure in which the surgeon uses a laser to cut through the clouded part of the capsule.

Risks

The risks of extracapsular cataract extraction include:

- Edema (swelling) of the cornea.
- A rise in intraocular pressure (IOP).
- Uveitis, which refers to inflammation of the layer of eye tissue that includes the iris.
- Infection of the external eye may develop into endophthalmitis, or infection of the interior of the eye.
- Hyphema, which refers to the presence of blood inside the anterior chamber of the eye and is most common within the first two to three days after cataract surgery.
- Leaking or rupture of the incision.
- Retinal detachment (RD) or tear. The risk of RD appears to be increased in patients for as long as 20 years after extracapsular cataract extraction.
- Malpositioning of the IOL. This complication can be corrected by surgery.
- Cystoid macular edema (CME). The macula is a small yellowish depression on the retina that may be affected after cataract surgery by fluid collecting within the tissue layers. The typical symptoms are blurring or distortion of central vision. CME rarely causes loss of sight, but may take between two and 15 months to resolve completely.

Normal results

Extracapsular cataract extraction is one of the safest and most successful procedures in contemporary eye surgery; about 95% of patients report that their vision is substantially improved after the operation.

Morbidity and mortality rates

Mortality as a direct result of cataract surgery is very rare. On the other hand, several studies have indicated that patients over the age of 50 who undergo cataract extraction have higher rates of mortality in the year following surgery than other patients in the same age group who have other types of **elective surgery**. Some researchers have interpreted these data to imply that cataracts related to the aging process reflect some kind of systemic weakness rather than a disorder limited to the eye.

About 23% of patients who have undergone cataract extraction have a postoperative complication. The majority of these, however, are not vision-threatening. The most common complication is swelling of the cornea (9.5%), followed by raised IOP (7.9%); uveitis (5.6%); leaking from the incision (1.2%); hyphema (1.1%); external eye infection (0.06%); endophthalmitis (0.03%); retinal detachment (0.03%); retinal tear (0.02%), and CME (0.017%). Of these complications, only endophthalmitis and retinal detachment or tear are considered potentially vision-threatening.

Standard ECCE and phacoemulsification have similar success rates and complication rates when performed by surgeons of comparable skill and length of experience, although a meta-analysis of 17 trials of these two methods reported in 2006 that phacoemulsification gives a better long-term outcome than standard ECCE with sutures.

Alternatives

Medical treatment

As of 2007, there are no medications that can prevent or cure cataracts. Many ophthalmologists, however, recommend a well-balanced diet as beneficial to the eyes as well as the rest of the body, on the grounds that some studies suggest that poor nutritional status is a risk factor for cataract. While vitamin supplements do not prevent cataracts, there is some evidence that an adequate intake of vitamins A, C, and E helps to slow the rate of cataract progression. Elderly people who may be at risk of inadequate vitamin intake due to loss of appetite and other reasons may benefit from supplemental doses of these vitamins.

Watchful waiting

Not all cataracts need to be removed. A patient whose cataracts are not interfering with his or her normal activities and are progressing slowly may choose to postpone surgery indefinitely. It is important, however, to have periodic checkups to make sure that the cataract is not growing in size or density. In the recent past, surgeons often advised patients to put off surgical treatment until the cataract had "ripened," which meant that the patient had to wait until the cataract had caused significant vision loss and was interfering with reading, driving, and most daily activities. At present, ophthalmologists prefer to remove cataracts before they get to this stage because they are harder and consequently more difficult to remove. In addition, a rapidly growing cataract that is not treated surgically may lead to swelling of the lens, secondary

WHO PERFORMS THE PROCEDURE AND WHERE IS IT PERFORMED?

Cataract surgery is performed by ophthalmologists, who are physicians that have completed four to five years of specialized training following medical school in the medical and surgical treatment of eye disorders. Ophthalmology is one of 24 specialties recognized by the American Board of Medical Specialties.

If cataract surgery is being considered, it is a good idea to find out how many extracapsular extractions the surgeon performs each year. The greatest single factor in the success rate of ECCE procedures is not whether the surgeon performs a standard extraction or phacoemulsification, but the volume of operations that he or she performs. Surgeons who perform between 200 and 400 extracapsular extractions per year have higher rates of successful outcomes than those who perform fewer than 200.

Extracapsular cataract extractions are done as outpatient procedures, either in the ophthalmologist's office or in an ambulatory surgery center.

glaucoma, and eventual blindness. In most cases, however, it is up to the patient to decide when the cataract is troublesome enough to schedule surgery.

Surgical alternatives

The major surgical alternative to ECCE is intracapsular cataract extraction, or ICCE. It is rarely performed at present in Europe and North America, but is still done in countries where operating microscopes and high-technology equipment are not always available. In ICCE, the surgeon makes an incision about 150 degrees of arc, or about half the circumference of the cornea, in order to extract the lens and its capsule in one piece. The surgeon then inserts a cryoprobe, which is an instrument for applying extreme cold to eye tissue. The cryoprobe is placed on the lens capsule, where it freezes into place. It is then used to slowly pull the capsule and lens together through the long incision around the cornea. Because of the length of the incision needed to perform ICCE and the pressure placed on the vitreous body, the procedure has a relatively high rate of complications. In addition, the recovery period is much longer than for standard ECCE or phacoemulsification.

- What type of cataract do I have and how fast is it developing?
- Would you recommend watchful waiting to see if surgery is necessary?
- How many cataract extractions do you perform each year, and what technique do you use?
- What is your success rate with cataract extractions?

Resources

BOOKS

Henderson, Bonnie An, ed. *Essentials of Cataract Surgery.* Thorofare, NJ: SLACK, 2007.

Malhotra, Raman, ed. *Cataract: Assessment, Classification, and Management.* New York: Elsevier, Butterworth Heinemann, 2007.

PERIODICALS

Erie, J. C., M. E. Raecker, K. H. Baratz, et al. "Risk of Retinal Detachment after Cataract Extraction, 1980–2004: A Population-based Study." *Transactions of the American Ophthalmological Society* 104 (2006): 167–175.

Guzek, J. P., and A. Ching. "Small-Incision Manual Extracapsular Cataract Surgery in Ghana, West Africa." *Journal of Cataract and Refractive Surgery* 29 (January 2003): 57–64.

Kalpadakis, P., et al. "A Comparison of Endophthalmitis After Phacoemulsification or Extracapsular Cataract Extraction in a Socio-Economically Deprived Environment: A Retrospective Analysis of 2,446 Patients." *European Journal of Ophthalmology* 12 (September–October 2002): 395–400.

Menabuoni, L., R. Pini, F. Rossi, et al. "Laser-assisted Corneal Welding in Cataract Surgery: Retrospective Study." *Journal of Cataract and Refractive Surgery* 33 (September 2007): 1608–1612.

Riaz, Y., J. S. Mehta, R. Wormald, et al. "Surgical Interventions for Age-Related Cataract." *Cochrane Database of Systematic Reviews*, October 18, 2006: CD001323.

Rowden, A., and R. Krishna. "Resident Cataract Surgical Training in United States Residency Programs." *Journal of Cataract and Refractive Surgery* 28 (December 2002): 2202–2205.

Smith, J. H. "Teaching Phacoemulsification in US Ophthalmology Residencies: Can the Quality Be Maintained?" *Current Opinion in Ophthalmology* 16 (February 2005): 27–32.

Thomas, R., T. Kuriakose, and R. George. "Towards Achieving Small-Incision Cataract Surgery 99.8% of the Time." *Indian Journal of Ophthalmology* 48 (June 2000): 145–151.

ORGANIZATIONS

American Academy of Ophthalmology. P. O. Box 7424, San Francisco, CA 94120-7424. (415) 561-8500. http://www.aao.org (accessed March 22, 2008).

American Optometric Association. 243 North Lindbergh Blvd., St. Louis, MO 63141. (314) 991-4100.

American Society of Cataract and Refractive Surgery (ASCRS). 4000 Legato Road, Suite 700, Fairfax, VA 22033. (703) 591-2220. http://www.ascrs.org (accessed March 22, 2008).

Canadian Ophthalmological Society (COS). 610-1525 Carling Avenue, Ottawa ON K1Z 8R9. http://www.eyesite.ca (accessed March 22, 2008).

National Eye Institute. 2020 Vision Place, Bethesda, MD 20892-3655. (301) 496-5248. http://www.nei.nih.gov (accessed March 22, 2008).

Prevent Blindness America. 211 West Wacker Drive, Suite 1700, Chicago, IL 60606. (800) 331-2020. http://www.prevent-blindness.org (accessed March 22, 2008).

Wills Eye Institute. 840 Walnut Street, Philadelphia, PA 19107. (877) 289-4557. http://www.willseye.org (accessed March 22, 2008).

OTHER

D'Ocampo, Vicente Victor, and C. Stephen Foster. "Cataract, Senile." *eMedicine* September 15, 2005 [January 1, 2008]. http://www.emedicine.com/oph/topic49.htm (accessed March 22, 2008).

National Eye Institute (NEI). *Are You at Risk for Cataract?* Bethesda, MD: NEI, 2001. NIH Publication No. 94-3463.

National Eye Institute (NEI). *Cataract.* Bethesda, MD: NEI, 2007. NIH Publication No. 03-201.

Royal College of Ophthalmologists. *Cataract Surgery Guidelines.* London, UK: Royal College of Ophthalmologists, 2005. http://www.rcophth.ac.uk/docs/publications/CataractSurgeryGuidelinesMarch2005Updated.pdf (accessed March 22, 2008).

Rebecca Frey, PhD

Extracorporeal shock-wave therapy *see* **Lithotripsy**

Eye muscle surgery

Definition

Eye muscle surgery is performed to weaken, strengthen, or reposition any of the extraocular muscles (small muscles) located on the surface of the eye that move the eyeball in all directions.

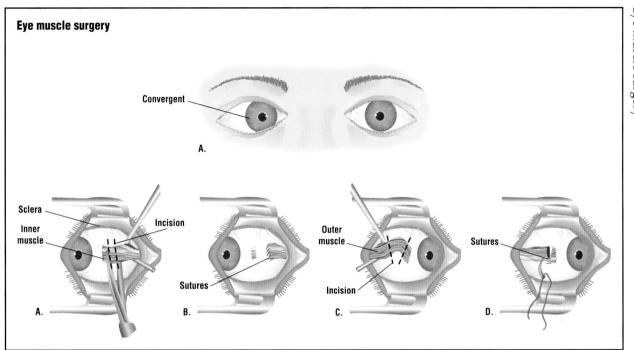

Eye muscle surgery

To repair a convergent gaze, the ophthalmogist cuts the muscles that move the eye from side to side (A). On one side, the muscles are attached further back on the eyeball (B). On the other, the muscle is shortened (C) and stitched (D). *(Illustration by GGS Information Services. Cengage Learning, Gale.)*

Purpose

The extraocular muscles attach via tendons to the sclera (the white, opaque, outer protective covering of the eyeball) at different places just behind an imaginary equator circling the top, bottom, left, and right of the eye. The other end of each of these muscles attaches to a part of the orbit (the eye socket in the skull). These muscles enable the eyes to move up, down, to one side or the other, or any angle in between.

Normally, both eyes move together, receiving the same image on corresponding locations on both retinas. The brain fuses these matching images into one three-dimensional image. The exception is in strabismus, which is a disorder where one or both eyes deviate out of alignment, most often outwardly (exotropia) or toward the nose (esotropia). In this case, the brain receives two different images, and either suppresses one or allows the person to see double (diplopia). By weakening or strengthening the appropriate muscles to center the eyes, a person can correct this deviation. For example, if an eye turns upward, the muscle at the bottom of the eye could be strengthened.

The main purpose of eye muscle surgery is thus to restore straight eye alignment. The surgery is performed to align both eyes so that they gaze in the same direction and move together as a team; to improve appearance; and to promote the development of binocular vision in a young child. To achieve binocular vision, the eyes must align so that the location of the image on the retina of one eye corresponds to the location of the image on the retina of the other eye.

In addition to being used to correct strabismus, eye muscle surgery is also performed to treat other eye disorders such as nystagmus or special types of congenital strabismus such as Duane syndrome. Nystagmus is a condition in which one or both eyes move rapidly or oscillate; this condition can be improved by moving the eyes to the position of least oscillation. Duane syndrome is a disorder in which there is limited horizontal eye movement; it can sometimes be relieved by surgery that weakens an eye muscle.

Demographics

According to doctors at the Wills Eye Hospital, Philadelphia, the most common divergent strabismus in childhood has a variable onset, often between six months and four years. The disorder occurs in 1.2% of children by seven years of age and occurs equally in males and females.

Duane syndrome commonly affects girls more often than boys, and the left eye more often than the right eye.

Congenital nystagmus is thought to be present at birth, but is usually not apparent until the child is a few months old. Acquired nystagmus occurs later than six months of age, and can be caused by stroke, diseases such as multiple sclerosis, or even a heavy blow to the head. It is not known how many people suffer from nystagmus, but it is thought to be one in 1,000 adults, and one in 640 children in the United States, according to the Nystagmus Network.

Description

The procedure used by the surgeon depends on the condition that needs correcting. During surgery, eye muscles can be:

- Weakened. This usually involves recessing the eye muscle or moving it posteriorly on the eye to elongate the muscle and allow the muscle tissue to relax.
- Tightened. Muscles are tightened by resection, which involves removing a piece of the muscle near its point of insertion and then reinserting the muscle into its original location. By removing a piece of muscle, the muscle is shortened and therefore strengthened.

- Repositioned. For some forms of strabismus, the eye muscles are neither weakened nor strengthened, but repositioned: i.e., the muscle's point of insertion is moved to a different location.

There are two methods to alter extraocular muscles. Traditional surgery can be used to strengthen, weaken, or reposition an extraocular muscle. The surgeon first makes an incision in the conjunctiva (the clear membrane covering the sclera), then puts a suture into the muscle to hold it in place, and loosens the muscle from the eyeball with a surgical hook. During a resection, the muscle is detached from the sclera, a piece of muscle is removed so that the muscle is now shorter, and the muscle is reattached to the same place. This strengthens the muscle. In a recession, the muscle is made weaker by repositioning it. More than one extraocular eye muscle might be operated on at the same time.

Eye muscle surgery is performed with the eye in its normal position and usually takes an hour and a half. At no time during the operation is the eye removed from the socket. The surgeon determines where to reattach the muscles based on eye measurements taken before surgery. Most of the time, it can hardly be seen except with magnification.

Diagnosis/Preparation

Depth perception (stereopsis) in humans develops around the age of three months. For successful development of binocular vision and the ability to perceive three-dimensionally, eye muscle surgery should not be postponed past the age of four years. The earlier the surgery, the better the outcome, so an early diagnosis is important. Surgery may even be performed before the child is two years old.

Patients (or their caregivers) should make sure their doctors are aware of any medications that they are taking, even over-the-counter medications. Patients should not take **aspirin**, or any other blood-thinning medications for 10 days prior to surgery, and should not eat or drink after midnight the night before.

Aftercare

After surgery, the eyes feel scratchy, but not very painful. Patients must be kept from rubbing their eyes. The eyes are also a little red and watery. There may be some hemorrhage under the conjunctival membrane over the white of the eye that usually settles over a period of two to three weeks. It usually takes on a yellowish discoloration similar to a bruise as it clears. Sometimes there is some thickening of the membranes over the eye, which can take several more weeks to clear. Very fine dissolving sutures are used to reposition the conjunctival membrane at the end of surgery and, until these sutures dissolve, there may be some scratchiness in the eyes. This feeling usually disappears after two or three weeks.

There will also be some swelling and discharge after the surgery. The swelling is usually minor, and patients should be able to open their eyes within the next two days, as the swelling should gradually disappear.

Patients will need someone to drive them home after the operation. They should continue to avoid aspirin and other nonsteroidal anti-inflammatory agents for an additional three days, but they can take **acetaminophen** (e.g., Tylenol). Patients should discuss what medications they can or cannot take with the surgeon. Pain will subside after two or three days, and patients can resume most normal activities within a few days. Again, the period of recovery may vary with the patient, and the patient can discuss with the surgeon when to return to normal activities. Patients should not get their eyes wet for three to four days and should refrain from swimming for 10 days. Eyes receiving surgery will be red for about two weeks.

Adults and children over the age of six often experience double vision for a limited period of time after surgery. Children younger than six sometimes will have double vision for a short period of time. Double vision is rarely permanent.

Patients generally do not have to wear patches after surgery, although occasionally a temporary patch may be recommended. They are usually required to use eye drops for a week until the follow-up examination. If the eye is healing on schedule, then the eye drops are usually discontinued at that stage. A further postoperative appointment is usually made for six to eight weeks later, by which time the eye will have stabilized.

After surgery for strabismus, the patient usually needs corrective lenses and eye exercises (vision therapy) if binocular vision is to develop.

Risks

As with any surgery, there are risks involved. Eye muscle surgery is relatively safe, but very rarely a cut muscle cannot be retrieved. This, and other serious reactions, including those caused by anesthetics, can result in vision loss in the affected eye. Occasionally, retinal or nerve damage occurs. Permanent double vision is also a risk of eye muscle surgery. The success rate of this surgery varies from person to person and depends on each person's particular condition.

Some infrequent complications include, but are not limited to, allergy to the sutures, bleeding, and change in pupil size.

The major risk of eye muscle surgery is failure to achieve a satisfactory alignment of the eyes. This may be an under-correction or an over-correction, with the eyes turning the other way after the operation. Surgeons aim to achieve perfect alignment, but this is not always possible. If the alignment is still unsatisfactory at the final postoperative visit, then a second operation may be required.

Infection is an unusual postoperative complication and can be treated with antibiotic drops.

Because an incision is made through the conjunctiva and muscle, there is always some residual scarring. Usually, this is detectable only under a microscope, although it may be possible to see it on close examination.

As with any eye surgery, there is a potential risk of visual loss from strabismus operations, but this is a very rare complication.

Normal results

Normal results of eye muscle surgery are an improved alignment of the eyes and improved cosmetic appearance without complications. The surgery usually has a very good outcome.

Morbidity and mortality rates

Cosmetic improvement is likely with success rate estimates varying from about 65–85%. According to the latest statistics from 1998, binocular vision is improved in young children about 35% of the time following eye muscle surgery. Between 15% and 35% of patients have either no improvement or a worsening of their condition. A second operation may rectify less-than-perfect outcomes.

Alternatives

Surgery is not the only treatment to correct eye muscle disorders. Options and outcomes vary considerably based on several factors such as the presence of double vision. Nonsurgical treatment is also available, such as orthoptics and vision therapy.

Orthoptics

Orthoptics is a medical term for the eye muscle training programs provided by orthoptists and optometrists. Vision therapy programs include orthoptics, but there are broad differences between vision therapy and orthoptics. Orthoptics dates back to the 1850s and is limited in scope to eye muscle training and the cosmetic straightening of eyes. Orthoptics treat muscle problems by considering only strength; it does not focus on neurological and visual-motor factors as vision therapy does. Treatment is home based.

Vision therapy

Vision therapy is an individualized, supervised, non-surgical treatment program designed to correct eye movements and visual-motor deficiencies. Vision therapy sessions include procedures designed to enhance the brain's ability to control:

- eye alignment
- eye teaming
- eye focusing abilities
- eye movements
- visual processing

Visual-motor skills and endurance may be developed through the use of specialized computer and optical devices, including therapeutic lenses, prisms, and filters. During the final stages of therapy, the patient's newly acquired visual skills are reinforced and made automatic through repetition and by integration with motor and cognitive skills.

Resources

BOOKS

Dyer, J. A., and D. A. Lee. *Atlas of Extraocular Muscle Surgery.* Westport, CT: Praeger Publishers, 1984.

Good, William V., and Craig S. Hoyt. *Strabismus Management.* Boston: Butterworth-Hienemann, 1996.

Roth, A., and C. Speeg-Schatz, eds. *Eye Muscle Surgery.* Lisse, The Netherlands: Swets & Zeitlinger, 2001.

Salmans, Sandra. *Your Eyes: Questions You Have...Answers You Need.* Allentown, PA: People's Medical Society, 1996.

von Noorden, Gunter K. *Binocular Vision and Ocular Motility: Theory and Management of Strabismus,* 5th edition. St. Louis: Mosby-Year Book, 1996.

PERIODICALS

Bosman, J., M. P. ten Tusscher, I. de Jong, J. S. Vles, and H. Kingma. "The Influence of Eye Muscle Surgery on Shape and Relative Orientation of Displacement Planes: Indirect Evidence for Neural Control of 3D Eye Movements." *Strabismus* 10 (September 2002): 199–209.

Mayr, H. "Virtual Eye Muscle Surgery Based upon Biomechanical Models." *Studies in Health and Technology Information* 81 (2001): 305–311.

Murray, T. "Eye Muscle Surgery." *Current Opinion in Ophthalmology* 11 (October 2000): 336–341.

Rubsam, B., W. D. Schafer, B. Schulte, and N. Roewer. "Preliminary Report: Analgesia with Remifentanil for Complicated Eye Muscle Surgery." *Strabismus* 8 (December 2000): 287–289.

Watts, J. C. "Total Intravenous Anesthesia Without Muscle Relaxant for Eye Surgery in a Patient with Kugelberg-Welander Syndrome." *Anaesthesia* 58 (January 2003): 96.

ORGANIZATIONS

American Academy of Ophthalmology. 655 Beach Street, P.O. Box 7424, San Francisco, CA 94120-7424. http://www.eyenet.org.

American Academy of Pediatric Ophthalmology and Strabismus (AAPOS). <http://med-aapos.bu.edu>.

OTHER

Olitsky, Scott E., and Leonard B. Nelson. *Strabismus Web Book.*www.members.aol.com/scottolitsky/webbook.htm.

*Kellogg Eye Center: Eye Muscle Surgery.*www.kellogg.umich.edu/patient/surg/eyemuscle.html.

*Pediatric Ophthalmic Consultants Webpage: Strabismus Surgery.*www.pedseye.com/StrabSurg.htm.

Lorraine Lica, PhD
Monique Laberge, PhD

Eye surgery *see* **Ophthalmologic surgery**
Eyeball removal *see* **Enucleation, eye**
Eyelid plastic surgery *see* **Blepharoplasty**
Eyelid surgery *see* **Tarsorrhaphy**

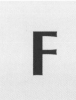

F

Face lift

Definition

Face lift surgery is a cosmetic procedure that involves removing sagging skin and tightening muscle tissue of the face and neck to counter signs of aging. The procedure is also called facialplasty, rhytidoplasty, and cervicofacial rhytidectomy.

Purpose

The purpose of face lift surgery is to improve the appearance of the face by repositioning the skin and tightening some of the underlying muscle and tissue. The procedure is designed to counter sagging and looseness in skin and muscle tissue that becomes more pronounced as individuals age. Face lift surgery will not eliminate all facial wrinkles. For example, wrinkles around the mouth and eyes may benefit little from face lift surgery. Also, additional procedures including **blepharoplasty**, chemical peel, botox injections, or **dermabrasion** may be necessary to achieve desired results.

Demographics

The American Society for Aesthetic Plastic Surgery estimated that nearly 6.9 million cosmetic surgical and nonsurgical procedures were performed in the United States in 2002. The number of face lift procedures increased by 6% from the previous year (2001). Among members of the American Academy of Cosmetic Surgery, 15,478 face lift procedures were performed. The average fee for a face lift in 2002 was $7,000. The American Society of Plastic Surgeons reported that a total of 1,852,012 cosmetic procedures and 9,138,275 nonsurgical procedures were performed in the United States in 2006, totaling almost 11 million procedures. Of that number, 104,055 were face lift procedures.

Description

A face lift takes about two hours and may be performed as an outpatient procedure or it may require hospitalization. General or local anesthetics will be used to sedate the patient. Typically, patients receiving **local anesthesia** will augment it with "twilight anesthesia," an intravenous sedative that helps to lower their awareness of the procedure being performed. An anesthesiologist will be present to administer the anesthetics and assist in monitoring and maintaining the patient's vital life functions.

The surgeon makes an incision within the hairline just above the ear. The incision continues down along the front edge of the ear, around the earlobe, and then up and behind the ear extending back into the hairline. The location of this incision is designed to hide any sign of the procedure later. The same procedure is repeated on the other side of the face. The surgeon separates the skin of the face from its underlying tissue, moving down to the cheek and into the neck area and below the chin. Fat deposits over the cheeks and in the neck may be removed surgically or with **liposuction** at this time. The surgeon tightens certain bands of muscle and tissue that extend up from the shoulder, below the chin, and up and behind the neck. If these muscles and tissue are not tightened, the looseness and sagging appearance of the skin will return. The surgeon trims excess skin from the edges of the original incision and the skin is pulled back into place. The incision is closed with sutures or **staples**.

Diagnosis/Preparation

Prior to the procedure, candidates meet with the surgeon to discuss the procedure, clarify the results that can be achieved, and the potential problems that can occur. Having realistic expectations is important in any cosmetic procedure. People will learn, for example, that although a face lift can improve the contour of the face and neck, other procedures will be necessary to reduce the appearance of many wrinkles. Candidates will be advised to stop taking **aspirin**, birth control pills or female hormones, and other medications affecting blood clotting two weeks before the procedure. Some physicians prescribe vitamin C and K to promote healing. Candidates are advised to stop smoking and to avoid exposure to passive smoke at least two weeks before and after the procedure. Some surgeons also recommend taking **antibiotics** prior to surgery to limit the risk of infection. Often a steroid injection is administered before or after the procedure to reduce swelling.

Aftercare

A pressure bandage is applied to the face to reduce the risk of hematoma, which is a pocket of blood below the skin. The person may spend a few hours resting in a **recovery room** to ensure that no bleeding has occurred. The individual then returns home. Some surgeons recommend that people stay in a reclining position for the 24 hours immediately following surgery, consuming a liquid diet, and avoiding flexing or bending the neck. Ice packs for the first few days can help to reduce swelling and lower the risk of hematoma. Individuals continue taking antibiotics until the first **stitches** come out about five days after the procedure. The remaining sutures are removed seven to ten days later. Many people return to work and limited activities within two weeks of the procedure.

Risks

Candidates with other medical conditions should consult with their primary care physician before undergoing a face lift. Lung problems, heart disease, and certain other conditions can lead to a higher risk of complications. Persons who use medications that affect blood clotting (including female hormones, aspirin, and some non-aspirin pain relievers) should stop taking these medications prior to surgery to lower the risk that a hematoma will form. A hematoma is the most frequent complication of face lifts. Most hematomas

form within 48 hours of surgery. The typical sign is pain or swelling affecting one side of the face but not the other.

Another risk is nerve damage. Sometimes it can affect a person's ability to raise an eyebrow, or distort the smile, or result in limited sensation in the earlobe; however, most of these nerve injuries repair themselves within two to six months.

Normal results

Some swelling and bruising is normal following a face lift. There should be a noticeable improvement in the contour of the face and neck. Some fine wrinkling of the skin may be improved, but deep wrinkles are likely to require another cosmetic procedure to improve their appearance.

Morbidity and mortality rates

In general, mortality and morbidity rates for face lifts and similar facial cosmetic procedures are very low. Almost all cases of mortality following facial **cosmetic surgery** involve patients who were treated for facial disfigurement because they had been severely burned or attacked by animals. Moreover, many plastic surgeons do not consider morbidity and mortality rates to be as significant as other factors in evaluating the success of facial cosmetic procedures. One group of researchers at the University of Washington maintains that "[t]he most important measures of outcome in facial cosmetic surgery are quality of life and patient satisfaction, in contrast to other, more objective measures such as complications or mortality rates."

Alternatives

Isometric exercises are recommended as non-surgical alternatives to face lift procedures.

Injections of Botox (botulinum toxin) have been used to achieve the same results as a face lift. Botulinum toxin is a compound produced by the spores and

QUESTIONS TO ASK THE DOCTOR

- How will I be evaluated as a potential candidate for a facelift?
- What will I look like after the surgery?
- When will I be able to resume normal activities after my procedure?
- Will my incisions be noticeable and how long will they take to heal?
- Is the surgeon board certified in plastic and reconstructive surgery?
- How many face lifts has the surgeon performed?
- May I see some before and after photos of the surgeon's facelift procedures?
- What is the surgeon's complication rate?

growing cells of the organism that causes botulism, *Clostridium botulinum*. The toxin causes muscle paralysis. It was first used clinically in the 1960s to treat neurological disorders but also proved to be effective in paralyzing the facial muscles that cause crow's feet and frown wrinkles. Botulinum toxin, or Botox, was approved by the U.S. Food and Drug Administration (FDA) in April 2002 as a treatment for facial lines and wrinkles. Botox treatments must be repeated in approximately six months.

Coherent ultrapulse carbon dioxide laser treatment is a promising new treatment alternative to traditional face lift procedures. As of 2003, this equipment has been used by a few major institutions.

Some plastic surgeons have used a procedure called fat rebalancing to achieve outcomes similar to a traditional face lift procedure. Fat rebalancing involves relocation of fatty tissue from distant sites on the body to the face.

Resources

BOOKS

Engler, Alan M. *BodySculpture: Plastic Surgery of the Body for Men and Women,* 2nd ed. New York: Hudson Publishing, 2000.

Irwin, Brandith, and Mark McPherson. *Your Best Face Without Surgery.* Carlsbad, CA: Hay House Inc., 2002.

Man, Daniel. *New Art of Man.* New York: BeautyArt Press, 2003.

Papel, I. D., J. Frodel, G. R. Holt, W. F. Larrabee, N. Nachlas, S. S. Park, J. M. Sykes, and D. Toriumi. *Facial Plastic and Reconstructive Surgery,* 2nd ed. New York: Thieme Medical Publishers, 2002.

PERIODICALS

Bisson, M. A., R. Grover, and A. O. Grobbelaar. "Long-term results of facial rejuvenation by carbon dioxide laser resurfacing using a quantitative method of assessment." *British Journal of Plastic Surgery* 55, no. 8 (December 2002): 652–656.

Byrd, H. S., and J. D. Burt. "Achieving aesthetic balance in the brow, eyelids, and midface." *Plastic and Reconstructive Surgery* 110, no. 3 (September 2002): 926–939.

Donofrio, L. M. "Fat rebalancing: the new 'Facelift.'" *Skin Therapy Letter* 7, no. 9 (November 2002): 7–9.

Morgenstern, K. E. and J. A. Foster. "Advances in cosmetic oculoplastic surgery." *Current Opinion in Ophthalmology* 13, no. 5 (October 2002): 324–330.

OTHER

Atisha, Dunya. "Face Lift." Online Surgery. http://www.onlinesurgery.com/procedures/face_lift.php (March 23, 2003).

"Cosmetic Surgery." Mayo Clinic. http://www.mayoclinic.org/cosmetic-surgery/ (March 30, 2008).

"Plastic and Cosmetic Surgery." Medline Plus. March 24, 2008. http://www.nlm.nih.gov/medlineplus/plasticcosmeticsurgery.html (March 23, 2003).

ORGANIZATIONS

American Academy of Facial Plastic and Reconstructive Surgery, 310 S. Henry Street, Alexandria, VA, 22314, (703) 229-9291, http://www.aafprs.org/.

American Board of Plastic Surgery, Seven Penn Center, Suite 400 1635 Market Street, Philadelphia, PA, 19103-2204, (215) 587-9322, http://www.abplsurg.org/.

American College of Surgeons, 633 North Saint Claire Street, Chicago, IL, 60611, (312) 202-5000, http://www.facs.org/.

American Society for Aesthetic Plastic Surgery, 11081 Winners Circle, Los Alamitos, CA, 90720, (888) 272-7711, http://www.surgery.org/.

American Society for Dermatologic Surgery, 5550 Meadowbrook Drive, Suite 120, Rolling Meadows, IL, 60008, (847) 956-0900, http://www.asds.net.

American Society of Plastic and Reconstructive Surgeons, 444 E. Algonquin Road, Arlington Heights, IL, 60005, (847) 228-9900, http://www.plasticsurgery.org.

L. Fleming Fallon, Jr., M.D., Dr.P.H.
Laura Jean Cataldo, R.N., Ed.D.

Fallopian tube implants

Definition

In the female reproductive tract there are two ovaries and two fallopian tubes. The fallopian tube is the path through which the egg passes after ovulation and potentially on the way to fertilization. If the fallopian tube is blocked, then the egg cannot pass through to become fertilized. One method of contraception is the use of fallopian tube implants. These are tiny metal springs that are placed in each fallopian tube. Scar tissue forms around these springs and blocks the transport of the egg through the fallopian tube.

Purpose

The purpose of fallopian tube implants is to create a permanent method of contraception. Many women who choose tubal implants for permanent contraception do so because they do not desire the side effects or risks of other methods of birth control.

Precautions

After tubal implant surgery another method of birth control needs to be used until it is confirmed that the fallopian tubes are in fact blocked, which is usually confirmed approximately three months after the fallopian tube implants are inserted.

Description

Fallopian tube implants are inserted without surgery. The procedure is done on an outpatient basis and does not usually take more than 30-60 minutes. During the procedure, the woman is placed in the same position as during a yearly pelvic exam. On occasion a physician may insert laminaria into the cervix several hours prior to the procedure, to gradually open the cervix. Laminaria are small sticks of dehydrated seaweed that slowly absorb moisture and gradually expand to open the cervix. If laminaria is not used prior to the procedure, then during the procedure, instruments are used to gradually open the cervix. A catheter is placed through the cervical opening and into the fallopian tube where the small metal spring is placed. This is repeated for the other fallopian tube. After the procedure an x ray is performed to make sure that both implants are properly placed.

Preparation

No special preparation for the procedure is needed. It is important, however, to make certain that the decision to have fallopian tube implants has been thoroughly discussed because this method of contraception is permanent.

Aftercare

After the procedure menstrual-like cramping may occur. As stated above, an x ray is performed after the procedure to make sure that the implants are properly placed. Approximately three months after the procedure, a follow-up visit should be planned. During this follow-up visit, a hysterosalpingogram will be performed. For a hysterosalpingogram, dye is injected into the uterus as the physician watches on the x ray to see if the dye is able to flow through the fallopian tubes. If the fallopian tube implants work, then the dye will be stopped in each fallopian tube, showing that the tubes have been blocked. On occasion, fallopian tube implants may be difficult to insert, or the hysterosalpingogram shows that the implant did not block the fallopian tube, in which case, the fallopian tube implant procedure would need to be repeated. Until it is verified that the fallopian tubes are blocked, another method of birth control needs to be used.

Risks

Fallopian tube implants are a new method of birth control that became available in 2002, therefore, there are no long-term statistics available on how effective they are at preventing pregnancy. Other methods of tubal contraception are not 100% effective at preventing pregnancy. There has been one reported confirmation of a pregnancy after a tubal implant and after confirmation by hysterosalpingram that the fallopian tube were blocked. If a tubal implant fails, there is an increased risk for ectopic pregnancy. An ectopic pregnancy occurs when the fertilized egg implants in the fallopian tube or in a place other than the uterus. Fallopian tube implants do not affect the menstrual cycle, and therefore, if a woman misses her menstrual period, or has other symptoms of pregnancy, she should contact her physician immediately.

Resources

BOOKS

Caughey, Aaron B., Arzou Ahsan, et al. *Blueprints Obstetrics and Gynecology,* 4th edition: Lippincott, Williams and Wilkins, 2006.

PERIODICALS

Ory, E. M., Hines, R. S., Cleland, W. H., Rehberg, J. F. "Pregnancy after microinsert sterilization with tubal occlusion confirmed by hysterosalpingogram." *Obstetrics and Gynecology.* 111 (2 PT 2) (2008): 508–510.

Wittmer, M. H., Famuyide, A. O., Creeden, D. J., Hartman, R. P. "Hysterosalpingography for assessing efficacy of Essure microinsert permanent birth control device." *American Journal of Roentgenology* 187, no. 4 (2006): 955–958.

ORGANIZATIONS

Our Bodies Ourselves Health Resource Center, 34 Plympton Street, Boston, MA 02118. (617) 451-3666. http:// www.ourbodiesourselves.org/.

Renee Laux, M.S.

Fallopian tube ligation *see* **Tubal ligation**

Fallopian tube removal *see* **Salpingostomy**

Fasciotomy

Definition

Fasciotomy is a surgical procedure that cuts away the fascia to relieve tension or pressure.

Purpose

Fascia is thin connective tissue covering, or separating, the muscles and internal organs of the body. It varies in thickness, density, elasticity, and composition, and is different from ligaments and tendons.

The fascia can be injured either through constant strain or through trauma. Fasciitis is an inflammation of the fascia. The most common condition for which fasciotomy is performed is plantar fasciitis, an inflammation of the fascia on the bottom of the foot that is sometimes called a heel spur or stone bruise.

Plantar fasciitis is caused by long periods on one's feet, being overweight, or wearing shoes that do not support the foot well. Teachers, mail carriers, runners, and others who make heavy use of their feet are especially likely to suffer from plantar fasciitis.

Plantar fasciitis results in moderate to disabling heel pain. If nine to 12 months of conservative treatment (reducing time on feet, **nonsteroidal anti-inflammatory drugs**, arch supports) under the supervision of a doctor does not result in pain relief, a fasciotomy may be performed. Fasciotomy removes a small portion of the fascia to relieve tension and pain. Connective tissue grows back into the space left by the incision, effectively lengthening the fascia.

When a fasciotomy is performed on other parts of the body, the usual goal is to relieve pressure from a compression injury to a limb. This type of injury often occurs during contact sports or after a snake bite. Blood vessels of the limb are damaged. They swell and leak, causing inflammation. Fluid builds up in the area contained by the fascia. A fasciotomy is performed to relieve this pressure and prevent tissue **death**. Similar injury occurs in high voltage electrical burns but cause deep tissue damage.

Demographics

People who are likely to need a fasciotomy include the following:

- athletes who have sustained one or more serious impact injuries;
- people who spend long periods of time on their feet;
- people with severe burns;

KEY TERMS

Endoscope—A tube that contains a tiny camera and light, that is inserted in the body to allow a doctor to see inside without making a large incision.

Fascia—Thin connective tissue covering or separating internal organs of the body; it is different from ligaments and tendons.

Plantar fasciitis—An inflammation of the fascia on the bottom of the foot.

- persons who are overweight; and
- snakebite victims.

There is a slight male predominance among people undergoing a fasciotomy.

Description

Fasciotomy in the limbs is usually performed by a surgeon under general or regional anesthesia. An incision is made in the skin, and a small area of fascia is removed where it will best relieve pressure. Then the incision is closed.

Plantar fasciotomy is an endoscopic (performed with the use of an endoscope) procedure. The doctor makes two small incisions on either side of the heel. An endoscope is inserted in one incision to guide the doctor. A tiny knife is inserted in the other. A portion of the fascia near the heel is removed. The incisions are then closed.

Diagnosis/Preparation

In the case of injury, fasciotomy is performed on an emergency basis, and the outcome of the surgery depends largely on the general health of the injured person. Plantar fasciotomies are appropriate for most people whose foot problems cannot be resolved in any other way.

Little preparation is needed before a fasciotomy. When the fasciotomy is related to burn injuries, the fluid and electrolyte status of the affected person are constantly monitored.

Aftercare

Aftercare depends on the reason for the fasciotomy. People who have endoscopic plantar fasciotomy can walk without pain almost immediately, return to wearing their regular shoes within three to five days, and return to normal activities within three weeks. Most will need to wear arch supports in their shoes.

Persons who require fasciotomy as a result of an injury or snake bite are usually able to resume their normal activities in a few weeks.

Risks

The greatest risk with endoscopic plantar fasciotomy is that the arch will drop slightly as a result of this surgery, causing other foot problems. Risks involved with other types of fasciotomy are those associated with the administration of anesthesia and the development of blood clots or postsurgical infections.

Normal results

Fasciotomy in the limbs reduces pressure, thus reducing tissue death. Endoscopic plantar fasciotomy has a success rate in excess of 95%.

Morbidity and mortality rates

The most common morbidity in a fasciotomy is an incomplete response that requires a repeat fasciotomy procedure. Mortality is very rare and usually due to a problem related to the original condition.

Alternatives

Conservative, non-operative treatment for plantar fasciitis consists of nonsteroidal anti-inflammatory drugs for several weeks. For persons who spend excessive time on their feet, a change of occupation or the use of arch supports may be useful. Overweight individuals may consider weight reduction to reduce the stress placed on their feet. For persons bitten by a poisonous snake, there are no acceptable alternatives to a fasciotomy, and there are rarely acceptable alternatives to fasciotomy for a person who has been burned.

Resources

BOOKS

Bland, K. I., W. G. Cioffi, and M. G. Sarr. *Practice of General Surgery*. Philadelphia: Saunders, 2002.

Canale, S. T. *Campbell's Operative Orthopedics*, 10th ed. St. Louis, MO: Mosby, 2002.

Schwartz, S. I., J. E. Fischer, F. C. Spencer, G. T. Shires, and J. M. Daly. *Principles of Surgery*, 7th ed. New York: McGraw-Hill, 1998.

Townsend, C., R. D. Beauchamp, B. M. Evers, and K. L. Mattox. *Sabiston Textbook of Surgery: Board Review*, 17th ed. Philadelphia: Saunders, 2004.

PERIODICALS

Cook, S., and G. Bruce. "Fasciotomy for Chronic Compartment Syndrome in the Lower Limb." *Australia New Zealand Journal of Surgery* 72, no. 10 (October 2002): 720–723.

Fulkerson, E., A. Razi, and N. Tejwani. "Review: Acute Compartment Syndrome of the Foot." *Foot and Ankle International* 24, no. 2 (February 2003): 180–187.

Lin, Y. M. "Will Fasciotomy Help in the Patients with Crush Syndrome?" *American Journal of Kidney Diseases* 41, no. 1 (January 2003): 265–266.

Watson, T. S., R. B. Anderson, W. H. Davis, and G. M. Kiebzak. "Distal Tarsal Tunnel Release with Partial Plantar Fasciotomy for Chronic Heel Pain: An Outcome Analysis." *Foot and Ankle International* 23, no. 6 (June 2002): 530–537.

OTHER

Swain, R., and D. Ross. "Lower Extremity Compartment Syndrome." *Postgraduate Medicine Online*. March 1999. http://www.postgradmed.com/issues/1999/03_99/swain.shtml (April 2, 2003).

"What Are the Signs of Compartment Syndrome?" Yale University School of Medicine. Department of Surgery. http://yalesurgery.med.yale.edu/surgery/sections/plastics/Core%20Curriculum%20Pages/Lower%20Extremity%20Page/LegAns2.html (April 2, 2003).

ORGANIZATIONS

American Academy of Orthopaedic Surgeons, 6300 N. River Road, Rosemont, IL, 60018-4262, (847) 823-7186, (800) 346-AAOS, (847) 823-8125, http://www.aaos.org.

American College of Foot and Ankle Surgeons, 8725 West Higgins Road, Suite 555, Chicago, IL, 60631-2724, (773) 693-9300, (800) 421-2237, info@acfas.org, http://www.acfas.org/.

American College of Surgeons, 633 North Saint Claire Street, Chicago, IL, 60611, (312) 202-5000, http://www.facs.org/.

American Orthopaedic Foot and Ankle Society, 6300 N. River Road, Suite 510, Rosemont, IL, 60018, (800) 235-4855 , aofas@aofas.org, http://www.aofas.org.

American Podiatric Medical Association, 9312 Old Georgetown Road, Bethesda, MD, 20814, (301) 581-9200, http://www.apma.org.

L. Fleming Fallon, Jr., M.D., Dr.P.H.
Laura Jean Cataldo, R.N., Ed.D.

Femoral hernia repair

Definition

A femoral hernia repair, or herniorrhaphy, is a surgical procedure performed to reposition tissue that has come out through a weak point in the abdominal wall near the groin. In general, a hernia is a protrusion of a loop or piece of tissue through a weak spot or opening in the abdominal wall. There are several different kinds of hernias; they are named according to their location. A femoral hernia is one that occurs in a person's groin near the thigh. In a child, a femoral hernia is usually the result of incomplete closing of this area during development in the womb.

Purpose

Femoral hernia repair is done to reduce the patient's risk of a future surgical emergency. A hernia may be congenital (present at birth) or may develop later in life because of a weakness in the abdominal wall. If the opening is very small, the amount of tissue that can push through it is small, and the person may barely be aware of the problem. One complication that may arise, however, is that the tissue that comes out through the opening can become incarcerated, or trapped. If the herniated tissue has its blood supply diminished because of pressure from other nearby organs or structures, it is referred to as strangulated. Strangulation may lead to gangrene, which means that the affected tissue can die and be invaded by bacteria.

Femoral hernias are more likely than other hernias to become incarcerated or strangulated because the affected tissue pushes through a relatively small and closely confined space. Because of the increased risk of eventual strangulation and gangrene, the patient's doctor may recommend surgical repair of the hernia.

Demographics

Femoral hernias are a relatively uncommon type, accounting for only 3% of all hernias. While femoral hernias can occur in both males and females, almost all of them develop in women because of the wider bone structure of the female pelvis. Femoral hernias usually grow larger over time; any activity that involves straining, such as heavy lifting or a chronic cough, may cause the hernia to enlarge. Poor abdominal muscle tone, obesity, and pregnancy also increase a woman's risk of developing a femoral hernia. Most femoral hernias develop on only one side of the patient's abdomen, but about 15% of femoral hernias are bilateral. These bilateral hernias are more likely to become strangulated. An additional 20% of femoral hernias become incarcerated.

Femoral hernias are more common in adults than in children. Those that do occur in children are more likely to be associated with a connective tissue disorder or with conditions that increase intra-abdominal pressure. Seventy percent of pediatric cases of femoral hernias occur in infants under the age of one.

Description

Femoral hernia repair may be performed under either general or **local anesthesia**. The repair of the hernia involves a cut, or incision, in the groin area (near the thigh, adjacent to the femoral artery). The surgeon locates the hernia, and reduces it by pushing the protruding tissue back inside the abdominal cavity. A hernia is referred to as reducible when the tissue that has come out through the opening can be pushed back and the opening closed. If incarceration or strangulation has occurred, the hernia is referred to as irreducible.

The procedure may be performed using the traditional open method, which requires a larger surgical incision, or by a laparoscopic approach. A laparoscopic procedure is performed through a few very small incisions. The hole in the abdominal wall may be closed with sutures, or by the use of a fine sterile **surgical mesh**. The mesh, which provides additional strength, is sewn into the abdominal wall with very small **stitches**. Some surgeons may choose to use the

Femoral hernia repair

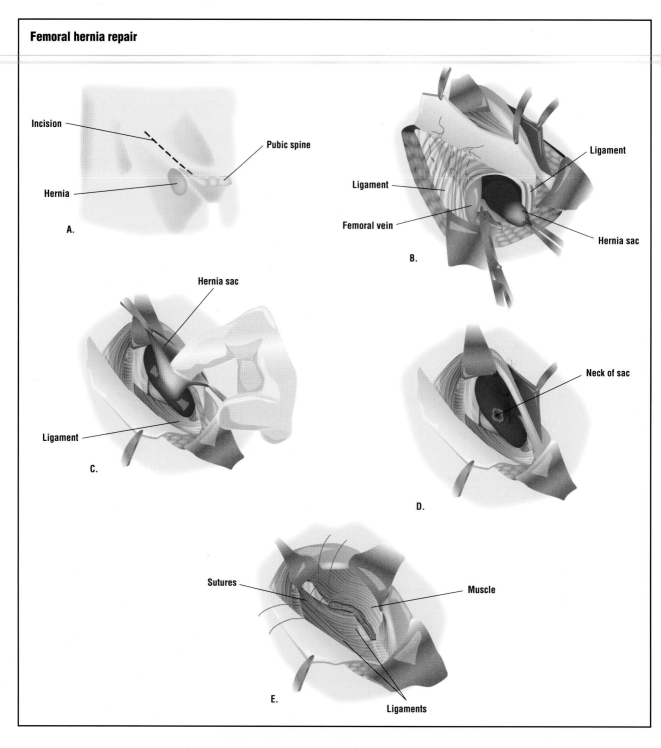

To repair a femoral hernia, an incision is made in the groin area near the hernia (A). Skin and ligaments are pulled aside to expose the hernia (B). The hernia sac is opened, and the contents are pushed back into the abdominal cavity (C). The neck of the sac is tied off, and excess tissue is removed (D). Layers of skin and tissues are repaired (E). *(Illustration by GGS Information Services. Cengage Learning, Gale.)*

mesh when repairing a larger hernia. A hernia repair done with a mesh insert is called a tension-free procedure because the surgeon does not have to put tension on the layer of muscle tissue in order to bring the edges of the hole together. A laparoscopic hernia repair takes about 40 minutes to complete.

KEY TERMS

Bilateral—Occurring on both the right and left sides of the body.

Femoral—Pertaining to the thigh region.

Gangrene—The death of a considerable mass of tissue, usually associated with loss of blood supply and followed by bacterial infection.

Hernia—The protrusion of a loop or piece of tissue through an incision or abnormal opening in other tissues. A femoral hernia is one that develops near the upper thigh in the groin area.

Herniorrhaphy—The medical term for a hernia repair.

Incarceration—The abnormal confinement of a section of the intestine or other body tissues. A femoral hernia may lead to incarceration of part of the intestine.

Intra-abdominal pressure—Pressure that occurs within the abdominal cavity. Pressure in this area builds up with coughing, crying, and the pressure exerted when bearing down with a bowel movement.

Reduction—The correction of a hernia, fracture, or dislocation.

Strangulation—A condition in which a vessel, section of the intestine, or other body part is compressed or constricted to the point that blood cannot circulate.

Diagnosis/Preparation

Diagnosis

A femoral hernia is usually diagnosed during a **physical examination**. In many cases, the patient will consult the doctor because of pain in the groin area or the inside of the upper thigh. The pain or discomfort of a femoral hernia may come and go, increasing when the person coughs or strains. If the pain is severe, the patient may go to an emergency room. In young children, symptoms of an incarcerated femoral hernia include severe irritability, abdominal pain, cramping, and vomiting. Adult patients may have also felt a mass in the groin that may be tender when it is pressed. Patients in severe pain may be given a sedative or pain-killing medication so that the doctor can examine the groin area and try to guide the herniated tissues back through the abdominal opening with gentle manual pressure.

In adult patients, the doctor will rule out the possibility that the pain is caused by an enlarged lymph node, a lipoma, or an inguinal hernia. Imaging studies are not generally used in diagnosing a hernia unless the doctor suspects that the hernia is incarcerated or strangulated. A strangulated hernia can be distinguished from an incarcerated hernia by the presence of fever, pain that persists after the doctor has reduced the hernia manually, and pain that is more severe than warranted by the examination findings.

Preparation

If the doctor suspects that the hernia is strangulated, he or she will give the patient a broad-spectrum antibiotic (usually cefoxitin) intravenously before the patient is taken to the **operating room**.

Adults scheduled for a nonemergency herniorraphy are given standard blood tests and a **urinalysis**. They should not eat breakfast on the morning of the procedure, and they should wear loose-fitting, comfortable clothing that they can easily pull on after the surgery without straining their abdomen.

Aftercare

Aftercare depends on several factors: the patient's age and general health status; the type of surgery (open or laparoscopic); and the type of anesthesia administered. Immediately after the procedure, the patient will be taken to the recovery area of the surgical center and monitored for signs of excessive bleeding, infection, uncontrolled pain, or shock. An uncomplicated femoral hernia repair is usually performed on an outpatient basis, which allows the patient to go home within a few hours of the surgery.

The patient will be given instructions about **incision care**, which will depend on the type of surgery and the way in which the incision was closed. Sometimes a transparent dressing is placed on the wound that the patient can remove about three days after the procedure. Very small incisions, such as those used for laparoscopic surgery, may be closed with Steri-strips ® instead of sutures. The incision should be kept dry, so patients should take a sponge bath rather than a shower or tub bath for several days after surgery.

Adults should avoid heavy lifting for several weeks after a hernia repair. The surgeon can give the patient advice about specific weight limits on lifting. Contact sports and vigorous **exercise** should be avoided for about three weeks after a femoral hernia repair. Many patients will be able to return to most of their daily activities in a few days, with complete recovery taking about a month in patients without other medical conditions.

Risks

All surgical procedures have associated risks, both surgical and anesthesia-related. Bleeding and infection are the two primary surgical risks. The risk of infection for an uncomplicated femoral hernia repair is about 1%. Anesthesia-related risks include reactions to the anesthetic agents, including interactions with over-the-counter and herbal preparations, as well as potential respiratory problems. There is a small risk of recurrence of a femoral hernia. In addition, female patients are at some risk of injury to the nerves and blood supply of their reproductive organs, because femoral hernias develop in a part of the abdominal wall that is close to the uterus and ovaries.

Normal results

Normal results with timely diagnosis and repair of a femoral hernia are a smooth recovery with no recurrence of the hernia.

Morbidity and mortality rates

The mortality rate following an uncomplicated femoral hernia repair is essentially zero. The mortality rate for repair of a strangulated hernia that has necessitated a **bowel resection** is higher, however, ranging from 5–19%. Morbidity following an uncomplicated herniorraphy is low; one Danish study reported that the most common complication, reported by 8% of patients, was pain during procedures performed under local anesthesia. A British study of laparoscopic hernia repairs found that only 22 out of 3017 patients reported recurrence of the hernia. The incidence of postoperative swelling and bruising was 8%.

Alternatives

There are no medical or surgical alternatives to a femoral hernia repair other than watchful waiting. There is some risk that the hernia will enlarge, however, which increases the risk of incarceration or strangulation. Moreover, the complications and risks of surgery increase with incarcerated or strangulated hernias. Once a hernia is suspected or diagnosed, it should be evaluated by a surgeon within a month to lower the risk of complications.

Resources

BOOKS

Ashcraft, Keith W. *Pediatric Surgery*. Philadelphia, PA: W. B. Saunders Company, 2000.

Delvin, David. *Coping with a Hernia*. London, UK: Sheldon Press, 1998.

PERIODICALS

Callesen, T., K. Bech, and H. Kehlet. "Feasibility of Local Infiltration Anaesthesia for Recurrent Groin Hernia Repair." *European Journal of Surgery* 167 (November 2001): 851-854.

Kapiris, S. A., W. A. Brough, C. M. Royston, et al. "Laparoscopic Transabdominal Preperitoneal (TAPP) Hernia Repair. A 7-Year Two-Center Experience in 3017 Patients." *Surgical Endoscopy* 15 (September 2001): 972-975.

Kulah, B., A. P. Duzgun, M. Moran, et al. "Emergency Hernia Repairs in Elderly Patients." *American Journal of Surgery* 182 (November 2001): 455-459.

Manthey, David, MD. "Hernias." *eMedicine*, June 22, 2001 [June 6, 2003]. www.emedicine.com/EMERG/topic251.htm.

ORGANIZATIONS

American Academy of Family Physicians. 11400 Tomahawk
Creek Parkway, Leawood, KS 66211-2672. (913) 906-
6000. E-mail: fp@aafp.org. www.aafp.org.

American Academy of Pediatrics. 141 Northwest Point
Boulevard, Elk Grove Village, IL 60007-1098. (847)
434-4000. Fax: (847) 434-8000. E-mail: kidsdoc@aap.
org. www.aap.org.

American College of Surgeons. 633 North St. Clair Street,
Chicago, IL 60611-3231. (312) 202-5000. Fax: (312)
202-5001. www.facs.org.

OTHER

Hernia Resource Center. www.herniainfo.com.
National Library of Medicine. www.nlm.nih.gov.

Esther Csapo Rastegari, RN, BSN, EdM

Femoropopliteal bypass *see* **Peripheral vascular bypass surgery**

Fetal lung maturity test *see* **Lipid tests**

Fetal surgery

Definition

Fetal surgery allows doctors to treat certain abnormalities of the fetus that might otherwise be fatal or cause significant problems if permitted to progress.

Purpose

Approximately 3% of babies born in the United States each year have a complex birth defect. Parents are often left with the options of choosing to abort the fetus or treat the condition after birth. Certain birth defects, however, are complicated by the labor and delivery process; others may progress quickly after birth to cause significant disability or **death**. Fetal surgical techniques offer early intervention in order to treat such defects before they become more serious. The first open fetal surgery took place at the University of California at San Francisco (UCSF) in 1981.

Some of the fetal abnormalities that may be treated by fetal surgery are:

- Myelomeningocele. Also called spina bifida, myelomeningocele is a condition in which the spine fails to close properly during early fetal development. The spinal cord may protrude or be exposed through an opening in the lower back. Paralysis, neurological problems, bowel and bladder problems, and hydrocephalus (fluid buildup in the brain) may result.

Myelomeningocele affects one out of every 1,000 babies born in the United States.

- Congenital diaphragmatic hernia (CDH). In babies with CDH, the diaphragm (the thin muscle that separates the chest from the abdomen) doesn't develop properly. The abdominal organs may enter the chest cavity through a hole (hernia) and cause pulmonary hyperplasia (underdeveloped lungs). CDH occurs in about one out of every 2,000 births.

- Urinary tract obstruction. The urethra (the tube that carries urine from the bladder to the outside of the body) may become obstructed *in utero* or fail to develop normally. When this happens, urine can back up into the kidneys and destroy tissue or cause the bladder to become enlarged. The amount of amniotic fluid also decreases because fetal urine is its major component. Pulmonary hypoplasia usually results because the lungs rely on amniotic fluid in their development.

- Congenital cystic adenomatoid malformation of the lung (CCAM). CCAM is a large mass of malformed lung tissue that does not function properly. As a result of its large size, it may put pressure on the heart and lead to heart failure. Lung development is also affected, and pulmonary hyperplasia may result.

- Twin/twin transfusion syndrome (TTTS). In some twin pregnancies, the two fetuses will share a placenta. TTTS occurs in approximately 15% of these twins when blood volume between the fetuses is unequal, causing abnormally low blood volume in the donor twin and abnormally high blood volume in the "recipient" twin. There is often a large difference in size between the twins. Approximately 70–80% of fetuses suffering from TTTS will die without intervention.

- Sacrococcygeal teratoma (SCT). This usually benign fetal tumor develops at the base of the spine (coccyx) and affects approximately one in 35,000 to 40,000 newborns in the United States. The tumor may become very large (sometimes as large as the fetus) and filled with blood vessels, causing stress on the heart.

Description

What fetal surgical technique is used depends on the specific condition of the fetus and its severity. The fetoscopic temporary tracheal occlusion procedure is used to treat CDH. The trachea is temporarily blocked (occluded) by a small balloon to trap fluid in the lungs (that normally escapes into the amniotic fluid); buildup of the fluid enlarges the lungs and stimulates their growth, pushing any abdominal organs that have moved into the chest cavity back into the abdomen. The occlusion is removed immediately after birth of the baby. The procedure is performed endoscopically. Rather than make a large incision into the abdomen and uterus, the surgeon inserts telescopic instruments through a tiny 1 in (2.5 cm) incision and uses them to perform the surgery. Other conditions that are treated with fetoscopic surgery are TTTS (to remove abnormal connections between blood vessels with a laser) and urinary tract obstruction (to insert a wire mesh tube called a stent into the bladder to allow urine to exit the body).

Open fetal surgery is used for conditions that cannot be treated endoscopically. An incision is made through the abdomen and the uterus is partially removed from the body. Amniotic fluid is drained from the uterus and kept in a warmer for replacement after completion of the surgery. An incision is made in the uterus (called a hysterotomy). In order to minimize bleeding of the uterus, an instrument called a uterine stapler is used to make an incision while simultaneously placing **staples** around the perimeter of the incision to prevent bleeding. Surgery is then performed on the fetus through the opening in the uterus to locate the abnormality and remove or fix it. Open fetal surgery is used for CCAM (to remove the cystic mass), myelomeningocele (to close the exposed spine), and SCT (to remove the tumor). Because of the nature of open fetal surgery, delivery for this child and all subsequent children of the mother will have to be performed by **cesarean section**.

Diagnosis/Preparation

Detection of many birth defects is possible through the use of sophisticated imaging and diagnostic techniques such as:

- Ultrasound. This imaging technique uses a machine that transmits high frequency sound waves to visualize structures in the human body, including the uterus and fetus. Ultrasound is used to determine the size, position, and age of the fetus; to measure the amount of amniotic fluid; and to assess the fetus for any congenital abnormalities.
- Chorionic villus sampling (CVS). Cells are collected from the placenta with a thin plastic tube inserted through the cervix (opening to the uterus) or a needle inserted through the abdomen. The cells may then be analyzed for possible genetic disorders.
- Alpha-fetoprotein (AFP) testing. AFP is a protein made by the developing fetus. Large amounts of AFP in the mother's bloodstream may indicate certain fetal abnormalities.
- Amniocentesis. A needle is inserted through the woman's abdomen and into the uterus to procure a sample of amniotic fluid. Fetal cells in the fluid are then analyzed for possible genetic disorders.

Once a congenital abnormality has been diagnosed, the condition will be assessed to determine if the fetus is eligible for fetal surgery. Generally only the most severe conditions that are certain to cause fetal death or significant disability are treated with fetal surgery. If fetal surgery is indicated, the parents will meet with the team of health care providers that will be involved in the surgery.

To prepare for the surgery, the steroid betamethasone will be given in order to speed up the development of the fetus's lungs. A complete history and **physical examination** will be performed. A monitor will be used to track uterine contractions and fetal heart rate. The patient will be instructed to refrain from eating and drinking after midnight the day of surgery, and will sign a surgical consent. Blood samples may be taken for laboratory tests and to type match the patient's blood in case a blood **transfusion** is necessary. An intravenous (IV) catheter will be used to infuse fluids and/or medications to the patient.

Aftercare

Postoperative recovery generally takes from five to 10 days. The patient will be closely monitored to ensure that she does not go into premature labor. She may be put on bed rest to minimize this risk. Some signs of premature labor include contractions, cramping, lower back or abdominal pain or pressure, vaginal bleeding,

WHO PERFORMS THE PROCEDURE AND WHERE IS IT PERFORMED?

Fetal surgery is a highly specialized procedure that is offered at only a handful of hospitals around the United States. Among those health care providers who will have a role in the surgery are:

- a perinatologist (a medical doctor specializing in the care and treatment of the fetus/infant during the time shortly before and after birth)
- a pediatric surgeon (a surgeon specializing in the treatment of children)
- a fetal treatment coordinator (a nurse who will coordinate the patient's care, including communication with the medical team and arranging various tests)
- a sonographer (a person who is trained to perform ultrasounds and interpret their results)
- an anesthesiologist (a medical doctor specializing in the science and application of techniques to decrease or eliminate pain)
- operating room nurses
- clinical nurses

QUESTIONS TO ASK THE DOCTOR

- Why is fetal surgery recommended in my case?
- What alternatives to fetal surgery are available to me?
- What are the costs associated with fetal surgery? Will my insurance cover the procedure?
- What will be the results if there is no medical intervention?
- Will my own obstetrician be able to care for me for the rest of my pregnancy or will I have to remain near the surgical center?

and leaking of fluid from the vagina. Tocolytics are drugs given to delay or stop labor; some commonly administered tocolytics are terbutaline, indocin, and magnesium sulfate. **Antibiotics** will usually be administered to prevent postsurgical infection.

Risks

Some risks associated with fetal surgery include infection of the incision or lining of the uterus, premature labor and delivery, bleeding, gestational diabetes, leakage of amniotic fluid, and infertility, as well as those complications associated with anesthesia.

Normal results

The results of fetal surgery depend on the reason for the procedure. Successful results of fetal surgery generally include halting the progression of the congenital malformation and perhaps reversing some of the potential complications that would arise without intervention.

Morbidity and mortality rates

One study of open fetal surgery used to repair myelomeningocele indicated that the risk of going into premature labor was significantly increased among women who had had the procedure (50% compared to 9% of similar cases with no fetal surgery performed). There was also an increased risk of oligohydramnios or low amniotic fluid (48% compared to 4% of similar cases with no fetal surgery performed). Because of the high risk of premature labor associated with fetal surgery, some fetuses have died during premature birth.

Alternatives

There are some alternative procedures that are offered for treating specific birth defects, depending on their severity. Fetal surgery is generally recommended only for the most severe defects. For example, myelomeningocele may be treated by closing of the lesion soon after delivery. SCTs and CCAMs may also be removed soon after the baby is born. Parents are often given the option of aborting the fetus (termed therapeutic abortion); or they may decide to refrain from medical intervention.

Resources

PERIODICALS

Bruner, Joseph, Noel Tulipan, Ray Paschall, Frank Boehm, William Walsh, Sandra Silva, Marta Hernanz-Schulman, Lisa Lowe, and George Reed. "Fetal Surgery for Myelomeningocele and Incidence of Shunt-Dependent Hydrocephalus." *Journal of the American Medical Association* 282, no. 19 (November 17, 1999): 1819–25.

ORGANIZATIONS

Center for Fetal Diagnosis and Treatment, Children's Hospital of Philadelphia. 34th Street and Civic Center Boulevard, Philadelphia, PA 19104-4399. (800) IN-UTERO. http://fetalsurgery.chop.edu.

Fetal Diagnosis & Therapy, Vanderbilt University Medical Center. B-1100 Medical Center North, Nashville, TN 37232. (615) 343-5227.

Fetal Treatment Center, University of California at San Francisco. 513 Parnassus Ave., HSW 1601, San Francisco, CA 94143-0570. (800) RX-FETUS. http://www.fetus.ucsf.edu.

Spina Bifida Association of America. 4590 MacArthur Blvd., SW, Washington, DC 20007. (800) 621-3141. http://www.sbaa.org.

OTHER

Danielpour, Moise, and Diana L. Farmer. "Fetal Surgery for Congenital CNS Abnormalities." *Cedars-Sinai Net Journal*. 2002 [cited February 28, 2003]. http://www.cedars-sinai.edu/mdnsi/images/fetalsurg.pdf.

"The Fetal Treatment Center: Our Treatments." *University of California at San Francisco*. 2001 [cited February 28, 2003]. http://www.fetus.ucsf.edu/ourtreatments.htm.

Iannelli, Vincent. "Surgery Before Birth?" *Pediatrics*. January 29, 2000 [cited February 28, 2003]. <http://pediatrics.about.com/library/weekly/aa012900.htm>.

Stephanie Dionne Sherk

Fetoscopy

Definition

Fetoscopy is a procedure to evaluate or treat the fetus during pregnancy.

Purpose

There are two different types of fetoscopy: external and endoscopic.

External fetoscopy

An external fetoscope resembles a **stethoscope**, but with a headpiece. It is used externally on the mother's abdomen to auscultate (listen to) the fetal heart sounds after about 18 weeks gestation (18 weeks gestation is the twentieth week of pregnancy). It also allows a birth attendant to monitor the fetus intermittently and ensure that the baby is tolerating labor without the mother having to be attached to a continuous fetal monitor.

Endoscopic fetoscopy

The second type of fetoscope is a fiber-optic endoscope. An endoscope is a thin fiber-optic tube with a tiny camera and a surgical tool at the end. The fetoscope is inserted into the uterus either transabdominally (through the abdomen) or transcervically (through the cervix) to visualize the fetus, to obtain fetal tissue samples, or to perform **fetal surgery**.

Approximately 3% of babies born in the United States each year have a complex birth defect. The labor and delivery process complicate certain birth defects, while others may progress quickly after birth to cause significant disability or **death**. Fetal surgical techniques using the endoscopic fetoscope (sometimes called an operative fetoscopy) offer early intervention

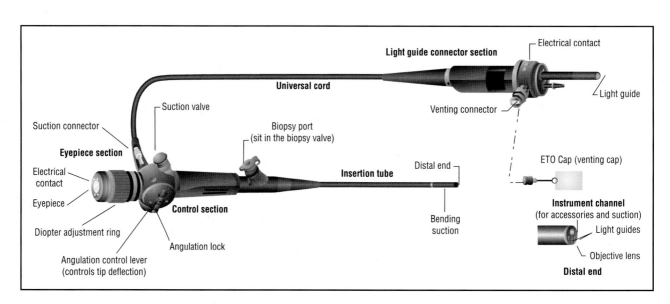

A modern fetoscope, much like an endoscope, allows physicians to hear, see, and manipulate what is going on inside many parts of the body. *(Illustration by GGS Information Services. Cengage Learning, Gale.)*

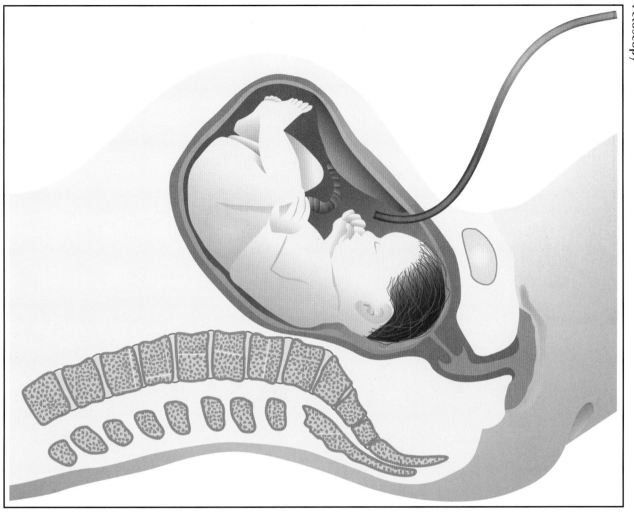

The insertion tube of a fetoscope inside the uterus. *(Illustration by GGS Information Services. Cengage Learning, Gale.)*

in order to treat such defects before they are life-threatening.

Some of the fetal abnormalities that may be treated by endoscopic fetoscopy include:

- Congenital diaphragmatic hernia (CDH). In babies with CDH, the diaphragm (the thin muscle that separates the chest from the abdomen) does not develop properly. The abdominal organs may enter the chest cavity through a hole (hernia) and cause pulmonary hyperplasia (underdeveloped lungs). CDH occurs in about one out of every 2,000–3,000 births and accounts for about 8% of all major congenital defects.

- Urinary tract obstruction. The urethra (the tube that carries urine from the bladder to the outside of the body) may become blocked *in utero* or fail to develop normally. When this happens, urine can back up into the kidneys and destroy tissue or cause the bladder to

become enlarged. The amount of amniotic fluid also decreases because fetal urine is its major component. Pulmonary hypoplasia usually results because the lungs rely on amniotic fluid in their development.

- Twin/twin transfusion syndrome (TTTS). In about 75% of twin pregnancies, the two fetuses share a single placenta (called a monochorionic pregnancy). TTTS occurs in approximately 15% of these twins when blood volume between the fetuses is unequal. This causes abnormally low blood volume in the donor twin and abnormally high blood volume in the recipient twin. There is often a large difference in physical size between the twins. Approximately 70–80% of fetuses with TTTS will die without intervention.

- Acardiac twin. This condition also occurs in monochorionic pregnancies, but one twin develops normally while the other develops without a heart. The twin without a heart receives its blood supply from the normal twin, whose heart must now work harder to pump blood through both fetuses. Approximately 50–75% of acardiac twins will die as a result. An acardiac twin occurs in 1% of monochorionic pregnancies or one out of 35,000 pregnancies.

Demographics

External fetoscopy may be used to determine the fetal heart rate in any woman with a viable pregnancy, although certain circumstances may compromise its quality (a noisy environment, an obese mother, or hydramnios [excess amniotic fluid]).

No demographic data are available regarding patients undergoing operative fetoscopy, since it is a relatively new procedure being performed at only a handful of hospitals around the United States. In the developed world, external fetoscopies have in many cases been replaced by diagnostic **ultrasound** tests.

Description

The external fetoscope is used to listen to fetal heart tones for rate and rhythm. The earpieces and the headpiece allow auscultation via both air and bone conduction. External fetoscopy is inexpensive, noninvasive, and does not require electricity. It is difficult, however, to clearly hear the fetal heart tones before 18–20 weeks gestation. Doppler ultrasound can detect fetal heart tones around weeks 10–12.

Endoscopic fetoscopy uses a very thin fiber-optic scope. Developed in the 1970s, the endoscope was originally inserted transabdominally to visualize the fetus for gross abnormalities suspected by ultrasound or to obtain tissue and blood samples. The procedure was performed after about 18 weeks gestation. Even

with practitioner expertise, associated fetal loss was 3–7%. During the 1980s, ultrasound-guided needle sampling of cord blood replaced fetoscopy when samples of fetal blood were required.

As laparoscopic and microsurgical techniques have become more common and the instrumentation has become more advanced technologically, fetoscopy has improved for fetal diagnostic and therapeutic purposes. Fetal surgery performed through an open maternal abdomen has a higher risk of complications, such as infection, premature rupture of membranes, preterm labor, or fetal death. If surgery is performed via fetoscopy, which requires a very small transabdominal incision, the risks are much smaller. Techniques have advanced enough to allow some fetoscopy to be performed in the first trimester via the mother's cervix. The term "obstetrical endoscopy" may be used for surgery on the placenta, umbilical cord, or on the fetal membranes. The term "endoscopic fetal surgery" is used for procedures such as the repair of a fetal congenital diaphragmatic hernia or obstructed bladder.

Diagnosis/Preparation

The use of external fetoscopy requires access to the maternal abdomen, with the mother lying supine or in a semi-seated position. Afterwards, the mother is able to get up and resume a normal activity level.

Preparation for endoscopic fetoscopy depends on the extent of the procedure and whether it is performed transcervically or transabdominally. For example, obtaining a small fetal tissue sample is a smaller procedure than fetal surgery. Other factors include outpatient versus inpatient stay and anesthesia (both maternal and fetal). For some procedures medication may be administered to temporarily decrease fetal movement to lower the risk of fetal injury. Maternal anesthesia may be local, regional, or general.

Aftercare

External fetoscopy does not require aftercare. The care following fetal endoscopic use will depend on the extent of the procedure and the type of anesthesia used. If the procedure is done on an outpatient basis, the mother and fetus will be monitored for a period before discharge. More extensive surgery will require inpatient hospital **postoperative care**.

Risks

The only potential complication with external fetoscopy is the possibility of missing an abnormal

WHO PERFORMS THE PROCEDURE AND WHERE IS IT PERFORMED?

Healthcare professionals who may use the external fetoscope include a nurse practitioner, nurse midwife, and obstetrician. External fetoscopy may be performed in any setting with the pregnant woman lying supine or in a semi-sitting position. Endoscopic fetoscopy requires a high level of skill and experience by fetal surgeons and is performed in a hospital setting. During the procedures, a radiology technician may perform an ultrasound, and a laboratory technician may be involved in blood sampling. Nurses will participate in both outpatient and inpatient procedures.

heart rate or rhythm. Its usefulness and accuracy depend on the skill of the practitioner.

Endoscopic fetoscopy has the potential for causing infection in the fetus and/or mother, premature rupture of the amniotic membranes, premature labor, and fetal death. When endoscopic fetal surgery is done instead of open-uterus fetal surgery, the risks to the mother and fetus are decreased. This reduction occurs because the incision is significantly smaller, with less potential blood loss, decreased uterine irritability, and decreased risk of early miscarriage.

Normal results

The normal fetal heart rate is 120–160 beats per minute, regardless of the method used for auscultation (external fetoscopy or Doppler ultrasound). Some variability of fetal heart rate is expected, as the heart rate increases with fetal activity and slows with fetal rest.

Results expected using endoscopic fetoscopy will vary depending on the procedure undertaken. The goal is for the maximum benefit with the minimum of risk or complication to both the mother and fetus.

Morbidity and mortality rates

There is no morbidity or mortality associated with external fetoscopy. In the case of endoscopic fetoscopy, the risk of fetal loss is estimated to be between 3% and 5%. The procedure is therefore usually recommended only for the more severe cases of fetal disorders that may be treated during pregnancy.

QUESTIONS TO ASK THE DOCTOR

- Why is fetoscopy recommended in my case?
- What alternatives to fetoscopy are available to me?
- For endoscopic fetoscopy, what will be the results if there is no medical intervention?
- For endoscopic fetoscopy, will the procedure be performed on an outpatient basis? What type of anesthesia will be used?

Alternatives

A healthcare provider may listen to the fetal heart rate by means of a handheld Doppler device, which uses ultrasound to amplify the heartbeat. A continuous electronic fetal monitor may also be used to track the fetal heart rate and maternal uterine contractions. It is held against the mother's abdomen by means of elastic straps.

Open fetal surgery is an alternative to internal fetoscopy. It is used for conditions that cannot be treated endoscopically. An incision is made through the abdomen and the uterus is partially removed from the body. Amniotic fluid is drained from the uterus and kept in a warmer for replacement after completion of the surgery. An incision is made in the uterus, a procedure called a hysterotomy. In order to minimize bleeding of the uterus, an instrument called a uterine stapler is used to make an incision while simultaneously placing **staples** around the perimeter of the incision to prevent bleeding. Surgery is then performed on the fetus through the opening in the uterus to locate the abnormality and remove or repair it. There is a greater risk of infection, premature labor, and leakage of amniotic fluid with open fetal surgery than there is with fetoscopy.

Resources

BOOKS

Van Vugt, John M. G., and Lee Schulman, eds. *Prenatal Medicine.* New York Taylor & Francis, 2006.

PERIODICALS

de Keersmaecker, B. and Y. Ville. "Fetoscopy and Fetal Endoscopic Surgery: A Review of the Literature." *Fetal and Maternal Medicine Review* 12(2001): 177–190.

Greco, P. A. Vimercati, S. Bettocchi, et al. "Endoscopic Examination of the Fetus in Early Pregnancy." *Journal of Perinatal Medicine.* 28 no. 1 (January 2000): 34–38. (2001): 151–159.

ORGANIZATIONS

American College of Obstetricians and Gynecologists. 409 12th St., SW, PO Box 96920. Washington, DC 20090-6920. (202) 638-5577. http://www.acog.com (accessed March 22, 2008).

Fetal Treatment Center, University of California San Francisco. 513 Parnassus Ave., HSW 1601, San Francisco, CA 94143-0570. (800) RX-FETUS or (415) 353-8489. http://www.fetus.ucsf.edu (accessed March 22, 2008).

OTHER

"The Fetal Treatment Center: Techniques of Fetal Intervention." *University of California at San Francisco* July 2, 2007 [cited January 4, 2008]. http://fetus.ucsfmedicalcenter.org/our_team/fetal_intervention.asp (accessed March 22, 2008).

Singh, Daljit and J. R. Singh. "Prenatal Testing for Congenital Malformations and Genetic Disorders." *eMedicine.* October 17, 2005 [cited January 4, 2008]. http://www.emedicine.com/oph/TOPIC485.htm (accessed March 22, 2008).

Esther Csapo Rastegari, RN, BSN, EdM
Stephanie Dionne Sherk
Tish Davidson, AM

Fibrin sealants

Definition

Fibrin sealants are a type of surgical tissue adhesive derived from human and animal blood products. The ingredients in these sealants interact during application to form a stable clot composed of a blood protein called fibrin. Fibrin sealants are also called fibrin glues. They have been used in Japan and Western Europe since the 1980s, but were not approved for use in the United States until 1998 due to the Food and Drug Administration's (FDA) concerns about virus contamination. As of 2007, all fibrin sealants used in the United States are made from blood plasma taken from carefully screened donors and rigorously tested to eliminate hepatitis viruses, HIV-1, and parvovirus.

Purpose

Originally developed during World War II to stop bleeding from battle injuries, fibrin sealants are presently used during surgery for several different purposes, including:

- to control bleeding in the area where the surgeon is operating
- to speed wound healing

- to seal off hollow body organs or cover holes made by standard sutures
- to provide slow-release delivery of medications to tissues exposed during surgery
- to reduce blood loss from skin grafting during operations to treat severe burns
- to deliver localized doses of antibiotics to lower the risk of infection after surgery

Fibrin sealants have several advantages over older methods of hemostasis (stopping bleeding): they speed up the formation of a stable clot; they can be applied to very small blood vessels and to areas that are difficult to reach with conventional sutures; they reduce the amount of blood lost during surgery; they lower the risk of postoperative inflammation or infection; and they are conveniently absorbed by the body during the healing process. They are particularly useful to minimize blood loss during surgery for severe burns, for minimally invasive procedures, and for treating patients with blood clotting disorders. Fibrin sealants are being replaced for some specialized purposes by newer wound adhesives known as cyanoacrylates. Fibrin sealants have a major advantage over cyanoacrylates, however, in that they are less likely to cause allergic reactions or inflammation that slows wound healing.

Description

All fibrin sealants in use as of 2007 have two major ingredients: purified fibrinogen (a protein) and purified thrombin (an enzyme) derived from human or bovine (cattle) blood. Many sealants have two additional ingredients: human blood factor XIII and a substance called aprotinin, which is derived from cows' lungs. Factor XIII is a compound that strengthens blood clots by forming cross-links between strands of fibrin. Aprotinin is a protein that inhibits the enzymes that break down blood clots.

Preparation

The preparation and application of fibrin sealants are somewhat complicated. The thrombin and fibrinogen are freeze-dried and packaged in vials that must be warmed before use. The two ingredients are then dissolved in separate amounts of water. Next, the thrombin and fibrinogen solutions are loaded into a double-barreled syringe that allows them to mix and combine as they are sprayed on the incision. Pieces of surgical gauze or fleece may be moistened with the sealant solutions to cover large incisions or stop heavy bleeding.

KEY TERMS

Aprotinin—A protein derived from cows' lungs included in some fibrin sealants to prevent the fibrin clot from dissolving.

Coagulation cascade—The process of blood clotting. The cascade itself is a series of chemical reactions involving blood proteins and enzymes that occurs wherever there is a break in a blood vessel. The end product of the cascade is a protein called fibrin.

Collagen—A fibrous protein found in the skin and other connective tissues of mammals. It is used to make patches coated with fibrinogen and thrombin as a wound sealant.

Factor XIII—A substance found in blood that forms cross-links between strands of fibrin during the process of blood coagulation. Factor XIII is an ingredient in some types of fibrin sealants. It is also known as fibrin stabilizing factor.

Fibrin—A blood protein formed as the end result of the coagulation cascade. Fibrin is formed from fibrinogen when it interacts with thrombin.

Fibrinogen—A blood protein made in the liver that is broken up into shorter molecules by the action of thrombin to form fibrin.

Hemostasis—Stopping bleeding from a wound or incision. Fibrin sealants are used to speed up hemostasis.

Plasma—The liquid part of blood. Plasma is a clear pale yellow fluid composed primarily of water and dissolved minerals.

Thrombin—An enzyme found in blood plasma that helps to convert fibrinogen into fibrin.

Fibrin sealants can also be applied in the form of a patch made from collagen, a protein found in the connective tissues of humans and other mammals. The collagen is coated with fibrinogen and thrombin to make a ready-to-use rapid-acting wound sealant. The coated patches are used in **neurosurgery** as well as cardiovascular, liver, and kidney surgery.

As the thrombin and fibrinogen solutions combine, a clot develops in the same way that it would form during normal blood clotting through a series of chemical reactions known as the coagulation cascade. At the end of the cascade, the thrombin breaks up the fibrinogen molecules into smaller segments of a second blood protein called fibrin. The fibrin molecules arrange themselves into strands that are then cross-linked by a blood factor known as Factor XIII to form a lattice or net-like pattern that stabilizes the clot.

Fibrin sealants are undergoing rapid refinement as the result of recent advances in tissue adhesives in general. In 1997, the Tissue Adhesive Center (TAC) was founded at University of Virginia Health Sciences Center in order to develop and test new fibrin sealants and other surgical glues. As of 2007, the TAC has been reorganized as a specialty center within the university's Surgical Therapeutic Advancement Center (STAC). Recent developments include a delivery system that forms a fibrin sealant from the patient's own blood within a 30-minute cycle, and uses a spray pen rather than a double-barreled syringe for applying the sealant. The use of the patient's own blood lowers the risk of allergic reactions to blood products derived from animal or donated blood.

Normal results

Reports that have been published between 2003 and 2007 indicate that fibrin sealants are a safe and highly effective form of surgical adhesive. A survey done in 2000 at the University of Virginia hospital found that over 90% of the surgeons who had tried fibrin sealants were pleased with the results. Several American studies have reported that fibrin sealants have improved surgical outcomes significantly by shortening the time required for operations; lowering the rate of infections and other complications; minimizing blood loss during surgery; and reducing the amount of scar tissue formed over incisions. German researchers have found that fibrin sealants containing Factor XIII generally give better results than those that do not.

Resources

BOOKS

Colman, Robert W., et al., eds. *Hemostasis and Thrombosis: Basic Principles and Clinical Practice*, 5th ed. Philadelphia: Lippincott Williams and Wilkins, 2006.

PERIODICALS

Albala, D.M. "Fibrin Sealants in Clinical Practice." *Cardiovascular Surgery* 11 (August 2003): Suppl 1, 5–11.

Dodd, R. A., R. Cornwell, N. E. Holm, et al. "The Vivostat Application System: A Comparison with Conventional Fibrin Sealant Application Systems." *Technology and Health Care* 10 (2002): 401–411.

Erdogan, D., and T. M. van Gulik. "Evolution of Fibrinogen-Coated Collagen Patch for Use as a Topical Hemostatic Agent: A Review." *Journal of Biomedical Materials Research, Part B, Applied Biomaterials*, September 5, 2007 [E-publication ahead of print].

Fortelny, R. H., A. H. Petter-Puchner, N. Walder, et al. "Cyanoacrylate Tissue Sealant Impairs Tissue Integration of Macroporous Mesh in Experimental Hernia Repair." *Surgical Endoscopy* 21 (October 2007): 1781–1785.

Foster, K. "The Use of Fibrin Sealant in Burn Operations." *Surgery* 142 (October 2007): 4 Suppl, S50–S54.

Tredwell, S., J. K. Jackson, D. Hamilton, et al. "Use of Fibrin Sealants for the Localized, Controlled Release of Cefazolin." *Canadian Journal of Surgery* 49 (October 2006): 347–352.

ORGANIZATIONS

Center for Biologics Evaluation and Research (CBER), U.S. Food and Drug Administration (FDA). 1401 Rockville Pike, Rockville, MD 20852-1448. (800) 835-4700 or (301) 827-1800. http://www.fda.gov/cber (accessed March 22, 2008).

Tissue Adhesive Center, Surgical Therapeutic Advancement Center. P. O. Box 801370, Charlottesville, VA 22908. (434) 243-0315. http://www.healthsystem.virginia.edu/internet/stac/overview/home.cfm (accessed March 22, 2008).

OTHER

Smith, Andrew. "Use of Surgical Glue Takes Hold at Temple." *Temple Times*, May 18, 2000 [cited February 18, 2003]. http://www.temple.edu/temple_times_archives/2000/5-18-00/glue.html (accessed March 22, 2008).

Rebecca Frey, PhD

Fibroid surgery *see* **Myomectomy**

Finding a surgeon

Definitions

Finding a surgeon refers to the process of choosing a doctor with specialized training in one or more branches of surgery to perform a specific procedure. It is almost always done in the context of **elective surgery** rather than emergency operations.

Description

Changes in the healthcare professions

Choosing a surgeon is a relatively new development in health care. Until the end of the twentieth century, many people, particularly in rural areas in the United States and Canada, relied on one doctor who treated all members of the family for most illnesses and some common surgical procedures, including **tooth extraction** and childbirth. These general practitioners often treated the same patients over a

period of many years and consequently knew their medical histories quite well. Most hospitals were so-called general hospitals, and admitted patients for a wide variety of surgical procedures. Since World War II, however, advances in medical knowledge and technology have led to increasing specialization of both health care professionals and the facilities they work in. As of 2008, three members of a family, each scheduled for a different surgical procedure, might be sent to three different hospitals and have three different surgeons perform the operations. Under these circumstances, choosing a surgeon can seem both complicated and confusing.

Referral to a surgeon

In the United States, most people with health insurance belong to a **health maintenance organization (HMO)** or similar health care plan that either assigns them to a doctor or asks them to choose from a list of primary care physicians (PCPs). PCPs are usually family practitioners, pediatricians, or internists, although some health care plans allow women to choose a gynecologist/obstetrician as their PCP. The PCP is sometimes referred to as a gatekeeper, because he or she makes decisions about referring patients to surgeons and other specialists. In some **managed care plans**, the PCP simply assigns patients to specific surgeons; in others, the patient may be given a list of surgeons to choose from. Many people use the PCP's list as a starting point for choosing their surgeon, and may ask the PCP for his or her opinion of the surgeons on the list. Some procedures, such as **cosmetic surgery**, are not covered by HMOs, however, many people consult their primary care physician about this type of surgery to obtain procedure information and a list of competant cosmetic surgeons.

In Canada, Australia, and other countries with publicly financed health care systems, patients usually have two options when surgery is considered. They may have the operation performed in a public hospital, in which case they are not likely to be able to choose their surgeon or even the date of the operation. Patients with private insurance, however, have the option of treatment in private clinics that give them some voice in selecting their surgeon. Private patients also do not have to wait as long for treatment; some estimates find that the average wait for surgery for private patients was about five weeks, but that the wait for surgery in a public hospital could be three times that long or longer. Canadian medical journals have reported advertisements promoting surgery in

KEY TERMS

Elective procedure—A surgical procedure that is a matter of choice rather than emergency treatment.

Malpractice—A doctor or lawyer's failure in his or her professional duties through ignorance, negligence, or criminal intent.

Primary care physician (PCP)—A family practitioner, pediatrician, internist, or gynecologist who takes care of a patient's routine medical needs and refers him or her to a surgeon or other specialist when necessary.

Referral—The process of directing a patient to a specialist for further diagnostic evaluation or treatment.

the United States to Canadians who are frustrated by long waiting lists for certain operations.

Basic considerations in choosing a surgeon

TYPE OF PROCEDURE. Surgical procedures vary considerably in complexity and the length of specialized training needed to perform them. Some can be carried out by a general surgeon, who is a physician who has completed residency training and passed an examination given by the American Board of Surgery (ABS). The ABS, which is one of 24 certifying boards that comprise the American Board of Medical Specialties (ABMS), provides a lengthy definition of the training and experience required of general surgeons. According to the ABS, a general surgeon should be competent to perform basic procedures in all of the following areas, though not necessarily the "full range and complexity of procedures" in each field.

The ABS defines the following fields as "essential in the comprehensive education of a broadly based surgeon":

- alimentary (digestive) tract;
- abdomen and its contents;
- breast, skin, and soft tissue;
- the endocrine system;
- head and neck surgery;
- pediatric surgery;
- critical care surgery;
- surgical oncology (surgery to treat cancer);
- organ transplantation;
- trauma and burns; and
- vascular surgery.

After certification by the ABS, a surgeon may undergo additional training in one of 10 surgical specialties as defined by the American Board of Medical Specialties (ABMS):

- colon and rectal surgery;
- neurological (brain and nervous system) surgery;
- obstetrics and gynecology;
- ophthalmology (eye surgery);
- orthopedic (bone and joint) surgery;
- otolaryngology (ear, nose, and throat surgery);
- pediatric surgery;
- plastic surgery;
- thoracic (chest) surgery; and
- urology.

To complicate the picture even further, some surgical specialties are further divided into subspecialties. For example, plastic surgeons may specialize in **plastic surgery** of the hand, or plastic surgery of the face and neck. Similarly, some ear, nose, and throat specialists specialize further in pediatric otolaryngology. For this reason, one of the first questions patients should ask their primary care provider when choosing a surgeon is the degree of specialization required to perform the specific procedure. Among other considerations, specialization will affect the range of choices available to the patient regarding the hospital or clinic where the operation is performed as well as choosing the operating surgeon. Some highly specialized procedures may require patients to travel long distances to a hospital or surgical center in another city.

ALTERNATIVES TO SURGERY. The Agency for Healthcare Quality and Research (formerly the Agency for Health Care Policy and Research) publishes a booklet called *Questions to Ask Your Doctor Before You Have Surgery,* which can be downloaded from the Agency's web site, www.ahrq.gov. One question discussed in the booklet concerns such nonsurgical treatments as medications or changes in diet and lifestyle. Elective surgical procedures have potential risks as well as benefits, and patients should ask about both before committing themselves to having an operation. Some health care professionals advise exploring medical options first before agreeing to surgery when both types of treatments are available for a given condition and there is time to try nonsurgical approaches.

CREDENTIALS AND SKILL LEVEL. It is important for patients to check a surgeon's credentials and length and depth of experience. After a doctor has received his or her M.D. or D.O. from an accredited school of medicine or osteopathy, he or she must pass a national licensure examination and a set of licensing procedures set by each state in order to practice general medicine or surgery in that state. Most surgeons have their medical school diploma and state licensing certificate framed and displayed on an office wall where patients can see them. A patient should never hesitate to ask questions about a surgeon's credentials, a good surgeon will be happy to answer them.

The American College of Surgeons recommends that patients look for the following credentials when they consult or are referred to a surgeon:

- Board certification. Board certification means that the surgeon has passed a rigorous examination administered by one of the specialty boards belonging to the ABMS. The ABMS publishes an annual directory of board certified medical specialists that can be found in many hospital libraries as well as university or medical school libraries. Patients can also call their local county medical society to verify a surgeon's specialty credentials.

- Fellowship in the American College of Surgeons. A surgeon with the letters FACS after his or her name is a Fellow of the ACS and is a board-certified surgeon.

- Approval for practice in accredited hospitals or other health care facilities. Patients can verify the accreditation status of the facility where the operation is to be performed by contacting the Joint Commission on Accreditation of Healthcare Organizations (JCAHO) for hospitals, or the Accreditation Association for Ambulatory Health Care (AAAHC) for outpatient surgery centers. These organizations are listed below under Resources.

An additional consideration is the number of procedures of a specific type that the surgeon performs on a regular basis. The more specialized the procedure, the more important it is for the surgeon to practice his or her skills. For example, the Johns Hopkins urology website states that a surgeon consulted for prostate surgery should have performed at least 150 prostate operations, and that it is preferable if he or she performs the same operation every day or several days a week. For some types of surgery, including joint replacement and cancer surgery, patients should look for a surgeon in high-volume medical centers where specialists have acquired a great deal of experience performing the specific procedure that the patient needs.

PERSONALITY ISSUES. In addition to a surgeon's level of skill and experience, his or her personality should be taken into consideration. Many operations require dietary changes, certain types of **exercise**, or other detailed preparations, therefore, the patient should feel comfortable about talking to the surgeon—particularly when it comes to asking important questions about the operation itself or the surgeon's length of experience. Some patients are afraid to talk to surgeons because they have heard that surgeons have a reputation among other health professionals for being impatient, bossy, and generally lacking in "people skills." One popular article on doctors' personality styles describes the typical surgeon as fitting the "dictator" pattern, and several studies have reported that over 50% of doctors advised to seek anger management counseling are surgeons. As of 2008, however, a growing number of surgeons are recognizing that patients who take an active role in their treatment have better outcomes, and that a well-informed patient is their best ally. Patients should not hesitate to talk to several different surgeons in order to find one whose personality is a good fit with their own.

DISCIPLINARY HISTORY. Although only a small percentage of doctors in the United States have ever been disciplined by a professional peer review, sued for malpractice, or had their licenses suspended—about 0.5% per year—patients who are considering surgery should find out if any of the surgeons they are considering have a history of disciplinary actions taken against them. The Federation of State Medical Boards has compiled a database called DocInfo that can be searched on the Federation's web site, www.fmsb.org, for information about a specific practitioner's record.

Preparation

Gathering information

Patients considering elective surgery should collect some information about the procedure in question and the qualifications required to perform it before they talk to a specific surgeon. People with Internet access can obtain information about surgical operations as well as credentialing processes on the web sites of the various surgical specialty associations. Links to these associations can be found on the ABMS web site, www.abms.org. Many surgical specialty groups have patient education brochures and other informational material available for downloading free of charge. Most of these materials can also be obtained by writing, telephoning, or e-mailing the associations.

Other useful sources of information include hospital and **outpatient surgery** center web sites. These sites often have reader-friendly descriptions of specific procedures as well as information about the hospital or clinic's accreditation, location, and other important features.

Another good source of information about choosing a surgeon is first-person accounts of surgical procedures. There are a growing number of patient guides to plastic surgery, joint replacement surgery, oral and facial surgery, cancer surgery, and other procedures written by people who have had these operations. Most of these books include advice on finding one's way through the referral process as well as a list of specific questions to ask surgeons in particular specialties.

Getting recommendations

The next step in choosing a surgeon is asking other health professionals to recommend specific practitioners. As mentioned above, most patients begin with their primary care doctor. Patients who have been treated recently by a medical specialist should also ask him or her for recommendations about surgeons. For example, someone who has been seeing a specialist in pulmonary (lung) medicine for asthma treatment should ask him or her for the names of good thoracic surgeons if an operation is recommended. Many authors suggest asking the PCP or medical specialist who they would ask to do the surgical operation if they or one of their family members needed it.

Other sources of recommendations include home health care nurses or physical therapists, who are often familiar with the work of local surgeons. One expert in sports medicine has been quoted as saying, "If you want a good surgeon, ask a physical therapist. We see patients from all the surgeons. I see the same good surgeries come from the same good surgeons and the same lousy surgeries come from the same lousy surgeons. You see it all the time."

A third source of recommendations is other people who have had the same procedure that the patient is considering and who were pleased with the results.

Advertisements

As recently as the 1960s, it was considered unprofessional for doctors or dentists to advertise themselves except for brief listings of their specialties in professional association and local telephone directories. The spread of high-pressure advertising techniques that originated in the business world and spread into medicine, however, has resulted in the production of web sites, radio announcements, and printed advertisements for doctors that can be confusing to patients who are looking for a surgeon. In particular, plastic surgeons who specialize in cosmetic procedures (face lifts, "tummy tucks," etc.) have been accused of exploiting people's vulnerabilities and fear of aging in their advertisements. The American Medical Association (AMA) has a set of guidelines, issued in 1996 and updated in 2002, that warn doctors against using publicity containing deceptive or misleading claims.

Patients looking for a surgeon should be wary of doctors who claim that they have unique skills, "secret" techniques, or an improbably large number of satisfied patients. In addition, an attractive web site or impressive advertisement should not be a substitute for a personal interview with the surgeon.

Second opinions

Patients who are considering surgery should not be shy about getting a **second opinion** if they feel unsure about having an operation after they talk to a surgeon. In fact, many health plans require patients to seek a second opinion for certain types of elective surgery before they will approve the procedure. Some insurance plans will reimburse patients for the cost of seeking a second opinion. The Centers for **Medicare** and **Medicaid** Services (CMS), formerly the Health Care Financing Administration (HCFA), publishes a brochure (Publication No. 02173) for Medicare patients on seeking second surgical opinions.

Resources

BOOKS

Miller, Craig A. *The Making of a Surgeon in the 21st Century.* Nevada City, CA: Blue Dolphin Publishing, 2004.

Raftery, Andrew T. *Applied Basic Science for Basic Surgical Training,* 2nd ed. New York: Churchill Livingstone, 2008.

Way, Lawrence W., and Gerard M. Doherty, eds. *Current Surgical Diagnosis & Treatment,* 11th ed. New York: McGraw-Hill, 2002.

PERIODICALS

Edelson, Edward. "Finding a Plastic Surgeon." *Woman's Day* (March 9, 1982): 36–37.

Helms, Sherry. "The Changing Face of Cosmetic Surgery." *Consumers Digest* 34, no. 4 (July–August 1995): 53–60.

ORGANIZATIONS

Accreditation Association for Ambulatory Health Care, 5250 Old Orchard Road, Suite 200, Skokie, IL, 60077, (847) 853-6060, (847) 853-9028, info@aaahc.org, http://www.aaahc.org.

Agency for Healthcare Research and Quality, 540 Gaither Road, Rockville, MD, 20850, (301) 427-1364, http://www.ahrq.gov.

American Board of Medical Specialties, 1007 Church Street, Suite 404, Evanston, IL, 60201-5913, (847) 491-9091, http://www.abms.org.

American Board of Surgery, 1617 John F. Kennedy Blvd., Suite 860, Philadelphia, PA, 19103-1847, (215) 568-4000, (215) 563-5718, http://www.absurgery.org.

American College of Surgeons, 633 N. Saint Clair St., Chicago, IL, 60611-3211, (312) 202-5000, (800) 621-4111, (312) 202-5001, postmaster@facs.org, http://www.facs.org.

Centers for Medicare and Medicaid Services, 7500 Security Boulevard, Baltimore, MD, 21244-1850, (410) 786-3000, (877) 267-2323, http://www.cms.hhs.gov.

Federation of State Medical Boards, P.O. Box 619850, Dallas, TX, 75261-9850, (817) 868-4000, (817) 868-4099, http://www.fsmb.org.

Health Canada/Santé Canada, A.L. 0900C2, Ottawa, Canada, K1A 0K9, (613) 957-2991, http://www.hc-sc.gc.ca.

Joint Commission on Accreditation of Healthcare Organizations, One Renaissance Boulevard, Oakbrook Terrace, IL, 60181, (630) 792-5000, (630) 792-5005, http://www.jointcommission.org.

Rebecca Frey, Ph.D.
Robert Bockstiegel

Finger reattachment

Definition

Finger reattachment (or replantation) is defined as reattachment of a finger that has been completely amputated. In general, a finger **amputation** may be defined as either complete (there is no connection between the amputated finger[s] and the rest of the hand) or incomplete (the finger is connected to the rest of the hand by tendons, skin fragments, or muscle tissue).

Purpose

Reattachment can be surgically performed for the finger and such other detached body parts as the hand or arm. The first successful replantation of a severed finger tip was performed in 1814 by William Balfour, a British surgeon. Replantation of amputated fingers was not attempted on a widespread basis, however, until the invention of the operating microscope in the early 1960s. The first successful replantation of an entire arm was performed in 1962 on a 12-year-old boy who had been injured in a train accident. The technique used in the early 2000s to reconstruct the blood vessels in an injured hand was developed in 1965 by two Japanese surgeons, Shigeo Komatsu and Susumu Tamai. Reattachment of an amputated finger can be carried out in most large hospitals in the early 2000s.

Demographics

There are about 30,000 cases of traumatic amputations in the United States each year; 65% of these involve the upper limbs (arms, hands, and fingers).

Most patients are between the ages of 15 and 40, and 80% are male. Good candidates for this procedure include persons with thumb or multiple digit amputation. Injury to multiple digits is an important patient selection criterion, since in some cases the least damaged digits may be moved to the least injured or most useful stump. Patient exclusion is neither clear-cut nor absolute; however, patients who have cut off their own fingers should receive a psychiatric evaluation before reattachment is attempted, as many of these patients later cut off the finger a second time. Generally, severe crushing or avulsing (tearing away) injuries to the fingers complicates replantation; however, venous grafts may help replace injured blood vessels. Additionally, older persons may have arteriosclerosis that frequently impairs function in blood vessels, especially in small vessels. Special efforts may be made to replant fingers if the person's livelihood (such as professional music performance) depends on absolute finger control.

Description

To increase efficiency, the replantation team splits into two smaller teams. One sub-team in the **operating room** cleans the amputated finger with sterile solutions, places it on ice, and identifies and tags (with special surgical clips) nerves and blood vessels. Dead or damaged tissue is surgically removed with a procedure called **debridement**. The emergency room (ER) sub-team will assess the patient during a physical exam with x rays of the injured area, blood analysis, and cardiac (heart) monitoring. The patient is given fluids intravenously (IV), a tetanus injection (to prevent infection by *Clostridium tetani*, a bacterium that can invade the body through crush injuries or penetrating wounds and release a potent neurotoxin), and **antibiotics**. Usually, most finger reattachments are performed with a local anesthetic such as bupivacaine and a nerve block to numb the affected arm. Maintaining a warm **body temperature** can enhance blood flow to the affected limb.

The surgical procedure consists of several stages. The bone in the amputated finger must be shortened and fixed, which means that the bone end is trimmed. After this process, the bone is stabilized with special sutures called K-wires, and fixed pins are placed in the bone after drilling a space to insert them. This process connects the two amputated bone fragments. After bone stabilization and fixation, the extensor and flexor tendons are repaired. This step is vital, since arteries, veins, and nerves should never be surgically connected under tension. Next, the surgeon must repair (suture) severed tendons, arteries, veins, and

Finger reattachment

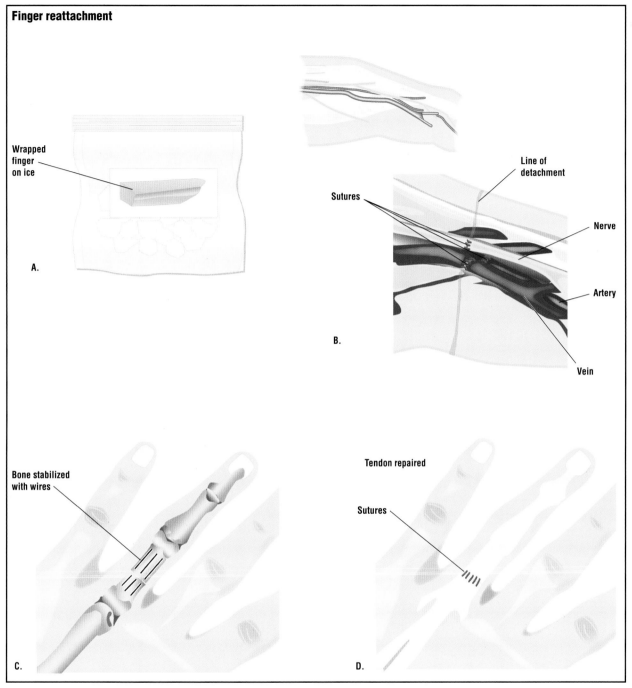

To save a detached finger for reattachment surgery, it should be wrapped in a moist paper towel and put on ice (A). First the surgeon will reattach the blood vessels and nerves of the finger (B). The bone may be repaired with wires (C), and tendons are repaired (D). Skin and muscle wounds are also closed during the procedure. *(Illustration by GGS Information Services. Cengage Learning, Gale.)*

nerves. Healthy arteries and veins are sutured together without tension. A vein graft is used for blood vessels that cannot be reattached.

Nerve repair for finger reattachment is not complicated. Since the reattached bone parts are shorter than the original length, nerves can be reattached without tension. A microscope is used for magnified visualization of finger nerves during reattachment. When the severed ends of the nerve cannot be reattached, a primary nerve graft is performed. Finally, it is vital to cover superficial veins on the affected finger (dorsal veins) with a skin flap to prevent death of the venous vessels. The skin over the surgical field is loosely sutured with a few sutures. Any damaged tissue that may die (necrotic tissue) is removed. No tension should be placed on the skin fields during closure of the wound. Wounds are covered with small strips of gauze impregnated with petrolatum. The upper extremity is immobilized, and compression hand dressing and plaster splints are arranged to prevent slipping and movement of the affected arm.

Diagnosis/Preparation

The diagnosis is easily made by visual inspection. The reattachment procedure is complex and involves the expertise and skill of a highly trained surgeon. There are several important factors necessary to successful replantation, including special instrumentation and transportation of the amputated finger. Surgical loupes (binocular-type eyepieces used by surgeons to magnify small structures during surgery) are necessary

for this procedure. Instruments should be at least 3.9 in (10 cm) long to allow for proper positioning in the surgeon's hands. Special clips are used to help suture blood vessels together. The best method of saving and transporting the amputated finger is to wrap it with moistened cloth (Ringer's lactate solution or saline solution) and place it on ice. Generally, the tissues will survive for about six hours without cooling. If the part is cooled, tissue survival time is approximately 12 hours. Fingers have the best outcome for transportation survival, since digits (fingers) do not have a large percentage of muscle tissue.

Aftercare

Postoperative care is vital for successful finger reattachment. The hand is wrapped in a bulky compression dressing and usually elevated. If arterial flow is impaired, then the hand should be lowered, since this maneuver will promote blood flow from the heart to the reattached finger. If venous outflow is slow, the hand must be elevated. Medications to increase blood flow (peripheral vasodilators) and an anticoagulant (heparin) are used. A tranquilizer may be given to reduce unnecessary blood vessel movement (vasospasm) that can occur due to anxiety. Careful examination of the reattached digit(s) is necessary. The surgeon frequently monitors color, the capacity of blood vessels, capillary refill, and warmth to monitor replant progress. The YSI telethermometer monitors the digital (finger) temperature with small surface probes. Skin temperature falling below 86°F (30°C) indicates poor blood perfusion (poor blood and oxygen delivery to the affected area) of the replant. The cause of poor blood circulation must be investigated and corrected, if possible. The patient's room should be warm, and bed rest for two to three days is recommended. Patients must refrain from smoking and take antibiotics for one week after surgery. Follow-up consultations are necessary for continued **wound care** and rehabilitation.

Some patients may need additional surgery at a later date to free tendons from scar tissue, transfer muscle tissue to the affected finger, or improve the functioning of the nerves in the finger. In a few cases the reattached finger may have to be removed because of complete loss of function or intractable pain.

Risks

The experienced surgeon can estimate the likelihood of complications based on the nature of the injury. Replantations that are risky, such as those with circulatory perfusion problems, have lower success rates. Generally, the most difficult replantations are those that involve children under 10, injuries caused by a ring catching in machinery (ring avulsion injury), and crush-and-tear injuries. Management of the

WHO PERFORMS THE PROCEDURE AND WHERE IS IT PERFORMED?

The reattachment procedure itself is usually performed in a hospital operating room by a microsurgeon, who may be a plastic surgeon with five years of general surgery training, plus two years of plastic surgery training and another one or two years of training in microneurovascular surgery; or an orthopedic surgeon with one year of general surgery training, five years of orthopedic surgery training, and additional years in microsurgery training.

The patient may be cared for by a variety of emergency medical technicians, nurses, and physicians at the scene of the accident or in the hospital emergency department before replantation is performed. These health professionals may cleanse or splint the injured limb, administer pain medications, and perform other procedures to prepare the patient for surgery.

difficult replant typically includes intravenous heparin to prevent clotting of the blood, and providing a continuous nerve block in either the median or ulnar nerve (depending on which fingers are reattached). A nerve block will cause vasodilation, or expansion of the blood vessels. Vasodilation will increase blood flow, bringing with it fresh oxygenated blood. Further evaluation should include checking the patient's dressing for constriction (i.e., if the dressing was placed too snugly and is constricting local blood vessels).

There are some psychological risks to replantation, as patients are often distressed by loss of function in the affected finger(s) or by the appearance of the injured hand. Since 100% of function cannot be restored, patients may find that there are some activities or hobbies that they can no longer enjoy. In some cases, they may not be able to do the work they did before their injury and may have to seek another type of employment. Some patients may need counseling in order to deal with the changes in their life that may be forced on them by loss of function in the injured hand.

Normal results

Normal results depend on several factors: how much of the finger was cut off; whether any joints were affected, or only the tip; whether the wound was a guillotine amputation (a clean cut by a sharp-edged object) or involved crushing or tearing; and the patient's age. In general, younger patients and non-smokers recover more function and sensation in the

QUESTIONS TO ASK THE DOCTOR

- Are there any special precautions I should take with my pain medication?
- How should I care for the wound?
- When will I regain feeling and function in the affected finger(s)?
- Will I need physical therapy for the injury?
- How much function can I expect to regain?
- Will I be able to go back to my old job?

reattached finger. Reattachment following a guillotine amputation has a higher rate of success (more than 80%) than reattachment following a crush or avulsion amputation (55%).

There are two types of nerves involved in recovering the use of the fingers: sensory nerves (which detect heat, cold, roughness, and other sensations) and motor nerves (which govern the movement of muscles). Nerves in the fingers grow about an inch per month. The number of inches from the injury to the tip of the injured finger gives the minimum number of months after which the patient may begin to notice sensations in that fingertip. Results usually include good nerve recovery and 60–80% recovery of range of motion; cold intolerance (usually reversed in about two years); and acceptable cosmetic appearance.

Morbidity and mortality rates

Most finger replantations involving guillotine amputations in patients younger than 40 years are successful. Replantations in patients with crush or avulsion injuries are more likely to have complications after surgery. Smokers and patients with diabetes also have poorer outcomes. Mortality from finger reattachment is very low; fatal outcomes are almost always in patients with multilevel injuries involving the head or chest as well as amputation of a finger or hand.

Alternatives

According to the American Society for Surgery of the Hand, the surgeon will explain to the patient how much function the patient can expect to have after replantation and allow the patient to decide whether the operation itself, time spent in the hospital, and a long period of rehabilitation are worth that degree of recovery. One alternative to replantation is a prosthesis for the missing finger.

Resources

BOOKS

Berger, Richard A., and Arnold-Peter C. Weiss, eds. *Hand Surgery*. Philadelphia: Lippincott Williams and Wilkins, 2004.

Green, David P. *Green's Operative Hand Surgery*, 5th ed. Philadelphia: Elsevier Churchill Livingstone, 2005.

Trumble, Thomas E., and Jeffrey E. Budoff. *Hand Surgery Update IV*, 4th ed. Rosemont, IL: American Society for Surgery of the Hand, 2007.

PERIODICALS

Brooks, D., R. F. Buntic, G. M. Kind, et al. "Ring Avulsion: Injury Pattern, Treatment, and Outcome." *Clinics in Plastic Surgery* 34 (April 2007): 187–195.

Datiashvili, R. O., K. R. Knox, and G. M. Kaplan. "Solutions to Challenging Digital Replantations." *Clinics in Plastic Surgery* 34 (April 2007): 167–175.

Molski, M. "Replantation of Fingers and Hands after Avulsion and Crush Injuries." *Journal of Plastic, Reconstructive and Aesthetic Surgery* 60 (July 2007): 748–754.

Morrison, W. A., and D. McCombe. "Digital Replantation." *Hand Clinics* 23 (February 2007): 1–12.

ORGANIZATIONS

American Association for Hand Surgery. 20 North Michigan Avenue, Suite 700, Chicago, IL 60602. (321) 236-3307; Fax: (312) 782-0553. E-mail: contact@handsurgery.org. http://www.handsurgery.org (accessed March 22, 2008).

American College of Emergency Physicians (ACEP). 1125 Executive Circle, Irving, TX 75038-2522. (800) 798-1822 or (972) 550-0911. http://www.acep.org/ (accessed March 22, 2008).

American Society for Surgery of the Hand (ASSH). 6300 North River Road, Suite 600, Rosemont, IL 60018. (847) 384-8300. http://www.assh.org/AM/Template.cfm (accessed March 22, 2008).

OTHER

American Society for Surgery of the Hand (ASSH). *Replantation*. http://www.assh.org/Content/NavigationMenu/PatientsPublic/HandConditions/Replantation/Replantation.htm (accessed January 15, 2008).

Kazzi, Zian M. "Replantation." *eMedicine*, September 4, 2007 [cited January 15, 2008]. http://www.emedicine.com/emerg/topic502.htm (accessed March 22, 2008).

Murphy, Paul, Chris Colwell, Gilbert Pineda, and Tamara Bryan. "Traumatic Amputations: How EMS Providers Can Manage Amputations in the Field." August 22, 2006. *EMSResponder.com*.http://publicsafety.com/article/article.jsp?id=3541&siteSection=4 (accessed January 15, 2008).

"Superficial Fingertip Avulsion." National Center for Emergency Medicine Informatics. [cited June 2003] http://www.ncemi.org/cse/cse1002.htm (accessed March 22, 2008).

"The V-Y Plasty in the Treatment of Fingertip Amputations." American Academy of Family Physicians. [cited June 2003] http://www.aafp.org/afp/20010801/455.html (accessed March 22, 2008).

Wilhelmi, Bradon J., and W. P. Andrew Lee. "Hand, Amputations and Replantation." eMedicine, June 28, 2006 [cited January 15, 2008]. http://www.emedicine.com/plastic/topic536.htm (accessed March 22, 2008).

Laith Farid Gulli, MD, MS
Bilal Nasser, MD, MS
Robert Ramirez, BS
Rebecca Frey, PhD

Fluoroquinolones

Definition

Fluoroquinolones are a subgroup of quinolones, which are medications that kill bacteria or prevent their growth. The parent drug of the group is nalidixic acid (NegGram), a synthetic drug used to treat urinary tract infections caused by gram-negative bacteria. Bacteria are one-celled disease-causing microorganisms that commonly multiply by cell division.

Purpose

Fluoroquinolones are a class of antimicrobials, which are medications used to treat infections caused by microorganisms. Physicians prescribe these drugs for bacterial infections in many parts of the body. For example, they are used to treat bone and joint infections, skin infections, urinary tract infections, inflammation of the prostate, serious ear infections, bronchitis, pneumonia, tuberculosis, some sexually transmitted diseases (STDs), and some infections that affect people with AIDS. Some fluoroquinolones, such as enrofloxacin (Baytril), were developed for use in veterinary practice to treat infections in household pets and farm animals but are not given to humans.

Although fluoroquinolones are normally used only to treat infections, and not for prophylaxis (prevention of infection), some of these compounds have been used before surgery, particularly if the patient is allergic to the **antibiotic** that is usually given. Fluoroquinolones have also been studied for their usefulness in eye surgery and surgery of the biliary tract.

Description

Fluoroquinolones are available only with a physician's prescription; they are sold in tablet and injectable forms. Examples of these medicines are moxifloxacin (Avelox), ciprofloxacin (Cipro), ofloxacin (Floxin), levofloxacin (Levaquin), lomefloxacin (Maxaquin), norfloxacin (Noroxin), enoxacin (Penetrex), and sparfloxacin (Zagam).

Newer (so-called fourth-generation) fluoroquinolones include gatifloxacin (Zymar) and gemifloxacin (Factive). Another new drug in this class, prulifloxacin, is still in clinical trials as of early 2008.

Recommended dosage

The recommended dosage depends on the type and strength of the specific fluoroquinolone and the kind of infection for which it is being taken. Patients should consult the physician who prescribed the drug or the pharmacist who filled the prescription for the correct dosage.

To make sure an infection clears up completely, patients should take the full course of fluoroquinolone that their doctor prescribed. It is important to not stop taking the drug just because the symptoms begin to diminish.

Fluoroquinolones work best when they are at constant levels in the blood. To help keep blood levels constant, patients should take the medicine in doses spaced evenly through the day and night without missing any doses. For best results, these medications should be taken with a full glass of water, and the patient should drink several more glasses of water every day. Drinking plenty of water will help prevent some of the medicine's side effects. Some fluoroquinolones should be taken on an empty stomach; others may be taken with meals. Patients should read the directions on the package very carefully or ask the physician or pharmacist for instructions on the best way to take a specific medicine.

Precautions

Other than allergic reactions, few patients experience significant problems when they are given a single dose of a fluoroquinolone for surgical prophylaxis. The external use of these drugs—for example, eye drops—is also generally safe.

An important precaution to observe with any antimicrobial drug is that the unnecessary use or abuse of these medications can encourage drug-resistant strains of bacteria to develop and spread. These drug-resistant strains then become difficult or even impossible to treat. Bacteria found in hospitals appear to have become especially resilient, and are causing increasing difficulty for patients and the doctors treating them.

KEY TERMS

Bacterium (plural, bacteria)—A microscopic one-celled form of life that causes many diseases and infections.

Biliary tract—The part of the digestive system that conveys or stores bile, consisting of the bile ducts and the gallbladder.

Bronchitis—Inflammation of the air passages in the lungs.

Digestive tract—The stomach, intestines, and other parts of the body through which food passes.

Inflammation—A condition characterized by pain, redness, swelling, and warmth. Inflammation usually develops in response to an injury or infection.

Microorganism—An organism that is too small to be seen with the naked eye.

Pneumonia—A disease characterized by inflammation of the lungs. Pneumonia may be caused by bacteria, viruses, or other organisms, or by physical or chemical irritants.

Prophylaxis—A medical intervention intended to prevent disease.

Prostate—A donut-shaped gland in males below the bladder that contributes to the production of semen.

Sexually transmitted disease (STD)—A disease that is passed from one person to another through sexual intercourse or other intimate sexual contact.

Tendon—A tough band of tissue that connects muscle to bone.

Tuberculosis (TB)—An infectious disease that usually affects the lungs, but may also affect other parts of the body. Its symptoms include fever, weight loss, and coughing up blood.

Urinary tract—The passage through which urine flows from the kidneys to the outside of the body.

One fear is that the overuse of fluoroquinolone medications could reduce their effectiveness against such infections as typhoid fever, hospital-acquired pneumonia, and others.

Research suggests that fluoroquinolones may cause bone development problems in children and teenagers. Infants, children, teenagers, pregnant women, and women who are breastfeeding should not take these drugs unless directed to do so by a physician.

Although such side effects are rare, some people have had severe and life-threatening reactions to fluoroquinolones. Several drugs in this class have been withdrawn in the United States because of severe reactions. One drug, temafloxacin (Omniflox), was withdrawn less than six months after its approval in 1992 because of three patient deaths related to liver damage and destruction of red blood cells. Another fluoroquinolone, trovafloxacin (Trovan), was withdrawn from the market in 2000 when it was found to cause liver damage. The tablet form of gatifloxacin, sold under the trade name Tequin, was withdrawn in 2006 after a Canadian study published in the *New England Journal of Medicine* showed that it could produce diabetes as a side effect. Gatifloxacin is presently available only in the form of eye drops (Zymar).

Patients should call their physician at once if they have any of the following signs:

- swelling of the face and throat
- problems swallowing
- shortness of breath
- rapid heartbeat
- tingling in the fingers or toes
- itching or hives
- loss of consciousness

Some fluoroquinolones may weaken the tendons in the shoulder, hand, or heel, making these fibrous bands of tissue more likely to tear. In 2004, the Food and Drug Administration (FDA) upgraded the warnings included in package inserts for these drugs to note the possibility of tendon damage or peripheral nerve damage. Anyone who notices pain or inflammation in the shoulder, heel, or other joints should stop taking the medicine immediately and call their physician. They should rest and avoid athletic activity or vigorous **exercise** until the physician determines whether the tendons have been damaged. Tendons that are torn may require surgical repair.

Fluoroquinolones make some people feel drowsy, dizzy, lightheaded, or less alert. Anyone who takes these drugs should not drive, use machines, or do anything else that requires a high level of alertness until they have found out how the drugs affect them.

Fluoroquinolones may increase the skin's sensitivity to sunlight. Even brief exposure to sun can cause severe sunburn or a rash. During treatment with these drugs, patients should avoid exposure to direct sunlight, especially high sun between 10 A.M. and 3 P.M.; wear a hat and tightly woven clothing that covers the arms and legs; use a sunscreen with a skin protection factor (SPF) of at least 15; protect the lips with a lip balm containing sun block; and avoid the use of tanning beds, tanning booths, or sunlamps.

Patients should not take antacids that contain aluminum, calcium, or magnesium at the same time as fluoroquinolones. The antacids may keep the fluoroquinolones from working as they should. If antacids are needed, they should be taken at least two hours before or two hours after taking norfloxacin or ofloxacin, and at least four hours before or two hours after taking ciprofloxacin. Patients who are taking sucralfate (Carafate), a medicine used to treat stomach ulcers and other irritations in the digestive tract and mouth, should follow the same instructions as for taking antacids.

People who have had unusual reactions to fluoroquinolones or such related compounds as cinoxacin (Cinobac) or nalidixic acid (NegGram) in the past should let their physician know before taking the drugs again. The physician should also be told about any allergies to foods, dyes, preservatives, or other substances.

People with any of these medical problems should make sure their physicians are aware of their conditions before using fluoroquinolones:

- kidney disease
- liver disease together with kidney disease
- diseases that affect the brain or spinal cord, including hardening of the arteries in the brain; epilepsy; and other seizure disorders

Taking fluoroquinolones with certain other drugs may affect the way the drugs work or may increase the chance of side effects.

Side effects

The most common side effects are mild diarrhea, nausea, vomiting, stomach or abdominal pain, dizziness, drowsiness, lightheadedness, nervousness, sleep problems, and headache. These side effects occur in about 5% of patients taking fluoroquinolones. They usually go away as the body adjusts to the drug and do not require medical treatment unless they are bothersome.

More serious side effects are not common, but may occur. If any of the following side effects occur, the patient should consult a physician immediately:

- skin rash or such other skin problems as itching, peeling, hives, or redness
- fever
- agitation or confusion
- hallucinations
- shakiness or tremors
- seizures or convulsions

- tingling in the fingers or toes
- pain at the injection site that persists after the drug was injected
- pain in the calves that spreads to the heel area
- swelling of the calves or lower legs
- swelling of the face or neck
- difficulty swallowing
- rapid heartbeat
- shortness of breath
- loss of consciousness

Other rare side effects may occur. People who have unusual symptoms after taking fluoroquinolones should consult their physician at once.

Interactions

Fluoroquinolones may interact with other medicines. When an interaction occurs, the effects of one or both of the drugs may change or the risk of side effects may be greater. Anyone who takes fluoroquinolones should give the doctor a list of all other medications that they take on a regular basis, including over-the-counter (OCT) drugs, herbal preparations, and traditional Chinese or other alternative medicines. Drugs that may interact with fluoroquinolones include:

- antacids containing aluminum, calcium, or magnesium
- medicines that contain iron or zinc, including multi-vitamin and mineral supplements
- sucralfate (Carafate)
- caffeine
- such blood-thinning drugs as warfarin (Coumadin)
- drugs given to open the airway (bronchodilators), including aminophylline, theophylline (Theo-Dur and other brands), and oxtriphylline (Choledyl and other brands)
- didanosine (Videx), a drug used to treat HIV infection

The list above does not include every drug that may interact with fluoroquinolones. Patients should check with a physician or pharmacist before combining fluoroquinolones with any other prescription or nonprescription (over-the-counter) medicine.

Resources

BOOKS

Abrams, Anne Collins, Carol Barnett Lammon, and Sandra Smith Pennington. *Clinical Drug Therapy: Rationales for Nursing Practice*. Philadelphia: Lippincott Williams and Wilkins, 2007.

Karch, A. M. *Lippincott's Nursing Drug Guide*. Springhouse, PA: Lippincott Williams & Wilkins, 2003.

Neal, Michael J. *Medical Pharmacology at a Glance*, 5th ed. Malden, MA: Blackwell Publishing, 2005.

PERIODICALS

Bayes, M., X. Rabasseda, and J. R. Prous. "Gateways to Clinical Trials." *Methods and Findings in Experimental and Clinical Pharmacology* 29 (October 2007): 547–583.

Park-Wyllie, Laura Y., David N. Juurlink, Alexander Kopp, et al. "Outpatient Gatifloxacin Therapy and Dysglycemia in Older Adults." *New England Journal of Medicine* 354 (March 30, 2006): 1352–1361.

Petersen, Melody. "Unforeseen Side Effects Ruined One Blockbuster." *New York Times*, August 27, 2000, p. 3.

Prats, G., et al. "Prulifloxacin: A New Antibacterial Fluoroquinolone." *Expert Review of Anti-Infective Therapy* 4 (February 2006): 27–41.

Zhanel, G. G., S. Fontaine, H. Adam, et al. "A Review of New Fluoroquinolones: Focus on their Role in Respiratory Tract Infections." *Treatments in Respiratory Medicine* 5 (2006): 437–465.

ORGANIZATIONS

American Society of Health-System Pharmacists (ASHP). 7272 Wisconsin Avenue, Bethesda, MD 20814. (866) 279-0681. http://www.ashp.org (accessed March 22, 2008).

United States Food and Drug Administration (FDA). 5600 Fishers Lane, Rockville, MD 20857-0001. (888) INFO-FDA. http://www.fda.gov (accessed March 22, 2008).

OTHER

Food and Drug Administration (FDA). Press release, June 5, 1992. Recall of temafloxacin (Omniflox) tablets. http://www.fda.gov/bbs/topics/NEWS/NEW00279. html [cited January 8, 2008, accessed March 22, 2008].

Rosalyn Carson-DeWitt, MD
Samuel Uretsky, PharmD
Rebecca Frey, PhD

Forehead lift

Definition

A forehead lift is a **cosmetic surgery** procedure intended to improve a person's appearance by correcting the shape of the eyebrows and reducing horizontal wrinkles or furrows in the skin of the forehead. It is also known as a brow lift.

Purpose

The purpose of a forehead lift is improvement of the patient's external appearance, particularly with regard to the upper third of the face. Some people have clearly marked frown lines or drooping of the eyebrows or eyelid caused by loosening of the tissues and muscles around the eyes during the aging process. The drooping of the eyelid is sometimes referred to as ptosis, which comes from a Greek word meaning "fall." In some cases, these signs of aging make the person look angry, anxious, or sad. A forehead lift is not done to cure disease or repair a major wound or injury.

Demographics

Like other cosmetic surgery procedures, forehead lifts are performed much more frequently than they were even a decade ago. According to the American Society of Plastic Surgeons (ASPS), the number of forehead lifts performed in the United States has risen 172% since 1992. These changes are attributed in part to concerns about appearance in the so-called baby boomer generation. Adults born between 1945 and 1960 are generally more image-conscious than previous generations of Americans. In addition, newer surgical techniques have made forehead lifts less painful, easier to perform, and less likely to have complications.

Most plastic surgeons recommend that a forehead lift should be done when the patient is between 40 and 60 years old, although it is sometimes done on younger patients who have very deep frown lines due to stress or have inherited very low and heavy brows. In addition, people whose facial skin has aged prematurely due to sun exposure or heavy smoking may be candidates for a forehead lift in their mid-30s. In 2002, the average age of patients of either sex who had forehead lifts done in the United States was 47.

Statistics published by the American Academy of Cosmetic Surgery (AACS) in January 2003 indicate that although more men are choosing to have cosmetic surgery than in the past, the female:male ratio for forehead lifts is still 6:1. In 2002, surgeons who are AACS members performed 7,882 forehead lifts on women compared to 1,139 procedures on men. Forehead lifts account for a little less than 1% (0.96%) of all cosmetic surgery procedures performed each year in the United States and Canada.

The American Society of Plastic Surgeons reported that a total of 1,852,012 cosmetic procedures and 9,138,275 nonsurgical procedures were performed in the United States in 2006, totaling almost 11 million procedures. Of that number, 52,525 were forehead lift procedures.

Although most forehead lifts and other facial cosmetic procedures are still performed on Caucasian patients, this type of surgery is gaining rapidly in popularity among Hispanics, Asian Americans, and African

Americans. Between 1999 and 2002, the proportion of cosmetic procedures performed on Hispanics has increased by 200%, on African Americans by 323%, and on Asian Americans by 340%. As of 2003, Caucasians account for only 77% of patients having elective facial surgery, compared to 83% in 1999.

Description

There are two main types of forehead lifts. The classic, or open, forehead lift involves a long incision along the top of the forehead and lifting of the skin of the forehead. The second type of forehead lift, known as an endoscopic lift, is performed with special instruments inserted through four or five small incisions behind the hairline.

In some cases, a forehead lift is combined with **plastic surgery** on the eyelids (**blepharoplasty**) or with a **face lift**.

KEY TERMS

Blepharoplasty—Plastic surgery performed on the eyelids.

Body dysmorphic disorder (BDD)—A psychiatric condition marked by excessive preoccupation with an imaginary or minor defect in a facial feature or localized part of the body. Many people with BDD seek cosmetic surgery as a treatment for their perceived flaw.

Botulinum toxin—A toxin produced by the spores and growing cells of *Clostridium botulinum*. It causes muscle paralysis, therefore this toxin can be used to reduce frown lines by temporarily paralyzing the muscles in the face that contract when a person frowns or squints.

Collagen—A type of protein found in connective tissue that gives it strength and flexibility. Collagen derived from cattle can be injected into wrinkles or lines in the face as an alternative to cosmetic surgery.

Cosmetic surgery—Surgery that is intended to improve a patient's appearance or correct disfigurement. It is also called aesthetic surgery.

Endoscope—An instrument that allows a surgeon to look underneath skin or inside a hollow organ while performing surgery.

Ptosis—The medical term for drooping of the upper eyelid.

Classic forehead lift

The classic forehead lift takes about one to two hours and may be performed with either general or **local anesthesia**. After the patient has been anesthetized, the surgeon makes a long incision across the top of the scalp from ear to ear. The exact location of the incision depends on the condition of the facial muscles to be removed or modified and the position of the patient's hairline. The most common type of incision in an open forehead lift is a coronal incision, which is made slightly behind the hairline. A second type of incision is called a pretrichial incision. It is similar to the coronal incision except that the central part of the incision lies directly on the hairline. A third type of incision, which is used mostly on male patients with very deep forehead creases, is placed directly inside the creases in the mid-forehead.

After the incision has been made, the surgeon lifts the skin of the forehead very carefully and cuts away excess underlying tissue. Some of the muscles that cause frowning may be loosened (released) or altered. If necessary, the brows will be lifted and excess skin along the line of the incision will be trimmed away. The incision is usually closed with **stitches** or **staples**, although some surgeons use tissue glues to hold the skin in place. The patient's face is then carefully washed to prevent infection and irritation. Some surgeons prefer to cover the incision with a gauze dressing held in place by an elastic bandage, but others do not apply any dressing.

One disadvantage of the classic forehead lift from the standpoint of male patients is that men's hairstyles will not usually cover the incision scar. It is easier for women, even those who prefer to wear their hair very short, to let the hair grow for several weeks before the procedure so that it will be long enough to cover the scar.

Endoscopic forehead lift

An endoscopic forehead lift is performed with the help of an endoscope, which is an instrument designed to allow the surgeon to see the tissues and other structures underneath the skin of the forehead. Instead of making one long incision, the surgeon makes four or five shorter incisions, each less than an inch (2.5 cm) long. The endoscope is inserted through one of these incisions; the others are used for the insertion of instruments for removing excess tissue and reshaping the facial muscles. If the eyebrows are being lifted, they may be kept in place in their new position by tiny stitches under the skin or fixation tacks placed behind the hairline. The incisions are closed and the patient's face washed and dressed in the same way as in the classic forehead lift.

Diagnosis/Preparation

Diagnosis

It is somewhat misleading to speak of diagnosis on the context of forehead lifts and similar procedures because cosmetic surgery is unique in one respect—it is the only type of surgery in which the patient initiates "treatment" rather than the doctor. This difference means that many plastic surgeons now screen patients for psychological stability as well as general physical fitness for surgery. Beginning in the 1970s and 1980s, psychiatrists began to see patients who were obsessed with a particular facial feature or other small part of their body, as distinct from over-concern about weight or general body shape. This condition, which is called body dysmorphic disorder (BDD), became an official psychiatric diagnostic category in 1987. Patients with BDD frequently seek plastic surgery as a solution for their dissatisfaction with their looks; however, in many cases, the "flaw" that the patient sees in his or her face is either exaggerated or nonexistent. Ironically, although men are less likely than women to request facial surgery, a higher percentage of male cosmetic surgery patients are emotionally disturbed; one survey of plastic surgeons estimated that six out of every 100 female patients and seven out of every 100 male patients meet the diagnostic criteria for BDD.

When a person consults a plastic surgeon about a forehead lift or similar procedure, the doctor will spend some time talking with the patient about his or her motives for facial surgery as well as taking a general medical and surgical history. Good candidates for facial surgery are people who have a realistic understanding of the risks as well as the benefits of this type of surgery, and equally realistic expectations of the outcome. On the other hand, the following are considered psychological warning signs:

- The patient is considering surgery to please someone else, most often a spouse or partner.
- The patient expects facial surgery to guarantee career advancement.
- The patient has a history of multiple cosmetic procedures and/or complaints about previous surgeons.
- The patient thinks that the surgery will solve all his or her life problems.
- The patient has an unrealistic notion of what he or she will look like after surgery.
- The patient seems otherwise emotionally unstable.

If the surgeon thinks that the patient is a good candidate in terms of motivation, he or she will continue the diagnostic assessment by examining the patient's face at close range. To make an initial evaluation of the possible results of a forehead lift, the surgeon will gently lift the skin at the outer edges of the eyes above the brows in an upward direction. He or she may also ask the patient to look in a mirror and describe what they don't like about their face. Next, the surgeon will ask the patient to frown, smile, or make a variety of other facial expressions. This technique allows the surgeon to observe the activity of the patient's facial muscles. Depending on the amount of loose skin in the upper eyelid, the height of the patient's hairline, and the relative position of the eyebrows, the surgeon may recommend a blepharoplasty or other procedure instead of a forehead lift.

Preparation

Preparation for a forehead lift involves practical as well as medical concerns.

FINANCIAL CONSIDERATIONS. Most cosmetic facial procedures are not covered by health insurance because they are regarded as nonessential elective procedures. As a result, many cosmetic surgeons request that fees be paid in full before the operation. According to the AACS, 13.4% of cosmetic surgery patients take out loans to finance their procedure. In 2002, the average cost of a forehead lift was $3,300.

MEDICAL AND HOME CARE ISSUES. A patient scheduled for a forehead lift will be asked to prepare for the operation by quitting smoking and discontinuing **aspirin** or any other medications that thin the blood. The surgeon will ask for a list of all medications that the patient is taking, including alternative herbal preparations and prescription drugs, to make sure that there will be no interactions with the anesthetic.

Patients are advised to have someone drive them home after the procedure and help them with routine chores for a day or two. If the forehead lift is combined with a face lift or blepharoplasty, the surgeon may have the patient remain in the hospital overnight. Although cosmetic surgery on the face does not interfere with walking or routine physical activity, most patients tire easily for the first few days after the procedure.

Aftercare

Classic forehead lift

Aftercare for a classic forehead lift is somewhat more complicated than for an endoscopic procedure. Pain or numbness around the incision is likely to last longer than for an endoscopic procedure. It is controlled with prescription medication. Patients are usually advised to keep the head elevated for two to three days after surgery to minimize swelling. **Bandages** are removed a day or two after the procedure; stitches or staples are taken out between 10 days and two weeks after surgery. The patient is asked to rest quietly for one or two days after surgery. Most patients can return to work after a week or 10 days.

Endoscopic forehead lift

Fixation devices around the eyebrows are usually removed within 10 days after endoscopic surgery. As of early 2003, new absorbable fixation tacks that do not require later removal are being used with good results.

Patients who have had either type of forehead lift should not wash their hair until the bandage or dressing is removed, usually within two days. Heavy lifting, vigorous athletic activity, sexual activity, or any type of exertion that raises the blood pressure should be avoided for five to six weeks after the surgery. The skin around the incision should be protected from direct exposure to the sun for at least six months, because the new tissue is much more vulnerable to sunburn than normal skin. Most surgeons advise patients to use a sunblock cream to protect the skin even after the first six months.

Patients can use a special camouflage makeup to cover the bruising or swelling that often occurs after surgery, although they should be careful to keep the makeup away from the incision. Most of the bruising and other signs of surgery will fade within about three weeks.

Risks

Major complications of a forehead lift are unusual. The most common risks from the procedure are as follows:

- Headaches for a day or two after surgery. This complication is much more common with a classic forehead lift than with endoscopic surgery.
- Mild pain around the incision for a few days after surgery.
- Numbness or itching sensations on the top of the scalp. These may last for as long as six months after surgery.
- Mild bruising or swelling around the eyelids and cheeks.
- Hair loss or thinning in the area of the incision. The hair will usually regrow within a few weeks or months.
- A feeling of numbness or dryness in the eye.
- Loss of function of the eyelid. This complication is corrected by another operation.
- Bleeding or infection. These are rare complications with forehead lifts.

WHO PERFORMS THE PROCEDURE AND WHERE IS IT PERFORMED?

A forehead lift is a specialized procedure performed only by a qualified plastic surgeon. Plastic surgeons are doctors who have completed three years of general surgical training followed by two to three years of specialized training in plastic surgery after completing their M.D. or D.O. degree.

A forehead lift may be performed either in a hospital or in an outpatient clinic that specializes in cosmetic surgery. Most endoscopic forehead lifts are performed in outpatient facilities.

Normal results

Normal results of a forehead lift are an improvement in appearance that is satisfying to the patient. Specifically, the forehead should look less creased or wrinkled and frown lines should be lighter. The cosmetic effects of a forehead lift last between five and 10 years, depending on the person's age and the condition of their skin when the procedure was performed.

Morbidity and mortality rates

In general, mortality and morbidity rates for forehead lifts and similar facial cosmetic procedures are very low. Almost all cases of mortality following facial cosmetic surgery involve patients who were treated for facial disfigurement because they had been severely burned or attacked by animals. Moreover, many plastic surgeons do not consider morbidity and mortality rates to be as significant as other factors in evaluating the success of facial cosmetic procedures. One group of researchers at the University of Washington maintains that "[t]he most important measures of outcome in facial cosmetic surgery are quality of life and patient satisfaction, in contrast to other, more objective measures such as complications or mortality rates."

Several American studies have reported that the rate of complications is no higher when a forehead lift is done in combination with other facial procedures than when it is done by itself.

Alternatives

Soft tissue fillers

Alternatives to surgical treatment for frown lines and wrinkles of the forehead include injections of filler materials under the skin to smooth wrinkles or injections of botulinum toxin to paralyze the facial muscles

QUESTIONS TO ASK THE DOCTOR

- How many forehead lifts have you performed?
- Should I consider combining the forehead lift with a face lift?
- Am I a candidate for an endoscopic forehead lift?
- Would I benefit from nonsurgical alternatives to a forehead lift?
- How long can I expect the effects of this surgery to last?

involved in frowning or brow wrinkling. The most commonly used filler materials are collagen and fat. Collagen is a protein found in human and animal connective tissue that makes the tissue strong and flexible. Most collagen that is used for cosmetic injections is derived from cattle, which produces allergic reactions in some people. Fat injections use fat taken from the patient's abdomen, thighs, or buttocks. The fat is then reinjected under the skin of the forehead to smooth out lines and wrinkles.

One drawback of both collagen and fat injections is that the effects are not permanent. Some new injectable filler substances are said to be permanent wrinkle removers. They include Artecoll, which contains small plastic particles that supposedly stimulate the body to produce its own collagen; and Radiance, which is made of a chemical called calcium hydroxylapatite. Still other injectable tissue fillers are made from synthetic hyaluronic acid, which has been used for a number of years to treat joint pain. Since hyaluronic acid is produced naturally in the body, allergic reactions to this type of tissue filler are relatively rare.

Botulinum toxin

Botulinum toxin is a compound produced by the spores and growing cells of the organism that causes botulism, *Clostridium botulinum*. The toxin causes muscle paralysis. It was first used clinically in the 1960s to treat neurological disorders but also proved to be effective in paralyzing the facial muscles that cause crow's feet and frown wrinkles. Botulinum toxin, or Botox, was approved by the U.S. Food and Drug Administration (FDA) in April 2002 as a treatment for facial lines and wrinkles.

Both soft tissue fillers and Botox injections are regarded as effective though temporary alternatives to a forehead lift for reducing frown lines. Collagen injections must be repeated every three to six months, while Botox injections are effective for about four months.

Fracture repair

Resources

BOOKS

Engler, Alan M. *BodySculpture: Plastic Surgery of the Body for Men and Women,* 2nd ed. New York: Hudson Publishing, 2000.

Irwin, Brandith, and Mark McPherson. *Your Best Face Without Surgery.* Carlsbad, CA: Hay House Inc., 2002.

Man, Daniel. *New Art of Man.* New York: BeautyArt Press, 2003.

Papel, I. D., J. Frodel, G. R. Holt, W. F. Larrabee, N. Nachlas, S. S. Park, J. M. Sykes, and D. Toriumi. *Facial Plastic and Reconstructive Surgery,* 2nd ed. New York: Thieme Medical Publishers, 2002.

PERIODICALS

Dayan, S. H., S. W. Perkins, A. J. Vartanian, and I. M. Wiesman. "The Forehead Lift: Endoscopic Versus Coronal Approaches." *Aesthetic Plastic Surgery* 25, no. 1 (January–February 2001): 35–39.

De Cordier, B. C., J. I. de la Torre, M. S. Al-Hakeem, et al. "Endoscopic Forehead Lift: Review of Technique, Cases, and Complications." *Plastic and Reconstructive Surgery* 110, no. 6 (November 2002): 1558–1568.

Landecker, A., J. B. Buck, J. C. Grotting, and B. Guyuron. "A New Resorbable Tack Fixation Technique for Endoscopic Brow Lifts." *Plastic and Reconstructive Surgery* 111, no. 2 (February 2003): 880–890.

Morgenstern, K. E. and J. A. Foster. "Advances in cosmetic oculoplastic surgery." *Current Opinion in Ophthalmology* 13, no. 5 (October 2002): 324–330.

Most, S. P., R. Alsarraf, and W. F. Larrabee, Jr. "Outcomes of Facial Cosmetic Procedures." *Facial Plastic Surgery* 18, no. 2 (May 2002): 119–124.

Namazie, A. R., and G. S. Keller. "Current Practices in Endoscopic Brow and Temporal Lifting." *Facial Plastic Surgery Clinics of North America* 9, no. 3 (August 2001): 439–451.

Paul, M. D. "The Evolution of the Brow Lift in Aesthetic Plastic Surgery." *Plastic and Reconstructive Surgery* 108, no. 5 (October 2001): 1409–1424.

OTHER

"Browlift." American Society of Plastic Surgeons. http://www.plasticsurgery.org/public_education/procedures/Browlift.cfm (February 2008).

"Forehead Lift." American Society for Aesthetic Plastic Surgery. http://www.surgery.org/public/procedures/forehead_lift (February 2008).

Sclafani, Anthony P., and Kyle S. Choe, MD. "Psychological Aspects of Plastic Surgery." *eMedicine.* August 29, 2006. http://www.emedicine.com/ent/topic36.htm (February 28, 2003).

Siwolop, Sana. "Beyond Botox: An Industry's Quest for Smooth Skin." *New York Times* March 9, 2003. http://query.nytimes.com/gst/fullpage.html?res=9806EFD7103FF93AA35750C0A9659C8B63 (March 9, 2003).

ORGANIZATIONS

American Academy of Cosmetic Surgery, 737 North Michigan Avenue, Suite 820, Chicago, IL, 60611-5405, (312) 981-6760, http://www.cosmeticsurgery.org.

American Academy of Facial Plastic and Reconstructive Surgery, 310 S. Henry Street, Alexandria, VA, 22314, (703) 229-9291, http://www.aafprs.org/.

American Board of Plastic Surgery, Seven Penn Center, Suite 4001635 Market Street, Philadelphia, PA, 19103-2204, (215) 587-9322, http://www.abplsurg.org/.

American College of Surgeons, 633 North Saint Claire Street, Chicago, IL, 60611, (312) 202-5000, http://www.facs.org/.

American Society for Aesthetic Plastic Surgery, 11081 Winners Circle, Los Alamitos, CA, 90720, (888) 272-7711, http://www.surgery.org/.

American Society of Plastic and Reconstructive Surgeons, 444 E. Algonquin Road, Arlington Heights, IL, 60005, (847) 228-9900, http://www.plasticsurgery.org.

Rebecca Frey, Ph.D.
Laura Jean Cataldo, R.N., Ed.D.

Fracture repair

Definition

Bone is the hardest tissue in the human body, but when bones are subjected to forces that exceed their strength, they may break. The likelihood that a bone will break depends on the location of the bone in the body, the thickness of the bone, and the circumstances under which the force was applied. The most commonly broken bones are those in the wrist, hip, and ankle. The terms "break" and "fracture" mean the same thing. Fracture repair is the process of rejoining and realigning the ends of broken bones, usually performed by an orthopedist, general surgeon, or family doctor. In cases of an emergency, first aid measures should be used to provide temporary realignment and immobilization until proper medical help is available.

Purpose

Fracture repair is required when there is a need to restore the normal alignment and function of a broken bone. Throughout the stages of fracture healing, the bones must be held firmly in the correct position. In the event that a fracture is not properly repaired, misalignment of the bone may occur, resulting in possible physical dysfunction of the bone, adjacent joint, or region of the body.

Fracture repair

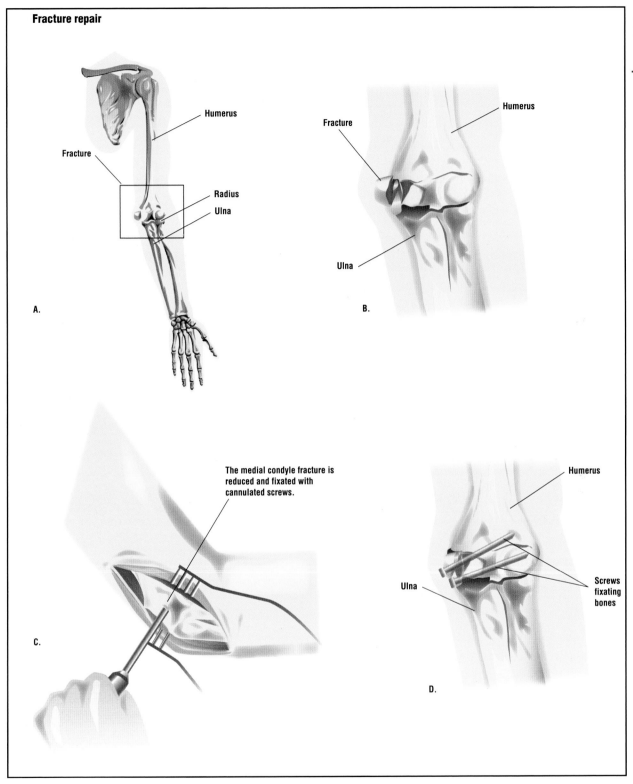

Humerus

Fracture

Radius

Ulna

A.

Humerus

Fracture

Ulna

B.

The medial condyle fracture is
reduced and fixated with
cannulated screws.

C.

Humerus

Screws
fixating
bones

Ulna

D.

In this patient, a fall has resulted in fractures in the bones of the elbow (B). To repair the fracture, and incision is made in the
elbow area (C), and the bones are fixed with screws to aid proper healing (D). *(Illustration by GGS Information Services. Cengage
Learning, Gale.)*

Demographics

The incidence of fractures that occur in the United States can only be estimated because fractures are not always reported. The average person sustains two to three fractured bones during the course of a lifetime. A reasonable estimate is approximately nine million fractures per year.

Fractures are slightly more common in children and adolescents than in young adults due to the levels and kinds of activities in which they engage. Fractures become more common in adults as they age due to changes in bone structure and generally diminished levels of physical activity.

Description

Fracture repair is accomplished by means of applied **traction**, surgery, and immobilizing affected bones. The bone fragments are aligned as closely as possible to their normal position without injuring the skin. Metal wires or screws may be needed to align smaller bone fragments. Once the broken ends of the bone are set, the affected area is immobilized for several weeks and kept rigid with a sling, plaster cast, brace, or splint. With the use of traction, muscles pulling on the fracture site are neutralized by weights attached to a series of ropes running over pulleys. Strategically implanted electrical stimulation devices have proven beneficial in healing a fracture site, especially when the fracture is healing poorly and repair by other means is difficult.

Diagnosis/Preparation

Fractures are commonly diagnosed on the basis of history of trauma or the presence of pain. An x ray is usually taken to confirm the diagnosis.

Precautions for fracture repair include any relevant factors in an individual's medical condition and history. These include allergic reactions to anesthesia and the presence of bleeding disorders that may complicate surgery.

Preparation often begins with emergency splinting to immobilize the body part or parts involved. When fracture repair is necessary, the procedure is often performed in a hospital, but can also be successfully done in an outpatient surgical facility, doctor's office, or emergency room. Before any surgery for fracture repair, blood and urine studies may be performed. X rays may be obtained. It must be noted, however, that not all fractures are immediately apparent on an initial x-ray examination. In such a case, when a fracture is highly suspected, the extent of the fracture can be properly diagnosed by repeating the x rays 10–14 days later. Depending upon the situation, local or **general anesthesia** may be used during fracture repair.

Aftercare

Immediately following surgical repair of a fracture, x rays may be again taken through the cast or splint to evaluate whether the rejoined pieces are in a good position for healing. The x ray can be performed either before the application of the splint or at least before an individual is awakened from the general anesthesia. Persons need to **exercise** caution and not place excess pressure on any part of the cast until it is completely dry. Excess pressure on the operative site should also be avoided until complete healing has taken place and the injury has been re-examined by the physician or surgeon. If the cast becomes exposed to moisture, it may soften and require repair. For this reason, plastic has largely replaced plaster as the casting material of choice. The injured region should be elevated or propped up whenever possible to reduce the possibility of swelling.

Risks

Surgical risks of fracture repair are greater in persons over 60 years of age because the bones often require more time to properly heal. Obesity may place extra stress on the fracture site, affecting healing and possibly increasing the risk of re-fracturing the same bone. The healing process after fracture repair may also be slowed by smoking, poor nutrition, alcoholism, and chronic illness. Some medications may affect the fracture site, causing poor union; such medications include anti-hypertensives and steroids such as cortisone.

WHO PERFORMS THE PROCEDURE AND WHERE IS IT PERFORMED?

Fracture repair is usually performed by an orthopedic surgeon, general surgeon, or family physician. In cases of an emergency, first aid measures should be used for temporary realignment and immobilization until proper medical help can be obtained. Relatively uncomplicated fractures may be immobilized in a physician's office. More commonly, fractures are treated in a hospital setting.

QUESTIONS TO ASK THE DOCTOR

Candidates for fracture repair should consider asking the following questions:

- What type of fracture do I have?
- Is the surgeon properly trained in the proposed method of fracture repair?
- How many similar procedures has the surgeon performed?

Possible complications following fracture repair include excessive bleeding, improper fit of joined bone ends, pressure on nearby nerves, delayed healing, and a permanent incomplete healing (union) of the fracture. If there is a poor blood supply to the fractured site and one of the portions of broken bone is not adequately supplied with blood, the bony portion may die and healing of the fracture will not take place. This complication is called aseptic necrosis. Poor immobilization of the fracture from improper casting that permits motion between the bone parts may prevent healing and repair of the bone, and result in possible deformity. Infection can interfere with bone repair. This risk is greater in the case of a compound fracture (a bone fracture involving a portion of bone that breaks through the surface of skin). Compound fracture sites provide ideal conditions for severe infections by *Streptococcus* and *Staphylococcus* bacteria. Occasionally, fractured bones in the elderly may never heal properly. The risk is increased when nutrition is poor.

Normal results

Once the procedure for fracture repair is completed, the body begins to produce new tissue to bridge the fracture site and rejoin the broken pieces. At first, this tissue (called a callus) is soft and easily injured. Later, the body deposits bone minerals (primarily compounds containing calcium) until the callus becomes a solid piece of bone. The fracture site is thus further strengthened with extra bone. It usually takes about six weeks for the pieces of a broken bone to knit (heal) together. The exact time required for healing depends on the type of fracture and the extent of damage. Before the use of x rays, fracture repair was not always accurate and frequently resulted in crippling deformities. With modern x-ray technology, physicians can view the extent of the fracture, check the setting following the repair, and be certain after the

procedure that the bones have not moved from their intended alignment. Children's bones usually heal more rapidly than do the bones of adults.

Morbidity and mortality rates

Morbidity associated with fracture repair includes damage to nerves or primary blood vessels that are adjacent to the fracture site. Improper alignment causing deformity is an abnormal outcome that is relatively rare due to presently available medical technology.

Mortality associated with fractures is also rare. It is usually associated with infections or contamination acquired during the fracture process.

Alternatives

There are no alternatives to proper fracture repair. Problems associated with allowing a fracture to heal without intervention include misalignment, deformity, loss of function, and pain.

Magnetic fields are occasionally used to stimulate healing when conventional techniques are not effective.

Resources

BOOKS

Browner, B., J. Jupiter, A. Levine, and P. Trafton. *Skeletal Trauma: Fractures, Dislocations, Ligamentous Injuries,* 3rd ed. Philadelphia: Saunders, 2002.

Canale, S. T. *Campbell's Operative Orthopedics,* 10th ed. St. Louis, MO: Mosby, 2002.

Dutton, Mark. *Orthopaedic Examination, Evaluation, and Intervention.* New York: McGraw-Hill, 2004.

Eiff, M. P., R. L. Hatch, and W. L. Calmbach. *Fracture Management for Primary Care,* 2nd ed. Philadelphia: Saunders, 2002.

Skinner, Harry.*Current Diagnosis & Treatment in Orthopedics.* New York: McGraw-Hill, 2006.

Staheli, L. T. *Fundamentals of Pediatric Orthopedics,* 4th ed. Philadelphia: Lippincott Williams & Wilkins, 2007.

PERIODICALS

Henry, B. J., et al. "The Effect of Local Hematoma Blocks on Early Fracture Healing." *Orthopedics* 25, no. 11 (2002): 1259–1262.

Ong, C. T., D. S. K. Choon, N. P. Cabrera, and N. Maffulli. "The Treatment of Open Tibial Fractures and of Tibial Non-union with a Novel External Fixator." *Injury* 33, no. 9 (2002): 829–834.

Sammarco, V. J., and L. Chang. "Modern Issues in Bone Graft Substitutes and Advances in Bone Tissue Technology." *Foot and Ankle Clinics of North America* 7, no. 1 (March 2002): 19–41.

Szczesny, G. "Molecular Aspects of Bone Healing and Remodeling." *Polish Journal of Pathology* 53, no. 3 (2002): 145–153.

OTHER

"Bone fracture repair." Medline Plus Medical Encyclopedia. October 23, 2006. http://www.nlm.nih.gov/medlineplus/ency/article/002966.htm (February 28, 2003).

International Society for Fracture Repair. Information on fracture repair research. http://www.fractures.com/ (February 28, 2003).

"Quality of Life After Hip Fracture Repair May Depend on the Type of Anesthesia Used, UM Medical Center Researchers Find." University of Maryland Medical Center. January 31, 2000. http://www.umm.edu/news/releases/hip.html (February 28, 2003).

ORGANIZATIONS

American Academy of Orthopaedic Surgeons, 6300 N. River Road, Rosemont, IL, 60018-4262, (847) 823-7186, (800) 346-AAOS, (847) 823-8125, http://www.aaos.org.

American College of Surgeons, 633 North Saint Claire Street, Chicago, IL, 60611, (312) 202-5000, http://www.facs.org/.

American Society for Bone and Mineral Research, 2025 M Street, NW, Suite 800, Washington, DC, 20036-3309, (202) 367-1161, http://www.asbmr.org/.

Orthopedic Trauma Association, 6300 N. River Road, Suite 727, Rosemont, IL, 60018-4226, (847) 698-1631, http://www.ota.org/links.htm.

L. Fleming Fallon, Jr., M.D., Dr.P.H.
Laura Jean Cataldo, R.N., Ed.D.

Functional endoscopic sinus surgery *see* **Endoscopic sinus surgery**

Fundoplication surgery *see* **Gastroesophageal reflux surgery**

Funnel chest repair *see* **Pectus excavatum repair**

Furosemide *see* **Diuretics**

G

Gallbladder removal *see* **Cholecystectomy**

Gallbladder ultrasound *see* **Abdominal ultrasound**

Gallstone removal

Definition

Also known as cholelithotomy, gallstone removal is a procedure that rids the gallbladder of calculus buildup.

Purpose

The gallbladder is not a vital organ. It is located on the right side of the abdomen underneath the liver. The gallbladder's function is to store bile, concentrate it, and release it during digestion. Bile is supposed to retain all of its chemicals in solution, but commonly one of them crystallizes and forms sandy or gravel-like particles, finally collecting into gallstones. The formation of gallstones causes gallbladder disease (cholelithiasis).

Chemicals in bile will form crystals as the gallbladder draws water out of the bile. The solubility of these chemicals is based on the concentration of three chemicals: bile acids, phospholipids, and cholesterol. If the chemicals are out of balance, one or the other will not remain in solution. Dietary fat and cholesterol are also implicated in crystal formation.

As the bile crystals aggregate to form stones, they move about, eventually blocking the outlet and preventing the gallbladder from emptying. This blockage results in irritation, inflammation, and sometimes infection (cholecystitis) of the gallbladder. The pattern is usually one of intermittent obstruction due to stones moving in and out of the way. Meanwhile, the gallbladder becomes more and more scarred. Sometimes,

infection fills the gallbladder with pus, which is a serious complication.

Occasionally, a gallstone will travel down the cystic duct into the common bile duct and get stuck there. This blockage will back bile up into the liver as well as the gallbladder. If the stone sticks at the ampulla of Vater (a narrowing in the duct leading to the pancreas), the pancreas will also be blocked and will develop pancreatitis.

Gallstones will cause a sudden onset of pain in the upper abdomen. Pain will last for 30 minutes to several hours. Pain may move to the right shoulder blade. Nausea with or without vomiting may accompany the pain.

Demographics

Gallstones are approximately two times more common in females than in males. Overweight women in their middle years constitute the vast majority of patients with gallstones in every racial or ethnic group. An estimated 10% of the general population has gallstones. The prevalence for women between ages 20 and 55 is about 20%, and is higher after age 50 (25–30%). Women between the ages of 20 and 60 years are three times more likely to have gallstones than are men. Certain people, in particular the Pima tribe of Native Americans in Arizona, have a genetic predisposition to forming gallstones. Scandinavians also have a higher than average incidence of this disease.

There seems to be a strong genetic correlation with gallstone disease, because stones are more than four times as likely to occur among first-degree relatives. Since gallstones rarely dissolve spontaneously, the prevalence increases with age. Obesity is a well-known risk factor since being overweight causes chemical abnormalities that lead to increased levels of cholesterol. Gallstones are also associated with rapid weight loss secondary to dieting. Pregnancy is a risk factor since increased estrogen levels result in an increased

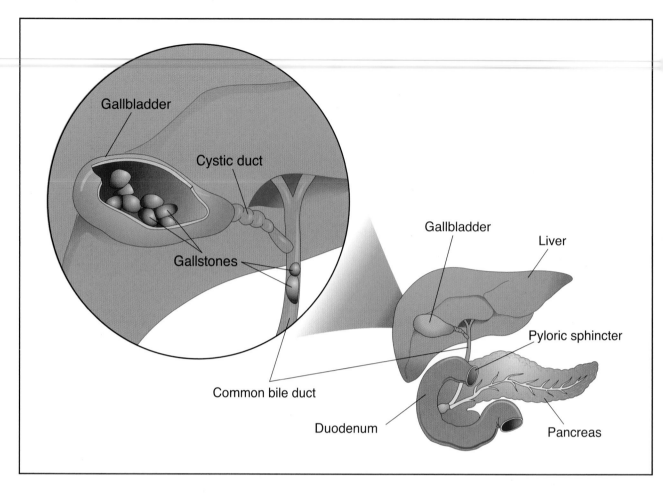

Gallstone removal, also known as cholelithotomy, usually involves the surgical removal of the entire gallbladder, but in recent years the procedure done by laparoscopy has resulted in smaller surgical incisions and faster recovery time. *(Illustration by Electronic Illustrators Group. Cengage Learning, Gale.)*

cholesterol secretion and abnormal changes in bile. However, while an increase in dietary cholesterol is not a risk factor, an increase in triglycerides is positively associated with a higher incidence of gallstones. Diabetes mellitus is also believed to be a risk factor for gallstone development.

Description

Surgery to remove the entire gallbladder with all its stones is usually the best treatment, provided the patient is able to tolerate the procedure. A relatively new technique of removing the gallbladder using a laparoscope has resulted in quicker recovery and much smaller surgical incisions than the 6-in (15-cm) gash under the ribs on the right that had previously been the standard procedure; however, not everyone is a candidate for this approach. If the procedure is not expected to have complications, laparoscopic **cholecystectomy** is performed. Laparoscopic surgery

requires a space in the surgical area for visualization and instrument manipulation. The laparoscope with attached video camera is inserted. Several other instruments are inserted through the abdomen to assist the surgeon to maneuver around other nearby organs during surgery. The surgeon must take precautions not to accidentally harm anatomical structures in the liver. Once the cystic artery has been divided and the gallbladder dissected from the liver, the gallbladder can be removed.

If the gallbladder is extremely diseased (inflamed, infected, or has large gallstones), the abdominal approach (open cholecystectomy) is recommended. This surgery is usually performed with an incision in the upper midline of the abdomen or on the right side of the abdomen below the rib (right subcostal incision).

If a stone is lodged in the bile ducts, additional surgery must be done to remove it. After surgery, the surgeon will ordinarily insert a drain to collect bile

KEY TERMS

Bilirubin—A pigment released from red blood cells.

Cholecystectomy—Surgical removal of the gallbladder.

Cholelithotomy—Surgical incision into the gallbladder to remove stones.

Contrast agent—A substance that causes shadows on x rays (or other images of the body).

Cystic artery—An artery that brings oxygenated blood to the gallbladder.

Endoscope—An instrument designed to enter body cavities.

Jaundice—A yellow discoloration of the skin and eyes due to excess bile that is not removed by the liver.

Laparoscopy—Surgery performed through small incisions with pencil-sized instruments.

Triglycerides—Chemicals made up mostly of fat that can form deposits in tissues and cause health risks or disease.

until the system is healed. The drain can also be used to inject contrast material and take x rays during or after surgery.

A procedure called endoscopic retrograde cholangiopancreatoscopy (ERCP) allows the removal of some bile duct stones through the mouth, throat, esophagus, stomach, duodenum, and biliary system without the need for surgical incisions. ERCP can also be used to inject contrast agents into the biliary system, providing finely detailed pictures.

Patients with symptomatic cholelithiasis can be treated with certain medications, a technique called oral bile acid litholysis or oral dissolution therapy. This technique is especially effective for dissolving small cholesterol-composed gallstones. Current research indicates that the success rate for oral dissolution treatment is 70–80% with floating stones (those predominantly composed of cholesterol). Approximately 10–20% of patients who receive medication-induced litholysis can have a recurrence within the first two or three years after treatment completion.

Extracorporeal shock wave **lithotripsy** is a treatment in which shock waves are generated in water by lithotripters (devices that produce the waves). There are several types of lithotripters available for gallbladder removal. One specific lithotripter involves the use of piezoelectric crystals, which allow the shock waves

to be accurately focused on a small area to disrupt a stone. This procedure does not generally require analgesia (or anesthesia). Damage to the gallbladder and associated structures (such as the cystic duct) must be present for stone removal after the shock waves break up the stone. Typically, repeated shock wave treatments are necessary to completely remove gallstones. The success rate of the fragmentation of the gallstone and urinary clearance is inversely proportional to stone size and number: patients with a small solitary stone have the best outcome, with high rates of stone clearance (95% are cleared within 12–18 months), while patients with multiple stones are at risk for poor clearance rates. Complications of shock wave lithotripsy include inflammation of the pancreas (pancreatitis) and acute cholecystitis. Gallstones do recur after lithotripsy; the rate of recurrence after the first year is 6–7%, and after five years the rate of recurrence is 31–44%.

A method called contact dissolution of gallstone removal involves direct entry (via a percutaneous transhepatic catheter) of a chemical solvent (such as methyl tertbutylether, MTBE). MTBE is rapidly removed unchanged from the body via the respiratory system (exhaled air). Side effects in persons receiving contact dissolution therapy include foul-smelling breath, dyspnea (difficulty breathing), vomiting, and drowsiness. Treatment with MTBE can be successful in treating cholesterol gallstones regardless of the number and size of stones. Studies indicate that the success rate for dissolution is well over 95% in persons who receive direct chemical infusions that can last 5–12 hours.

Diagnosis/Preparation

Diagnostically, gallstone disease, which can lead to gallbladder removal, is divided into four diseases: biliary colic, acute cholecystitis, choledocholithiasis, and cholangitis. Biliary colic is usually caused by intermittent cystic duct obstruction by a stone (without any inflammation), causing a severe, poorly localized, and intensifying pain on the upper right side of the abdomen. These painful attacks can persist from days to months in patients with biliary colic.

Persons affected with acute cholecystitis caused by an impacted stone in the cystic duct also suffer from gallbladder infection in approximately 50% of cases. These people have moderately severe pain in the upper right portion of the abdomen that lasts longer than six hours. Pain with acute cholecystitis can also extend to the shoulder or back. Since there may be infection inside the gallbladder, the patient may also have fever. On the right side of the abdomen below the last rib, there is usually tenderness with inspiratory (breathing in) arrest (Murphy's sign). In about 33% of cases of acute cholecystitis, the gallbladder may be felt in the abdomen with palpation (feeling for tenderness). Mild jaundice can be present in about 20% of cases.

Persons with choledocholithiasis, or intermittent obstruction of the common bile duct, often do not have symptoms; but, if present they are indistinguishable from the symptoms of biliary colic.

A more severe form of gallstone disease is cholangitis, which causes stone impaction in the common bile duct. In about 70% of cases, these patients present with Charcot's triad (pain, jaundice, and fever). Patients with cholangitis may have chills, mild pain, lethargy, and delirium, which indicate that infection has spread to the bloodstream (bacteremia). The majority of patients with cholangitis will have fever (95%), tenderness in the upper right side of the abdomen, and jaundice (80%).

In addition to a **physical examination**, preparation for laboratory (blood) and special tests is essential to gallstone diagnosis. Patients with biliary colic may have elevated bilirubin and should have an **ultrasound** study to visualize the gallbladder and associated structures. An increase in the **white blood cell count** (leukocytosis) can be expected for both acute cholecystitis and cholangitis (seen in 80% of cases). Ultrasound testing is recommended for acute cholecystitis patients, whereas ERCP is the test usually indicated to assist in a definitive diagnosis for both choledocholithiasis and cholangitis. Patients with either biliary colic or choledocholithiasis are treated with elective laparoscopic cholecystectomy. Open cholecystectomy is recommended for acute cholecystitis. For cholangitis, emergency ERCP is indicated for stone removal. ERCP therapy can remove stones produced by gallbladder disease.

Aftercare

Without a gallbladder, stones rarely recur. Patients who have continued symptoms after their gallbladder is removed may need an ERCP to detect residual stones or damage to the bile ducts caused by the original stones. Occasionally, the ampulla of Vater is too tight for bile to flow through and causes symptoms until it is opened up.

Risks

The most common medical treatment for gallstones is the surgical removal of the gallbladder

(cholecystectomy). Risks associated with gallbladder removal are low, but include damage to the bile ducts, residual gallstones in the bile ducts, or injury to the surrounding organs. With open cholecystectomy, bile duct damage occurs at a rate of 1 per 1,000 patients; for laparoscopic cholecystectomy, the bile duct damage rate is 1–5 per 1,000 patients.

Normal results

Most patients undergoing laparoscopic cholecystectomy may go home the same day of surgery, and may immediately return to normal activities and a normal diet, while most patients who undergo open cholecystectomy must remain in the hospital for five to seven days. After one week, they may resume a normal diet, and in four to six weeks they can expect to return to normal activities.

Morbidity and mortality rates

Cholecystectomy is generally a safe procedure, with an overall mortality rate of 0–1 per 1,000. Infections occur in less than 1 per 1,000 patients undergoing laparoscopic cholecystectomy. Heart problems during the procedures occur at a rate of 5 per 1,000 for arrythmias and 1 per 1,000 for actual heart attack. Pregnant women who must undergo cholecystectomy have a high rate of fetal loss: 40 per 1,000 when no pancreatitis is present and as high as 600 per 1,000 when pancreatitis is present. The improved technique of laparoscopic cholecystectomy accounts for 90% of all cholecystectomies performed in the United States; the improved technique reduces time missed away from work, patient hospitalization, and postoperative pain.

Alternatives

There are no other acceptable alternatives for gallstone removal besides surgery, shock wave fragmentation, or chemical dissolution.

QUESTIONS TO ASK THE DOCTOR

- How long must I remain in the hospital following gallstone removal?
- How do I care for the my incision site?
- How soon can I return to normal activities following gallstone removal?

Resources

BOOKS

Feldman, M, et al. *Sleisenger & Fordtran's Gastrointestinal and Liver Disease*, 8th ed. St. Louis: Mosby, 2005.

Khatri, V. P., and J. A. Asensio. *Operative Surgery Manual*, 1st ed. Philadelphia: Saunders, 2003.

Townsend, C. M., et al. *Sabiston Textbook of Surgery*, 17th ed. Philadelphia: Saunders, 2004.

Laith Farid Gulli, MD
Nicole Mallory, MS, PA-C
J. Polsdorfer, MD
Constance Clyde
Rosalyn Carson-DeWitt, MD

Ganglion cyst removal

Definition

Ganglion cyst removal, or ganglionectomy, is the removal of a fluid-filled sac on the skin of the wrist, finger, or sole of the foot. The cyst is attached to a tendon or a joint through its fibers and contains synovial fluid, which is the clear liquid that lubricates the joints and tendons of the body. The surgical procedure is performed in a doctor's office. It entails aspiration, or draining fluid from the cyst with a large hypodermic needle. The cyst may also be excised (removed by cutting).

Purpose

Ganglion cysts are sacs that contain the synovial fluid found in joints and tendons. They are the most common forms of soft tissue growth on the hand and are distinguished by their sticky liquid contents. The cystic structures are attached to tendon sheaths via a long thin tube-like arm. About 65% of ganglion cysts occur on the upper surface of the wrist, with another 20–25% on the volar (palm) surface of the hand. Most of the remaining 10–15% of ganglion cysts occur on the sheath of the flexor tendon. In a few cases, the cysts emerge on the sole of the foot.

Ganglion cysts have appeared in medical writing from the time of Hippocrates (c. 460–c. 375 B. C.). Their exact cause is unknown. There are some indications, however, that ganglion cysts result from trauma to or deterioration of the tissue lining in the joints that secretes synovial fluid.

Ganglion cysts can emerge quite quickly, and can disappear just as fast. They are benign growths, usually causing problems in the functioning of the joints or tendons of the hand or finger only when they are large. Many people do not seek medical attention for ganglion cysts unless they cause pain, affect the movement of the nearby tendons, or become particularly unsightly.

An old traditional treatment for a ganglion cyst was to hit it with a Bible, since the cysts can burst when struck. Today, cysts are removed surgically by aspiration but often reappear. Surgical excision is the most reliable treatment for ganglion cysts, but aspiration is the more common form of therapy.

Demographics

Ganglion cysts account for 50–70% of all soft tissue tumors of the hand and wrist. They are most likely to occur in adults between the ages of 20 and 50, with the female: male ratio being about three to one. Most ganglion cysts are visible; however, some are occult (hidden). Occult cysts may be diagnosed because the patient feels pain in that part of the hand or has noticed that the tendon cannot move normally. In about 10% of cases, there is associated trauma.

Description

Patients are given a local or regional anesthetic in a doctor's office. Two methods are used to remove the cysts. Most physicians use the more conservative procedure, which is known as aspiration.

Aspiration

- An 18- or 22-gauge needle attached to a 20–30-mL syringe is inserted into the cyst. The doctor removes the fluid slowly by suction.
- The doctor may inject a corticosteroid medication into the joint after the fluid has been withdrawn.
- A compression dressing is applied to the site.
- The patient remains in the office for about 30 minutes.

Ganglion cyst removal

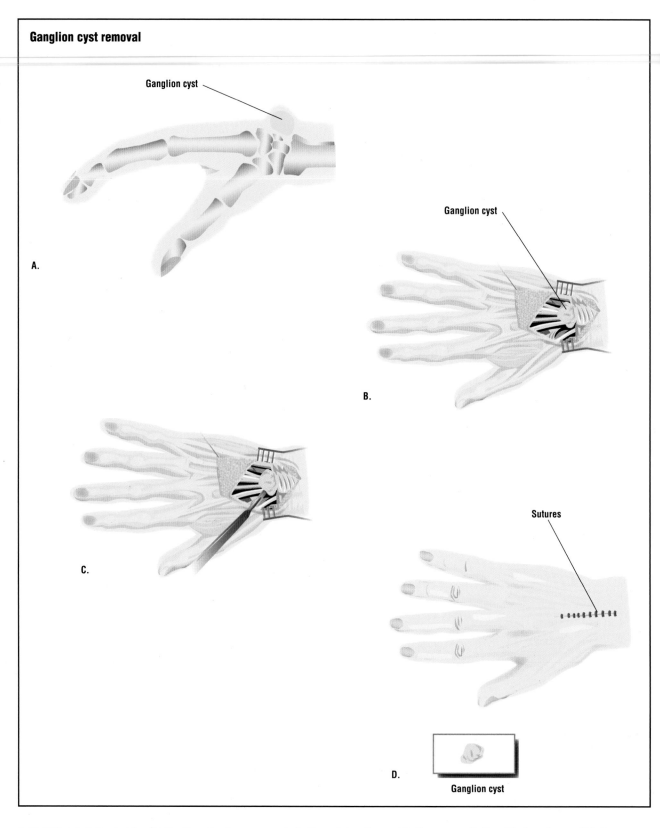

A ganglion cyst is usually attached to a tendon or muscle in the wrist or finger (A). To remove it, the skin is cut open (B), the growth is removed (C), and the skin is sutured closed (D). *(Illustration by GGS Information Services. Cengage Learning, Gale.)*

Excision

Some ganglion cysts are so large that the doctor recommends excision. This procedure also takes place in the physician's office with local or regional anesthetic.

Excision of a ganglion cyst is performed as follows:

- The physician palpates, or feels, the borders of the sac with the fingers and marks the sac and its periphery.
- The sac is cut away with a scalpel.
- The doctor closes the incision with sutures and applies a bandage.
- The patient is asked to remain in the office for at least 30 minutes.

Diagnosis/Preparation

Ganglion cysts are fairly easy to diagnose because they are usually visible and pliable to the touch. They are distinguished from other growths by their location near tendons or joints and by their fluid consistency. Ganglion cysts are sometimes confused with a carpal boss (a bony, non-mobile spur on the top of the wrist), but can usually be distinguished by the fact that they can be moved and are usually less painful for the patient.

The doctor may schedule one or more imaging studies of the hand and wrist. An x ray may reveal

bone or joint abnormalities. **Ultrasound** may be used to diagnose the presence of occult cysts.

Aftercare

Patients should avoid strenuous physical activity for at least 48 hours after surgery and report any signs of infection or inflammation to their physician. A follow-up appointment should be scheduled within three weeks of aspiration or excision. Excision may result in some stiffness after the surgery and some difficulties in flexing the hand because of scar tissue formation.

Risks

Aspiration has very few complications as a treatment for ganglion cysts; the most common aftereffects are infection or a reaction to the cortisone injection. Complications of excision include some stiffness in the hand and scar formation. Ganglion cysts recur after excision in about 5–15% of cases, usually because the cyst was not completely removed.

Normal results

Aspirated ganglion cysts disappear and cause no further symptoms in 27–67% of cases. They may, however, reoccur and require repeated aspiration. Aspiration combined with an injection of cortisone has more success than aspiration by itself. Excision is a much more reliable procedure, however, and the stiffness that the patient may experience after the procedure eventually goes away. The formation of a small scar is normal.

Morbidity and mortality rates

The only risks for ganglion cyst removal are infections or inflammation due to the cortisone injection. There is a small risk of damage to nearby nerves or blood vessels.

Alternatives

Alternatives to aspiration and excision in the treatment of ganglion cysts include watchful waiting and resting the affected hand or foot. It is quite common for ganglion cysts to fade away without any surgical treatment.

Resources

BOOKS

"Common Hand Disorders." Section 5, Chapter 61 in *The Merck Manual of Diagnosis and Therapy*, edited by Mark H. Beers, MD, and Robert Berkow, MD. Whitehouse Station, NJ: Merck Research Laboratories, 1999.

Ferri, Fred F. *Ferri's Clinical Advisor: Instant Diagnosis and Treatment*. St. Louis, MO: Mosby, Inc., 2003.

Ruddy, Shaun, et al. *Kelly's Textbook of Rheumatology*, 6th ed. Philadelphia, PA: W.B. Saunders, 2001.

PERIODICALS

Tallia, A. F., and D. A. Cardone. "Diagnostic and Therapeutic Injection of the Wrist and Hand Region." *American Family Physician* 67 (February 15, 2003): 745-750.

Nancy McKenzie, PhD

Gastrectomy

Definition

Gastrectomy is the surgical removal of all or part of the stomach.

Purpose

Gastrectomy is performed most often to treat the following conditions:

- stomach (gastric) cancer
- bleeding gastric ulcer
- perforation of the stomach wall
- noncancerous tumors

Demographics

According to the World Health Organization (WHO), stomach cancer is the second leading cause of cancer deaths in the world, accounting for about 8.8% of all deaths from cancer. (Lung cancer accounts for 17.8% of cancer deaths). Although stomach cancer is a worldwide problem, the incidence rates vary considerably in different countries. In the 2000s, the highest **death** rates from stomach cancer are found in Japan, South America, especially Chile, and parts of the former Soviet Union. In the United States, the American Cancer Society expected about 21,300 new cases of stomach cancer to be diagnosed and 11,000 deaths to be attributed to the disease. Since gastrectomy is most often done to treat stomach cancer, gastrectomy rates should mirror stomach cancer rates.

Description

Gastrectomy for cancer

Surgery is the only curative treatment for gastric (stomach) cancer. If the cancer is diagnosed early and limited to one part of the stomach, The tumor and only part of the stomach may be removed (partial or subtotal gastrectomy.) More often, the entire stomach is removed (total gastrectomy) along with the surrounding lymph nodes. When the entire stomach is removed, the esophagus is attached directly to the small intestine.

A gastrectomy is performed under **general anesthesia**. Once the patient is anesthetized, a urinary catheter is usually inserted to monitor urine output. A thin nasogastric tube is inserted into the nose, through the esophagus, and into the stomach. The abdomen is cleansed with an antiseptic solution. The surgeon makes a large incision from just below the breastbone down to the navel. The surgeon then removes all or part of the stomach and attaches connects either the remaining piece of stomach or the esophagus to the small intestine.

Gastrectomy for gastric cancer is almost always done using the traditional open surgery technique, which requires a wide incision to open the abdomen. However, some surgeons use a laparoscopic technique that requires only a small incision. The laparoscope is connected to a tiny video camera that relays a picture of the abdomen to a monitor to guide the surgeon who then operates through this incision.

Gastrectomy

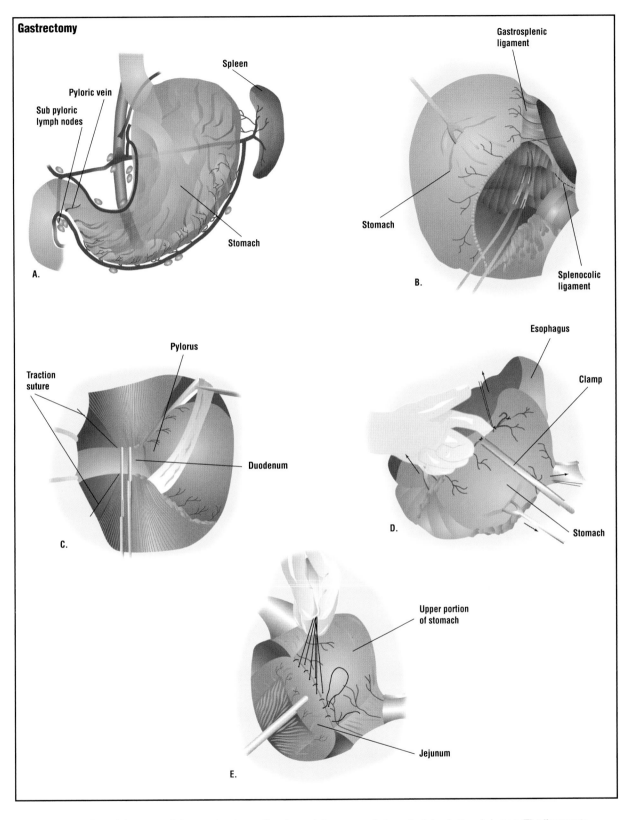

A.

Spleen

Pyloric vein

Sub pyloric lymph nodes

Stomach

B.

Gastrosplenic ligament

Stomach

Splenocolic ligament

C.

Pylorus

Traction suture

Duodenum

D.

Esophagus

Clamp

Stomach

E.

Upper portion of stomach

Jejunum

To remove a portion of the stomach in a gastrectomy, the stomach is accessed via an incision in the abdomen. The ligaments connecting the stomach to the spleen and colon are severed (B). The duodenum is clamped and separated from the bottom of the stomach, or pylorus (C). The end of the duodenum will be stitched closed. The stomach itself is clamped, and the portion to be removed is severed (D). The remaining stomach is attached to the jejunum, another portion of the small intestine (E). *(Illustration by GGS Information Services. Cengage Learning, Gale.)*

KEY TERMS

Adenocarcinoma—A form of cancer that involves cells from the lining of the walls of many different organs of the body.

Antrectomy—A surgical procedure for ulcer disease in which the antrum, a portion of the stomach, is removed.

Biopsy—Surgical removal of a small piece of tissue so that it can be examined under the microscope for malignancy (cancer).

Laparoscopy—The examination of the inside of the abdomen through a lighted tube (endoscope) inserted through a small incision, sometimes accompanied by surgery.

Lymphoma—Malignant tumor of lymphoblasts derived from B lymphocytes, a type of white blood cell.

The potential benefits of laparoscopic surgery include less postoperative pain, decreased hospitalization, and earlier return to normal activities. The use of laparoscopic gastrectomy is limited, however. Only patients with early-stage gastric cancers or those whose surgery is intended only as palliative treatment (pain and symptomatic relief rather than cure) are considered for this minimally invasive technique.

Gastrectomy for ulcers

Gastrectomy is also used occasionally in the treatment of severe peptic ulcer disease or its complications. While the vast majority of peptic ulcers (gastric ulcers in the stomach or duodenal ulcers in the duodenum) are managed with medication, partial gastrectomy is sometimes required for peptic ulcer patients who have complications. These include patients who do not respond satisfactorily to medical therapy, those who develop a bleeding or perforated ulcer, and those who develop pyloric obstruction (a blockage to the exit from the stomach). The surgical procedure for severe ulcer disease is also called an **antrectomy**. An antrectomy is a limited form of gastrectomy in which the antrum, or lower portion of the stomach that produces digestive juices, is removed.

Diagnosis/Preparation

Before undergoing gastrectomy, patients require a variety of tests such as x rays, computed tomography (CT) scans, ultrasonography, or endoscopic biopsies (microscopic examination of tissue) to confirm the diagnosis and localize the tumor or ulcer. **Laparoscopy** and tissue biopsy may be used to diagnose a malignancy or to determine the extent of a tumor that is already diagnosed. When a tumor is strongly suspected, laparoscopy is often performed immediately before the surgery to remove the tumor. This avoids the need to anesthetize the patient twice, and sometimes avoids the need for surgery completely if the tumor found through laparoscopy is deemed inoperable.

Aftercare

After gastrectomy surgery, patients are taken to the recovery unit and **vital signs** are closely monitored by the nursing staff until the anesthesia wears off. Patients commonly feel pain from the incision, and pain medication is prescribed to provide relief and is usually delivered intravenously (IV, directly into a vein). Upon waking from anesthesia, patients have an intravenous line, a urinary catheter, and a nasogastric tube in place. They cannot eat or drink immediately following surgery. In some cases, oxygen is delivered through a mask that fits over the mouth and nose. The nasogastric tube is attached to intermittent suction to keep what remains of the stomach empty.

If the whole stomach has been removed, the tube goes directly to the small intestine and remains in place until bowel function returns. This can take two to three days and is monitored by listening with a **stethoscope** for bowel sounds. When bowel sounds return, the patient can drink clear liquids. If the liquids are tolerated, the nasogastric tube is removed and the diet is gradually changed from liquids to soft foods, and then to more solid foods. Dietary adjustments may be necessary, as certain foods may now be difficult to digest. Overall, gastrectomy surgery usually requires a stay of 7–10 days in the hospital and recuperation time of at least several weeks.

Risks

Surgery for peptic ulcer is effective, but it may result in a variety of postoperative complications. Following gastrectomy surgery, as many as 30% of patients have significant symptoms. An operation called highly selective **vagotomy**, in which a nerve that stimulates the stomach is cut, is now preferred for ulcer management, as it is safer than gastrectomy.

After a gastrectomy, several abnormalities may develop that produce symptoms related to food intake. They happen largely because the stomach, which serves as a food reservoir, has been reduced in its capacity by the surgery. Other surgical procedures

WHO PERFORMS THE PROCEDURE AND WHERE IS IT PERFORMED?

A gastrectomy is performed by a board-certified surgeon trained in gastroenterology, the branch of medicine that deals with the diseases of the digestive tract. An anesthesiologist is responsible for administering anesthesia The operation is always performed in a hospital setting.

QUESTIONS TO ASK THE DOCTOR

- What happens on the day of surgery?
- What type of anesthesia will be used?
- How long will it take to recover from the surgery?
- When can I expect to return to work and/or resume normal activities?
- What are the risks associated with a gastrectomy?
- How many gastrectomies do you perform in a year?
- What is the rate of postsurgical complications among your patients?
- Will there be a scar?

that often accompany gastrectomy for ulcer disease can also contribute to later symptoms. These other surgical procedures include vagotomy, which lessens acid production and slows stomach emptying, and **pyloroplasty**, which enlarges the opening between the stomach and small intestine to facilitate emptying of the stomach.

Some patients experience lightheadedness, heart palpitations (racing heart), sweating, nausea, and vomiting after a meal. These may be symptoms of dumping syndrome, as food is rapidly moved into the small intestine from the remaining stomach or directly from the esophagus. Dumping syndrome is treated by adjusting the diet and pattern of eating, for example, eating smaller, more frequent meals, and limiting liquids.

Patients who have abdominal bloating and pain after eating, followed frequently by nausea and vomiting, may have afferent loop syndrome, a serious condition that must be corrected surgically. Patients who have early satiety (feeling of fullness after eating), abdominal discomfort, and vomiting may have bile reflux gastritis (also called bilious vomiting), which is also surgically correctable. Many patients experience weight loss after gastrectomy.

Reactive hypoglycemia is a condition that results when blood sugar levels become too high after a meal, stimulating the release of insulin, occurring about two hours after eating. Should this occur after gastrectomy, changing to a high-protein diet and smaller meals is advised.

Ulcers recur in a small percentage of patients after partial gastrectomy for peptic ulcer. Recurrence is usually within the first few years after surgery. Further surgery is usually necessary.

Vitamin and mineral supplementation is necessary after gastrectomy to correct certain deficiencies, especially vitamin B_{12}, iron, and folate. Vitamin D and calcium are also needed to prevent and treat the bone

problems that often occur. These include softening and bending of the bones, which can produce pain and osteoporosis, which is a loss of bone mass. According to one study, the risk for spinal fracture after gastrectomy may be as high as 50%.

Normal results

Overall, survival after gastrectomy for gastric cancer varies greatly by the stage of disease at the time of surgery. For early gastric cancer, the five-year survival rate is as high as 77%. For late-stage disease, the five-year survival rate is only 3%. The five-year survival rate for cancers in the lower stomach is better than for those found in the upper stomach, and the survival rate for gastric lymphoma is better than for gastric adenocarcinomas.

Most studies have shown that patients can have an acceptable quality of life after gastrectomy for a potentially curable gastric cancer. Many patients maintain a healthy appetite and eat a normal diet. Others lose weight and do not enjoy meals as much as before gastrectomy. Some studies show that patients who have total gastrectomies have more disease-related or treatment-related symptoms after surgery and poorer physical function than patients who have subtotal gastrectomies. There does not appear to be much difference, however, in emotional status or social activity level between patients who have undergone total versus subtotal gastrectomies.

Morbidity and mortality rates

Depending on the extent of surgery, the risk for postoperative death after gastrectomy for gastric cancer has been reported as 1–3%, and the risk of nonfatal complications as 9–18%.

Resources

BOOKS

Beers, Mark H., Robert S. Porter, and Thomas V. Jones, eds. "Disorders of the Stomach and Duodenum." In *The Merck Manual*, 18th ed. Whitehouse Station, NJ: Merck, 2007.

Feldman, Mark, et al., eds. "Stomach and Duodenum: Complications of Surgery for Peptic Ulcer Disease." In *Sleisenger's and Fordtran's Gastrointestinal and Liver Disease*, 8th ed. Philadelphia: W. B. Saunders Co., 2006.

ORGANIZATIONS

American College of Gastroenterology. P.O. Box 342260 Bethesda, MD 20827-2260. (301) 263-9000. http://www.acg.gi.org (accessed March 23, 2008).

American Gastroenterological Association (AGA). 4930 Del Ray Avenue, Bethesda, MD 20814. (301) 654-2055. http://www.gastro.org (accessed March 23, 2008).

Caroline A. Helwick
Monique Laberge, PhD
Tish Davidson, AM

Gastric acid inhibitors

Definition

Gastric acid inhibitors are medications that reduce the production of stomach acid. They are different from antacids, which act on stomach acid after it has been produced and released into the stomach.

Purpose

Gastric acid inhibitors are used to treat conditions that are either caused or made worse by the presence of acid in the stomach. These conditions include gastric ulcers; gastroesophageal reflux disease (GERD); and Zollinger-Ellison syndrome, which is marked by atypical gastric ulcers and excessive amounts of stomach acid. Gastric acid inhibitors are also widely used to protect the stomach from drugs or conditions that may cause stomach ulcers. Medications that may cause ulcers include steroid compounds and **nonsteroidal anti-inflammatory drugs** (NSAIDs), which are often used to treat arthritis. Gastric acid inhibitors offer some protection against the stress ulcers that are associated with some types of illness and with surgery.

Description

There are two types of gastric acid inhibitors, H_2-receptor blockers and **proton pump inhibitors**. H_2-receptor blockers are a type of antihistamine.

Histamine, in addition to its well-known effects in colds and allergies, also stimulates the stomach to produce more acid. The receptors (nerve endings) that respond to the presence of histamine are called H_2 receptors, to distinguish them from the H_1 receptors involved in causing allergy symptoms. The most common H_2-receptor blockers are cimetidine (Tagamet), famotidine (Pepcid), nizatidine (Axid), and ranitidine (Zantac).

The proton pump inhibitors (PPIs) are drugs that block an enzyme called hydrogen/potassium adenosine triphosphatase in the cells lining the stomach. Blocking this enzyme stops the production of stomach acid. These drugs are more effective in reducing stomach acid than the H_2-receptor blockers. The PPIs include such medications as omeprazole (Prilosec), esomeprazole (Nexium), lansoprazole (Prevacid), pantoprazole (Protonix) and rabeprazole (AcipHex).

Recommended dosages

The recommended dosage depends on the specific drug, the purpose for which it is being used, and the route of administration, whether oral or intravenous. Patients should check with the physician who prescribed the medication or the pharmacist who dispensed it. If the drug is an over-the-counter preparation, patients should read the package labeling carefully, and discuss the correct use of the drug with their physician or pharmacist. This precaution is particularly important with regard to the H_2-receptor blockers, because they are available in over-the-counter (OTC) formulations as well as prescription strength. The two are not interchangeable; OTC H_2-receptor blockers are only half as strong as the lowest available dose of prescription-strength versions of these drugs.

Patients should not use the over-the-counter preparations as an alternative to seeking professional care. For some conditions, particularly stomach ulcers, acid-inhibiting drugs may relieve the symptoms, but will not cure the underlying problems, which require both acid reduction and antibiotic therapy.

Gastric acid inhibitors work best when they are taken regularly, so that the amounts of stomach acid are kept low at all times. Patients should check the package directions or ask the physician or pharmacist for instructions on the best way to take the medicine.

Precautions

There are relatively few adverse reactions when gastric acid inhibitors are used for one to two doses before or just after surgery, The side effects listed below are most often seen with long-term use.

KEY TERMS

Enzyme—A biological compound that causes changes in other compounds.

Gastroesophageal reflux disease (GERD)—A condition in which the contents of the stomach flow backward into the esophagus. There is no known single cause.

Nonsteroidal anti-inflammatory drugs (NSAIDs)—Drugs that relieve pain and reduce inflammation but are not related chemically to cortisone. Common drugs in this class are aspirin, ibuprofen (Advil, Motrin), naproxen (Aleve, Naprosyn), ketoprofen (Orudis), and several others.

Platelets—Disk-shaped structures found in blood that play an active role in blood clotting. Platelets are also known as thrombocytes.

Receptor—A sensory nerve ending that responds to chemical or other stimuli of various kinds.

Stress ulcers—Stomach ulcers that occur in connection with some types of physical injury, including burns and invasive surgical procedures.

Thrombocytopenia—A disorder characterized by a drop in the number of platelets in the blood.

Zollinger-Ellison syndrome—A condition marked by stomach ulcers, with excess secretion of stomach acid and tumors of the pancreas.

H₂-receptor blockers

Although the H_2-receptor blockers are very safe drugs, they are capable of causing thrombocytopenia, a disorder in which there are too few platelets in the blood. This deficiency may cause bleeding problems, since platelets are essential for blood clotting. Platelet deficiencies can only be recognized by blood tests; there are no symptoms that the patient can see or feel. In addition to affecting platelet levels, the H_2-receptor blockers may cause changes in heart rate, making the heart beat either faster or slower than normal. Patients should call a physician immediately if any of these signs occur:

- tingling of the fingers or toes;
- difficulty breathing;
- difficulty swallowing;
- swelling of the face or lips;
- rapid heartbeat; or
- slow heartbeat.

In addition to these signs, the H_2-receptor blockers may cause the following unwanted reactions:

- headache;
- diarrhea;
- dizziness;
- drowsiness;
- nausea;
- depression;
- skin rash; or
- vomiting.

In addition, cimetidine is an inhibitor of male sex hormones; it may cause loss of libido, breast tenderness and enlargement, and impotence.

Ranitidine may cause loss of hair or severe skin rashes that require prompt medical attention. In rare cases, this drug may cause a reduction in the **white blood cell count**.

Before using H_2-receptor blockers, people with any of these medical problems should make sure their physicians are aware of their conditions:

- kidney disease;
- liver disease; or
- medical conditions associated with confusion or dizziness.

Proton pump inhibitors

The proton pump inhibitors are also very safe, but have been associated with rare but severe skin reactions. Patients should be sure to report any rash or change in the appearance of the skin when taking these drugs. The following adverse reactions are also possible:

- stomach cramps;
- weakness;
- chest pain;
- constipation;
- diarrhea;
- dizziness;
- drowsiness;
- gas pains;
- headache;
- nausea with or without vomiting;
- itching; and
- blood in urine.

The PPIs make some people feel drowsy, dizzy, lightheaded, or less alert. Anyone who takes these drugs should not drive, use heavy machinery, or do anything else that requires full alertness until they have found out how the drugs affect them.

Before using proton pump inhibitors, people with liver disease should make sure their physicians are aware of their condition.

Taking gastric acid reducers with certain other drugs may affect the way the drugs work or may increase the chance of side effects.

Side effects

The most common side effects of both types of gastric acid reducer are mild diarrhea, nausea, vomiting, stomach or abdominal pain, dizziness, drowsiness, lightheadedness, nervousness, sleep problems, and headache. The frequency of each type of problem varies with the specific drug selected and the dose. These problems usually go away as the body adjusts to the drug and do not require medical treatment unless they are bothersome.

Serious side effects are uncommon with these medications, but may occur. Patients should consult a physician immediately if they notice any of the following:

- skin rash or such other skin problems as itching, peeling, hives, or redness;
- fever;
- agitation or confusion;
- hallucinations;
- shakiness or tremors;
- seizures or convulsions;
- tingling in the fingers or toes;
- pain at the injection site that lasts for some time after the injection;
- pain in the calves that spreads to the heels;
- swelling of the calves or lower legs;
- swelling of the face or neck;
- difficulty swallowing;
- rapid heartbeat;
- shortness of breath; or
- loss of consciousness.

Other side effects may occur in rare instances. Anyone who has unusual symptoms after taking gastric acid inhibitors should get in touch with his or her physician.

Interactions

Gastric acid inhibitors may interact with other medicines. When an interaction occurs, the effects of one or both of the drugs may change or the risk of side effects may be increased. Anyone who takes gastric acid inhibitors should give their physician a list of all the other medicines that he or she is taking.

Of the drugs in this class, cimetidine has the highest number of drug interactions, and specialized reference works should be consulted for guidance about this medication.

The drugs that may interact with H_2-receptor blockers include:

- itraconazole (Sporanox);
- ketoconazole (Nizoral);
- warfarin (Coumadin);
- dofetilide (Tikosyn); and
- drugs given to open the airway (bronchodilators), including aminophylline, theophylline (Theo-Dur and other brands), and oxtriphylline (Choledyl and other brands).

Drugs that may interact with proton pump inhibitors include:

- itraconazole (Sporanox);
- ketoconazole (Nizoral);
- phenytoin (Dilantin) and other anticonvulsant drugs;
- cilostazol (Pletal); and
- voriconazole (Vfend).

The preceding lists do not include every drug that may interact with gastric acid inhibitors. Patients should consult a physician or pharmacist before combining gastric acid inhibitors with any other prescription or nonprescription (over-the-counter) medicine.

Resources

BOOKS

Beers, M. H., R. S. Porter, T. V. Jones, J. L. Kaplan, and M. Berkwits, eds. *The Merck Manual of Diagnosis and Therapy,* 18th ed. Whitehouse Station, NJ: Merck Research Laboratories, 2006.

Parkman, Henry, and Robert S. Fisher, eds. *The Clinician's Guide to Acid/Peptic Disorders and Motility Disorders of the Gastrointestinal Tract,* 1st ed. Thorofare, NJ: Slack Inc., 2006.

Sweetman, Sean C., ed. *Martindale: The Complete Drug Reference,* 35th ed. London: The Pharmaceutical Press, 2007.

Udall, Kate Gilbert. *Managing Acid Reflux.* North Orem, UT: Woodland Health, 2007.

Wilson, Billie Ann, Carolyn L. Stang, and Margaret T. Shannon. *Nurses Drug Guide 2000.* Stamford, CT: Appleton and Lange, 1999.

PERIODICALS

Gardner, J. D., S. Rodriguez-Stanley, and M. Robinson. "Integrated Acidity and the Pathophysiology of Gastroesophageal Reflux Disease." *American Journal of Gastroenterology* 96, no. 5 (May 2001): 1363–1370.

OTHER

"Cimetidine." Medline Plus. July 1, 2003. www.nlm.nih.gov/medlineplus/druginfo/medmaster/a682256.html (March 31, 2008).

"Esomeprazole." Medline Plus. January 1, 2008. http://www.nlm.nih.gov/medlineplus/druginfo/medmaster/a699054.html (March 31, 2008).

"Ranitidine." Medline Plus. July 1, 2003. www.nlm.nih.gov/medlineplus/druginfo/medmaster/a601106.html (March 31, 2008).

ORGANIZATIONS

American Society for Gastrointestinal Endoscopy, 1520 Kensington Road, Suite 202, Oak Brook, IL, 60523, (630) 573-0600 , http://www.asge.org.

American Society of Health-System Pharmacists, 7272 Wisconsin Avenue, Bethesda, MD, 20814, (301) 657-3000, http://www.ashp.org.

Society for Gastroenterology Nurses and Associates, 401 North Michigan Avenue, Chicago, IL, 60611-4267, (800) 245-7462, http://www.sgna.org.

U.S. Food and Drug Administration, 5600 Fishers Lane, Rockville, MD, 20857-0001, (888) INFO-FDA, http://www.fda.gov.

Samuel Uretsky, Pharm.D.
Laura Jean Cataldo, R.N., Ed.D.

Gastric bypass

Definition

A gastric bypass is one type of elective bariatric (weight-loss) surgery done on the digestive system to help morbidly obese people lose weight. Gastric bypass surgery is also called malabsorptive surgery because it creates an alternate route for food traveling through the digestive system that bypasses a section of the small intestine where many nutrients are absorbed.

Purpose

Gastric bypass surgery is intended to treat severe (morbid) obesity in people who have tried unsuccessfully to lose weight and whose excess weight threatens their health and well being. Obesity is defined by the body mass index (BMI). The BMI calculation compares weight to height. Adults age 20 and older are evaluated as follows:

- BMI below 18.5: underweight
- BMI 18.5–24.9: normal weight
- BMI 25.0–29.9: overweight

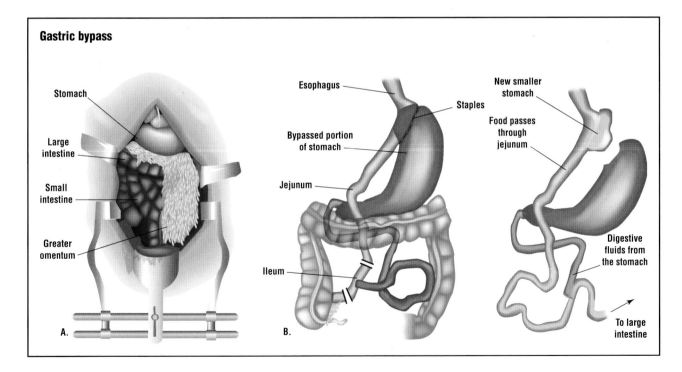

Gastric bypass

In this Roux-en-Y gastric bypass, a large incision is made down the middle of the abdomen (A). The stomach is separated into two sections. Most of the stomach will be bypassed, so food will no longer go to it. A section of jejunum (small intestine) is then brought up to empty food from the new smaller stomach (B). Finally, the surgeon connects the duodenum to the jejunum, allowing digestive secretions to mix with food further down the jejunum. *(Illustration by GGS Information Services. Cengage Learning, Gale.)*

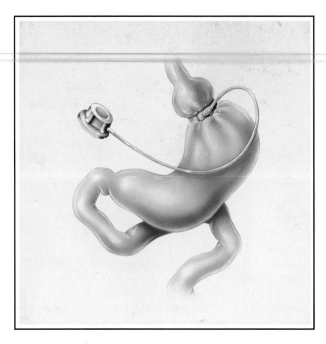

An adjustable gastric band. *(Kevin A. Somerville / Phototake. Reproduced by permission.)*

- BMI 30 and above: obese
- BMI 40 and above: morbidly or severely obese

Obesity is linked to an increased likelihood of developing over 20 different diseases and disorders, including high blood pressure (hypertension), type 2 diabetes, heart disease, stroke, deep vein blood clots, fatty liver disease, sleep apnea, heartburn, gastroesophageal reflux disease (GERD), gallstone disease, arthritis, colon cancer, breathing problems, and depression. Gastric bypass surgery reduces the amount of nutrients that are absorbed from food. It is performed in conjunction with bariatric restriction surgery in which the size of the stomach is reduced through surgical application of a band or stomach **staples** that close off a portion of the stomach. People who have had restriction surgery can eat only small amounts at a time before feeling full. Reduced food intake along with reduced nutrient absorption can lead to dramatic weight loss.

Demographics

Obesity is the second leading cause (after tobacco use) of preventable **death** in the United States. The number of overweight and obese Americans has steadily increased since 1960. According to the National Institutes of Health, in 2006, 34% of Americans were overweight and 27% were obese. Of these, 15 million were morbidly obese, however, less than 1% chose to undergo a surgical weight-loss procedure.

The number of all surgical weight-loss procedures has increased rapidly. In 1995, only 20,000 weight-loss surgeries were performed in the United States. By 2006, 170,000 of these surgeries were done, and the number is expected to continue to increase. In 2006, the United States government agreed to pay for certain bariatric surgeries for individuals who qualified for **Medicare**. At that time, about 395,000 Americans ages 65–69 were medically eligible for obesity surgery. This number is expected to grow to 475,000 persons by 2010. With Medicare coverage, it is likely that more older people will have weight-loss surgery. In 2006, the average patient having bariatric surgery was a woman in her late 30s who weighed about 300 pounds (135 kg).

Description

There are several different variations on gastric bypass, all of which are malabsorptive surgeries designed to lower caloric intake by reducing the amount of nutrients absorbed by the digestive system. These include:

- gastric bypass with long gastrojejunostomy
- Roux-en-Y (RNY) gastric bypass
- transected (Miller) RNY bypass
- laparoscopic RNY bypass
- vertical (Fobi) gastric bypass
- distal RNY bypass
- biliopancreatic (BPD) diversion

All bariatric procedures create an alternate route for food through the digestive system so that the food bypasses part of the intestine. These procedures are accompanied by a procedure to reduce the size of the stomach so that less food can be comfortably consumed. Choice of procedure relies on the patient's overall health status and on the surgeon's judgment and experience.

In the **operating room**, the patient is put under **general anesthesia** by the anesthesiologist. Once the patient is asleep, an endotracheal tube is placed through the mouth into the trachea (windpipe) to connect the patient to a respirator during surgery. A urinary catheter is also placed in the bladder to drain urine during surgery and for the first two days after surgery. This also allows the surgeon to monitor the patient's hydration. A nasogastric (NG) tube is also placed through the nose to drain secretions and is typically removed the morning after surgery.

The most common gastric bypass operation is the Roux-en-Y (RNY) gastric bypass. In this surgery, a small stomach pouch is created by stapling and banding the stomach. The pouch is about the size of an egg

KEY TERMS

Gastrojejunostomy—A surgical procedure in which the stomach is surgically connected to the jejunum (middle portion of the small intestine).

Gastroesophageal reflux disease (GERD)—A condition in which gastric juice from the stomach backs up into the bottom of the esophagus and causes irritation, inflammation, or erosion of the cells lining the esophagus.

Heartburn—A pain in the center of the chest behind the breastbone caused by the contents of the stomach flowing backwards (refluxing) into the lower end of the esophagus and causing irritation.

Hernia—The protrusion of a loop or section of an organ or tissue through an abnormal opening.

Laparoscopy—The examination of the inside of the abdomen through a lighted tube (endoscope), sometimes accompanied by surgery done through a small incision.

Malabsorption—Poor absorption of materials in the digestive system.

Morbidly obese—Definition of a person who is 100 lb (45 kg) or more than 50% overweight and has a body mass index above 40.

Osteoporosis—A condition found in older individuals in which bones decrease in density and become fragile and more likely to break. It can be caused by lack of vitamin D and/or calcium in the diet.

Sleep apnea—A temporary interruption in breathing during sleep.

Small intestine—Consists of three sections: duodenum (nearest the stomach), jejunum, and ileum (nearest the colon or large intestine). Different nutrients are absorbed in different sections of the small intestine.

Type 2 diabetes—Sometimes called adult-onset diabetes, this disease prevents the body from properly using glucose (sugar), but can often be controlled with diet and exercise.

and initially can hold 1–2 oz (30–60 ml), as compared to the 40–50 oz (1.2–1.5 l) held by a normal stomach. It is created along the more muscular side of the stomach, which makes it less likely to stretch over time.

Next, a Y-shaped piece of intestine is attached to the pouch on one end, and the jejunum, or middle part of the small intestine, on the other. This allows food to bypass the duodenum, or first part of the small intestine, where nutrients are absorbed. The food then continues normally through the rest of the small intestine and the large intestine.

The RNY gastric bypass can also be performed laparoscopically. The result is the same as an open surgery RNY, except that instead of opening the patient with a long incision on the stomach, surgeons make a small incision and insert a pencil-thin optical instrument called a laparoscope, to project a picture to a TV monitor. The laparoscopic RNY results in smaller scars, as usually only three to four small incisions are made. The average time required to complete the laparoscopic RNY gastric bypass is approximately two hours.

The great advantage of Roux-en-Y gastric bypass is that individuals lose, on average, 60–70% of their excess weight and are able to maintain the weight loss for 10 years or more. As a result, most obesity-related health problems are substantially reduced or cured when weight is lost and that weight loss is maintained. As of 2006, Medicare would usually pay for this surgery.

However, Roux-en-Y surgery also has some serious disadvantages, including:

- This surgery is more difficult for the surgeon than restrictive surgeries, and involves permanently altering the digestive system.
- Many vitamins and minerals are absorbed in the part of the small intestine bypassed by this surgery. The individual must commit to a lifetime of taking nutritional supplements to prevent serious vitamin and mineral deficiencies.
- Tearing, bleeding, and infection at the sites where the incisions and reconnections are potentially fatal complications.
- Dumping syndrome may occur in response to meals high in sugar. Dumping occurs when food moves too fast through the intestine and causes symptoms of nausea, bloating, weakness, sweating, fainting, and diarrhea.

Biliopancreatic diversion (BPD), another type of malabsorptive surgery, bypasses an even longer section of the small intestine. In BPD, about two-thirds of the stomach is surgically withdrawn, leaving a pouch that can hold about 3 cups of food. A bypass is then created to the ileum, or final portion of the small intestine. In all, about 9 ft (3 m) of intestine are bypassed. As a result, many fewer calories and nutrients are absorbed. The main advantage of BPD is the large amount of excess weight—between 75% and 80%—that is lost over the first two years and the health benefits that this loss brings. As of 2006, Medicare would usually pay for this surgery. Disadvantages are the same as for Roux-en Y surgery, but nutrient deficiencies are greater. Because fat is poorly digested as a result of this surgery, bowel movements are frequent and stools are especially foul smelling.

Diagnosis/Preparation

A diagnosis of obesity relies on a body weight assessment based on the body mass index (BMI) and waist circumference measurements. Waist circumference exceeding 40 in (101 cm) in men and 35 in (89 cm) in women increases disease risk. Gastric bypass as a weight-loss treatment is considered only for morbidly obese patients whose health is impaired by their obesity. To be candidates for gastric bypass surgery, individuals need to have failed at serious attempts to lose weight in the past, be in good mental health, demonstrate an understanding of the risks associated with this surgery, and be willing to make a lifetime commitment to changing eating habits.

Before the surgery, the patient will undergo a physical and psychological examination and receive nutritional counseling. To prepare for the surgery itself, an intravenous (IV) line is placed, and the patient may be given a sedative to help relax before going to the operating room.

Aftercare

Patients experience postoperative pain and the other common discomforts of major surgery, such as the NG tube and a dry mouth. Pain is managed with medication. A large dressing covers the surgical incision on the abdomen of the patient and is usually removed by the second day in the hospital. Short showers 48 hours after surgery are usually allowed. Patients are also fitted with special socks to improve blood flow in their legs and prevent blood clot formation. At the surgeon's discretion, some patients may have a **gastrostomy** tube (g-tube) inserted during surgery to drain secretions from the larger bypassed portion of the stomach. After a few days, it will be clamped and will remain closed. When inserted, the g-tube usually remains for another four to six weeks. It is kept in place in the unlikely event that the patient may need direct feeding into the stomach.

By the evening after surgery or the next day at the latest, patients are usually able to sit up or walk around. Gradually, physical activity may be increased, with normal activity resuming three to four weeks after surgery. Patients are also taught breathing exercises and are asked to cough frequently to clear their lungs of mucus. Postoperative pain medication is prescribed to ease discomfort and initially administered by an epidural. At the time patients are discharged from the hospital, they will be given oral medications for pain. Most patients will typically have a three-day hospital stay if their surgery is uncomplicated.

After gastric bypass or BPD, the individual does not eat anything for one or two days, giving the bowel time to rest. During this time, all nutrition is given intravenously. Once the person begins eating, the diet will include:

- liquids such as juice, broth, milk, or diluted cooked cereal for two or three days
- pureed foods that have the texture of baby food for two or three weeks while the stomach heals; these foods must be smooth and contain no large pieces
- soft foods such as ground meat and soft-cooked fruits and vegetables for about eight weeks
- regular food can be eaten in very small amounts

Most people begin by eating six tiny meals a day. These meals should be high in protein. Food must be chewed thoroughly. Liquids are drunk between meals, not with them. Vitamin and mineral supplements are essential.

Risks

Gastric bypass surgery has many of the same risks associated with other major abdominal operations. Life-threatening complications or death are rare, occurring in less than 1% of patients. Significant side effects, such as wound healing problems, difficulty in swallowing food, infections, and extreme nausea, can occur in 10–20% of patients. Blood clots after major surgery are rare, but extremely dangerous; if they occur, they may require re-hospitalization and anticoagulants (blood-thinning medications).

Some risks are specific to gastric bypass surgery, including:

- Dumping syndrome. Usually occurs when sweet foods are eaten or when food is eaten too quickly. When the food enters the small intestine, it causes cramping, sweating, and nausea.
- Abdominal hernias. These are the most common complications, requiring follow-up surgery. Incisional hernias occur in 10–20% of patients and require follow-up surgery.
- Narrowing of the stoma. The stoma, or opening between the stomach and intestines, can sometimes become too narrow, causing vomiting. The stoma can be repaired by an outpatient procedure that uses a small endoscopic balloon to stretch it.
- Gallstones. They develop in more than a third of obese patients undergoing gastric surgery. Gallstones

are clumps of cholesterol and other matter that accumulate in the gallbladder. Rapid or major weight loss increases a person's risk of developing gallstones.

- Leakage of stomach and intestinal contents. Leakage of stomach and intestinal contents from the staple and suture lines into the abdomen can occur. This is a rare occurrence and sometimes seals itself. If not, another operation is required.

Nutritional deficiencies. People who have gastric bypass surgery or BPD need extensive nutritional counseling and must take vitamin and mineral supplements for the rest of their lives. Most iron and calcium is absorbed in the duodenum, the first part of the intestine that is bypassed by these operations. Calcium deficiency can lead to osteoporosis, and iron deficiency can cause anemia.

In BPD, only 25% of the fat in food is absorbed because so much of the small intestine is bypassed. The fat-soluble vitamins A, D, E, and K are absorbed along with fat. When the body absorbs too little fat, inadequate amounts of these fat-soluble vitamins are absorbed, so dietary supplements containing these vitamins must be taken. Other vitamins that may not be absorbed in adequate amounts are vitamin B_{12}, folic acid, and vitamin B_1 (thiamine). Research published in the journal *Neurology* in March 2007 found that a very small number of people developed a brain disorder called Wernicke encephalopathy 4–12 weeks after bariatric surgery. This disorder is caused by a deficiency of vitamin B_1. Most of the people who developed the disorder had failed to take their vitamin supplements as prescribed after surgery.

Normal results

Most people who have surgery for obesity lose anywhere from 50–80% of their excess weight. However, quite a few put pounds back on beginning several years after surgery. The main reason for weight gain is noncompliance with their nutrition and **exercise** plan. Also, over time the size of the stomach pouch in restrictive surgeries tends to stretch, allowing people to eat more and still feel comfortable. On the positive side, people who lose weight through surgery almost always see great improvement in any obesity-related diseases they have.

Alternatives

Surgical alternatives

Lap-band and adjustable gastric band restrictive surgery used alone represent alternatives to gastric bypass surgery. Lap-Band surgery achieves restriction by placing a saline (salt water) filled bag around the stomach, pinching off a portion of it leaving only a small pouch at the top. The exit to the pouch is narrowed so that the rate at which the pouch empties is slowed. Because the pouch is so small, the individual can only eat about half a cup of food at a time without feeling nauseated. Since there is no cutting, stapling, or stomach rerouting involved, the procedure is the least invasive of all weight-loss surgeries. Patients generally experience less pain and scarring, and their hospital stay is shorter than with malabsorptive surgeries. In addition, a port allows access to the saline bag, so that the size of the stomach pouch can be adjusted without additional surgery. This surgery is reversible; the band or saline bag can be removed and the digestive system will function normally. Weight loss averages 50–65% of the excess body weight during the first two years. The procedure is often covered by Medicare.

Gastric band surgery uses a different technique to reduce the size of the stomach. The United States Food and Drug Administration (FDA) approved this surgery in 2001. Its long-term effects have not been studied.

Vertical banded gastroplasty (VBG) is also known as stomach stapling. This surgery is performed less often than lap-band surgery. With VBG, part of the stomach is stapled shut, making it smaller so that individuals feel full sooner. The advantage of VBG is that the procedure is quick and has few complications. Disadvantages are that average weight loss is less than with other weight-loss surgeries, and staples can pull out allowing small leaks between the stomach and the abdomen to develop. Infection is possible, but rare (less than 1%).

Nonsurgical alternatives

Diet and nutrition counseling is the main nonsurgical method of weight loss. Diet therapy involves instruction on how to adjust a diet to reduce the number of calories eaten. Reducing calories moderately is essential in achieving gradual and steady weight and in maintaining the loss. Strategies of diet and nutrition therapy include teaching individuals about the calorie content of different foods, food composition (fats, carbohydrates, and proteins), reading nutrition labels, types of foods to buy, and how to prepare foods. To be healthful, a diet must provide balanced nutrition along with calorie reduction.

WHO PERFORMS THE PROCEDURE AND WHERE IS IT PERFORMED?

A board-certified bariatric surgeon or a general surgeon who has specialized in the surgical treatment of obese patients performs gastric bypass surgery. An anesthesiologist is responsible for administering anesthesia. The operation is performed in a hospital setting. A registered dietitian usually provides dietary counseling before and after the procedure.

QUESTIONS TO ASK THE DOCTOR

- What type of bariatric surgery is best for me?
- What benefits can I expect from this surgery?
- When can I expect to return to work and/or resume normal activities?
- What are the risks associated with a the type of gastric bypass surgery I plan to have?
- How many gastric bypass surgery do you perform in a year?
- What is the rate of post-surgery complications among your patients?
- Will my insurance cover this procedure?
- What are the alternatives to this surgery?

Physical activity, especially when combined with a healthy low-calorie diet is another nonsurgical way to lose weight. Moderate physical activity, progressing to 30 minutes or more five or more days a week, is recommended for weight loss. Physical activity has also been reported to be a key part of maintaining weight loss. Abdominal fat and, in some cases, waist circumference can be modestly reduced through physical activity. Strategies of successful weight loss through long-term physical activity involve selecting enjoyable activities that can be scheduled into a regular daily routine.

Behavior therapy aims to improve diet and physical activity patterns and develop habits and new behaviors that promote weight loss. Behavioral therapy strategies for weight loss and maintenance include keeping a food and exercise diary, identifying high-risk situations such as having high-calorie foods in the house and learning to avoiding these situations, using non-food rewards for specific actions such as exercising regularly, developing realistic goals and modifying false beliefs about weight loss and body image, developing a social support network (family, friends, or colleagues), and joining a support group that will encourage weight loss in a positive and motivating manner.

Drug therapy is another nonsurgical alternative option for treating obesity. The United States Food and Drug Administration (FDA) has approved three prescription drugs for treating obesity: orlistat (Xenical), phentermine (an appetite suppressant available under more than a dozen trade names), and sibutramine (Meridia in the United States, Reductil in Europe). In 2007, orlistat became available in the United States as an over-the-counter (nonprescription) drug under the name Alli. These drugs alone are not magic bullets for weight loss and should be used in addition to calorie reduction and regular exercise.

Resources

BOOKS

Apple, Robin F. James Lock, and Rebecka Peebles. *Is Weight Loss Surgery Right for You?* New York: Oxford University Press, 2006.

Furtado, Margaret M. and Lynette Schultz. *Recipes for Life after Weight-Loss Surgery: Delicious Dishes for Nourishing the New You.* Gloucester, MA: Fair Winds Press, 2007.

Kurian, Marina S., Barbara Thompson, and Brian K. Davidson. *Weight Loss Surgery for Dummies* Hoboken, NJ: Wiley, 2005.

Leach, Susan M. *Before &amp: After, Revised Edition: Living and Eating Well After Weight-Loss Surgery.* New York: Morrow Cookbooks, 2007.

ORGANIZATIONS

American Obesity Association. 1250 24th Street, NW, Suite 300, Washington, DC 20037. (202) 776-7711. http://www.obesity.org (accessed March 30, 2008).

American Society for Bariatric Surgery. 7328 West University Avenue, Suite F, Gainesville, FL 32607. (352) 331-4900. http://www.asbs.org (accessed March 30, 2008).

Weight-control Information Network (WIN). 1 WIN Way, Bethesda, MD 20892-3665. Telephone: (877)946-4627 or (202) 828-1025. Fax: (202) 828-1028. http://win.niddk.nih.gov (accessed March 30, 2008).

OTHER

"Calculate Your Body Mass Index." *United States Department of Health and Human Services*, March 26, 2007 [cited January 5, 2008]. http://www.nhlbisupport.com/bmi (accessed March 30, 2008).

" Gastric Bypass Surgery: What Can You Expect?" *Mayo Clinic*, October 5, 2007 [cited January 5, 2008]. http://

www.mayoclinic.com/health/gastric-bypass/HQ01465 (accessed March 30, 2008).

"Gastrointestinal Surgery for Severe Obesity." *Weight-control Information Network (WIN)*, December 2004 [cited January 5, 2008]. http://win.niddk.nih.gov/publications/gastric.htm (accessed March 30, 2008).

Monique Laberge, PhD
Tish Davidson, AM

Gastroduodenostomy

Definition

A gastroduodenostomy is a surgical reconstruction procedure by which a new connection between the stomach and the first portion of the small intestine (duodenum) is created.

Purpose

A gastroduodenostomy is a gastrointestinal reconstruction technique. It may be performed in cases of stomach cancer, a malfunctioning pyloric valve, gastric obstruction, and peptic ulcers.

As a gastrointestinal reconstruction technique, it is usually performed after a total or partial **gastrectomy** (stomach removal) procedure. The procedure is also referred to as a Billroth I procedure. For benign diseases, a gastroduodenostomy is the preferred type of reconstruction because of the restoration of normal gastrointestinal physiology. Several studies have confirmed the advantages of the procedure, because it preserves the duodenal passage. Compared to a gastro-jejunostomy (Billroth II) procedure, meaning the surgical connection of the stomach to the jejunum, gastroduodenostomies have been shown to result in less modification of pancreatic and biliary functions, as well as in a decreased incidence of ulceration and inflammation of the stomach (gastritis). However, gastroduodenostomies performed after gastrectomies for cancer have been the subject of controversy. Although there seems to be a definite advantage of performing gastroduodenostomies over gastrojejunostomies, surgeons have become reluctant to perform gastroduodenostomies because of possible obstruction at the site of the surgical connection due to tumor recurrence.

As for gastroduodenostomies specifically performed for the surgical treatment of malignant gastric tumors, they follow the general principles of oncological surgery, aiming for at least 0.8 in (2 cm) of margins around the tumor. However, because gastric adenocarcinomas tend to metastasize quickly and are locally invasive, it is rare to find good surgical candidates. Gastric tumors of such patients are thus only occasionally excised via a gastro-duodenostomy procedure.

Gastric ulcers are often treated with a distal gastrectomy, followed by gastroduodenostomy or gastro-jejunostomy, which are the preferred procedures because they remove both the ulcer (mostly on the lesser curvature) and the diseased antrum.

Demographics

Stomach cancer was the most common form of cancer in the world in the 1970s and early 1980s. The incidence rates show substantial variations worldwide. Rates are currently highest in Japan and eastern Asia, but other areas of the world have high incidence rates, including eastern Europesan countries and parts of Latin America. Incidence rates are generally lower in western European countries and the United States. Stomach cancer incidence and mortality rates have been declining for several decades in most areas of the world.

Description

After removing a piece of the stomach, the surgeon reattaches the remainder to the rest of the bowel. The Billroth I gastroduodenostomy specifically joins the upper stomach back to the duodenum.

Typically, the procedure requires ligation (tying) of the right gastric veins and arteries as well as of the blood supply to the duodenum (pancreatico-duodenal vein and artery). The lumen of the duodenum and stomach is occluded at the proposed site of resection (removal). After resection of the diseased tissues, the stomach is closed in two layers, starting at the level of the lesser curvature, leaving an opening close to the diameter of the duodenum. The gastroduodenostomy is performed in a similar fashion as small intestinal end-to-end anastomosis, meaning an opening created between two normally separate spaces or organs. Alternatively, the Billroth I procedure may be performed with stapling equipment (ligation and thoraco-abdominal staplers).

Diagnosis/Preparation

If a gastroduodenostomy is performed for gastric cancer, diagnosis is usually established using the following tests:

- Endoscopy and barium x rays. The advantage of endoscopy is that it allows for direct visualization

Gastroduodenostomy

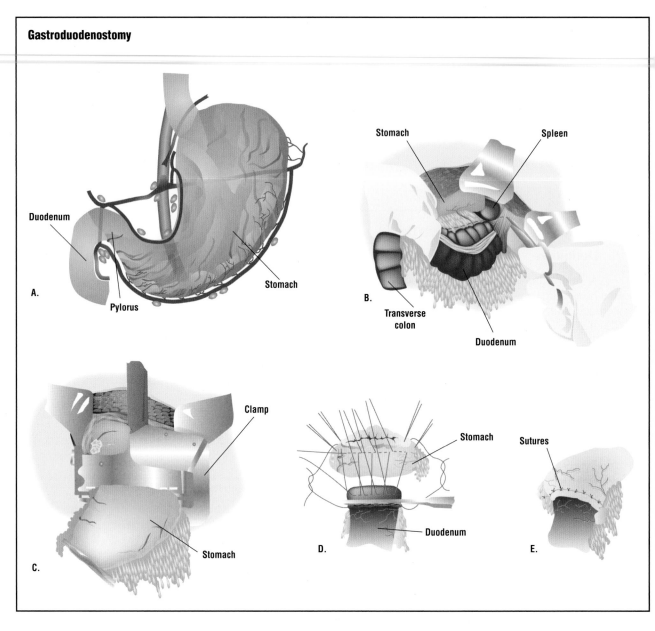

An abdominal incision exposes the stomach and duodenum (small intestine) (A). The duodenum is freed from connecting materials (B), and is clamped and severed. The stomach is also clamped and severed (C). The remaining stomach is then connected to the duodenum with sutures (D and E). *(Illustration by GGS Information Services. Cengage Learning, Gale.)*

of abnormalities and directed biopsies. Barium x rays do not facilitate biopsies, but are less invasive and may give information regarding motility.

- Computed tomagraphy **(CT) scan**. A CT scan of the chest, abdomen, and pelvis is usually obtained to help assess tumor extent, nodal involvement, and metastatic disease.

- Endoscopic ultrasound (EUS). EUS complements information gained by CT. Specifically, the depth of tumor invasion, including invasion of nearby organs, can be assessed more accurately by EUS than by CT.

- Laparoscopy. This technique allows examination of the inside of the abdomen through a lighted tube.

The diagnosis of gastric ulcer is usually made based on a characteristic clinical history. Routine laboratory tests such as a complete blood cell count and iron studies can help detect anemia, which is indicative of the condition. By performing high-precision endoscopy and by obtaining multiple mucosal biopsy specimens, the diagnosis of gastric ulcer can be confirmed. Additionally, upper gastrointestinal tract radiography tests are usually performed.

KEY TERMS

Adenocarcinoma—The most common form of gastric cancer.

Anastomosis—An opening created by surgical, traumatic, or pathological means between two normally separate spaces or organs.

Barium swallow—An upper gastrointestinal series (barium swallow) is an x-ray test used to define the anatomy of the upper digestive tract; the test involves filling the esophagus, stomach, and small intestines with a white liquid material (barium).

Computed tomography (CT) scan—An imaging technique that creates a series of pictures of areas inside the body, taken from different angles. The pictures are created by a computer linked to an x-ray machine.

Duodenum—The first part of the small intestine that connects the stomach above and the jejunum below.

Endoscopy—The visual inspection of any cavity of the body by means of an endoscope.

Gastrectomy—A surgical procedure in which all or a portion of the stomach is removed.

Gastroduodenostomy—A surgical procedure in which the doctor creates a new connection between the stomach and the duodenum.

Gastrointestinal—Pertaining to or communicating with the stomach and intestine.

Gastrojejunostomy—A surgical procedure where the stomach is surgically connected to the jejunum.

Laparoscopy—The examination of the inside of the abdomen through a lighted tube, sometimes accompanied by surgery.

Lumen—The cavity or channel within a tube or tubular organ.

Small intestine—The small intestine consists of three sections: duodenum, jejunum, and ileum. All are involved in the absorption of nutrients.

Preparations for the surgery include nasogastric decompression prior to the administration of anesthesia, intravenous or intramuscular administration of **antibiotics**, insertion of intravenous lines for administration of electrolytes, and a supply of compatible blood. Suction provided by placement of a nasogastric tube is necessary if there is any evidence of obstruction. Thorough medical evaluation, including hematological studies, may indicate the need for preoperative transfusions. All

WHO PERFORMS THE PROCEDURE AND WHERE IS IT PERFORMED?

A gastroduodenostomy is performed by a surgeon trained in gastroenterology, the branch of medicine that deals with the diseases of the digestive tract. An anesthesiologist is responsible for administering anesthesia, and the operation is performed in a hospital setting.

patients should be prepared with systemic antibiotics, and there may be some advantage in washing out the abdominal cavity with tetracycline prior to surgery.

Aftercare

After surgery, the patient is brought to the **recovery room** where **vital signs** are monitored. Intravenous fluid and electrolyte therapy is continued until oral intake resumes. Small meals of a highly digestible diet are offered every six hours, starting 24 hours after surgery. After a few days, the usual diet is gradually introduced. Medical treatment of associated gastritis may be continued in the immediate postoperative period.

Risks

A gastroduodenostomy has many of the same risks associated with any other major abdominal operation performed under **general anesthesia**, such as wound problems, difficulty swallowing, infections, nausea, and blood clotting.

More specific risks are also associated with a gastroduodenostomy, including:

- Duodenogastric reflux, resulting in persistent vomiting.

- Dumping syndrome, occurring after a meal and characterized by sweating, abdominal pain, vomiting, lightheadedness, and diarrhea.

- Low blood sugar levels (hypoglycemia) after a meal.

- Alkaline reflux gastritis marked by abdominal pain, vomiting of bile, diminished appetite, and iron-deficiency anemia.

- Malabsorption of necessary nutrients, especially iron, in patients who have had all or part of the stomach removed.

Normal results

Results of a gastroduodenostomy are considered normal when the continuity of the gastrointestinal tract is reestablished.

Morbidity and mortality rates

For gastric obstruction, a gastroduodenostomy is considered the most radical procedure. It is recommended in the most severe cases and has been shown to provide good results in relieving gastric obstruction in most patients. Overall, good to excellent gastroduodenostomy results are reported in 85% of cases of gastric obstruction. In cases of cancer, a median survival time of 72 days has been reported after gastroduodenostomy following the removal of gastric carcinoma, although a few patients had extended survival times of three to four years.

Alternatives

In the case of ulcer treatment, the need for a gastroduodenostomy procedure has diminished greatly over the past 20–30 years due to the discovery of two new classes of drugs and the presence of the responsible germ (*Helicobacter pylori*) in the stomach. The drugs are the H_2 blockers such as cimetidine and ranitidine and the **proton pump inhibitors** such as omeprazole; these effectively stop acid production. *H. pylori* can be eliminated from most patients with combination therapy that includes antibiotics and bismuth.

If an individual requires gastrointestinal reconstruction, there is no alternative to a gastroduodenostomy.

Resources

BOOKS

Benirschke, R. *Great Comebacks from Ostomy Surgery.* Rancho Santa Fe, CA: Rolf Benirschke Enterprises Inc, 2002.

Magnusson, B. E. O. *Iron Absorption after Antrectomy with Gastroduodenostomy: Studies on the Absorption from Food and from Iron Salt Using a Double Radio-iron Isotope Technique and Whole-Body Counting.* Copenhagen: Blackwell-Munksgaard, 2000.

PERIODICALS

Kanaya, S., et al. "Delta-shaped Anastomosis in Totally Laparoscopic Billroth I Gastrectomy: New Technique of Intra-Abdominal Gastroduodenostomy." *Journal of the American College of Surgeons* 195 (August 2002): 284–287.

Kim, B. J., and T. O'Connell T. "Gastroduodenostomy after Gastric Resection for Cancer." *American Surgery* 65 (October 1999): 905–907.

Millat, B., A. Fingerhut, and F. Borie. "Surgical Treatment of Complicated Duodenal Ulcers: Controlled Trials." *World Journal of Surgery* 24 (March 2000): 299–306.

Tanigawa, H., H. Uesugi, H. Mitomi, K. Saigenji, and I. Okayasu. "Possible Association of Active Gastritis, Featuring Accelerated Cell Turnover and p53 Overexpression, with Cancer Development at Anastomoses after Gastrojejunostomy. Comparison with Gastroduodenostomy." *American Journal of Clinical Pathology* 114 (September 2000): 354–363.

ORGANIZATIONS

American College of Gastroenterology. 4900-B South 31st St., Arlington, VA 22206. (703) 820-7400. www.acg.gi.org.

American Gastroenterological Association (AGA). 4930 Del Ray Avenue, Bethesda, MD 20814. (301) 654-2055. www.gastro.org.

United Ostomy Association, Inc. (UOA). 19772 MacArthur Blvd., Suite 200, Irvine, CA 92612-2405. (800) 826-0826. http://www.uoa.org.

OTHER

"Gastroduodenostomy After Gastric Resection for Cancer." *Nursing Hands* [cited June 2003] www.nursinghands.com/news/newsstories/1004031.asp.

Monique Laberge, PhD

Gastroenterologic surgery

Definition

Gastroenterologic surgery includes a variety of surgical procedures performed on the organs and conduits of the digestive system. These procedures include the repair, removal, or resection of the esophagus, liver, stomach, spleen, pancreas, gallbladder, colon, anus, and rectum. Gastroenterologic surgery is performed for diseases ranging from appendicitis, gastroesophageal reflux disease (GERD), and gastric ulcers; to the life-threatening cancers of the stomach, colon, liver, and pancreas; and ulcerative conditions like ulcerative colitis and Crohn's disease.

Purpose

Scientific understanding, treatment, and diagnostic advances, combined with an aging population, have made this century the golden age of gastroenterology. Modern gasteroenterologic surgery's success in treating conditions of the digestive system by removing obstructions, diseased or malignant tissue, or by enlarging and augmenting conduits for digestion is largely due to the ability to view and work on the various critical organs through video representation and by biopsy. The word abdomen is derived from the Latin *abdere,* meaning concealed or un-seeable. The use of gastrointestinal endoscopy, **laparoscopy**, computer tomography **(CT) scan**, and **ultrasound** has made the inspection of inaccessible organs possible without surgery, and sometimes treatable with only minor surgery. Advances in other diagnostics, such as the fecal occult blood test known as the Guaiac test, have made it possible to quickly determine the need for bowel surgery without expensive tests. This is especially important for colon cancer, which is the leading cause of cancer mortality in the United States, with about 56,000 Americans **dying** from it each year.

Some prominent surgical procedures included in gasteroentologic surgery are:

- Fundoplication to prevent reflux acids in the stomach from damaging the esophagus.
- Appendectomy for removal of an inflamed or infected appendix.
- Cholecystectomy for removal of an inflamed gallbladder and the crystallized salts called gallstones.
- Vagotomy, antrectomy, pyloroplasty are surgeries for gastric and peptic ulcers and are very rare in the twenty-first century. In the last 10 years, medical research has confirmed that gastric and peptic ulcers are due primarily to *Heliobacter pylori*, which causes more than 90% of duodenal ulcers and up to 80% of gastric ulcers. The most frequent surgeries today for ulcers of the stomach and duodenum are for complications of ulcerative conditions, largely perforation.
- Colostomy, ileostomy, and ileoanal reservoir surgery are done to remove part of the colon by colostomy, part of the colon as it enters the small intestine by

ileostomy, and removal of part of the colon as it enters the rectal reservoir by ileonal reservoir surgery. These surgeries are required to relieve diseased tissue and allow for the continuation of waste to be removed from the body. Inflammatory bowel disease includes two severe conditions: ulcerative colitis and Crohn's disease. In both cases, portions of the bowel must be resected. Crohn's disease affects the small intestine and ulcerative colitis affects the lining of the colon. Cancers in the area of the colon and rectum can also necessitate the resection of the colon, intestine, and/or rectum.

Demographics

Gasteroentologic diseases disproportionately affect the elderly, with prominent disorders including diverticulosis and other diseases of the bowel, and fecal and urinary incontinence. Many diseases, like gastrointestinal malignancies and liver diseases, occur more frequently as people age. The number of Americans age 65 and above is expected to rise from 35 million in 2000 to 78 million by 2050, with those over 85 rising from four million in 2000 to almost 18 million by 2050, therefore gastroenterologic surgeries are greatly in need, not only to prolong life but to relieve suffering. It is not surprising that the elderly account for approximately 60% of health care expenditures, 35% of hospital discharges, and 47% of hospital days.

Sixty to 70 million Americans are affected by digestive diseases, according to the National Digestive Diseases Clearinghouse. Digestive diseases accounted for 13% of all hospitalizations in the United States in 1985 and 16% of all diagnostic procedures. The most costly digestive diseases are gastrointestinal disorders such as diarrhea infections ($4.7 billion); gallbladder disease ($4.5 billion); colorectal cancer ($4.5 billion); liver disease ($3.2 billion); and peptic ulcer disease ($2.5 billion). **Appendectomy** is the fourth most frequent intra-abdominal operation performed in the United States. Appendicitis is one of the most common causes of emergency abdominal surgery in children. Appendectomies are more common in males than females, with incidence peaking in the late teens and early twenties. Each year in the United States, four appendectomies are performed per 1,000 children younger than 18 years of age. Gallstones are responsible for about half of the cases of acute pancreatitis in the United States. More than 500,000 Americans have gallbladder surgery annually. The most common procedure is the laparoscopic **cholecystectomy**. Women 20–60 years of age have twice the rate of gallstones as men, and individuals over 60 develop gallstones at higher rates than those who are younger. Those at highest risk for gallstones are individuals who are obese and those with elevated estrogen levels, such as women who take birth control pills or hormone replacement therapy.

According to the U.S. Centers for Disease Control and Prevention, 25 million Americans suffer from peptic ulcer disease some time in their life. Between 500,000 and 850,000 new cases of peptic ulcer disease and more than one million ulcer-related hospitalizations occur each year. Ulcers cause an estimated one million hospitalizations and 6,500 deaths per year. According to the American College of Gastroenterology Bleeding Registry, patients tend to be elderly; male; and users of alcohol, tobacco, **aspirin**, nonsteroidal anti-inflammatory drugs (NSAIDs), and anticoagulants. According to the National Institute of Diabetes and Digestive and Kidney Diseases (NIDDK), about 25–40% of ulcerative colitis patients must eventually have their colons removed because of massive bleeding, disease, rupture, or the risk of cancer. The use of **corticosteroids** to control inflammation can destroy tissue and require removal of the colon. According to the Society of American Gastrointestinal Endoscopic Surgeons, 600,000 surgical procedures alone are performed in the United States each year to treat a colon disease.

The incidence of gasteroenterologic diseases differs among ethnic groups. For instance, while gastroesophageal reflux disease (GERD) is common in Caucasians, its incidence is lower among African Americans. This is true for the incidence of esophageal and gastric-cardio adenocarcinoma. On the other hand, African Americans, Hispanics, and Asians have a different form of cancer of the esophagus called squamous cell carcinoma, seen also in new immigrants from northern China, India, and northern Iran. While gastric and peptic ulcerative incidence due to *Heliobacter pylori* ranges in rates from 70–80% for African Americans and Hispanics, the rate for Caucasians in only 34%. Caucasians, on the other hand, have higher rates of intestinal gastric cancer. Finally, there are differences in colon cancer mortality between African Americans and Caucasians. African Americans with colon cancer have a 50% higher mortality risk than Caucasians. Advanced cancer stage at presentation accounts for half of this increased risk. Restricted access to health care, especially screening innovations, may account for much of this disparity.

Description

Advances in laparoscopy allow the direct study of large portions of the liver, gallbladder, spleen, lining of the stomach, and pelvic organs. Many biopsies of these organs can be performed by laparoscopy. Increasingly, laparoscopic surgery is replacing open abdomen surgery for many diseases, with some procedures performed on an outpatient basis. Gastrointestinal applications have resulted in startling changes in surgeries for appendectomy, gallbladder, and adenocarcinoma of the esophagus, the fastest increasing cancer in North America. Significant other diseases include liver, colon, stomach, and pancreatic cancers; ulcerative conditions in the stomach and colon; and inflammations and/or irritations of the stomach, liver, bowel, and pancreas that cannot be treated with medications or other therapies. Research has shown that laparoscopy is useful in detecting small (<0.8 in [<2 cm]) cancers not seen by imaging techniques and can be used to stage pancreatic or esophageal cancers, averting surgical removal of the organ wall in a high percentage of cases. There are also indications, however, that some laparoscopic procedures may not have the long-lasting efficacy of open surgeries and may involve more complications. This drawback has proven true for laparoscopic fundoplication for GERD disease.

Advances in gastrointestinal fiber-optic endoscopic technology have made endoscopy mandatory for gastrointestinal diagnosis, therapy, and surgery. Especially promising is the use of endoscopic techniques in the diagnosis and treatment of bowel diseases, **colonoscopy**, and **sigmoidoscopy**, particularly with acute and chronic bleeding. Combined with laparoscopic techniques, endoscopy has substantially reduced the need for open surgical techniques for the management of bleeding.

For most gasteroenterologic surgeries, whether laparoscopic or open, preoperative medications are given as well as **general anesthesia**. Food and drink are not allowed after midnight before the surgery the next morning. Surgery proceeds with the patient under general anesthetics for open surgery and local or regional anesthetics for laparoscopic surgery. Specific diseases require specific procedures, with resection and repair of abdomen, colon and intestines, liver, and pancreas considered more serious than other organs. The level of complication of the procedure dictates whether laparoscopic procedures may be used.

Diagnosis/Preparation

The need for surgery of the esophagus, duodenum, stomach, colon, and intestines is assessed by medical history, general physical, and X-ray after the patient swallows barium for maximum visibility. Diagnosis and preparation for gasteroentological surgery involve some very advanced techniques. Upper and lower gastrointestinal endoscopies are more accurate in spotting abnormalities than X-ray and can be used in treatment. Endoscopy utilizes a long, flexible plastic tube with a camera to look at the stomach and bowel. Quite often, physicians will also use a CT scan for procedures like appendectomy. Upper esophagogastroduodenal endoscopy is considered the reference method of diagnosis for ulcers of the stomach and duodenum. Colonoscopy and sigmoidoscopy are mandatory for diseases and cancers of the colon and large intestine.

Aftercare

For simple procedures like appendectomy and gallbladder surgery, patients stay in the hospital the night of surgery and may require extra days in the hospital, but they usually go home the next day. Postoperative pain is mild, with liquids strongly recommended in the diet, followed gradually with solid foods. Return to normal activities usually occurs in a short period. For more involved procedures on organs like the stomach, bowel, pancreas, and liver, open surgery usually dictates a few days of hospitalization with a slow recovery period.

Risks

The risks in gastroenterologic surgery are largely confined to wound or injuries to adjacent organs, infection, and the general risks of open surgery that involve thrombosis and heart difficulties. With some laparoscopic procedures such as fundoplication with injury or laceration of other organs, the return of symptoms within two to three years may occur. With appendectomy, the rates of infection and wound

complications range between 10% and 18% in patients. The institution of new clinical practice guidelines that include wound guidelines and directed management of postoperative infectious complications are substantially reducing patient mortality. Gallbladder surgery, especially laparoscopic cholecystectomy, is one of the most common surgical procedures in the United States; however, injuries to adjacent organs or structures may occur, requiring a second surgery to repair it. Stomach surgical procedures carry risks, generally in proportion to their benefits. In the 2000s, surgery for peptic ulcer disease is largely restricted to the treatment of complications such as bleeding for ulcer perforation. Research indicates that surgery for bleeding is 90% effective using endoscopic techniques. Laparoscopic surgery for ulcer complications has not been found to be better than regular surgery. Stomach and intestinal surgery risks include diarrhea, reflux gastritis, malabsorption of nutrients, especially iron, as well as the general surgical risks associated with abdominal surgery. The risks of colon surgery are tied to both the general risks of surgical procedures—thrombosis and heart problems—and to the specific disease being treated. For instance, in Crohn's disease, resection of the colon may not be effective in the long run and may require repeated surgeries. Colon surgery in general has risks for bowel obstruction and bleeding.

Morbidity and mortality rates

According to a study published by the *British Journal of Surgery*, a small minority of patients undergoing gastroenterologic surgery are at high risk for postoperative complications that may lead to prolonged hospital stays. In a study of 235 patients, 47% had at least one postoperative complication, with the **length of hospital stay** at 11 days compared to those without complications with length of stay at six days.

QUESTIONS TO ASK THE DOCTOR

- How often do you perform this surgery?
- Is this surgery one that can be done laparoscopically?
- How long will it take for me to heal postoperatively?
- What are the risks involved for this type of procedure?
- How long have you been performing this surgery laparoscopically?

Resources

BOOKS

Pagana, Kathleen D., and Timothy J. Pagana. *Diagnostic Testing and Nursing Implications,* 5th ed. St. Louis, MO: Mosby, 1999.

PERIODICALS

Cappell, M. S. "Fifty Landmark Discoveries in Gastroenterology during the Past 50 Years." *Gastroenterology Clinics of North America* 29, no. 1 (June 2000): 223–263.

Cappell, M. S. "Recent Advances in Gastroenterology." *Medical Clinics of North America* 86, no. 6 (November 2002): xiii–xv.

Eisen G. M., et al. "Ethnic Issues in Endoscopy." *Gastrointestinal Endoscopy* 53, no. 7, (June 2001): 874–875.

Farrell, J. J., and L. S. Friedman. "Gastrointestinal Bleeding in the Elderly." *Gastroenterology Clinics of North America* 30, no. 2, (June, 2001): 377–407.

Lang, M., M. Niskanen, P. Miettinen, E. Alhava, and J. Takala. "Outcome and Resource Utilization in Gastroenterological Surgery." *British Journal of Surgery* 88, no. 7 (July 2001): 1006–1014.

OTHER

"The Role of Laparoscopy in the Diagnosis and Management of Gastrointestinal Disease." Society of American Gastrointestinal and Endoscopic Surgeons. http://www.sages.org/sg_asgepub1015.html (March 31, 2008).

ORGANIZATIONS

American Society for Gastrointestinal Endoscopy, 1520 Kensington Road, Suite 202, Oak Brook, IL, 60523, (630) 573-0600 , http://www.asge.org.

Crohn's & Colitis Foundation of America, 386 Park Avenue South, 17th Floor, New York, NY, 10016-8804, (800) 932-2423, <info@ccfa.org>, http://www.ccfa.org.

International Foundation for Functional Gastrointestinal Disorders, P.O. Box 170864, Milwaukee, WI, 53217, (414) 964-1799, (888) 964-2001, http://www.iffgd.org.

National Institute of Diabetes and Digestive and Kidney Diseases, 31 Center Drive, MSC 2560, Bethesda, MD, 20892-2560, (301) 496-3583, http://www.niddk.nih.gov.

Society for Gastroenterology Nurses and Associates, 401 North Michigan Avenue, Chicago, IL, 60611-4267, (800) 245-7462, http://www.sgna.org.

Nancy McKenzie, Ph.D.
Laura Jean Cataldo, R.N., Ed.D.

Gastroesophageal reflux scan

Definition

Gastrointestinal reflux imaging refers to several methods of diagnostic imaging used to visualize and diagnose gastroesophageal reflux disease (GERD). GERD is one of the most common gastrointestinal problems among children or adults. It is defined as the movement of solid or liquid contents from the stomach backward into the esophagus.

Purpose

The purpose of gastroesophageal reflux scanning is to allow the doctor to visualize the interior of the patient's upper stomach and lower esophagus. This type of visual inspection helps the doctor make an accurate diagnosis and plan appropriate treatment.

Description

A brief description of gastroesophageal reflux disease is helpful in understanding the scanning methods used to diagnose it. Gastroesophageal reflux disease is the term used to describe the symptoms and damage caused by the backflow (reflux) of the contents of the stomach into the esophagus. The contents of the human stomach are usually acidic. Because of their acidity, they have the potential to cause chemical burns in such unprotected tissues as the lining of the esophagus.

Gastrointestinal reflux is common in the general American population. Approximately one adult in three reports experiencing some occasional reflux, commonly referred to as heartburn. About 10% of these persons experience reflux on a daily basis. Most persons, however, have only very mild symptoms. Occasionally, someone may experience a burning sensation as a result of gastrointestinal reflux. This symptom is described as reflux esophagitis when it occurs in association with inflammation.

Gastroesophageal reflux scan

KEY TERMS

Barrett's esophagus—An abnormal condition of the esophagus in which normal mucous cells are replaced by changed cells. This condition is often a prelude to cancer.

Clearance—The process of removing a substance or obstruction from the body.

Dysphagia—Difficulty in swallowing.

Endoscope—An instrument with a light source attached that allows the doctor to examine the inside of the digestive tract or other hollow organ.

Erosion—A gradual breakdown or ulceration of the uppermost layer of tissue lining the esophagus or stomach.

Erythema—Redness.

Esophageal varices —Varicose veins at the lower-most portion of the esophagus. Esophageal varices are easily injured, and bleeding from them is often difficult to stop.

Esophagus—The muscular tube that connects the mouth to the stomach.

Heartburn—A sensation of warmth or burning behind the breastbone, rising upward toward the neck. It is often caused by stomach acid flowing upward from the stomach into the esophagus.

Hematemesis—Vomit that contains blood, usually seen as black specks in the vomitus.

Incompetent—In a medical context, insufficient. An incompetent sphincter is one that is not closing properly.

pH—A measure of acidity; technically, a measure of hydrogen ion concentration. The stomach contents are more acidic than the tissues of the esophagus.

Raynaud's disease—A disease of the arteries in hands or feet.

Reflux—Backflow, also called regurgitation.

Sjögren's syndrome—An autoimmune disorder characterized by dryness of the eyes, nose, mouth, and other areas covered by mucous membranes.

Sphincter—A circular band of muscle fibers that constricts or closes a passageway in the body. The esophagus has sphincters at its upper and lower ends.

Visualize—To achieve a complete view of a body structure or area.

Gastroesophageal reflux has several possible causes:

- An incompetent lower esophageal sphincter. Acid reflux can occur when the ring of muscular tissue at the boundary of the esophagus and stomach is weak and relaxes too far. Sphincter incompetence is the most common cause of gastroesophageal reflux. The acid juices from the stomach are most likely to flow backward through a weak sphincter when a person bends, lifts a weight, or strains. People with esophageal strictures or Barrett's esophagus are more likely to experience gastroesophageal reflux than are others.

- Acid irritation. Gastric contents are acidic, with a pH lower than 3.9. This degree of acidity is very caustic to the lining of the esophagus; repeated exposures may lead to scarring. If the exposure is sufficiently severe or prolonged, strictures can develop. Occasionally, pancreatic enzymes or bile may also flow backward into the stomach and lower esophagus. These fluids are extremely acidic, with a pH lower than 2.0.

- Abnormal esophageal clearance. Clearance refers to the process of removing a substance from a part of the body, in this case the removal of stomach acid from the esophagus. Acid reflux is ordinarily washed out of the esophagus by the saliva that a person swallows over the course of a day. Saliva also contains some bicarbonate, which helps to neutralize the acidity of the stomach juices. During sleep, however, people swallow less frequently, which results in a longer period of contact between the acid contents of the stomach and the tissues that line the esophagus. The net result is a chemical injury. Sjögren's syndrome, radiation to the oral cavity, and some medications (anticholinergics) also decrease the flow of saliva and can result in chemical injury. Such other medical conditions as Raynaud's disease and scleroderma are often associated with abnormal esophageal clearance. Hiatal hernia is present in more than 90% of persons with erosive disease.

- Delayed gastric emptying. When outflow from the stomach is blocked or the stomach's contractions are weakened, the partially digested food does not leave the stomach in a timely manner. This delay makes gastric reflux more likely to occur.

Heartburn associated with gastroesophageal reflux occurs 30–60 minutes after eating. It also occurs when a person is lying down. Most people who

GALE ENCYCLOPEDIA OF SURGERY AND MEDICAL TESTS, 2ND EDITION

665

experience gastroesophageal reflux can obtain relief from heartburn with baking soda, bismuth subsalicylate (Pepto-Bismol), or antacid tablets. A pattern of symptom relief following a dose of one of these nonprescription remedies is usually enough to make the diagnosis of gastroesophageal reflux. Under these conditions, the results of a **physical examination** and laboratory tests are usually within normal limits.

Persons with complicated GERD, or those who do not respond to nonprescription heartburn remedies, require special examinations. There are several imaging methods used in the diagnosis of GERD:

Upper endoscopy

Upper endoscopy is the standard procedure for diagnosing GERD, determining the degree of tissue damage, and documenting the findings. A barium esophagography may be performed in addition to an upper endoscopy. Between 50% and 75% of all patients diagnosed with GERD will have abnormalities in the mucous lining of the esophagus, usually erosion, tissue fragility, and erythema. Upper endoscopy is also used to document esophageal strictures and Barrett's esophagus. Patients with such symptoms as hematemesis (vomiting blood), iron deficiency anemia, guaiac-positive stools, or dysphagia should have an upper endoscopy.

To perform this study, the doctor passes an endoscope, which is a thin instrument with a light source attached, through the patient's mouth into the esophagus. The endoscope allows the doctor to visualize the mucosal lining of the esophagus, the junction between the esophagus and the stomach, and the lining of the upper portion of the stomach. He or she can take biopsy specimens at the same time.

Ambulatory esophageal pH monitoring

This test provides information concerning the frequency and duration of episodes of acid reflux. It can also provide information related to the timing of these episodes. Ambulatory esophageal monitoring is the standard procedure for documenting abnormal acid reflux; however, it is not necessary for most persons with GERD as they can be adequately diagnosed on the basis of their history or by performing an upper endoscopy.

To perform this test, the doctor passes a tiny catheter (about 2 mm wide) with two electrodes through the patient's nose and throat. One electrode is positioned about 2 in (5 cm) above the esophageal sphincter. The other electrode is positioned just below the esophageal sphincter. Data related to pH level are obtained every four seconds for 24 hours. The patient is instructed to keep a diary of his or her symptoms, and to record coughing episodes, meal times, bedtime, and time of rising. The electrodes are removed after 24 hours and the patients' diary is reviewed.

Barium esophagography

In a barium esophagograph, the patient is given a solution of water and barium sulfate to drink slowly. X rays are taken at intervals as the patient swallows the mixture; the images are analyzed for signs of reflux, inflammation, dysmotility, strictures, and other abnormalities. Barium esophagography provides important information about a number of disorders involving esophageal function, including cricopharyngeal achalasia (a swallowing disorder of the throat); decreased or reverse peristalsis; and **hiatal hernia**.

Esophageal manometry

Esophageal manometry is a useful test for patients who may need surgery because it provides data about esophageal peristalsis and the minimum closing pressure of the esophageal sphincter by measuring the pressure within the esophagus. To perform this test, the doctor passes a thin soft tube through the patient's nose or mouth. When the patient swallows, the tip of the tube enters the esophagus and is positioned at the desired location. The patient then swallows air or water while a technician records the pressure at the tip of the tube.

Preparation

Upper endoscopy

Persons are instructed not to eat or drink for 6 hours before an upper endoscopy. A mild sedative may be given to patients who are unusually nervous.

Ambulatory esophageal pH monitoring

No special preparations are needed for this test. A short-acting anesthetic spray is sometimes used to relieve any discomfort associated with placing the electrodes.

Barium esophagography

The patient should not eat or drink for 6 hours before a barium test.

Esophageal manometry

The patient should take nothing by mouth for 8 hours prior to the test. The doctor may use an anesthetic spray to reduce the throat irritation caused by the manometry tube.

Aftercare

Upper endoscopy

After an upper endoscopy, a friend or relative should drive the patient home because of the lingering effects of the sedative.

Other esophageal scans

There are no special aftercare instructions for patients who have had ambulatory esophageal **pH monitoring**, barium esophagography, or esophageal manometry.

Risks

Upper endoscopy

Patients sometimes feel as if they are choking as the doctor passes the endoscope down the throat. This feeling is uncommon, however, if the patient has been given a sedative.

Ambulatory esophageal pH monitoring

There are no common complications following this test.

Barium esophagography

Constipation after the test is an infrequent side effect that is treated by giving the patient a laxative.

Esophageal manometry

Complications following this test are very rare.

Normal results

Upper endoscopy

An upper endoscopy documents the condition of the mucous lining of the lower esophagus and upper stomach, thus allowing the doctor to evaluate the progression of GERD.

Ambulatory esophageal pH monitoring

Measurements of pH are used to evaluate the degree of GERD.

Barium esophagography

Barium esophagography can detect many structural and functional abnormalities, including the presence of acid reflux, inflammation, tissue masses, or strictures in the esophagus.

Esophageal manometry

This test documents the ability of the esophageal sphincter to close adequately and keep the contents of the stomach from flowing backward into the esophagus.

Resources

BOOKS

Bentley D., M. Lawson, and C. Lifschitz. *Pediatric Gastro-enterology and Clinical Nutrition.* New York, NY: Oxford University Press, 2001.

Davis, M., and J.D. Houston. *Fundamentals of Gastroenterology.* Philadelphia, PA: Saunders, 2001.

Herbst, J. J. "Gastroesophageal Reflux (Chalasia)," in Richard E. Behrman et al., eds., *Nelson Textbook of Pediatrics,* 16th ed. Philadelphia, PA: Saunders, 2000.

Isselbacher, K. J., and D. K. Podolsky. "Approach to the Patient with Gastrointestinal Disease," in A. S. Fauci et al., eds., *Harrison's Principles of Internal Medicine,* 14th ed. New York, NY: McGraw-Hill, 1998.

Murry, T., and R. L. Carrau. *Clinical Manual for Swallowing Disorders.* Albany, NY: Delmar, 2001.

Orlando, R. *Gastroesophageal Reflux Disease.* New York, NY: Marcel Dekker, 2000.

Owen, W. J., A. Adam, and R. C. Mason. *Practical Management of Oesophageal Disease.* Oxford, UK: Isis Medical Media, 2000.

Richter, J. E. *Gastroesophageal Reflux Disease: Current Issues and Controversies.* Basel, SWI: Karger Publishing, 2000.

Wuittich, G. R. "Diagnostic Imaging Procedures in Gastroenterology," in Lee Goldman and J. Claude Bennett, eds., *Cecil Textbook of Medicine,* 21st ed. Philadelphia, PA: W. B. Saunders, 2000.

PERIODICALS

Carr, M. M., M. L. Nagy, M. P. Pizzuto, et al. "Correlation of Findings at Direct Laryngoscopy and Bronchoscopy with Gastroesophageal Reflux Disease in Children: A Prospective Study." *Archives of Otolaryngology, Head and Neck Surgery* 127 (April 2001): 369-374.

Carr, M. M., A. Nguyen, C. Poje, et al. "Correlation of Findings on Direct Laryngoscopy and Bronchoscopy with Presence of Extraesophageal Reflux Disease." *International Journal of Pediatric Otorhinolaryngology* 54, (August 11, 2000): 27-32.

Mercado-Deane, M. G., E. M. Burton, S. A. Harlow, et al. "Swallowing Dysfunction in Infants Less Than 1 Year of Age." *Pediatric Radiology* 31 (June 2001): 423-428.

Stordal, K., E. A. Nygaard, and B. Bentsen. "Organic Abnormalities in Recurrent Abdominal Pain in Children." *Acta Paediatrica* 90 (June 2001): 638-642.

ORGANIZATIONS

American College of Gastroenterology. 4900 B South 31st Street, Arlington, VA, 22206. (703) 820-7400. www.acg.gi.org.

American College of Radiology. 1891 Preston White Drive, Reston, VA, 20191. (703) 648-8900. www.acr.org.

American Osteopathic College of Radiology. 119 East Second St., Milan, MO 63556. (660) 265-4011. www.aocr.org.

OTHER

American Academy of Family Physicians. www.aafp.org/afp/990301ap/1161.html.

American College of Gastroenterology. www.acg.gi.org/phyforum/gifocus/2evi.html.

American Medical Association. www.ama-assn.org/special/asthma/library/readroom/40894.htm.

National Digestive Diseases Clearinghouse. www.niddk.nih.gov/health/digest/pubs/heartbrn/heartbrn.htm.

L. Fleming Fallon, Jr., MD, DrPH
Lee A. Shratter, M.D.

Gastroesophageal reflux surgery

Definition

Gastroesophageal reflux surgery is typically performed in patients with serious gastroesophageal reflux disease that does not respond to drug therapy.

Gastroesophageal reflux is classified as the symptoms produced by the inappropriate movement of stomach contents back up into the esophagus. Nissen fundoplication is the most common surgical approach in the correction of gastroesophageal reflux. The laparoscopic method of Nissen fundoplication is becoming the standard form of surgical correction.

Purpose

Gastroesophageal reflux surgery, including Nissen fundoplication and laparoscopic fundoplication, has two essential purposes: heartburn symptom relief and reduced backflow of stomach contents into the esophagus.

Heartburn symptom relief

Because Nissen fundoplication is considered surgery, it is usually considered as a treatment option only when drug treatment is only partially effective or ineffective. Nissen fundoplication is often used in patients with a particular anatomic abnormality called

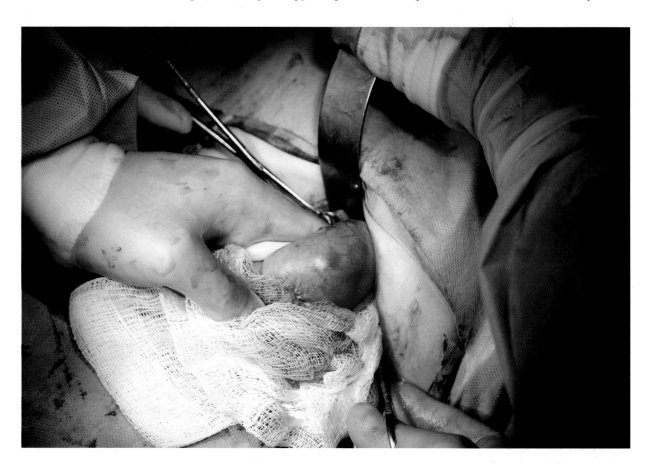

A pediatric surgeon performing gastroesophageal reflux surgery (stomach stapling) on an 8-year-old with GERD. *(Barry Slaven, MD, PhD / Phototake. Reproduced by permission.)*

Gastroesophageal reflux surgery (Fundoplication)

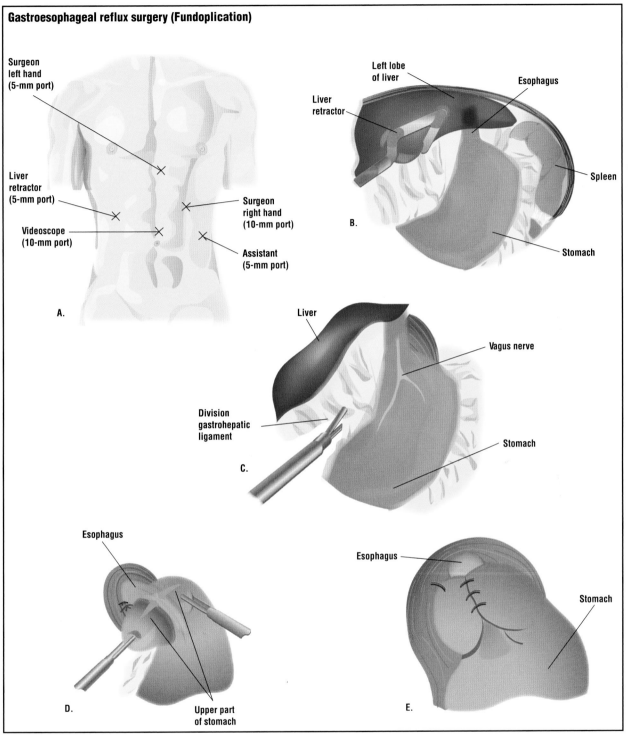

A.
- Surgeon left hand (5-mm port)
- Liver retractor (5-mm port)
- Videoscope (10-mm port)
- Surgeon right hand (10-mm port)
- Assistant (5-mm port)

B.
- Left lobe of liver
- Liver retractor
- Esophagus
- Spleen
- Stomach

C.
- Liver
- Division gastrohepatic ligament
- Vagus nerve
- Stomach

D.
- Esophagus
- Upper part of stomach

E.
- Esophagus
- Stomach

In a laparoscopic surgery to alleviate gastroesophageal reflux, the surgeon makes several incisions to gain access to the stomach and esophagus (A). Using the videoscope, the stomach is visualized (B), and the ligament connecting the stomach to the liver is divided (C). The upper part of the stomach is brought up around the base of the esophagus (D), and stitched to place (E). *(Illustration by GGS Information Services. Cengage Learning, Gale.)*

hiatal hernia that causes significant gastroesophageal reflux. In some cases, Nissen fundoplication is also used when the patient cannot or does not want to take reflux medication. Surgery is also more likely to be considered when it is obvious that the patient will need to take reflux drugs on a permanent basis. Reflux

Barrett's esophagus—Changes in the cells lining the esophagus that result from constant exposure to refluxed stomach acid.

Esophagitis—Inflammation of the esophagus.

Hiatal hernia—Protrusion of the stomach upward into the mediastinal cavity through the esophageal hiatus of the diaphragm.

Motility—Gastrointestinal movement.

drugs, like virtually all drugs, may produce side effects, especially when taken over a period of years.

One of the biggest problems in diagnosing and controlling gastroesophageal reflux disease is that the severity of disease is not directly related to the presence or intensity of symptoms. There is also no consistent relationship between the severity of disease and the degree of tissue damage in the esophagus. When reflux occurs, stomach acid comes into contact with the cells lining the esophagus. This contact can produce a feeling of burning in the esophagus and is commonly called heartburn. Some of the other symptoms associated with this condition include:

- chest pain
- swallowing problems
- changes in vocal qualities

Reduced reflux

The reduction or elimination of reflux is as important, and sometimes more important, than the elimination of symptoms. This leads to one of the most important points in gastroesophageal reflux disease. Long-term exposure to acid in the esophagus tends to produce changes in the cells of the esophagus. These changes are usually harmful and can result in very serious conditions, such as Barrett's esophagus and cancer of the esophagus. Because of this, all persons with gastroesophageal reflux disease symptoms need to be evaluated with a diagnostic instrument called an endoscope. An endoscope is a long, flexible tube with a camera on the end that is inserted down the throat and passed all the way down to the esophageal/stomach region.

All gastroesophageal reflux surgery, including Nissen fundoplication, attempts to restore the normal function of the lower esophageal sphincter (LES). Malfunction of the LES is the most common cause of gastroesophageal reflux disease. Typically, the LES opens during swallowing but closes quickly thereafter

to prevent the reflux of acid back into the esophagus. Some patients have sufficient strength in the sphincter to prevent reflux, but the sphincter opens and closes at the wrong times. However, this is not the case in most individuals with gastroesophageal reflux disease. These individuals usually have insufficient sphincter strength. In a small number of cases, the muscles of the upper esophagus region are too weak and are not appropriately coordinated with the process of swallowing.

The development of heartburn does not necessarily suggest the presence of gastroesophageal reflux disease, which is a more serious condition. Gastroesophageal reflux disease is often defined as the occurrence of heartburn more than twice per week on a long-term basis. Gastroesophageal reflux disease can lead to more serious health consequences if left untreated. The primary symptoms of gastroesophageal reflux disease are chronic heartburn and acid regurgitation, or reflux. It is important to note that not all patients with gastroesophageal reflux disease have heartburn. Gastroesophageal reflux disease is most common in adults, but it can also occur in children.

The precise mechanism that causes gastroesophageal reflux disease is not entirely known. It is known that the presence of a hiatal hernia increases the likelihood that gastroesophageal reflux disease will develop. Other factors that are known to contribute to gastroesophageal reflux disease include:

- smoking
- alcohol ingestion
- obesity
- pregnancy

The following foods and drinks are known to increase the production of stomach acid and the resulting reflux into the esophagus:

- caffeinated drinks
- high-fat foods
- garlic
- onions
- citrus fruits
- chocolate
- fried foods
- foods that contain tomatoes
- foods that contain mint
- spicy foods

Most patients take over-the-counter antacids initially to relieve the symptoms of acid reflux. If antacids do not help, the physician may prescribe drugs called H_2 blockers, which can help those with mild-to-moderate disease. If these drugs are not effective, more powerful acid-inhibiting drugs called **proton-pump inhibitors** may be prescribed. If these drugs are not effective in controlling gastroesophageal reflux disease, then the patient may require surgery.

Demographics

It has been estimated that heartburn occurs in more than 60% of adults. About 20% of the population take antacids or over-the-counter H_2 blockers at least once per week to relieve heartburn. In addition, about 80% of pregnant women have significant heartburn. Hiatal hernia is believed to develop in more than half of all persons over the age of 50 years. Hiatal hernia is present in about 70% of patients with gastroesophageal reflux disease, but the majority of patients with hiatal hernia do not have symptoms of gastroesophageal reflux disease. In addition, about 7-10% of the population has daily episodes of heartburn. It is these individuals who are likely to be classified as having gastroesophageal reflux disease.

Description

The most common type of gastroesophageal reflux surgery to correct gastroesophageal reflux disease is Nissen fundoplication. Nissen fundoplication is a specific technique that is used to help prevent the reflux of stomach contents back into the esophagus. When Nissen fundoplication is successful, symptoms and further damage to tissue in the esophagus are significantly reduced. Prior to Nissen fundoplication, open surgery was required to access to the lower esophageal region. This approach required a large external incision in the abdomen of the patient.

Fundoplication involves wrapping the upper region of the stomach around the lower esophageal sphincter to increase pressure on the LES. This procedure can be understood by visualizing a bun being wrapped around a hot dog. The wrapped portion is then sewn into place so that the lower part of the esophagus passes through a small hole in the stomach muscle. When the surgeon performs the fundoplication wrap, a large rubber dilator is usually placed inside the esophagus to reduce the likelihood of an overly tight wrap. The goal of this approach is to strengthen the sphincter; to repair a hiatal hernia, if present; and to prevent or significantly reduce acid reflux.

Fundoplication was greatly improved with the development of the laparoscope. The laparoscope is a long, thin, flexible instrument with a camera and tiny surgical tools on the end. Laparoscopic fundoplication (sometimes called "telescopic" or "keyhole" surgery) is performed under **general anesthesia** and usually includes the following steps:

- Several small incisions are created in the abdomen.
- The laparoscope is passed into the abdomen through one of the incisions. The other incisions are used to admit instruments to manipulate structures within the abdomen.
- The abdomen is inflated with carbon dioxide. The contents of the abdomen can now be viewed on a video monitor that receives its picture from the laparoscopic camera.
- The stomach is freed from its attachment to the spleen.
- An esophageal dilator is passed through the mouth into the esophagus. This dilator keeps the stomach from being wrapped too tightly around the esophagus.
- The portion of the esophagus in the abdomen is freed of its attachments.
- The top portion of the stomach (the fundus) is passed behind the esophagus, wrapped around it 360°, and sutured in place.
- If a hiatal hernia is present, the hiatus (the hole in the diaphragm through which the esophagus passes) is made smaller with one to three sutures so that it fits around the esophagus snugly. The sutures keep the fundoplication from protruding into the chest cavity.
- The laparoscope and instruments are removed and the incisions are closed.

Diagnosis/Preparation

The diagnosis of gastroesophageal reflux disease can be straightforward in cases where the patient has the classic symptoms of regurgitation, heartburn, and/or swallowing difficulties. Gastroesophageal reflux disease can be more difficult to diagnose when these classic symptoms are not present. Some of the less common symptoms associated with reflux disease include asthma, nausea, cough, hoarseness, and chest pain. Symptoms such as severe chest pain and weight loss may be an indication of disease more serious than gastroesophageal reflux disease.

The most accurate test for diagnosing gastroesophageal reflux disease is ambulatory **pH monitoring**. This is a test of the pH (a measurement of acids and bases) above the lower esophageal sphincter over a 24-hour period. Endoscopies can be used to diagnose the complications of gastroesophageal reflux disease, such as esophagitis, Barrett's esophagus, and esophageal cancer, but only about 50% of patients with gastroesophageal reflux disease have changes that are evident using this diagnostic tool. Some physicians prescribe omeprazole, a proton-pump inhibiting drug, to persons suspected of having gastroesophageal reflux disease to see if the person improves over a period of several weeks.

Aftercare

Patients should be able to participate in light physical activity at home in the days following **discharge from the hospital**. In the days and weeks following surgery, anti-reflux medication should not be necessary. Pain following this surgery is usually mild, but some patients may need pain medication. Some patients are instructed to limit food intake to a liquid diet in the days following surgery. Over a period of days, they are advised to gradually add solid foods to their diet. Patients should ask the surgeon about the post-operative diet. Normal activities, such as lifting, work, driving, showering, and sexual intercourse, can usually be resumed within a short period of time. If pain is more than mild and pain medication is not effective, then the surgeon should be consulted in a follow-up appointment.

The patient should call the doctor if any of the following symptoms develop:

- drainage from the incision region
- swallowing difficulties
- persistent cough
- shortness of breath
- chills
- persistent fever
- bleeding
- significant abdominal pain or swelling
- persistent nausea or vomiting

Risks

Risks or complications that have been associated with fundoplication include:

- heartburn recurrence
- swallowing difficulties caused by an overly tight wrap of the stomach on the esophagus
- failure of the wrap to stay in place so that the LES is no longer supported
- normal risks associated with major surgical procedures and the use of general anesthesia
- increased bloating and discomfort due to a decreased ability to expel excess gas

Complications, though rare, can occur during fundoplication. These complications can include injury to

surrounding tissues and organs, such as the liver, esophagus, spleen, and stomach. One of the major drawbacks to fundoplication surgery, whether it is open or laparoscopic, is that the procedure is not reversible. In addition, some of the symptoms associated with complications are not always treatable. One study showed that about 10% to 20% of patients who receive fundoplication have a recurrence of gastroesophageal reflux disease symptoms or develop other problems, such as bloating, intestinal gas, vomiting, or swallowing problems, following the surgery. In addition, some patients may develop altered bowel habits following the surgery.

Normal results

One research study found that fundoplication is successful in 50–90% of cases. This study found that successful surgery typically relieves the symptoms of gastroesophageal reflux disease and esophagus inflammation (esophagitis). However, the researchers in this study provided no information on the long-term stability of the procedure. Fundoplication does not always eliminate the need for medication to control gastroesophageal reflux disease symptoms. A different study found that 62% of patients who received fundoplication continued to need medication to control reflux symptoms. However, these patients required less medication than before fundoplication.

QUESTIONS TO ASK THE DOCTOR

Questions to ask the primary care physician:

- What are my alternatives?
- Is surgery the answer for me?
- Can you recommend a surgeon who performs the laparoscopic procedure?
- If surgery is appropriate for me, what are the next steps?

QUESTIONS TO ASK THE SURGEON:

- How many times have you performed Nissen or laparoscopic fundoplication?
- Are you a board-certified surgeon?
- What types of outcomes have you had?
- What are the most common side effects or complications?
- What should I do to prepare for surgery?
- What should I expect following the surgery?
- Can you refer me to one of your patients who has had this procedure?
- What type of diagnostic procedures are performed to determine if patients require surgery?
- Will I need to see another specialist for the diagnostic procedures?
- Do you use endoscopy, motility studies, and/or pH studies for your pre-operative evaluation?

Two studies demonstrated that laparoscopic fundoplication improved reflux symptoms in 76% and 98% of the treated populations, respectively. In an additional study, researchers evaluated 74 patients with reflux disease who received Nissen fundoplication after failure of medical therapy. The researchers concluded that 93.8% of the patients had complete resolution of symptoms and did not require anti-reflux medications approximately 14 months after fundoplication. Researchers have found that when fundoplication is successful, the resting pressure in the LES increases. This reflects a return to more normal LES functioning where the LES keeps stomach acid in the stomach through increased pressure.

Overall, studies have suggested that the vast majority of patients who receive laparoscopic reflux surgery have positive results. These patients are either symptom-free or have significant improvements in reflux symptoms. The laparoscopic approach has a few advantages over other forms of fundoplication. These advantages include:

- decreased postoperative pain
- more rapid return to work
- decreased hospital stay
- better cosmetic results

Morbidity and mortality rates

Mortality is extremely rare during or following fundoplication. Complications and side effects are not common following fundoplication, especially using the laparoscopic approach, and are usually mild. A review of 621 laparoscopic fundoplication procedures performed in Italy found no cases of mortality and complications in 7.3% of cases. The most serious complication was acute dysphagia (difficulty swallowing) that required a re-operation in 10 patients. In general, long-term complications resulting from this procedure are uncommon.

Alternatives

There are several variations of fundoplication that may be performed. In addition, laparoscopic fundoplication may require conversion to an open, or traditional, surgical fundoplication in a small percentage of cases. The most common alternative to fundoplication is simply a continuation of medical therapy. Typically, patients receive medication for a period prior to being evaluated for surgery. A review of nine studies found that omeprazole, a proton-pump inhibitor, was as effective as surgery. However, this same review found that the other commonly used anti-reflux drugs, histamine H_2-antagonists, were not as effective as surgery.

Resources

BOOKS

Current Medical Diagnosis & Treatment. New York: McGraw-Hill, 2003.

Ferri, Fred F. *Ferri's Clinical Advisor.* St. Louis, MO: Mosby, 2001.

PERIODICALS

Allgood, P. C., and M. Bachmann. "Medical or Surgical Treatment for Chronic Gastroesophageal Reflux: A Systematic Review of Published Effectiveness." *European Journal of Surgery* 166 (2000): 9.

Kahrilas, P. J. "Management of GERD: Medical vs. Surgical." *Seminars in Gastrointestinal Disease* 12 (2001): 3–15.

Scott, M., et al. "Gastroesophageal Reflux Disease: Diagnosis and Management." *American Family Physician* 59 (March 1, 1999): 1161–1172.

Society of American Gastrointestinal Endoscopic Surgeons. "Guidelines for Surgical Treatment of Gastroesophageal Reflux Disease (GERD)." *Surgical Endoscopy* 12 (1998): 186–188.

Spechler, S. J., et al. "Long-term Outcome of Medical and Surgical Therapies for Gastroesophageal Reflux Disease: Follow-Up of a Randomized Controlled Trial." *Journal of the American Medical Association* 285 (May 9, 2001): 2331–2338.

Triadafilopoulos, G., et al. "Radiofrequency Energy Delivery to the Gastroesophageal Junction for the Treatment of GERD." *Gastrointestinal Endoscopy* 53 (2001): 407–415.

Zaninotto, G., D. Molena, and E. Ancona. "A Prospective Multicenter Study on Laparoscopic Treatment of Gastroesophageal Reflux in Italy." *Surgical Endoscopy* 14 (2000): 282–288.

OTHER

National Digestive Diseases Information Clearinghouse. *Heartburn, Hiatal Hernia, and Gastroesophageal Reflux Disease (GERD).* 2003.

Society of American Gastrointestinal Endoscopic Surgeons. *Patient Information from Your Surgeon and SAGES.* 1997.

Mark Mitchell, M.D., M.P.H., M.B.A.

Gastrostomy

Definition

Gastrostomy is a surgical procedure for inserting a tube through the abdomen wall and into the stomach. The tube, called a "g-tube," is used for feeding or drainage.

Purpose

Gastrostomy is performed because a patient temporarily or permanently needs to be fed directly through a tube in the stomach. Reasons for feeding by gastrostomy include birth defects of the mouth, esophagus, or stomach, and neuromuscular conditions that cause people to eat very slowly due to the shape of their mouth or a weakness affecting their chewing and swallowing muscles.

Gastrostomy is also performed to provide drainage for the stomach when it is necessary to bypass a longstanding obstruction of the stomach outlet into the small intestine. Obstructions may be caused by peptic ulcer scarring or a tumor.

Demographics

In the United States, gastrostomies are more frequently performed on older individuals.

Description

Gastrostomy, also called gastrostomy tube (g-tube) insertion, is surgery performed to give an external opening into the stomach. Surgery is performed either when the patient is under **general anesthesia** or under **local anesthesia**.

Fitting the g-tube usually requires a short surgical operation that lasts about 30 minutes. During the surgery, an opening (stoma) about the diameter of a small pencil is cut in the skin and into the stomach; the stomach is then carefully attached to the abdominal wall. The g-tube is then fitted into the stoma. It is a special tube held in place by a disc or a water-filled balloon that has a valve inside allowing food to enter, but nothing to come out. The hole can be made using two different methods. The first uses a tube called an endoscope that has a light at the end, which is inserted into the mouth and fed down the esophagus and into the stomach. The light shines through the skin, showing the surgeon where to perform the incision. The other procedure does not use an endoscope. Instead, a small incision is made on the left side of the abdomen; an incision is then made through the stomach. A small, flexible, hollow tube, usually made of polyvinyl chloride or rubber, is inserted into the stomach. The stomach is stitched tightly around the tube, and the incision is closed.

The length of time the patient needs to remain in the hospital depends on the age of the patient and the patient's general health. In some cases, the hospital stay can be as short as one day, but often is longer. Normally, the stomach and abdomen heal in five to seven days.

The cost of the surgery varies, depending on the age and health of the patient. Younger patients are usually sicker and require more intensive, and thus more expensive, care. The procedure is normally covered by medical insurance.

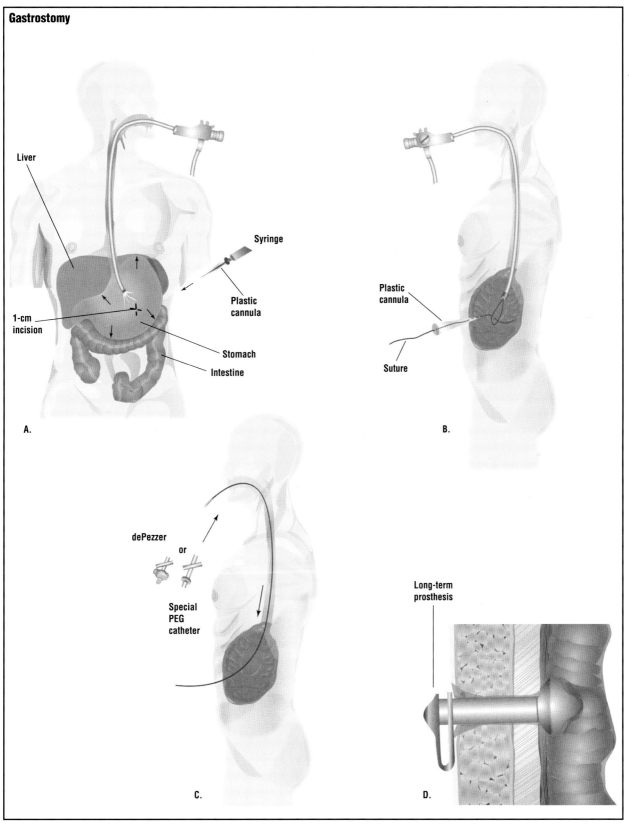

Gastrostomy

Liver

Syringe

Plastic
cannula

1-cm
incision

Stomach

Intestine

A.

Plastic
cannula

Suture

B.

dePezzer

or

Special
PEG
catheter

C.

Long-term
prosthesis

D.

For a percutaneous endoscopic gastrostomy procedure, the stomach is inflated with air (A). An incision is made into the abdomen and the stomach, and a plastic cannula is inserted (B). A catheter is inserted into the patient's mouth, pulled down the esophagus, and into the stomach (C). When the catheter is in place, access to the stomach is maintained (D). *(Illustration by GGS Information Services. Cengage Learning, Gale.)*

Preparation

Before the operation, the doctor will perform an endoscopy and take x rays of the gastrointestinal tract. Blood and urine tests will also be performed, and the patient will meet with the anesthesiologist to evaluate any special conditions that might affect the administration of anesthesia.

Aftercare

Immediately after the operation, the patient is fed intravenously (through a vein) for at least 24 hours. Once bowel sounds are heard, indicating that the gastrointestinal system is working, the patient can begin clear liquid feedings through the tube. The volume of the feedings is gradually increased.

Patient education concerning use and care of the gastrostomy tube is very important. Patients and their families are taught how to recognize and prevent infection around the tube, how to insert food through the tube, how to handle tube blockage, what to do if the tube pulls out, and what normal activities can be resumed.

Risks

There are few risks associated with this surgery. The main complications are infection, bleeding, dislodgment of the tube, stomach bloating, nausea, and diarrhea.

Gastrostomy is a relatively simple procedure. As with any surgery, however, patients are more likely to experience complications if they are smokers, obese, use alcohol heavily, or use illicit drugs. In addition,

some prescription medications may increase risks associated with anesthesia.

Normal results

The patient is able to eat through the gastrostomy tube, or the stomach can be drained through the tube.

Morbidity and mortality rates

The mortality rate of people who have had a gastrostomy is relatively high, however, the cause of **death** is almost always related to the illness or conditions that necessitated the insertion of the tube rather than to the actual surgical procedure.

Alternatives

There are no alternatives to a gastrostomy because the decision to perform it is made when a person is unable to take in enough calories to meet the demands of the body.

Resources

PERIODICALS

Angus, F., and R. Burakoff. "The Percutaneous Endoscopic Gastrostomy Tube. Medical and Ethical Issues in Placement." *American Journal of Gastroenterology* 98 (February 2003): 272–277.

Pontieri-Lewis, V. "Basics of Ostomy Care." *MedSurg Nursing* 15 no. 4 (August 1, 2006): 199—203.

ORGANIZATIONS

American College of Gastroenterology. P.O. Box 342260 Bethesda, MD 20827-2260. (301) 263-9000. http://www.acg.gi.org (accessed March 31, 2008).

American Gastroenterological Association (AGA). 4930 Del Ray Avenue, Bethesda, MD 20814. (301) 654-2055. http://www.gastro.org (accessed March 31, 2008).

United Ostomy Association of America. (UOAA). P. O. Box 66, Fairview, TN 37062-0066 (800) 826-0826. http://www.uoaa.org (accessed March 31, 2008).

QUESTIONS TO ASK THE DOCTOR

- What happens on the day of surgery?
- What type of anesthesia will be used?
- What happens after g-tube insertion?
- What are the risks associated with the procedure?
- How is the g-tube insertion done?
- Will there be a scar?
- Will I be able to eat normal food?
- Will people notice that I have a g-tube?
- Will it be there forever?

OTHER

"Feeding Tube Insertion." Medline Plus. December 13, 2006 [cited January 5, 2008]. http://www.nlm.nih.gov/medlineplus/ency/article/002937.htm (accessed March 31, 2008).

Tish Davidson, AM
Monique Laberge, PhD

GE surgery *see* **Gastroenterologic surgery**

General anesthetia *see* **Anesthesia, general**

General surgery

Definition

General surgery is the treatment of injury, deformity, and disease using operative procedures.

Purpose

General surgery is frequently performed to alleviate suffering when a cure is unlikely through medication alone. It can be used for routine procedures performed in a physician's office, such as **vasectomy**, or for more complicated operations requiring a medical team in a hospital setting, such as laparoscopic **cholecystectomy** (removal of the gallbladder). Areas of the body treated by general surgery include the stomach, liver, intestines, appendix, breasts, thyroid gland, salivary glands, some arteries and veins, and the skin. The brain, heart, lungs, eyes, feet, kidneys, bladder, and reproductive organs—to name only a few—are areas that require specialized surgical repair.

KEY TERMS

Appendectomy—Removal of the appendix.

Endoscope—Instrument for visual examination of the inside of a body canal or a hollow organ such as the stomach, colon, or bladder.

Hysterectomy—Surgical removal of part or all of the uterus.

Laparoscopic cholecystectomy—Removal of the gallbladder using a laparoscope, a fiber-optic instrument inserted through the abdomen.

Microsurgery—Surgery on small body structures or cells performed with the aid of a microscope and other specialized instruments.

Portal—An entrance or a means of entrance.

New methods and techniques are less invasive than older practices, permitting procedures that were considered impossible in the past. For example, **microsurgery** has been used in reattaching severed body parts by successfully reconnecting small blood vessels and nerves. Laparoscopic techniques are more efficient, promote more rapid healing, leave smaller scars, and have lower postoperative infection rates.

Demographics

All surgeons receive similar training in the first two years of their residency (post-medical school) training. General surgeons are the surgical equivalent of family practitioners. General surgeons typically differ from other surgical specialties in the operations that they perform. This difference is most easily understood by exclusion. For example, procedures involving nerves or the brain are usually performed by neurosurgeons. Surgeons having specialized training during the final three years of their residency period similarly focus on other regions of the body. General surgeons may perform such procedures in the absence of other surgeons with specialized training; however, these situations are the exception rather than the rule.

In the United States, there are approximately 850,000 physicians licensed to practice medicine and surgery. Experts estimate that fewer than 5% of these physicians (approximately 42,000) restrict their practices to general surgery.

Description

In earlier times, surgery was a dangerous and dirty practice. Through the middle of the nineteenth century, the number of people who died from surgery approximately equaled the number of those who were cured. With the discovery and development of **general anesthesia** in the mid-nineteenth century, surgery became more humane. As knowledge about infections grew and sterile practices were introduced into the **operating room**, surgery became more successful. The last 50 years have brought continued advancements.

General surgery experienced major advances with the introduction of the endoscope. This is an instrument for visualizing the interior of a body canal or a hollow organ. Endoscopic surgery relies on this pencil-thin instrument, equipped with its own lighting system and small video camera. The endoscope is inserted through tiny incisions called portals. While viewing the procedure on a video screen, the surgeon then operates with various other small, precise instruments inserted through one or more of the portals. The specific area of the body to be treated determines the type of endoscopic surgery performed. For example, **colonoscopy** uses an endoscope, which can be equipped with a device for obtaining tissue samples for visual examination of the colon. Gastroscopy uses an endoscope inserted through the mouth to examine the interior of the stomach. Arthroscopy refers to joint surgery. Abdominal procedures are called laparoscopies.

Endoscopy is frequently used in both treatment and diagnosis involving the digestive and female reproductive systems. Endoscopy has advantages over many other surgical procedures, resulting in a quicker recovery and shorter hospital stays. This non-invasive technique is used for appendectomies, gallbladder surgery, hysterectomies, and the repair of shoulder and knee ligaments; however, endoscopy has limitations such as complications and operating expense. Endoscopy does not offer advantages over conventional surgery in all procedures. Some literature states that, as general surgeons become more experienced in their prospective fields, additional non-invasive surgical procedures will become more common options.

One-day surgery is also termed same-day or **outpatient surgery**. Surgical procedures in this category usually require two hours or less and involve minimal blood loss and a short recovery time. In the majority of surgical cases, oral medications control postoperative pain. Cataract removal, **laparoscopy**, **tonsillectomy**, repair of broken bones, hernia repair, and a wide range of cosmetic procedures are common same-day surgical procedures. Many individuals prefer the convenience and atmosphere of one-day surgery centers, as there is less competition for attention with more serious surgical cases. These centers are accredited by the Joint Commission on Accreditation of Healthcare Organizations or the Accreditation Association for Ambulatory Health Care.

Diagnosis/Preparation

The preparation of persons for surgery has advanced significantly with improved diagnostic techniques and procedures. Before surgery, a candidate may be asked to undergo a series of tests, including blood and urine studies, X-rays, and specific heart studies if the person's past medical history or **physical examination** warrants this testing. Before any surgical procedure, the physician will explain the nature of the surgery needed, the reason for the procedure, and the anticipated outcome. The risks involved will be discussed, along with the types of anesthesia to be utilized. The expected length of recovery and limitations imposed during the recovery period are also explained in detail before any surgical procedure.

Surgical procedures most often require some type of anesthetic. Some procedures require only **local anesthesia**, produced by injecting the anesthetic agent into the skin near the site of the operation. The person remains awake with this form of medication. Injecting anesthetic agents near a primary nerve located adjacent to the surgical site produces block anesthesia (also known as regional anesthesia), which is a more extensive local anesthesia. The person remains conscious, but is usually sedated. General anesthesia involves injecting anesthetic agents into the blood stream or inhaling medicines through a mask placed over the person's face. During general anesthesia, an individual is asleep and an airway tube is usually placed into the windpipe (trachea) to help keep the airway open.

As part of the preoperative preparation, surgical patients will receive printed educational material and may be asked to review audio or videotapes. They will be instructed to shower or bathe the evening before or morning of surgery and may be asked to scrub the operative site with a special antibacterial soap. Instructions will also be given to eat or drink nothing by mouth for a determined period of time prior to the surgical procedure.

Precautions

Persons who are obese, smoke, have bleeding tendencies, or are over 60 must follow special precautions, as do persons who have recently experienced illnesses, including pneumonia or a heart attack. People taking medications such as heart and blood pressure medicine, blood thinners, **muscle relaxants**, tranquilizers, anticonvulsants, insulin, or sedatives may require special laboratory tests prior to surgery and special monitoring during surgery. Extra precautions may be necessary for persons using mind-altering drugs such as narcotics, psychedelics, hallucinogens, marijuana, sedatives, or cocaine since these drugs may interact with the anesthetic agents used during surgery.

Risks

A risk associated with general surgery is the potential for postoperative complications. These complications include, but are not limited to, pneumonia, internal bleeding, and wound infection as well as adverse reactions to anesthesia.

Normal results

Advances in diagnostic and surgical techniques have greatly increased the success rate of general surgery. Contemporary procedures are less invasive than those practiced a decade or more ago. The results include reduced length of hospital stays, shortened recovery times, decreased postoperative pain, and decreases in the size and extent of surgical incisions. The length of time required for a full recovery varies with the procedure.

Morbidity and mortality rates

Mortality from general surgical procedures is uncommon. The most common causes of mortality are adverse reactions to anesthetic agents or drugs used to control pain, postsurgical clot formation in the veins, and postsurgical heart attacks or strokes.

Abnormal results from general surgery include persistent pain, swelling, redness, drainage, or bleeding in the surgical area and surgical wound infection, resulting in slow healing.

Alternatives

For the removal of diseased or nonvital tissue, there is no alternative to surgery. Alternatives to general surgery depend on the condition being treated. Medications, acupuncture, or hypnosis are used to relieve pain. Radiation is an occasional alternative for shrinking growths. Chemotherapy may be used to treat cancer. Some foreign bodies may remain in the body without harm.

Resources

BOOKS

Brunicardi, F. C., D. K. Anderson, D. L. Dunn, J. G. Hunter, and R. E. Pollock. *Schwartz's Manual of Surgery,* 8th ed. New York: McGraw Hill, 2006.

Ellis, H., R. Caine, and C. Watson. *General Surgery: Lecture Notes,* 11th ed. New York: Wiley, 2006.

Lawrence, P. F. *Essentials of General Surgery,* 4th ed. Philadelphia: Lippincott Williams & Wilkins, 2005.

Townsend, C.M., R. D. Beauchamp, B. M. Evers, and K. Mattox. *Sabiston Textbook of Surgery,* 17th ed. Philadelphia: Saunders, 2004.

Toy, E. C., T. H. Liu, and A. R. Campbell. *Case Files: Surgery.* New York: McGraw Hill, 2006.

PERIODICALS

Allen, T. K., A. S. Habib, G. L. Dear, W. White, D. A. Lubarsky, and T. J. Gan. "How much are patients willing to pay to avoid postoperative muscle pain associated with succinylcholine?" *Journal of Clinical Anesthesia* 19, no. 8 (December 2007): 601–608.

Gurusamy, K. S., and K. Samraj. "Early versus delayed laparoscopic cholecystectomy for acute cholecystitis." *Cochran Database of Systematic Reviews* 18, no. 4 (October 2006).

Halpern, L. R., and S. Feldman. "Perioperative risk assessment in the surgical care of geriatric patients." *Oral and*

Maxillofacial Surgery Clinics of North America 18, no. 1 (February 2006): 19–34.

Vergis, A., L. Gillman, S. Minor, M. Taylor, and J. Park. "Structured assessment format for evaluating operative reports in general surgery." *American Journal of Surgery* 195, no. 1 (January 2008): 24–29.

OTHER

Archives of Surgery. American Medical Association. http://archsurg.ama-assn.org/ (December 23, 2007).

General Surgery. MedScape. http://www.medscape.com/generalsurgery (December 23, 2007).

Journal of Surgery. National Medical Society. http://www.medical-library.org/j_surg.htm (December 23, 2007).

Online Atlas of Surgery. Wake Forest University School of Medicine. http://www.bgsm.edu/surg-sci/atlas/atlas.html (December 23, 2007).

ORGANIZATIONS

American Board of Surgery, 1617 John F. Kennedy Boulevard, Suite 860, Philadelphia, PA, 19103, (215) 568-4000, (215) 563-5718, http://www.absurgery.org.

American College of Surgeons, 633 North Saint Claire Street, Chicago, IL, 60611, (312) 202-5000, http://www.facs.org/.

American Medical Association, 515 N. State Street, Chicago, IL, 60610, (800) 621-8335, http://www.ama-assn.org.

American Society for Aesthetic Plastic Surgery, 11081 Winners Circle, Los Alamitos, CA, 90720, (888) 272-7711, http://www.surgery.org/.

American Society for Dermatologic Surgery, 5550 Meadowbrook Drive, Suite 120, Rolling Meadows, IL, 60008, (847) 956-0900, http://www.asds.net.

American Society of Plastic and Reconstructive Surgeons, 444 E. Algonquin Road, Arlington Heights, IL, 60005, (847) 228-9900, http://www.plasticsurgery.org.

L. Fleming Fallon, Jr., M.D., Dr.P.H.

GERD scan *see* **Gastroesophageal reflux scan**

GERD surgery *see* **Gastroesophageal reflux surgery**

Gingivectomy

Definition

Gingivectomy is periodontal surgery that removes and reforms diseased gum tissue or other gingival buildup related to serious underlying conditions. For more chronic gingival conditions, gingivectomy is utilized after other nonsurgical methods have been tried, and before gum disease has advanced enough to jeopardize the ligaments and bone supporting the teeth. Performed in a dentist's office, the surgery is primarily done one quadrant of the mouth at a time under local anesthetic. Clinical attachment levels of the gum to teeth and supporting structures determine the success of the surgery. Surgery required beyond gingivectomy involves the regeneration of attachment structures through tissue and bone grafts.

Purpose

Periodontal surgery is primarily performed to alter or eliminate the microbial factors that create periodontitis, and thereby stop the progression of the disease. Periodontal diseases comprise a number of conditions that affect the health of periodontium. The factors include a variety of microorganisms and host conditions, such as the immune system, that combine to affect the gums and, ultimately, the support of the teeth. The primary invasive factor creating disease is plaque-producing bacteria. Once the gingiva are infected by plaque-making bacteria unabated due to immunosuppression or by oral hygiene, the bacterial conditions for periodontitis or gum infections are present. Unless the microorganisms and the pathological changes they produce on the gum are removed, the disease progresses. In the most severe cases, graft surgery may be necessary to restore tissue ligament and bone tissue destroyed by pathogens.

In healthy gums, there is very little space between the gum and tooth, usually less than 0.15 in (4 mm). With regular brushing and flossing, most gums stay healthy and firm unless there are underlying hereditary or immunosuppressive conditions that affect the gums. The continuum of progressive bacterial infection of the gums leads to two main conditions in the periodontium: gingivitis and periodontitis. External factors such as smoking and certain illnesses such as diabetes are associated with periodontal disease and increase the severity of disease in the gum tissue, support, and bone structures. Two types of procedures are necessitated by the severity of gum retreat from the teeth, represented by periodontal pockets. Both nonsurgical and surgical procedures are designed to eliminate these pockets and restore gum to the teeth, thereby ensuring the retention of teeth.

Gingivitis

Gingivitis occurs when gum tissue is invaded by bacteria that change into plaque in the mouth due to disease-fighting secretions. This plaque resides on the gums and hardens, becoming tartar, or crystallized plaque, known also as calculus. Brushing and flossing

KEY TERMS

Calculus—A term for plaque buildup on the teeth that has crystallized.

Gingivitis—Inflammation of the gingiva or gums caused by bacterial buildup in plague on the teeth.

Periodontitis—Generalized disease of the gums in which unremoved calculus has separated the gingiva or gum tissue from the teeth and threatens support ligaments of the teeth and bone.

Scaling and root planing—A dental procedure to treat gingivitis in which the teeth are scraped inside the gum area and the root of the tooth is planed to dislodge bacterial deposits.

cannot remove calculus. The gum harboring calculus becomes irritated, causing inflammation and a loss of a snug fit to the teeth. As the pockets between the gum and the teeth become more pronounced, more residue is developed, and the calculus becomes resistant to the cleaning ability of brushing and flossing. Gums become swollen and begin to bleed. A dentist or periodontist can reverse this form of gum disease through the mechanical removal of calculus and plaque. This cleaning is called curettage, which is a deep cleaning process that includes scraping the tartar off the teeth above and below the gum line and planing or smoothing the tooth at the root. Also known as dental **debridement**, this procedure is often accompanied by antibiotic treatment to stave off further microbe proliferation.

Periodontitis

Periodontitis is the generalized condition of the periodontium in which gums are so inflamed by bacteria-produced calculus that they separate from the teeth, creating large pockets (more than 0.23 in [6 mm] from the teeth), with increased destruction of periodontal structures and noticeable tooth mobility. Periodontitis is the stage of the disease that threatens significant ligament damage and tooth loss. If earlier procedures like scaling and root planing cannot restore the gum tissue to a healthy, firm state and pocket depth is still sufficient to warrant treatment, a gingivectomy is indicated. The comparative success of this surgery over nonsurgical treatments such as more debridement and more frequent use of **antibiotics** has not been demonstrated by research.

Demographics

According to a report by the U.S. Surgeon General in 2000, half of adults living in the United States have gingivitis, and about one in five have periodontitis. According to the same report, smokers are four times more likely than nonsmokers to have periodontitis, and three to four times more likely to lose some or all of their teeth. By region, individuals living in the Southern states have a higher rate of periodontal disease and tooth loss than other regions of the country. Severe gum disease affects about 14% of adults aged 45–54 years. One of the main risk factors for gum disease is lack of dental care. Initiatives by the Centers for Disease Control and Prevention have begun to study the relation between periodontal disease and general health. There is growing acknowledgment of the public health issues related to chronic periodontal disease.

The delivery of oral surgery, or even dental care, to individuals in the United States is difficult to determine. Race, ethnicity, and poverty level stratified individuals making dental visits in a year. While 70% of white individuals made visits, only 56% of non-Hispanic black individuals and only 50% of Mexican-American individuals made visits. Seventy-two percent of individuals at or above the federal poverty level made visits, while only 50% of those below the poverty level made visits. Since it is also estimated that more than 100 million Americans lack dental insurance, it is likely that periodontal surgery among the people most likely to have periodontal disease (low-income individuals with nutritional issues, with little or no preventive dental care, and who smoke) are the least likely to have periodontal surgery.

Description

Periodontal procedures for gingivitis involve gingival curettage, in which the surgeon cuts away some of the most hygienically unhealthy tissue, reducing the depth of the pocket. This surgery is usually done under a local anesthetic and is done on one quadrant of the mouth at a time.

Gingival or periodontal flap surgery (gingivectomy) is indicated in advanced periodontal disease, in which the stability of the teeth are compromised by infection, which displaces ligament and bone. In gingivectomy, the gingival flap is resected or separated from the bone, exposing the root. The calculus buildup on the tooth, down to the root, is removed. The surgery is performed under local anesthetic.

Small incisions are made in the gum to allow the dentist to see both tooth and bone. The surrounding alveolar, or exposed bone, may require reforming to ensure proper healing. Gum tissue is returned to the tooth and sutured. A putty-like coating spread over the teeth and gums protects the sutures. This coating serves as a kind of bandage and allows the eating of soft foods and drinking of liquids after surgery. The typical procedure takes between one and two hours and usually involves only one or two quadrants per visit. The sutures remain in place for approximately one week. Pain medication is prescribed and antibiotics treatment is begun.

Diagnosis/Preparation

Many factors contribute to periodontal disease, and the process that leads to the need for surgery may occur early or take many months or years to develop. Early primary tooth mobility or early primary tooth loss in children may be due to very serious underlying diseases, including hereditary gingival fibromatosis, a fibrous enlargement of the gingiva; conditions induced by drugs for liver disease; or gum conditions related to leukemia. Patient-related factors for chronic periodontal disease include systemic health, age, oral hygiene, various presurgical therapeutic options, and the patient's ability to control plaque formation and smoking. Another factor includes the extent and frequency of periodontal procedures to remove subgingival deposits. Gum inflammation can be secondary to many conditions, including diabetes, genetic predisposition, stress, immunosuppression, pregnancy, medications, and nutrition.

The most telling signs of early gum disease are swollen gums and bleeding. If gingivectomy is considered, consultation with the patient's physician is important, as are instruction and reinforcement with the patient to control plaque. Gingiva scaling and root planing should be performed to remove plaque and calculus to see if gum health improves.

The protective responses of the body and the use of dental practices to overcome the pathology of periodontal disease may be thwarted and the concentration of pathogens may be such that plaque below the gum line leads to tissue destruction. Refractory periodontitis, or the form of periodontal disease characterized by its resistance to repeated gingival treatments, and often also associated with diabetes mellitus and other systematic diseases, may require surgery to remove deep pockets and to offer regenerative procedures like tissue and bone grafts.

The level of damage is determined by signs of inflammation and by measuring the pocket depth.

Healthy pockets around the teeth are usually between 0.04–0.11 in (1–3 mm). The dentist measures each tooth and notes the findings. If the pockets are more than 0.19–0.23 in (5–6 mm), x rays may be taken to look at bone loss. After conferring with the patient, a decision will be made to have periodontal surgery or to try medications and/or more gingival scaling.

Risks for infection must be assessed prior to surgery. Certain conditions, including damaged heart valves, congenital heart defects, immunosuppression, liver disease, and artificial joints such as hip or **knee replacement**, put the oral surgery patient at higher risk for infection. Ultimately, the decision for surgery should be based upon the health of the patient, the quality of life with or without surgery, their willingness to change lifestyle factors such as smoking and bad nutrition, and the ability to incorporate oral hygiene into a daily regimen. Expense is also a factor since periodontal surgery is relatively expensive. Long-term studies are still needed to determine if medications such as antibiotic treatments are superior to surgery for severe chronic periodontal disease.

Aftercare

Surgery will take place in the periodontist's office and usually takes a few hours from the time of surgery until the anesthetic wears off. After that, normal activities are encouraged. It takes a few days or weeks for the gums to completely heal. Ibuprofen (Advil) or **acetaminophen** (Tylenol) is very effective for pain. Dental management after surgery that includes deep cleaning by a dental hygienist will be put in force to maintain the health of the gums. Visits to the dentist for the first year are scheduled every three months to remove plaque and tartar buildup. After a year, periodontal cleaning is required every six months.

Risks

Periodontal surgery has few risks. However, there is the risk of introducing infection into the bloodstream. Some surgeons require antibiotic treatment before and after surgery.

Normal results

The gold standard of periodontal treatment is the decrease of attachment loss, which is the decrease in tooth loss due to gingival conditions. Normal immediate results of surgery are short-term pain; some gum shrinkage due to the surgery, which over time takes on a more normal shape; and easier success with oral

WHO PERFORMS THE PROCEDURE AND WHERE IS IT PERFORMED?

Periodontal surgery involving gingivectomy and regenerative grafts are performed by a dentist specializing in diseases and surgery of the gums; the specialist is known as a periodontist. This is usually through a referral from the patient's general dentist. The procedure is performed in a dentist's office.

hygiene. Long-term results are equivocal. One study followed 600 patients in a private periodontal practice for more than 15 years. The study found tooth retention was more closely related to the individual case of disease than to the type of surgery performed. In another study, a retrospective chart review of 335 patients who had received non-surgical treatment was conducted. All patients were active cases for 10 years, and 44.8% also had periodontal surgery. The results of the study showed that those who received surgical therapy lost more teeth than those who received nonsurgical treatment. The factor that predicted tooth loss was neither procedure: it was earlier or initial attachment loss.

Morbidity and mortality rates

The most common complications of oral surgery include bleeding, pain, and swelling. Less common complications are infections of the gums from the surgery. Rarer still is a bloodstream infection from the surgery, which can have serious consequences.

Alternatives

Alternatives to periodontal surgery include other dental procedures concomitant with medication treatment as well as changes in lifestyle. Lifestyle changes included quitting smoking, nutritional changes, **exercise**, and better oral hygiene. There have been some medication advances for the gum infections that lead to inflammation and disease. Medication, combined with scaling and root planing, can be very effective. New treatments include antimicrobial mouthwashes to control bacteria; a gelatin-filled antibiotic "chip" inserted into periodontal pockets; and low doses of an antibiotic medication to keep destructive enzymes from combining with the bacteria to create plaque.

QUESTIONS TO ASK THE DOCTOR

- How many quadrants for surgery will be performed at each visit?
- Can the gum scaling and root planing be repeated with antibiotic treatment as an alternative to gingivectomy?
- How effective have you found antibacterial, antibiotic, or anti-microbial treatment in slowing down disease progression?
- How often must I return to have periodontal cleaning after the surgery? Can my regular dentist do that?
- Besides dental care and home hygiene, what can I do to keep the disease from reoccurring after surgery?

Resources

PERIODICALS

"Guidelines for Periodontal Therapy." *Journal of Periodontology* 72, nos. 11 and 16 (November 2001): 1624–1628.
Delaney, J. E., amd M. A. Keels. "Pediatric Oral Health." *Pediatric Clinics of North America* 47, no. 5 (October 2000).
Matthews, D. C., et al. "Tooth Loss in Periodontal Patients." *Journal of the Canadian Dental Association,* Vol. 67, (2001): 207–10.

ORGANIZATIONS

Periodontal (Gum) Diseases. National Institute of Dental and Craniofacial Research, National Institutes of Health. Bethesda, MD 20892-2190. (301) 496-4261. http://www.nidcrinfo.nih.gov.

OTHER

"Cigarette Smoking Linked to Gum Diseases." *National Center for Chronic Disease Prevention and Health Promotion.* http://www.cdc.gov/nccdphp.
"Gingivectomy for Gum Disease." *WebMD Health.* www.webmd.com.

Nancy McKenzie, PhD

Glaucoma cryotherapy *see*
Cyclocryotherapy

Glossectomy

Definition

A glossectomy is the surgical removal of all or part of the tongue.

Purpose

A glossectomy is performed to treat cancer of the tongue. Removing the tongue is indicated if the patient has a cancer that does not respond to other forms of treatment. In most cases, however, only part of the tongue is removed (partial glossectomy). Cancer of the tongue is considered very dangerous due to the fact that it can easily spread to nearby lymph glands. Most cancer specialists recommend surgical removal of the cancerous tissue.

Demographics

According to the Oral Cancer Foundation, 30,000 Americans will be diagnosed with oral or pharyngeal cancer in 2003, or about 1.1 persons per 100,000. Of these 30,000 newly diagnosed individuals, only half will be alive in five years. This percentage has shown little improvement for decades. The problem is much greater in the rest of the world, with over 350,000 to 400,000 new cases of oral cancer appearing each year.

The most important risk factors for cancer of the tongue are alcohol consumption and smoking. The risk is significantly higher in patients who use both alcohol and tobacco than in those who consume only one.

Description

Glossectomies are always performed under **general anesthesia**. A partial glossectomy is a relatively simple operation. If the "hole" left by the excision of the cancer is small, it is commonly repaired by sewing up the tongue immediately or by using a small graft of skin. If the glossectomy is more extensive, care is taken to repair the tongue so as to maintain its mobility. A common approach is to use a piece of skin taken from the wrist together with the blood vessels that supply it. This type of graft is called a radial forearm free flap. The flap is inserted into the hole in the tongue. This procedure requires a highly skilled surgeon who is able to connect very small arteries. Complete removal of the tongue, called a total glossectomy, is rarely performed.

Diagnosis/Preparation

If an area of abnormal tissue has been found in the mouth, either by the patient or by a dentist or doctor, a biopsy is the only way to confirm a diagnosis of cancer. A pathologist, who is a physician who specializes in the study of disease, examines the tissue sample under a microscope to check for cancer cells.

KEY TERMS

Biopsy—A diagnostic procedure that involves obtaining a tissue specimen for microscopic analysis to establish a precise diagnosis.

Fistula (plural, fistulae)—An abnormal passage that develops either between two organs inside the body or between an organ and the surface of the body. Fistula formation is one of the possible complications of a glossectomy.

Flap—A piece of tissue for grafting that has kept its own blood supply.

Lymph—The almost colorless fluid that bathes body tissues. Lymph is found in the lymphatic vessels and carries lymphocytes that have entered the lymph glands from the blood.

Lymph gland—A small bean-shaped organ consisting of a loose meshwork of tissue in which large numbers of white blood cells are embedded.

Lymphatic system—The tissues and organs (including the bone marrow, spleen, thymus and lymph nodes) that produce and store cells that fight infection, together with the network of vessels that carry lymph throughout the body.

Oncology—The branch of medicine that deals with the diagnosis and treatment of cancer.

If the biopsy indicates that cancer is present, a comprehensive **physical examination** of the patient's head and neck is performed prior to surgery. The patient will meet with the treatment team before **admission to the hospital** so that they can answer questions and explain the treatment plan.

Aftercare

Patients usually remain in the hospital for seven to 10 days after a glossectomy. They often require oxygen in the first 24–48 hours after the operation. Oxygen is administered through a face mask or through two small tubes placed in the nostrils. The patient is given fluids through a tube that goes from the nose to the stomach until he or she can tolerate taking food by mouth. Radiation treatment is often scheduled after the surgery to destroy any remaining cancer cells. As patients regain the ability to eat and swallow, they also begin speech therapy.

Risks

Risks associated with a glossectomy include:

WHO PERFORMS THE PROCEDURE AND WHERE IS IT PERFORMED?

A glossectomy is performed in a hospital by a treatment team specializing in head and neck oncology surgery. The treatment team usually includes an ear, nose & throat (ENT) surgeon, an oral-maxillofacial (OMF) surgeon, a plastic surgeon, a clinical oncologist, a nurse, a speech therapist, and a dietician.

- Bleeding from the tongue. This is an early complication of surgery; it can result in severe swelling leading to blockage of the airway.

- Poor speech and difficulty swallowing. This complication depends on how much of the tongue is removed.

- Fistula formation. Incomplete healing may result in the formation of a passage between the skin and the mouth cavity within the first two weeks following a glossectomy. This complication often occurs after feeding has resumed. Patients who have had radiotherapy are at greater risk of developing a fistula.

- Flap failure. This complication is often due to problems with the flap's blood supply.

Normal results

A successful glossectomy results in complete removal of the cancer, improved ability to swallow food, and restored speech. The quality of the patient's speech is usually very good if at least one-third of the tongue remains and an experienced surgeon has performed the repair.

Total glossectomy results in severe disability because the "new tongue" (a prosthesis) is incapable of movement. This lack of mobility creates enormous difficulty in eating and talking.

Morbidity and mortality rates

Even in the case of a successful glossectomy, the long-term outcome depends on the stage of the cancer and the involvement of lymph glands in the neck. Five-year survival data reveal overall survival rates of less than 60%, although the patients who do survive often endure major functional, cosmetic, and psychological burdens as a result of their difficulties in speaking and eating.

QUESTIONS TO ASK THE DOCTOR

- Will the glossectomy prevent the cancer from coming back?
- What are the possible complications of this procedure?
- How long will it take to recover from the surgery?
- How will the glossectomy affect my speech?
- What specific techniques do you use?
- How many new cancers of the head and neck do you treat every year?

Alternatives

An alternative to glossectomy is the insertion of radioactive wires into the cancerous tissue. This is an effective treatment but requires specialized surgical skills and facilities.

Resources

BOOKS

"Disorders of the Oral Region: Neoplasms." Section 9, Chapter 105 in *The Merck Manual of Diagnosis and Therapy*, edited by Mark H. Beers, MD, and Robert Berkow, MD. Whitehouse Station, NJ: Merck Research Laboratories, 1999.

Johnson, J. T., ed. *Reconstruction of the Oral Cavity*. Alexandria, VA: American Academy of Otolaryngology, 1994.

Shah, J. P., J. G. Batsakis, and J. Shah. *Oral Cancer*. Oxford, UK: Isis Medical Media, 2003.

PERIODICALS

Barry, B., B. Baujat, S. Albert, et al. "Total Glossectomy Without Laryngectomy as First-Line or Salvage Therapy." *Laryngoscope* 113 (February 2003): 373-376.

Chuanjun, C., Z. Zhiyuan, G. Shaopu, et al. "Speech After Partial Glossectomy: A Comparison Between Reconstruction and Nonreconstruction Patients." *Journal of Oral and Maxillofacial Surgery* 60 (April 2002): 404-407.

Furia, C. L., L. P. Kowalski, M. R. Latorre, et al. "Speech Intelligibility After Glossectomy and Speech Rehabilitation." *Archives of Otolaryngology - Head & Neck Surgery* 127 (July 2001): 877-883.

Kimata, Y., K. Uchiyama, S. Ebihara, et al. "Postoperative Complications and Functional Results After Total Glossectomy with Microvascular Reconstruction." *Plastic Reconstructive Surgery* 106 (October 2000): 1028-1035.

ORGANIZATIONS

American Academy of Otolaryngology - Head and Neck Surgery. One Prince Street, Alexandria, VA 22314. (703) 806-4444. www.entnet.org.

American Cancer Society. National Headquarters, 1599 Clifton Road NE, Atlanta, GA 30329. (800) ACS -2345. www.cancer.org

Oral Cancer Foundation. 3419 Via Lido, #205, Newport Beach, CA 92663. (949) 646-8000. www.oralcancer.org

OTHER

"Oral Cavity Cancer." *Cancer Information Network.* www. ontumor.com/oral/.

"Tongue Base and Tonsil Cancer." *Cancer Answers.com.* www.canceranswers.com/Tongue.Base.Tonsil.html.

Monique Laberge, Ph. D.

Blood glucose test (blood sugar, fasting blood sugar [FBS])

	Normal findings	Possible critical values
Cord	45–96 mg/dl (2.5–5.3 mmol/L)	
Premature infant	20–60 mg/dl (1.1–3.3 mmol/L)	
Newborn	30–60 mg/dl (1.7–3.3 mmol/L)	,30 and .300 mg/dl
Infant	40–90 mg/dl (2.2–5.0 mmol/L)	,40 mg/dl
Child ,2 years	60–100 mg/dl (3.3–5.5 mmol/L)	
Child ,2 years to adult	70–105 mg/dl (3.9–5.8 mmol/L)	Male: ,50 and .400 mg/dl Female: ,40 and .400 mg/dl
Elderly	increase in normal range after age 50 years	

SOURCE: Pagana, K.D. and T.J. Pagana. *Mosby's Diagnostic and Laboratory Test Reference.* 3rd ed. St. Louis: Mosby, 1997.

(Cengage Learning, Gale.)

Glucose tests

Definition

Glucose tests are used to determine the concentration of glucose in blood, urine, cerebrospinal fluid (CSF), and other body fluids. These tests are used to detect increased blood glucose (hyperglycemia), decreased blood glucose (hypoglycemia), increased glucose in the urine (glycosuria), and decreased glucose in CSF, serous, and synovial fluid glucose.

Purpose

The results of glucose tests are used in a variety of situations, including:

- Screening persons for diabetes mellitus. The American Diabetes Association (ADA) recommends that a fasting plasma glucose (fasting blood sugar) be used to diagnose diabetes. People without symptoms of diabetes should be tested when they reach the age of 45 years, and again every three years. People in high-risk groups should be tested before the age of 45, and then more frequently. If a person already has symptoms of diabetes, a blood glucose test without fasting (a casual plasma glucose test), may be performed. In difficult diagnostic cases, a glucose challenge test called a two-hour oral glucose tolerance test (OGTT) is recommended. If the result of any of these three tests is abnormal, it must be confirmed with a second test—performed on another day. The same test or a different test can be used. However, the result of the second test must be abnormal as well to establish a diagnosis of diabetes.

- Screening for gestational diabetes. Diabetes that occurs during pregnancy is called gestational diabetes. This condition is associated with hypertension, increased birth weight of the fetus, and a higher risk for preeclampsia. Women who are at risk are screened when they are 24–28 weekss pregnant. A woman is considered at risk if she is older than 25 years, is not at her normal body weight, has a parent or sibling with diabetes, or is in an ethnic group that has a high rate of diabetes (such as Hispanic, Native American, or African-American).

- Blood glucose monitoring. Daily measurement of whole blood glucose identifies persons with diabetes who require intervention to maintain their blood glucose within an acceptable range as determined

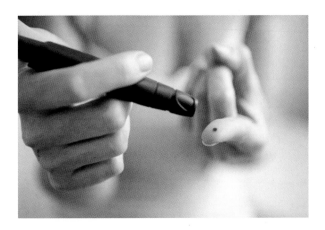

Testing blood sugar level. *(moodboard / Alamy)*

Normal findings for glucose tolerance test (GTT, oral glucose tolerance test [OGTT])	
Blood test	
Fasting	70–115 mg/dl (<6.4 mmol/L)
30 minutes	<200 mg/dl (<11.1 mmol/L)
1 hour	<200 mg/dl (<11.1 mmol/L)
2 hours	<140 mg/dl (<7.8 mmol/L)
3 hours	70–115 mg/dl (<6.4 mmol/L)
4 hours	70–115 mg/dl (<6.4 mmol/L)
Urine test	Negative

SOURCE: Pagana, K.D. and T.J. Pagana. *Mosbyís Diagnostic and Laboratory Test Reference.* 3rd ed. St. Louis: Mosby, 1997.

(Cengage Learning, Gale.)

by their doctors. The Diabetes Control and Complications Trial (DCCT) demonstrated that persons with diabetes who maintained blood glucose and glycated hemoglobin (hemoglobin with glucose bound to it) at or near normal decreased their risk of complications by 50–75%. Based on results of this study, the ADA recommends routine glycated hemoglobin testing to measure long-term control of blood sugar. The most common glycated hemoglobin test, is the HbA_{1c}, which provides the average, overall blood glucose levels over the prior two to three month period. A DCCT randomized study found that the knowledge alone that their glycated hemoglobin results were good improved blood glucose control in some patients.

- Diagnosis and differentiation of hypoglycemia. Low blood glucose may be associated with symptoms such as confusion, memory loss, and seizures. Demonstration that such symptoms are the result of hypoglycemia requires evidence of low blood glucose at the time of symptoms and reversal of the symptoms by glucose. In documented hypoglycemia, blood glucose tests are used along with measurements of insulin and C-peptide (a fragment of proinsulin) to differentiate between fasting and postprandial (after a meal) causes.

- Analysis of glucose in body fluids. High levels of glucose in body fluids reflect a hyperglycemic state and are not otherwise clinically significant. However, low body fluid glucose levels indicate increased glucose utilization, often caused by infection (meningitis causes a low CSF glucose); inflammatory disease (rheumatoid arthritis causes a low pleural fluid glucose); or malignancy (a leukemia or lymphoma, such as Hodgkin's disease infiltrating the CNS or serous cavity).

KEY TERMS

Diabetes mellitus—A disease in which a person can't effectively use glucose to meet the needs of the body. It is caused by a lack of the hormone insulin.

Glucose—The main form of sugar (chemical formula $C_6H_{12}O_6$) used by the body for energy.

Glycated hemoglobin—A test that measures the amount of hemoglobin bound to glucose. It is a measure of how much glucose has been in the blood during a two to three month period beginning approximately one month prior to sample collection.

Hyperglycemia—Abnormally increased amount of sugar in the blood.

Hypoglycemia—Abnormally decreased amount of sugar in the blood.

Ketones—Waste products in the blood that build up in uncontrolled diabetes.

Ketosis—Abnormally elevated concentration of ketones in body tissues. A complication of diabetes.

Precautions

Diabetes must be diagnosed as early as possible so that treatment can begin. If left untreated, it will result in progressive vascular disease that may damage the blood vessels, nerves, kidneys, heart, and other organs. Brain damage can occur from glucose levels below 40 mg/dL and coma from levels above 450 mg/dL. For this reason, plasma glucose levels below 40 mg/dL or above 450 mg/dL are commonly used as alert values. Point-of-care and home glucose monitors measure glucose in whole blood rather than plasma. They are accurate, for the most part, within a range of glucose concentration between 40 mg/dL and 450 mg/dL. In addition, whole blood glucose measurements are generally 10% lower than those of serum or plasma glucose.

Other endocrine disorders and a number of medications can cause both hyperglycemia and hypoglycemia. For this reason, abnormal glucose test results must be interpreted by a doctor.

Glucose is affected by heat; therefore, plasma or serum must be separated from the blood cells and refrigerated as soon as possible. **Splenectomy**, for example, can result in an increase in glycated hemoglobin, but hemolytic anemia can produce a decrease in it.

There are other factors that can also affect the OGTT, such as **exercise**, diet, anorexia, and smoking.

Drugs that decrease tolerance to glucose and affect the test include steroids, oral contraceptives, estrogens, and thiazide **diuretics**.

Description

The body uses glucose to produce most of the energy it needs to function. Glucose is absorbed from the gastrointestinal tract directly and is also derived from digestion of other dietary carbohydrates. It is also produced inside cells by the processes of glycogen breakdown (glycogenolysis) and reverse glycolysis (gluconeogenesis). Insulin is made by the pancreas and facilitates the movement of glucose from the blood and extracellular fluids into the cells. Insulin also increases the formation of glucose by cells.

Diabetes may result from a lack of insulin or a subnormal (below normal) response to insulin. There are three forms of diabetes: Type I or insulin-dependent (IDDM); type II or noninsulin dependent (NIDDM); and gestational diabetes (GDM). Type I diabetes usually occurs in childhood and is associated with low or absent blood insulin and production of ketones. It is caused by autoantibodies to the islet cells in the pancreas that produce insulin, and persons must be given insulin to control blood glucose and prevent ketosis. Type II accounts for 85% or more of persons with diabetes. It usually occurs after age 40, and is usually associated with obesity. Persons who have a deficiency of insulin may require insulin to maintain glucose, but those who have a poor response to insulin may not. Gestational diabetes is a form of glucose intolerance that first appears during pregnancy. It usually ends after delivery, but over a 10-year span approximately 30–40% of females with gestational diabetes go on to develop NIDDM.

There are a variety of ways to measure a person's blood glucose level.

Whole blood glucose tests

Whole blood glucose testing can be performed by a person at home, or by a member of the health care team outside the laboratory. The test is usually performed using a drop of whole blood obtained by finger puncture. Care must be taken to wipe away the first drop of blood because it is diluted with tissue fluid. The second drop is applied to the dry reagent test strip or device.

Fasting plasma glucose test

The fasting plasma glucose test requires an eight-hour fast. The person must have nothing to eat or drink except water. The person's blood is usually collected by a nurse or phlebotomist (person trained to draw blood) by insertion of a needle into a vein in the patient's arm. Either serum, the liquid portion of the blood after it clots, or plasma may be used. Plasma is the liquid portion of unclotted blood that is collected. The ADA recommends a normal range for fasting plasma glucose of 55–109 mg/dL. A glucose level equal to greater than 126 mg/dL is indicative of diabetes. A fasting plasma glucose level of 110–125 gm/dL is referred to as "impaired fasting glucose."

Oral glucose tolerance test (OGTT)

The OGTT is done to see how well the body handles a standard amount of glucose. There are many variations of this test. A two-hour OGTT as recommended by the ADA is described below. The person must have at least 150 grams of carbohydrate each day for at least three days before this test. The person must take nothing but water and abstain from exercise for 12 hours before the glucose is given. At 12 hours after the start of the fast, the person is given 75 grams of glucose to ingest in the form of a drink or standardized jelly beans. A health care provider draws a sample of venous blood two hours following the dose of glucose. A glucose concentration equal to or greater than 200 mg/dL is indicative of diabetes. A level below 140 mg/dL is considered normal. A level of 140–199 mg/dL is termed "impaired glucose tolerance."

Testing for gestational diabetes

The screening test for gestational diabetes is performed between 24 and 28 weeks of pregnancy. No special preparation or fasting is required. The patient is given an oral dose of 50 grams of glucose and blood is drawn one hour later. A plasma or **serum glucose level** less than 140 mg/dL is normal and requires no follow-up. If the glucose level is 140 mg/dL or higher, a three-hour OGTT is performed. The same pretest preparation is followed for the two-hour OGTT described previously, except that 100 grams of glucose are given orally. Blood is drawn at the end of the fast and at one-, two-, and three-hour intervals after the glucose is ingested. Gestational diabetes is diagnosed if two or more of the following results are obtained:

- fasting plasma glucose is greater than 105 mg/dL
- one-hour plasma glucose is greater than 190 mg/dL
- two-hour plasma glucose is greater than 165 mg/dL
- three-hour plasma glucose is greater than 145 mg/dL

Glycated hemoglobin blood glucose test (G-Hgb)

The glycated (glycosylated) **hemoglobin test** is used to diagnose diabetes and monitor the effectiveness of treatment. Glycated hemoglobin is a test that indicates how much glucose was in a person's blood during a two- to three-month window beginning about four weeks prior to sampling. The test is a measure of the time-averaged blood glucose over the 120-day lifespan of the red blood cells (RBCs). The normal range for glycated hemoglobin measured as HbA_{1c} is 3–6%. Values above 8% indicate that a hyperglycemic episode occurred sometime during the window monitored by the test (two to three months beginning four weeks prior to the time of blood collection).

The ADA recommends that glycated hemoglobin testing be performed during a person's first diabetes evaluation, again after treatment begins and glucose levels are stabilized, then repeated semiannually. If the person does not meet treatment goals, the test should be repeated quarterly.

A related blood test, fructosamine assay, measures the amount of albumin in the plasma that is bound to glucose. Albumin has a shorter halflife than RBCs, and this test reflects the time-averaged blood glucose level over a period of two to three weeks prior to sample collection.

Preparation

Blood glucose tests require either whole blood, serum, or plasma collected by vein puncture or finger puncture. No special preparation is required for a casual blood glucose test. An eight-hour fast is required for the fasting plasma or whole-blood glucose test. A 12-hour fast is required for the two-hour OGTT and three-hour OGTT tests. In addition, the person must abstain from exercise in the 12-hour fasting period. Medications known to affect carbohydrate metabolism should be discontinued three days prior to an OGTT test if possible (the doctor should provide guidance on this), and the patient must maintain a diet of at least 150 grams of carbohydrate per day for at least three days prior to the fast.

Aftercare

After the test or series of tests is completed (and with the approval of the doctor), the person should eat and drink as normal, and take any medications that were stopped for the test.

The patient may feel discomfort when blood is drawn from a vein. Pressure should be applied to the puncture site until the bleeding stops; this will help to reduce bruising. Warm packs can also be placed over the puncture site to relieve discomfort.

Risks

The patient may experience weakness, fainting, sweating, or other reactions while fasting or during the test. If any of these reactions occur, the patient should immediately inform the doctor or nurse.

Normal results

Normal values listed below are for children and adults. Results may vary slightly from one laboratory to another depending on the method of analysis used.

- fasting plasma glucose test: 55–109 mg/dL
- OGTT at two hours: less than 140 mg/dL.
- glycated hemoglobin: 3%–6%
- fructosamine: 1.6–2.7 mmol/L for adults (5% lower for children)
- gestational diabetes screening test: less than 140 mg/dL
- cerebrospinal glucose: 40–80 mg/dL
- serous fluid glucose: equal to plasma glucose
- synovial fluid glucose: within 10 mg/dL of the plasma glucose
- urine glucose (random semiquantitative): negative

For the person with diabetes, the ADA recommends an ongoing blood glucose level of less than or equal to 120 mg/dL.

The following results are suggestive of diabetes mellitus, and must be confirmed with repeat testing:

- fasting plasma glucose test: greater than or equal to 126 mg/dL
- OGTT at two hours: equal to or greater than 200 mg/dL
- casual plasma glucose test (nonfasting, with symptoms): equal to or greater than 200 mg/dL
- gestational diabetes three-hour oral glucose tolerance test: two or more of the limits following are exceeded fasting plasma glucose greater than 105 mg/dL; one-hour plasma glucose greater than 190 mg/dL; two-hour plasma glucose greater than 165 mg/dL; three-hour plasma glucose: greater than 145 mg/dL

Resources

BOOKS

Chernecky, Cynthia C., and Barbara J. Berger. *Laboratory Tests and Diagnostic Procedures,* 3rd ed. Philadelphia, PA: W. B. Saunders Company, 2001.

Henry, John B., ed. *Clinical Diagnosis and Management by Laboratory Methods,* 20th ed. Philadelphia: W. B. Saunders Company, 2001.

Kee, Joyce LeFever. *Handbook of Laboratory and Diagnostic Tests,* 4th ed. Upper Saddle River, NJ: Prentice Hall, 2001.

Wallach, Jacques. *Interpretation of Diagnostic Tests,* 7th ed. Philadelphia, PA: Lippincott Williams & Wilkens, 2000.

ORGANIZATIONS

American Diabetes Association (ADA), National Service Center. 1660 Duke St., Alexandria, VA 22314. (703) 549-1500. http://www.diabetes.org.

Centers for Disease Control and Prevention (CDC). Division of Diabetes Translation, National Center for Chronic Disease Prevention and Health Promotion. TISB Mail Stop K-13, 4770 Buford Highway NE, Atlanta, GA 30341-3724. (770) 488-5080. http://www.cdc.gov/diabetes.

National Diabetes Information Clearinghouse (NDIC). 1 Information Way, Bethesda, MD 20892-3560. (301) 907-8906. http://www.niddk.nih.gov/health/diabetes/ndic.htm.

National Institute of Diabetes and Digestive and Kidney Diseases (NIDDK). National Institutes of Health, Building 31, Room 9A04, 31 Center Drive, MSC 2560, Bethesda, MD 208792-2560. (301) 496-3583. http://www.niddk.nih.gov.

OTHER

National Institutes of Health. [cited April 4, 2003] http://www.nlm.nih.gov/medlineplus/encyclopedia.html.

Victoria E. DeMoranville
Mark A. Best

Goniotomy

Definition

A goniotomy is a surgical procedure primarily used to treat congenital glaucoma, first described in 1938. It is caused by a developmental arrest of some of the structures within the anterior (front) segment of the eye. These structures include the iris and the ciliary body, which produces the aqueous fluid needed to maintain the integrity of the eye. These structures do not develop normally in the eyes of patients with isolated congenital glaucoma. Instead, they overlap and block the trabecular meshwork, which is the primary drainage system for the aqueous fluid. As a result of this blockage, the trabecular meshwork itself becomes thicker and the drainage holes within the meshwork are narrowed. These

changes lead to an excess of fluid in the eye, which can cause pressure that can damage the internal structures of the eye and cause glaucoma.

All types of congenital glaucoma are caused by a decrease in or even a complete obstruction of the outflow of intraocular fluid. The ocular syndromes and anomalies that predispose a child to congenital glaucoma include the following: Reiger's anomaly; Peter's anomaly; Axenfeld's syndrome; and Axenfeld-Rieger's syndrome. Systemic disorders that affect the eyes in ways that may lead to glaucoma include Marfan's syndrome; rubella (German measles); and the phacomatoses, which include neurofibromatosis and Sturge-Weber syndrome. Since these disorders affect the entire body as well as the eyes, the child's pediatrician or family doctor will help to diagnose and treat these diseases.

Purpose

The purpose of a goniotomy is to clear the obstruction to aqueous outflow from the eye, which in turn lowers the intraocular pressure (IOP). Lowering the IOP helps to stabilize the enlargement of the cornea and the distension and stretching of the eye that often occur in congenital glaucoma. The size of the eye, however, will not return to normal. Most importantly, once the aqueous outflow improves, damage to the optic nerve is halted or reversed. The patient's visual acuity may improve after surgery.

Goniotomies are commonly performed to treat the following eye disorders:

- congenital glaucomas
- aniridia (Aniridia is a condition in which the patient lacks a visible iris. A goniotomy is performed as a preventive measure, as 50–75% of patients with aniridia will develop glaucoma.)
- uveitic glaucoma associated with juvenile rheumatoid arthritis
- maternal rubella syndrome
- juvenile-onset open angle glaucoma (JOAG)

Demographics

The congenital glaucomas affect one in 10,000 infants, with boys affected twice as often as girls. Both eyes are affected in 75% of patients. These glaucomas are differentiated from the secondary glaucomas caused by such medical conditions as juvenile rheumatoid arthritis (JRA), Marfan's syndrome, or diabetes; or caused by intraocular tumors, cataract surgery, or trauma. Many of the secondary glaucomas respond

KEY TERMS

Anomaly—A marked deviation from normal structure or function, particularly as the result of congenital defects.

Anterior chamber—The anterior part of the eye, bound by the cornea in front and the iris in the back, filled with aqueous fluid. The trabecular meshwork is located in a channel of the anterior chamber referred to as the angle.

Ciliary body—The structure of the eye, located behind the iris, that produces the aqueous fluid.

Congenital—Present at birth.

Cornea—The clear structure on the front of the eye that allows light to enter the eye.

Intraocular pressure (IOP)—A measurement of the degree of pressure exerted by the aqueous fluid in the eye. Elevated IOP is usually 21 mm/Hg or higher, but glaucoma can be present when the pressure is lower.

Miotics—Medications that cause the pupil of the eye to contract.

Optic nerve—A large nerve found in the posterior part of the eye, through which all the visual nerve fibers leave the eye on their way to the brain.

Schlemm's canal—A reservoir deep in the front part of the eye where the fluid drained from the trabecular meshwork collects prior to being send out to systemic or general circulation.

Trabecular meshwork—Canals of the eye through which the aqueous fluid is drained before it collects in Schlemm's canal.

better to medical treatment than to surgical treatment. Ninety-five percent of developmental or congenital glaucoma appears before age three. Another type of pediatric glaucoma is usually diagnosed between ages 10 and 35 and resembles the type of glaucoma seen in adults more closely than the congenital glaucomas, although some developmental anomalies may be present. This type of glaucoma is referred to as juvenile-onset open angle glaucoma (JOAG).

Congenital glaucoma is a polygenic disorder; that is, it involves more than one gene. Since this type of glaucoma is inherited and the genes for JOAG and congenital glaucoma have been mapped, genetic testing is available to determine whether a specific child is at risk for these disorders.

Description

Before the surgeon begins the procedure, the patient is given miotics, which are drugs that cause the pupil to contract. This partial closure improves the surgeon's view of and access to the trabecular meshwork; it also protects the lens of the eye from trauma during surgery. Other drugs are administered to lower the intraocular pressure.

Once the necessary drugs have been given and the patient is anesthetized, the surgeon uses a forceps or sutures to stabilize the eye in the correct position. The patient's head is rotated away from the surgeon so that the interior structures of the eye are more easily seen. Next, with either a knife-needle or a goniotomy knife, the surgeon punctures the cornea while looking at the interior of the eye through a microscope or a loupe. An assistant uses a syringe to introduce fluid into the eye's anterior chamber through a viscoelastic tube as the surgeon performs the goniotomy.

A gonioscopy lens is then placed on the eye. As the eye is rotated by an assistant, the surgeon sweeps the knife blade or needle through 90–120 degrees of arc in the eye, making incisions in the anterior trabecular meshwork, avoiding the posterior part of the trabecular meshwork in order to decrease the risk of damage to the iris and lens.

Once the knife and tubing are removed, saline solution is introduced through the hole to maintain the integrity of the eye and the hole is closed with sutures. The surgeon then applies **antibiotics** and **corticosteroids** to the eye to prevent infection and reduce inflammation. The head is then rotated away from the incision site so that blood cannot accumulate. The second eye may be operated on at the same time. If the procedure needs to be repeated, another area of the eye is treated.

Diagnosis/Preparation

Diagnosis

The clinical signs of congenital and infantile glaucoma may be detected within a few months after birth. They include an enlarged eye, called buphthalmos; corneal swelling; decreased vision; tearing; sensitivity to light; and blepharospasm, or uncontrolled twitching of the eyes. These signs, however, are usually absent in JOAG. As a result, glaucoma in the older child may go undetected until the child loses vision.

The examiner must take some measurements in order to confirm a diagnosis of glaucoma, including measurement of the corneal diameter and the axial length of the eye. The corneal diameter is usually less then 10 mm in an infant and only 11–12 mm in a one-year-old, but can be as large as 14 mm in a child with advanced glaucoma. The axial length is measured with an A-scan, which is a type of **ultrasound**. The doctor will also determine the intraocular pressure. An elevated intraocular pressure is not always present in congenital glaucoma; unless it is extremely high, it is only one factor in the diagnosis of glaucoma. Gonioscopy, a technique used to examine the interior structures of the eye, is performed by placing a special contact lens on the eye. This lens, used in combination with a biomicroscope, allows the surgeon to evaluate the structures of the anterior part of the eye. The condition of the optic nerve is also evaluated; photos or drawings may be taken for future comparison.

Since cooperation is difficult for infants and young children, these assessments may be done either under anesthesia or with the use of a sedative. Older children are examined in a manner similar to adults.

Preparation

Once the diagnosis of glaucoma is confirmed, goniotomy is often the first line of treatment. If goniotomy is determined to be the best procedure and there is a lot of corneal haze, the surgeon may treat the patient for several days pre-operatively with azetozolamide to lower the IOP and increase the clarity of the cornea. Or, he may elect to perform another procedure called a trabeculotomy, which is the preferred surgery if the corneal diameter is greater than 14 mm. The patient is given antibiotics for several days before surgery.

Obtaining the family's **informed consent** is another important part of preparing for a goniotomy. The surgeon tells the family that the child will need **general anesthesia**, and that several postoperative visits with anesthesia or sedation will be necessary after the goniotomy.

Aftercare

The patient will continue to be given antibiotics, corticosteroids, and miotics for one to two weeks after surgery. If the surgeon believes that the procedure was not successful, then he or she may give the patient acetazolamide by mouth in addition to these medications for up to 10 days to lower the IOP.

The patient will be anesthetized again three to six weeks after surgery for a reevaluation of the anterior chamber of the eye. This examination is repeated every three months for the first year; every six months during the second year; and once a year thereafter. Once the child is older, usually three to four years old, the physician can perform the follow-up examination in his or her office without anesthesia or sedation. Since a visual field test is difficult or impossible to do on an infant or young child, the doctor measures the cornea to assess progression of the disease. An increase in corneal diameter indicates that the glaucoma is getting worse. Visual field testing will be performed when the child is old enough to understand it. A visual field test can establish the extent of vision loss that has occurred because of glaucoma.

An important aspect of managing glaucoma patients after surgery is assessing the degree of nearsightedness and astigmatism, both of which result from the stretching of the eye caused by increased intraocular pressure. If the child needs eyeglasses, they should be given as early in life as possible to decrease the probability of amblyopia. Amblyopia is a condition in which the vision cannot be corrected completely, even with glasses, and is common for pediatric glaucoma patients. Although almost 80% of children with congenital glaucoma can have their vision corrected to 20/50 or better, patching of an eye and vision therapy is often required to achieve this level of correction.

About 10% of goniotomy patients will experience a recurrence of the glaucoma or have it develop in the unaffected eye. As a result, the patient will need periodic eye examinations for the rest of his/her life. If glaucoma does recur later in life, then either medical or surgical treatment is instituted depending on the cause.

Risks

Since goniotomy is performed under general anesthesia, there is some risk of a reaction to the anesthetic. The most common risk of general anesthesia in infants is cardiorespiratory arrest. This complication is not life-threatening, however, and occurs in fewer than 2% of goniotomies.

A hyphema (bleeding and formation of a blood clot in the anterior chamber) is the most common complication of a goniotomy. In most cases, however, the blood clots resolve within a few days.

If the cornea is not clear during surgery, the surgeon may accidentally sever the iris from the ciliary body or separate the ciliary body from the sclera of the eye. Both of these complications can lead to hypotony, a condition in which the integrity of the eye is compromised because of insufficient intraocular fluid.

Other complications of goniotomy are cataract formation; inflammation in the anterior chamber; scarring of the cornea; subluxation or dislocation of the lens; and retinal detachment. The risk of damage to the lens is greater when the patient is aniridic.

The intraocular pressure may increase in spite of, or due to complications of the procedure, and the goniotomy may have to be repeated. If the goniotomy is not successful after two or three attempts, the surgeon will perform a trabeculotomy.

Normal results

Goniotomy is considered to be successful when the measured IOP is below 21 mm/Hg, or below 16 mm/Hg if the patient is under anesthesia; when there is no increase in corneal diameter; and when damage to the optic nerve is stabilized or even reversed. Goniotomy is successful in about 94% of patients with primary congenital glaucoma in decreasing IOP, corneal haze, and corneal diameter. Tearing, sensitivity to light, and blepharospasm all decrease over time.

If a goniotomy is successful it will be apparent within three to six weeks. A repeat goniotomy is required for 50% of patients. Goniotomy is most successful when the child is between one month and three years of age; it is successful only a quarter of the time in patients younger than one month. It is also more successful when the corneal diameter is less than 14 mm and when the IOP is not extremely high. Even if the IOP has been lowered, anti-glaucoma medication or drops may still be needed after the goniotomy.

When a goniotomy is performed on patients with uveitic glaucoma, the success rate is 75–83%, although most of these patients need ongoing medication for glaucoma, and 30% require a repeat procedure.

Morbidity and mortality rates

Fifteen years after a goniotomy, one in seven patients will have such serious complications as corneal decompensation or detachment of the retina. Vision loss occurs in 50% of children with congenital glaucoma in spite of surgical and medical intervention. This is particularly true of infants diagnosed with glaucoma before two months of age. About 50% of children who undergo goniotomy require a repeat procedure. Complications are more common for patients treated as young infants and as older children.

Alternatives

Congenital glaucoma does not respond well to medical treatment, so the first line of treatment is usually surgical. Medical therapy is often initiated as adjunct therapy after surgery.

One alternative to goniotomy is trabeculotomy. Goniotomy has been the preferred procedure for treatment of congenital glaucoma, but trabeculotomy has been favored in recent years because of the surgeon's

WHO PERFORMS THE PROCEDURE AND WHERE IS IT PERFORMED?

A goniotomy is performed in a hospital by an ophthalmologist, or eye specialist, while the patient is under general anesthesia. Preoperative and postoperative evaluations are also done in a hospital setting if anesthesia is required. These evaluations can be done for older children in an office setting. An ophthalmologist qualified to perform a goniotomy has usually had advanced fellowship training in glaucoma surgery after completing a three-year residency in ophthalmology.

difficulty in seeing the structures in the eye when the cornea is hazy. A clear view of the cornea is required for goniotomy. In a trabeculotomy, the surgeon inserts a probe into the eye, passes it through Schlemm's canal, and rotates it inside the anterior chamber in order to tear a hole in the trabecular meshwork. This maneuver creates an alternative passageway for the aqueous fluid to leave the anterior chamber of the eye. In some cases the surgeon will perform a **trabeculectomy**, a procedure in which part of the trabecular meshwork is removed by cutting, at the same time as the trabeculotomy.

Another alternative procedure involves placement of a filtering shunt to direct the intraocular fluid out of the eye. A shunt is often placed if Schlemm's canal cannot easily be located, as in the case with infants. The safety profile for trabeculotomy and filtering surgery are comparable to goniotomy, but there is a higher rate of long-term success with goniotomies and trabeculotomies.

A newer variation of surgical goniotomy is laser goniotomy, in which the surgeon uses a Yag:Nd laser to cut into the trabecular meshwork. Laser goniotomies appear to be less effective than surgical goniotomies, but if a patient responds well to a laser procedure, then surgical goniotomy may be considered.

Other alternative treatments for pediatric glaucoma are the cyclodestructive techniques, which include cyclophotocoagulation, and the more commonly performed **cyclocryotherapy**. These procedures involve destruction of the ciliary body by using either freezing temperatures or lasers. These procedures have lower success rates and a higher risk of complications; they are usually performed as a last resort when other techniques have failed.

QUESTIONS TO ASK THE DOCTOR

- How many goniotomies have you performed?
- Have you had advanced training in glaucoma surgery?
- What are the chances that the procedure will need to be repeated?
- Is a goniotomy the best surgical procedure for my child?

Resources

BOOKS

Albert, Daniel M., MD, MS, et al. *Principles and Practice of Ophthalmology*, 2nd ed. Philadelphia, PA, W.B. Saunders Company, 2000.

Azuara-Blanco, Augusto, MD, PhD, et al. *Handbook of Glaucoma*. London, UK: Martin Dunitz Ltd., 2002.

Charlton, Judie F., MD, and George W. Weinstein, MD. *Ophthalmic Surgery Complications: Prevention and Management*. Philadelphia, PA: J. B. Lippincott Company, 1995.

Epstein, David L., MD, et al. *Chandler and Grant's Glaucoma*, 4th ed. Baltimore, MD: Williams and Wilkins, 1997

Kanski, Jack, MD, MS, FRCS, FRCOphthal, et al. *Glaucoma: A Colour Manual of Diagnosis and Treatment*, 2nd ed. Oxford, UK: Butterworth Heinemann, 1996.

Krupin, Theodore, MD, and Allan E. Kolker, MD. *Atlas of Complications in Ophthalmic Surgery*. London, UK: Wolfe, 1993.

Ritch, Robert, MD, et al. *The Glaucomas*. St. Louis, MO: Mosby, 1996.

Shields, M. Bruce, MD. *Textbook of Glaucoma*. Baltimore, MD: Williams and Wilkins, 1998.

Weinreb, Robert, et al. *Glaucoma in the 21st Century*. London, UK: Mosby International, 2000.

PERIODICALS

Bayraktar, Sukru, MD, and Taylan Koseoglu, MD. "Endoscopic Goniotomy with Anterior Chamber Maintainer: Surgical Technique and One-Year Results." *Ophthalmic Surgery and Lasers* 32 (November-December 2001): 496-502.

Beck, Allen D. "Diagnosis and Management of Pediatric Glaucoma." *Ophthalmology Clinics of North America* 32 (September 2001): 501-512.

Freedman, Sharon F., MD, et al. "Goniotomy for Glaucoma Secondary to Chronic Childhood Uveitis." *American Journal of Ophthalmology* 133 (May 2002): 617-621.

Kiefer, Gesine, et al. "Correlation of Postoperative Axial Length Growth and Intraocular Pressure in Congenital Glaucoma— A Retrospective Study in Trabeculotomy and Goniotomy." *Graefe's Archive for Clinical and Experimental Ophthalmology* 239 (December 2001): 893-899.

ORGANIZATIONS

American Academy of Ophthalmology. P.O. Box 7424, San Francisco, CA 94120-7424. (415) 561-8500. www.aao.org.

Canadian Ophthalmological Society (COS). 610-1525 Carling Avenue, Ottawa ON K1Z 8R9. www.eyesite.ca.

National Eye Institute. 2020 Vision Place, Bethesda, MD 20892-3655. (301) 496-5248. www.nei.nih.gov.

OTHER

Nova Southeastern University. *Congenital and Developmental Glaucoma*. www.nova.edu/~jsowka/congenglauc.html.

Martha Reilly, OD

Grafts and grafting *see* **Bone grafting; Coronary artery bypass graft surgery; Skin grafting**

Gum disease surgery *see* **Gingivectomy**

Gynecologic sonogram *see* **Pelvic ultrasound**

Gynecologic surgery *see* **Obstetric and gynecologic surgery**

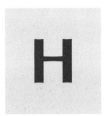

H2 reception blockers *see* **Gastric acid inhibitors**

Hair transplantation

Definition

Hair transplantation is a surgical procedure used to treat baldness or hair loss (alopecia). Typically, tiny patches of scalp are removed from the back and sides of the head and implanted in the bald spots in the front and top of the head.

Purpose

Hair transplantation is a cosmetic procedure performed on men and occasionally on women who have significant hair loss, thinning hair, or bald spots where hair no longer grows. In men, hair loss and baldness are most commonly due to genetic factors and age. Male pattern baldness, in which the hairline gradually recedes to expose more and more of the forehead, is the most common form. Men may also experience a gradual thinning of hair at the crown, or very top of the skull. For women, hair loss is more commonly due to hormonal changes and is more likely to be a thinning of hair from the entire head. Transplants can also be performed

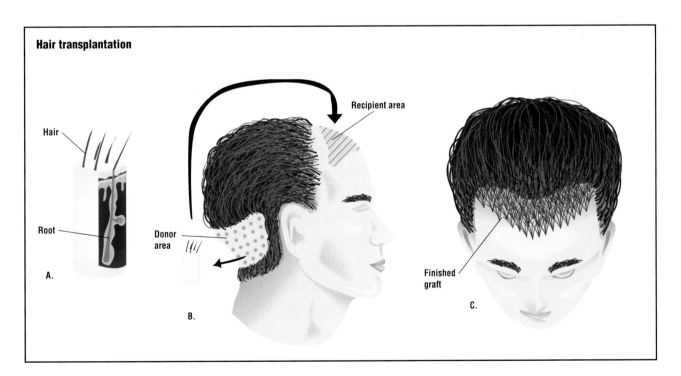

Hair transplantation

A. Hair / Root

B. Donor area / Recipient area

C. Finished graft

In a hair transplant, plugs of hair and supporting tissues are removed from a donor area at the back of the head (A and B). Pieces of skin are removed at the front of the head, and grafts are placed (C). *(Illustration by GGS Information Services. Cengage Learning, Gale.)*

KEY TERMS

Alopecia—Hair loss or baldness.

Hair follicle—A tube-like indentation in the skin from which a single hair grows.

Minigraft or micrograft—Transplantation of a small number of hair follicles, as few as one to three hairs, into a transplant site.

Transplantation—Surgically cutting out hair follicles and replanting them in a different spot on the head.

to replace hair lost due to burns, injury, or diseases of the scalp.

Demographics

An estimated 50,000 men receive hair transplants each year.

Description

Hair transplantation surgery is performed by a physician with specialty training in **plastic surgery** or, less commonly, dermatology. Each surgery lasts two to three hours during which approximately 250 grafts will be transplanted. A moderately balding man may require up to 1,000 grafts to get good coverage of a bald area; consequently, a series of surgeries scheduled three to four months apart is usually required. Individuals may be completely awake during the procedure with just a local anesthetic drug applied to numb the areas of the scalp. Some persons may be given a drug to help them relax or may be given an anesthetic drug that puts them to sleep.

The most common transplant procedure uses a thin strip of hair and scalp from the back of the head. This strip is cut into smaller clumps of five or six hairs. Tiny slits are made in the balding area of the scalp, and a clump is implanted into each slit. The doctor performing the surgery will attempt to recreate a natural-looking hairline along the forehead. Minigrafts, micrografts, or implants of single hair follicles can be used to fill in between larger implant sites and can provide a more natural-looking hairline. The implants will also be arranged so that thick and thin hairs are interspersed and the hair will grow in the same direction.

Another type of hair replacement surgery is called scalp reduction. This involves removing some of the skin from the hairless area and "stretching" some of the nearby hair-covered scalp over the cut-away area.

Health insurance will not pay for hair transplants that are performed for cosmetic reasons. Insurance plans may pay for hair replacement surgery to correct hair loss due to accidents, burns, or disease.

It is important to be realistic about what the final result of a hair transplant will look like. This procedure does not create new hair. Rather, it simply redistributes the hair that an individual still has. Chest hair has been experimentally transplanted onto the scalp. As of 2003, this procedure has not been widely used.

Diagnosis/Preparation

Although hair transplantation is a fairly simple procedure, some risks are associated with any surgery. It is important to inform the physician about any medications being used and about previous allergic reactions to drugs or anesthetic agents. People with blood-clotting disorders also need to inform their physician before the procedure is performed.

It is important to find a respected, well-established, experienced surgeon and discuss the expected results prior to the surgery. The candidate may need blood tests to check for bleeding or clotting problems and is usually asked not to take **aspirin** products before the surgery. The type of anesthesia used will depend on how extensive the surgery will be and the setting in which it will be performed. The candidate may be awake during the procedure, but is usually given medication to cause relaxation. A local anesthetic drug that numbs the area will be applied or injected into the skin at the surgery sites.

Aftercare

The areas involved in transplantation may need to be bandaged overnight. People can return to normal activities within a day. Strenuous activities should be avoided in the first few days after the surgery. On rare occasions, the implants can be ejected from the scalp during vigorous **exercise**. There may be some swelling, bruising, headache, and discomfort around the graft areas and around the eyes. These symptoms can usually be controlled with a mild pain reliever such as aspirin. Scabs may form at the graft sites and should not be scraped off. There may be some numbness at the sites, but it will diminish within two to three months.

Risks

Although there are rare cases of infection or scarring, the major risk is that the grafted area might not look the way the patient expects it to look.

WHO PERFORMS THE PROCEDURE AND WHERE IS IT PERFORMED?

Hair transplantation is performed by a physician with specialty training in plastic and cosmetic surgery or dermatology. It may be performed in a professional office, outpatient, or hospital setting.

Normal results

The transplanted hair will fall out within a few weeks; however, new hair will start to grow in the graft sites within about three months. A normal rate of hair growth is about 0.25–0.5 in (6–13 mm) per month.

Morbidity and mortality rates

Major complications as a result of hair transplantation are extremely rare. Occasionally, a person may have problems with delayed healing, infection, scarring, or rejection of the graft, but these are uncommon.

Alternatives

There are several alternatives to hair transplantation. The two most common include use of a lotion that contains a drug preparation, or the use of a wig.

As of 2003, only lotions containing minoxidil or finasteride actually grow any new hair. This does not occur for all users. The new hair minoxidil grows is usually only a light fuzz on the crown of the head. When minoxidil treatment is discontinued, the fuzz disappears, in addition to any hairs that were supposed to die during treatment. In some cases, finasteride does grow thick, strong, long-growing hair on the crown.

Wigs and hairpieces have been used for centuries. They are available in a wide price range, the more expensive ones providing a more realistic appearance than less expensive models.

Resources

BOOKS

Buchwach, K. A., and R. J. Konior. *Contemporary Hair Transplant Surgery*. New York: Thieme, 1997.

Harris, James, and Emanuel Marritt. *The Hair Replacement Revolution: A Consumer's Guide to Effective Hair Replacement Techniques*. Garden City Park, NY: Square One Publishers, 2003.

Man, Daniel, and L. C. Faye. *The New Art of Man: Faces of Plastic Surgery*, 3rd ed. New York: BeautyArt Press, 2003.

QUESTIONS TO ASK THE DOCTOR

Candidates for hair transplantation surgery should ask the following questions:

- What will be the resulting appearance?
- Is the doctor board certified in plastic and reconstructive surgery or dermatology?
- How many hair transplantation procedures has the doctor performed?
- What is the doctor's complication rate?

Papel, I. D., et al. *Facial Plastic and Reconstructive Surgery*, 2nd ed. New York: Thieme Medical Publishers, 2002.

PERIODICALS

Bernstein, R. M., W. R. Rassman, N. Rashid, and R. C. Shiell. "The Art of Repair in Surgical Hair Restoration—Part I: Basic Repair Strategies." *Dermatologic Surgery* 28, no. 9 (2002): 783–794.

Bernstein, R. M., W. R. Rassman, N. Rashid, and R. C. Shiell. "The Art of Repair in Surgical Hair Restoration—Part II: The Tactics of Repair." *Dermatologic Surgery* 28, no. 10 (2002): 873–893.

Epstein, J. S. "Hair Transplantation in Women: Treating Female Pattern Baldness and Repairing Distortion and Scarring from Prior Cosmetic Surgery." *Archives of Facial Plastic Surgery* 5, no. 1 (2003): 121–126.

Epstein, J. S. "Hair Transplantation for Men with Advanced Degrees of Hair Loss." *Plastic and Reconstructive Surgery* 111, no. 1 (2003): 414–421.

Swinehart, J. M. "Local Anesthesia in Hair Transplant Surgery." *Dermatologic Surgery* 28, no. 12 (2002): 1189–1190.

OTHER

"How Hair Replacement Works." How Stuff Works. http://people.howstuffworks.com/hair-replacement6.htm (April 13, 2008).

"Locate a Hair Loss Doctor in Your State with DocShop." DocShop.com http://www.docshop.com/hair_loss_specialists/states.html (April 13, 2008).

"UW Dermatologic Surgery: Hair Transplantation." University of Washington School of Medicine, Division of Dermatology. May 1, 2006. http://faculty.washington.edu/danberg/bergweb/page3.htm (April 13, 2008).

ORGANIZATIONS

American Academy of Cosmetic Surgery, 737 North Michigan Avenue, Suite 820, Chicago, IL, 60611-5405, (312) 981-6760, http://www.cosmeticsurgery.org.

American Academy of Dermatology, P.O. Box 4014, Schaumburg, IL, 60618-4014, (847) 330-0230, (866) 503-7546, (847) 240-1859, MRC@aad.org, http://www.aad.org/.

American Academy of Facial Plastic and Reconstructive Surgery, 310 S. Henry Street, Alexandria, VA, 22314, (703) 229-9291, http://www.aafprs.org/.

American Board of Plastic Surgery, Seven Penn Center, Suite 4001635 Market Street, Philadelphia, PA, 19103-2204, (215) 587-9322, http://www.abplsurg.org/.

American College of Surgeons, 633 North Saint Claire Street, Chicago, IL, 60611, (312) 202-5000, http://www.facs.org/.

American Society for Aesthetic Plastic Surgery, 11081 Winners Circle, Los Alamitos, CA, 90720, (888) 272-7711, http://www.surgery.org/.

American Society for Dermatologic Surgery, 5550 Meadowbrook Drive, Suite 120, Rolling Meadows, IL, 60008, (847) 956-0900, http://www.asds.net.

American Society of Plastic Surgeons, 444 E. Algonquin Road, Arlington Heights, IL, 60005, (847) 228-9900, http://www.plasticsurgery.org.

L. Fleming Fallon, Jr., M.D., Dr.P.H.
Laura Jean Cataldo, R.N., Ed.D.

Hammer, claw, and mallet toe surgery

Definition

Hammer, claw, and mallet toe surgery refers to a series of surgical procedures performed to correct deformed toes.

Purpose

There are three main forms of toe abnormalities in the human foot: hammer toes, claw toes, and mallet toes. A hammer toe, also called contracted toe, bone spur, rotated toe, or deformed toe, is a toe curled as the result of a bend in the middle joint. It may be either flexible or rigid, and may affect any of the four smaller toes. The joints in the toe buckle due to tightening of the ligaments and tendons, which points the toe upward at an angle. The patient's shoes then put pressure on the prominent portion of the toe, leading to inflammation, bursitis, corns, and calluses. Mallet toes and claw toes are similar to hammer toes, except that different joints on the toe are affected. The joint at the end of the toe buckles in a mallet toe, while a claw toe involves abnormal positions of all three joints in the toe.

Toe deformities are caused by a variety of factors:

- Genetic. All three toe deformities may be hereditary.
- Poorly fitted shoes. Claw toes are usually the result of wearing shoes that are too short. Many people have second toes that are longer than their big toes; if they wear shoes sized to fit the big toe, the second toe has to bend to fit into the shoe. High-heeled shoes with pointed toes are also a major cause of claw toes.
- Bunions. A bunion is an abnormal prominence of the first joint of the big toe that pushes the toe sideways toward the smaller toes. Hammer toes often develop together with bunion deformities, and they are often treated together.
- Flat feet. This condition is due to poor biomechanics of the foot and may lead to hammer toes.
- Highly arched feet.
- Rheumatoid arthritis.
- Tendon imbalance. When the foot cannot function normally, the tendons may stretch or tighten to compensate and lead to toe deformities.
- Traumatic injuries of the toes.

When the toe deformity is painful or permanent, surgical repair is performed to relieve pain, correct the problem, and provide a stable, functional toe.

Demographics

As of 2002, the incidence of claw and hammer toe deformities ranges from 2–20% of the population in the United States, with the frequency gradually increasing in the older age groups. Claw and hammer toes are most often seen in patients in the seventh and eighth decades of life. Women are affected four to five times more often than men. Little is known about the incidence of these deformities among people who usually wear sandals or go barefoot.

Description

Some of the most common surgical procedures used to repair hammer, claw, and mallet toes include:

- Tenoplasty and capsulotomy. These procedures release or lengthen tightened tendons and ligaments that have caused the toe joints to contract. In some patients with flexible hammer toes, the toe straightens out after these soft tissue structures are lengthened or relaxed.
- Tendon transfer. This procedure is used to correct a flexible hammer toe deformity. It involves the repositioning of a tendon to straighten the toe.
- Bone arthroplasty. In this procedure, the surgeon removes some bone and cartilage to correct the toe deformity. A small segment of bone is removed at the joint to eliminate pressure on the toe, relieve pain, and straighten the toe. The tendons and ligaments surrounding the joint may also be reconstructed.

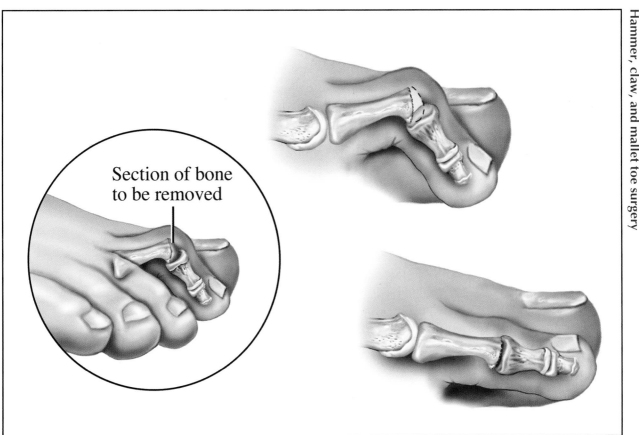

Surgical repair of hammertoe. *(Nucleus Medical Art, Inc/Phototake. Reproduced by permission.)*

- Derotation arthroplasty. In this technique, the surgeon removes a small wedge of skin and realigns the deformed toe. The surgeon may also remove a small section of bone, and repair tendons and ligaments if necessary.
- Implant arthroplasty. In this procedure, the surgeon inserts a silicone rubber or metal implant specially designed for the toe to replace the gliding surfaces of the joint and act as a joint spacer.

Diagnosis/Preparation

Patients usually consult a doctor about toe deformities because of pain or discomfort in the foot when walking or running. The physician takes several factors into consideration when examining a patient who may require surgery to correct a toe deformity. Some surgical procedures require only small amounts of cutting or tissue removal while others require extensive dissection. The blood supply in the affected toe is an important factor in planning surgery. It determines not only whether the toe will heal fully but also whether the surgeon can perform more than one procedure on the toe. In addition to a visual examination of the patient's

foot, the doctor will ask the patient to walk back and forth in the office or hallway in order to evaluate the patient's gait (habitual pattern of walking). This part of the office examination allows the doctor to identify static or dynamic forces that may be causing the toe deformity. Imaging tests are also performed, usually x-ray studies.

If the doctor considers it necessary to rule out systemic disorders, he or she may order the following laboratory tests: a fasting glucose test to evaluate or rule out diabetes, and a **sedimentation rate** test to evaluate the possibility of an underlying infection in the foot.

Before surgery, the patient receives an appropriate local anesthetic, and the foot is cleansed and draped.

Aftercare

The patient can expect moderate swelling, stiffness and limited mobility in the operated foot following toe surgery, sometimes for as long as eight to 12 weeks. Patients are advised to keep the operated foot elevated above heart level and apply ice packs to

KEY TERMS

Arthroplasty—The surgical repair of a joint.

Bunion—A swelling or deformity of the big toe, characterized by the formation of a bursa and a sideways displacement of the toe.

Bursa (plural, bursae)—A pouch lined with joint tissue that contains a small quantity of synovial fluid. Bursae are located between tendons and bone, or between bones and muscle tissue.

Bursitis—Inflammation of a bursa.

Callus—A localized thickening of the outer layer of skin cells, caused by friction or pressure from shoes or other articles of clothing.

Corn—A horny thickening of the skin on a toe, caused by friction and pressure from poorly fitted shoes or stockings.

Gait—A person's habitual manner or style of walking.

Orthopedics—The branch of medicine that deals with bones and joints.

Orthotics—Shoe inserts that are intended to correct an abnormal or irregular gait or walking pattern. They are sometimes prescribed to relieve gait-related foot pain.

Podiatrist—A physician who specializes in the care and treatment of the foot.

reduce swelling during the first few days after surgery. Many patients are able to walk immediately after the operation, although the podiatric surgeon may restrict any such activity for at least 24 hours. Crutches or walkers are not usually needed. There is no cast on the foot, but only a soft gauze dressing. Wearing a splint for the first two to four weeks after surgery is usually recommended. Special surgical shoes are also available to protect the foot and help to redistribute the patient's body weight. If the surgeon has used sutures, they must be kept dry until they are removed, usually seven to 10 days after the operation.

The patient's physician may also suggest exercises to be done at home or at work to strengthen the toe muscles. These exercises may include picking up marbles with the toes and stretching the toe muscles.

Risks

Risks associated with hammer, claw, and mallet toe surgery include:

- swelling of the toes for one to six months following surgery;
- recurrence of the deformity;
- infection;
- persistent pain and discomfort; and
- nerve injury.

Normal results

All corrective toe procedures usually have good outcomes in relieving pain and improving toe mobility. They restore appropriate toe length and anatomy while realigning and stabilizing the joints in the foot.

Morbidity and mortality rates

There are no reported cases of **death** following corrective surgery on the toes.

Alternatives

Conservative treatments may be tried by patients with minor discomfort or less serious toe deformities. These treatments include:

- trimming or wearing protective padding on corns and calluses;
- wearing supportive custom-made plastic or leather shoe inserts (orthotics) to help relieve pressure on toe deformities. Orthotics allow the toes and major joints of the foot to function more efficiently;
- using splints or small straps to realign the affected toe;
- wearing shoes with a wider toe box; and
- injecting anti-inflammatory medications to relieve pain and inflammation.

Resources

BOOKS

Adelaar, R. S., ed. *Disorders of the Great Toe*. Rosemont, IL: American Academy of Orthopaedic Surgeons, 1997.

Dutton, Mark. *Orthopaedic Examination, Evaluation, and Intervention*. New York: McGraw-Hill, 2004.

Holmes, G. B. *Surgical Approaches to the Foot and Ankle*. New York: McGraw-Hill, 1994.

Marcinko, D. E. *Medical and Surgical Therapeutics of Foot and Ankle*. Baltimore: Williams & Wilkins, 1992.

Skinner, Harry.*Current Diagnosis & Treatment in Orthopedics*. New York: McGraw-Hill, 2006.

PERIODICALS

American College of Foot and Ankle Surgeons. "Hammer Toe Syndrome." *Journal of Foot and Ankle Surgery* 38 (March–April 1999): 166–178.

Coughlin, M. J., J. Dorris, and E. Polk. "Operative Repair of the Fixed Hammertoe Deformity." *Foot & Ankle International* 21 (February 2000): 94–104.

Harmonson, J. K., and L. B. Harkless. "Operative Procedures for the Correction of Hammertoe, Claw Toe, and Mallet Toe: A Literature Review." *Clinical Podiatric Medical Surgery* 13 (April 1996): 211–220.

Hennessy, M. S., and T. S. Saxby. "Traumatic Mallet Toe of the Hallux: A Case Report." *Foot & Ankle International* 22 (December 2001): 977–978.

"What is a Hammer Toe, and What Causes It?" *Mayo Clinic Health Letter* 20, no. 7 (July 2002): 8.

Miller, S. J. "Hammer Toe Correction by Arthrodesis of the Proximal Interphalangeal Joint Using a Cortical Bone Allograft Pin." *Journal of the American Podiatric Medical Association* 92 (November–December 2002): 563–569.

OTHER

"Hammertoe and Mallet Toe." Ohio Health Online. August 21, 2006. http://www.birthofamom.com/bodymayo.cfm?id = 6&action = detail&ref = 1284 (April 14, 2008).

"Hammertoe Deformity." Foot Pain and Podiatry Online. 1999. http://www.footpain.org/Hammertoes.html (April 14, 2008).

ORGANIZATIONS

American Academy of Orthopaedic Surgeons, 6300 N. River Road, Rosemont, IL, 60018-4262, (847) 823-7186, (800) 346-AAOS, (847) 823-8125, http://www.aaos.org.

American College of Foot and Ankle Surgeons, 8725 West Higgins Road, Suite 555, Chicago, IL, 60631-2724, (773) 693-9300, (800) 421-2237, (773) 693-9304, info@acfas.org, http://www.acfas.org.

American Podiatric Medical Association, 9312 Old Georgetown Road, Bethesda, MD, 20814, (301) 581-9200, http://www.apma.org.

Monique Laberge, Ph.D.
Laura Jean Cataldo, R.N., Ed.D.

Hand surgery

Definition

Hand surgery refers to procedures performed to treat traumatic injuries or loss of function resulting from such diseases as advanced arthritis of the hand.

Purpose

The purpose of hand surgery is the treatment of a broad range of problems that affect the hand, whether they result from cuts, burns, crushing injuries, or disease processes. Hand surgery includes procedures that treat traumatic injuries of the hands, including closed-fist injuries; congenital deformities; repetitive stress injuries; deformities caused by arthritis and similar disorders affecting the joints; nail problems; and **tendon repair**.

The central priority of the hand surgeon is adequate reconstruction of the skin, bone, nerve, tendon, and joint(s) in the hand. Proper repair of any cuts, tears, or burns in the skin will help to ensure a wound free of infection and will provide cover for the anatomical structures beneath the skin. Early repair and grafting is an essential component of hand surgery. Nerve repair is important because a delay in reconnecting the nerve fibers may affect the recovery of sensation in the hand. Restoration of sensation in the hand is necessary if the patient is to recover a reasonable level of functionality. Next, the bones in the hand must be stabilized in a fixed position before the surgeon can repair joints or tendons. Joint mobility may be restored by specific tendon repairs or grafts. In some cases, the patient's hand may require several operations over a period of time to complete the repair.

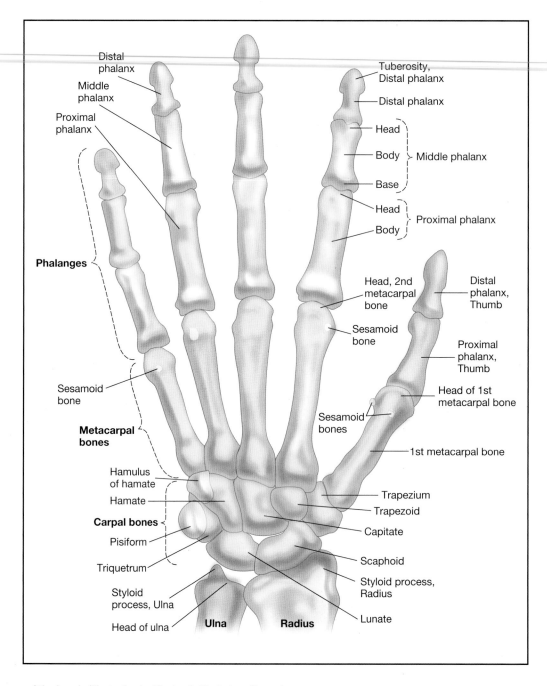

The bones of the hand. *(Illustration by Electronic Illustrators Group.)*

Demographics

The demographics of hand injuries and disorders depend on the specific injury or disorder in question. Repetitive stress injuries (RSIs) of the hands are often related to occupation; for example, nurse anesthetists, dental hygienists, keyboard instrumentalists, word processors, violinists, and some assembly-line workers are at relatively high risk of developing carpal tunnel syndrome or tendinitis of the fingers related to their work. Nearly 17% of all disabling work injuries in the United States involve the fingers, most often when the finger strikes or is jammed against a hard surface. Over 25% of athletic injuries involve the hand or wrist.

In terms of age groups, children under the age of six are the most likely to be affected by crushing or burning injuries of the hand. Closed-fist injuries, which frequently involve infection of the hand resulting from a human bite, are almost entirely found in

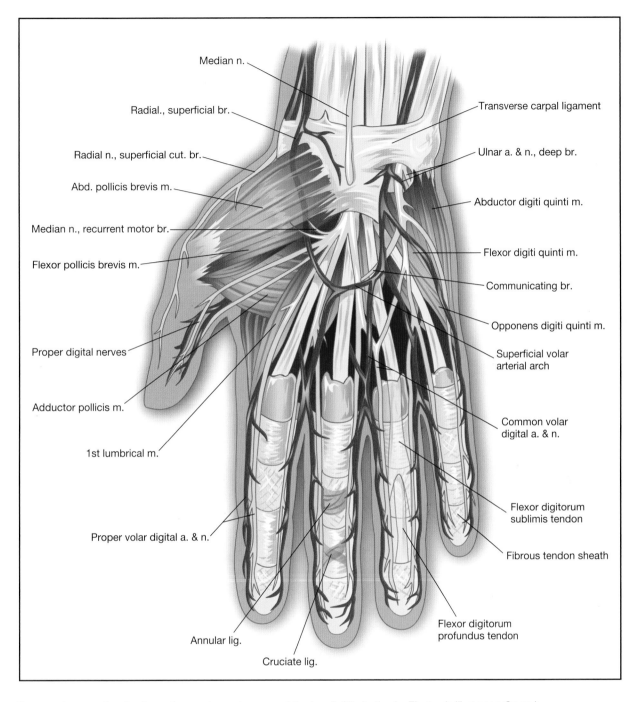

Median n.

Radial., superficial br.

Radial n., superficial cut. br.

Abd. pollicis brevis m.

Median n., recurrent motor br.

Flexor pollicis brevis m.

Proper digital nerves

Adductor pollicis m.

1st lumbrical m.

Proper volar digital a. & n.

Annular lig.

Cruciate lig.

Transverse carpal ligament

Ulnar a. & n., deep br.

Abductor digiti quinti m.

Flexor digiti quinti m.

Communicating br.

Opponens digiti quinti m.

Superficial volar arterial arch

Common volar digital a. & n.

Flexor digitorum sublimis tendon

Fibrous tendon sheath

Flexor digitorum profundus tendon

Some major muscles, tendons, ligaments, and nerves of the hand. *(Illustration by Electronic Illustrators Group.)*

males between the ages of 15 and 35. Pain or loss of function in the hands resulting from osteoarthritis, however, is found most often in middle-aged or older adults, and affects women as often as men.

Some specific categories of conditions that may require hand surgery include:

- Congenital malformations. The most common congenital hand deformity is syndactyly, in which two or

more fingers are fused together or joined by webbing; and polydactyly, in which the person is born with an extra finger, often a duplication of the thumb.

- Infections. Hand surgeons treat many different types of infections, including paronychia, an infection resulting from a penetrating injury to the nail; felon, an inflammation of the deeper tissue under the fingertip resulting in an abscess; suppurative tenosynovitis,

KEY TERMS

Congenital—Present at birth.

Felon—A very painful abscess on the lower surface of the fingertip, resulting from infection in the closed space surrounding the bone in the fingertip. It is also known as whitlow.

Hemostat—A small surgical clamp used to hold a blood vessel closed.

Lipoma—A type of benign tumor that develops within adipose or fatty tissue.

Loupe—A convex lens used to magnify small objects at very close range. It may be held on the hand, mounted on eyeglasses, or attached to a headband.

Paresthesia—An abnormal touch sensation, such as a prickling or burning feeling, often in the absence of an external cause.

Paronychia—Inflammation of the folds of tissue surrounding the nail.

Polydactyly—A developmental abnormality characterized by an extra digit on the hand or foot.

Skin flap—A piece of skin with underlying tissue that is used in grafting to cover a defect and that receives its blood supply from a source other than the tissue on which it is laid.

Syndactyly—A developmental abnormality in which two or more fingers or toes are joined by webbing between the digits.

an infection of the flexor tendon sheath of the fingers or thumb; and deeper infections that often result from human or animal bites.

- Tumors. The most common tumor of the hand is the ganglion cyst, which is a mass of tissue fluid arising from a joint or tendon space. Giant cell tumors are the second most common hand tumor. These tumors usually arise from joints or tendon sheaths and are yellow-brown in color. The third type of hand tumor is a lipoma, which is a benign tumor that occurs in fatty tissue.

- Nerve compression syndromes. These syndromes occur when a peripheral nerve is compressed, usually because of an anatomic or developmental problem, infection or trauma. For example, carpal tunnel syndrome develops when a large nerve in the arm called the median nerve is subjected to pressure building up inside the carpal tunnel, which is a passageway through the wrist. This pressure on the nerve may result from injury, overuse of the hand and wrist,

fluid retention during pregnancy, or rheumatoid arthritis. The patient may experience tingling or aching sensations, numbness, and a loss of function in the hand. The ulnar nerve is another large nerve in the arm that runs along the little finger. Compression of the ulnar nerve at the elbow can cause symptoms that typically include aching pain, numbness, and paresthesias.

- Amputation. Some traumatic injuries result in the loss of a finger or the entire hand, requiring reattachment or replantation. Crushing injuries of the hand have the lowest chance of a successful outcome. Children and young adults have the best chances for recovery following surgery to repair an accidental amputation.

- Fractures and dislocations. Distal phalangeal fractures (breaking the bone of a finger above the first joint towards the tip of the finger) are the most commonly encountered fractures of the hand. They often occur while playing sports.

- Fingertip injury. Fingertip injuries are extremely dangerous since they comprise the most common hand injuries and can lead to significant disability. Fingertip injuries can cause damage to the tendons, nerves, or veins in the hands.

Description

There are a number of different procedures that may be involved in hand surgery, with a few general principles that are applicable to all cases: operative planning; preparing and draping the patient; hair removal; tourniquet usage; the use of special **surgical instruments**; magnification (special visualization attachments); and **postoperative care**. The operative preplanning stage is vitally important since it allows for the best operative technique. The hand to be operated on is shaved and washed with an antiseptic for five minutes. A tourniquet will be placed on the patient's arm to minimize blood loss; special inflation cuffs are available for this purpose.

The four basic instruments used in hand surgery include a knife, small forceps, dissecting scissors, and mosquito hemostats. A standard drill with small steel points is used to drill holes in bone during reconstructive bone surgery. Additionally, visualization of small anatomical structures is essential during hand surgery. Frequently, the hand surgeon may use wire loupes (a special instrument held in place on top of the surgeon's head) or a double-headed binocular microscope in order to see the tendons, blood vessels, muscles, and other structures in the hand.

In most cases, the anesthesiologist will administer a regional nerve block to keep the patient comfortable during the procedure. The patient is usually positioned lying on the back with the affected arm extended on a hand platform. If the surgeon is performing a bone reconstruction, he or she may require such special instruments as a drill, metal plates and/or screws, and steel wires (K-wires). Arteries and veins should be reconnected without tension. If this cannot be done, the hand surgeon must take out a piece of vein from another place in the patient's body and use it to reconstruct the vein in the hand. This process is called a venous graft. Nerves damaged as a result of traumatic finger injuries can usually be reconnected without tension, since bone reconstruction prior to nerve surgery shortens the length of the bones in the hand. The surgeon may also perform skin grafts or skin flaps. After all the bones, nerves, and blood vessels have been repaired or reconstructed, the surgeon closes the wound and covers it with a dressing.

Diagnosis/Preparation

With the exception of emergencies requiring immediate treatment, the diagnosis of hand injuries and disorders begins with a detailed history and **physical examination** of the patient's hand. During the physical examination, the doctor evaluates the range of motion (ROM) in the patient's wrist and fingers. Swollen or tender areas can be felt (palpated) by the clinician. The doctor can assess sensation in the hand by very light pinpricks with a fine sterile needle. In cases of trauma to the hand, the doctor will inspect the hand for bite marks, burns, foreign objects that may be embedded, or damage to deeper anatomical structures within the hand. The tendons will be evaluated for evidence of tearing or cutting. Broken bones or joint injuries will be tender to the touch and are easily visible on x-ray imaging.

The doctor may order special tests, including radiographic imaging (x rays), **wound culture**, and special diagnostic tests. X rays are the most common and most useful diagnostic tools available to the hand surgeon for evaluating traumatic injuries. Wound cultures are important for assessing injuries involving bites (human or animal) as well as wounds that have been badly contaminated by foreign matter. Such other special tests as a Doppler flowmeter examination can be used to evaluate the patterns of blood flow in the hand.

Before a scheduled operation on the hand, the patient will be given standard blood tests and a physical examination to make sure that he or she does not suffer from a general medical condition that would be a contraindication to surgery.

WHO PERFORMS THE PROCEDURE AND WHERE IS IT PERFORMED?

Hand surgery is usually performed by a microsurgeon, who may be a plastic surgeon (a surgeon with five years of general surgery training plus two years of plastic surgery training and another one to two years of training in microneurovascular surgery) or an orthopedic surgeon (a surgeon with one year of general surgery training, five years of orthopedic surgery training and additional years in microsurgery training).

Hand therapists are usually occupational therapists who have received specialized training in hand rehabilitation and are certified in hand therapy.

Aftercare

Aftercare following hand surgery may include one or more of the following, depending on the specific procedure: oral painkilling medications; anti-inflammatory medications; **antibiotics**; splinting; **traction**; special **dressings** to reduce swelling; and heat or massage therapy. Because the hand is a very sensitive part of the body, the patient may experience severe pain for several days after surgery. The surgeon may prescribe injections of painkilling drugs to manage the patient's discomfort.

Exercise therapy is an important part of aftercare for most patients who are recovering from hand surgery. A rehabilitation hand specialist will demonstrate exercises for the hand, instruct the patient in proper **wound care**, massage the hand and wrist, and perform an ongoing assessment of the patient's recovery of strength and range of motion in the hand.

Risks

According to the American Society of Plastic Surgeons, the most common complications associated with hand surgery are the following:

- infection
- poor healing
- loss of sensation or range of motion in the hand
- formation of blood clots
- allergic reactions to the anesthesia

Complications are relatively infrequent with hand surgery, however, and most can be successfully treated.

QUESTIONS TO ASK THE DOCTOR

- Are there any alternatives to surgery for treating my hand?
- Is the disorder likely to recur?
- Will I need a second operation?
- How many patients with my condition have you treated, and what were their outcomes?
- Can I expect to recover full range of motion in my hand?
- What will my hand look like after surgery?

Normal results

Normal results for hand surgery depend on the nature of the injury or disorder being treated.

Morbidity and mortality rates

Mortality following hand surgery is virtually unknown. The rates of complications depend on the nature of the patient's disorder or injury and the specific surgical procedure used to treat it.

Alternatives

Some disorders that affect the hand, such as osteoarthritis and rheumatoid arthritis, may be managed with such nonsurgical treatments as splinting, medications, physical therapy, or heat. Fractures, amputations, burns, bite injuries, congenital deformities, and severe cases of compression syndromes usually require surgery.

Resources

BOOKS

Canale, S. T., ed. *Campbell's Operative Orthopaedics*, 10th ed. St. Louis: Mosby, 2003.

DeLee, J. C., and D. Drez. *DeLee and Drez's Orthopaedic Sports Medicine*, 2nd ed. Philadelphia: Saunders, 2005.

Khatri, V. P., and J. A. Asensio. *Operative Surgery Manual*, 1st ed. Philadelphia: Saunders, 2003.

Townsend, C. M., et al. *Sabiston Textbook of Surgery*, 17th ed. Philadelphia: Saunders, 2004.

ORGANIZATIONS

American Association for Hand Surgery. 20 North Michigan Avenue, Suite 700, Chicago, IL 60602. (321) 236-3307. http://www.handsurgery.org (accessed March 31, 2008).

American Society of Plastic Surgeons (ASPS). 444 East Algonquin Road, Arlington Heights, IL 60005. (847) 228-9900. http://www.plasticsurgery.org; (accessed March 31, 2008).

American Society for Surgery of the Hand. 6300 North River Road, Suite 600. Rosemont, IL 60018. (847) 384-1435. http://www.assh.org (accessed March 31, 2008).

OTHER

American Society of Plastic Surgeons. http://www.plastic surgery.org (accessed March 31, 2008).

Laith Farid Gulli, MD,MS
Bilal Nasser, MD, MS
Robert Ramirez, BS
Nicole Mallory, MS, PA-C
Rosalyn Carson-DeWitt, MD

HCT *see* **Hematocrit**

Head and neck surgery *see* **Ear, nose, and throat surgery**

Health care proxy

Definition

A health care proxy, or health care proxy form, is a legal document that allows a person to choose someone to make medical decisions on their behalf when they are unable to do so. In some states the person who is authorized may be called a proxy, in others the person may be called an agent.

Description

A health care proxy form is part of a set of legal documents that allows a person to appoint someone to make medical decisions for them if they cannot act on their own behalf, and to make sure that health care professionals follow their wishes regarding specific medical treatments at the end of life. These documents are referred to as advance directives. The document naming the person appointed to make the decisions is called a health care proxy. The document that lists acceptable and unacceptable measures of artificial life support is called a **living will**. Most states have passed laws that authorize people to draw up living wills, but it is important to get specific information about the laws in one's own state.

Any competent adult can appoint a health care proxy or agent. It is not necessary to hire a lawyer to draw up or validate the form. Most states, however, require two adult witnesses to sign a proxy form. Many hospitals provide proxy forms on request.

It is important to have a health care proxy in order to be able to choose the person who will be making

KEY TERMS

Advance directive—A general term for two types of documents, living wills and medical powers of attorney, that allow people to give instructions about health care in the event that they cannot speak for themselves.

Proxy—A person authorized or empowered to act on behalf of another; also, the document or written authorization appointing that person.

medical decisions on one's behalf. In addition to naming the specific person who will make those decisions, one should think about what life-sustaining treatments one would be willing to undergo in the event of a medical emergency or terminal illness.

A health care proxy form does not deprive a person of the right to make decisions about medical treatment as long as he or she is able to do so. It is put into effect only when the patient's health care team determines that the patient is unable to make decisions on his or her own. For example, a person may be in a coma following an automobile accident. The physician would document in the patient's medical record that the patient is unable to make his or her own medical decisions, the circumstances that led to the patient's present condition, the nature of the disease or injury, and the expected length of the patient's incapacitation.

The person named as proxy makes health care decisions only as long as the patient is unable to make them for him- or herself. If the person regains the ability to make his or her own decisions, the proxy will no longer make them. If the incapacitation is permanent, the proxy will continue to make health care decisions on the patient's behalf as long as the patient is alive, or until the proxy is no longer able to carry out the responsibility.

Any trusted adult can be named as a health care proxy. Most married people name their spouse, but it is not necessary to do so. In addition, it is important to select an alternate proxy, in the event that the person first named is unable to fulfill the responsibility. For example, if the spouse has been named as proxy, and both members of the couple were incapacitated in a house fire, then someone else should be empowered to act on their behalf. A married couple does not need to name the same individual as a proxy or as the alternate. It is best to choose someone who lives close enough to carry out the responsibilities of a proxy without having to travel across state lines.

One should consider whether a potential proxy will be able to ask the necessary questions of medical personnel in order to obtain information needed to make a decision. It is important to discuss with the proxy his or her own value system, and whether he or she could make a decision for someone else that he or she would not make for him or herself. It is a good idea to carry the name and contact information of the proxy in one's wallet in the event of an emergency or sudden incapacitation.

The purpose of a living will is to give specific instructions about emergency or end-of-life health care. In some states a living will may be part of the health care proxy document. But because it is impossible to plan for all possible situations, the health care proxy can interpret one's wishes to members of the health care team and make decisions that one could not foresee at the time of making a living will. This is why it is important for the proxy to understand one's value system, so that the proxy can use his or her judgment as to what one would want. The proxy should be given a written copy of all advance directives. Even if a living will is not legal in the state in which one resides, writing such a will is an opportunity to think through one's beliefs and health care preferences. The proxy or agent can then can use the living will as a guide in making health care decisions as need arises.

Completing a health care proxy form and living will is useful because it helps one to think through one's value system and one's definition of quality of life. Some areas to consider are:

- What makes my life meaningful?
- What religious or personal beliefs do I hold that affect my health care decisions?
- Do I want my proxy to make health care decisions on his or her own, or are there other people I would want him or her to consult? If so, who are these people? Is there anyone who should *not* be consulted?
- Who besides myself will be affected by these decisions? Are they aware of my value system? Would they try to interfere with the proxy's decisions?
- What do I want to do about organ donation?
- Have I informed my physician of my wishes?

Appointing a health care proxy is not an irrevocable decision. One can change or revoke the proxy at any time, usually by filling out a new form. In some states, one can specify that the health care proxy will expire on a certain date or if certain events occur. If one has named one's spouse as an agent, the proxy is no longer in effect in the event of separation or divorce. People who want a former spouse to continue as their agent must complete a new proxy form.

In addition to keeping a copy of the proxy form in one's own file of important documents, one should give copies to the proxy, the alternate, and one's physicians.

Resources

BOOKS

Haman, Edward A. *How to Write Your Own Living Will,* 4th ed. Naperville, IL: Sphinx Publishing, 2004.

Lynn, Joanne, et al. *Improving Care for the End of Life: a Sourcebook for Health Care Managers and Clinicians,* 2nd ed. New York: Oxford University Press, 2008.

Pettus, Mark C. *The Savvy Patient: the Ultimate Advocate for Quality Health Care.* Sterling, VA: Capital Books, 2004.

PERIODICALS

Gibbons, Muriel. "Health Care Proxy Registry Proposed; Would Allow NYers to Better Communicate End of Life Decisions." *Insurance Advocate* 118, no. 7 (March 26, 2007): 8–9.

Lyden, Martin. "Assessing Capacity to Execute a Health Care Proxy: a Rationale and Protocol." *Mental Health Aspects of Developmental Disabilities* 10, no. 4 (October–December 2007): 145–157.

Tergesen, Anne. "Power to the Proxy." *Business Week* 3885 (May 31, 2004): 101.

ORGANIZATIONS

American Association of Retired Persons, 601 E. Street NW, Washington, DC, 20049, (888) 687-2277, http://www.aarp.org.

American Medical Association, 515 N. State Street, Chicago, IL, 60610, (800) 621-8335, http://www.ama-assn.org.

Caring Connections, National Hospice Foundation, Dept 6058, Washington, DC, 20042-6058, (703) 516-4928, http://www.caringinfo.org.

National Cancer Institute, 6116 Executive Boulevard, Room 3036A, Bethesda, MD, 20892-8322, (800) 422-6237, http://www.cancer.gov.

National Library of Medicine, 8600 Rockville Pike, Bethesda, MD, 20894, (888) 346-3656, http://www.nlm.nih.gov.

Esther Csapo Rastegari, R.N., B.S.N., Ed.M.
Robert Bockstiegel

Health history

Definition

The health history is a current collection of organized information unique to an individual. Relevant aspects of the history include biographical, demographic,

physical, mental, emotional, sociocultural, sexual, and spiritual data.

Purpose

The health history aids both individuals and health care providers by supplying essential information that will assist with diagnosis, treatment decisions, and establishment of trust and rapport between lay persons and medical professionals. The information also helps determine an individual's baseline, or what is normal and expected for that person.

Demographics

Every person should have a thorough health history recorded as a component of a periodic **physical examination**. These occur frequently (monthly at first) in infants and gradually reach a frequency of once per year for adolescents and adults.

Description

The clinical interview is the most common method for obtaining a health history. When a person or a designated representative can communicate effectively, the clinical interview is a valuable means for obtaining information.

The information that comprises the health history may be obtained from a person's previous records, the individual, or, in some cases, significant others or caretakers. The depth and length of the history-taking process is affected by factors such as the purpose of the visit, the urgency of the complaint or condition, the person's willingness or ability to contribute information, and the environment in which information is sought. When circumstances allow, a history may be holistic and comprehensive, but at times only a cursory review of the most pertinent facts is possible. In cases where the history-gathering process needs to be abbreviated, the history focuses on a person's medical experiences.

Health histories can be organized in a variety of ways. Often a hospital or clinic will provide a form, template, or computer database that serves as a guide and documentation tool for the history. Generally, the first aspect covered by the history is identifying data.

Identifying or basic demographic data includes facts such as:

- name;
- gender;
- age;
- date of birth;
- occupation;
- family structure or living arrangements; and
- source of referral.

Once the basic identifying data is collected, the history addresses the reason for the current visit in expanded detail. The reason for the visit is sometimes referred to as the chief complaint or the presenting complaint. Once the reason for the visit is established, additional data is solicited by asking for details that provide a more complete picture of the current clinical situation. For example, in the case of pain, aspects such as location, duration, intensity, precipitating factors, aggravating factors, relieving factors, and associated symptoms should be recorded. The full picture or story that accompanies the chief complaint is often referred to as the history of present illness (HPI).

The review of systems is a useful method for gathering medical information in an orderly fashion. This review is a series of questions about the person's current and past medical experiences. It usually proceeds from general to specific information. A thorough record of relevant dates is important in determining relevance of past illnesses or events to the current condition. A review of systems typically follows a head-to-toe order.

The names for categories in the review of systems may vary, but generally consists of variations on the following list:

- head, eyes, ears, nose, throat (HEENT);
- cardiovascular;
- respiratory;
- gastrointestinal;
- genitourinary;
- integumentary (skin);
- musculoskeletal, including joints;
- endocrine;
- nervous system, including both central and peripheral components; and
- mental, including psychiatric issues.

Past and current medical history includes details on medicines taken by the person, as well as allergies, illness, hospitalizations, procedures, pregnancies, environmental factors such as exposure to chemicals, toxins, or carcinogens, and health maintenance habits such as breast or testicular self-examination or immunizations.

An example of a series of questions might include the following:

- How are your ears?
- Are you having any trouble hearing?
- Have you ever had any trouble with your ears or with your hearing?

If an individual indicates a history of auditory difficulties, this would prompt further questions about medicines, surgeries, procedures, or associated problems related to the current or past condition.

In addition to identifying data, chief complaint, and review of systems, a comprehensive health history also includes factors such as a person's family and social life, family medical history, mental or emotional illnesses or stressors, detrimental or beneficial habits such as smoking or **exercise**, and aspects of culture, sexuality, and spirituality that are relevant to each individual. The clinicians also tailor their interviewing style to the age, culture, educational level, and attitudes of the persons being interviewed.

Diagnosis/Preparation

The information obtained from the interview is subjective, therefore, it is important that the interviewer assess the person's level of understanding, education, communication skills, potential biases, or other information that may affect accurate communication. Thorough training and practice in techniques of interviewing such as asking open-ended questions, listening effectively, and approaching sensitive topics such as substance abuse, chemical dependency, domestic violence, or sexual practices assists a clinician in obtaining the maximum amount of information without upsetting the person being questioned or disrupting the interview. The interview should be preceded by a review of the chart and an introduction by the clinician. The health care professional should explain the scope and purpose of the interview and provide privacy for the person being interviewed. Others should only be present with the person's consent.

Aftercare

Once a health history has been completed, the person being queried and the examiner should review the relevant findings. A health professional should

WHO PERFORMS THE PROCEDURE AND WHERE IS IT PERFORMED?

A health history is best obtained by a physician who has the training to appreciate nuances and details that may be overlooked by those with less training. Other health care professionals such as physician assistants and nurse practitioners have similar but somewhat limited training. Health histories are usually obtained in professional offices or hospitals. Occasionally, they are obtained in private homes or in the field.

discuss any recommendations for treatment or follow-up visits. Suggestions or special instructions should be put in writing. This is also an opportunity for persons to ask any remaining questions about their own health concerns.

Risks

There are virtually no risks associated with obtaining a health history. Only information is exchanged. The risk is potential embarrassment if confidential details are inappropriately distributed. Occasionally, a useful piece of information or data may be overlooked. In a sense, complications may arise from the findings of a health history. These usually trigger further investigations or initiate treatment. They are usually far more beneficial than negative as they often begin a process of treatment and recovery.

Normal results

Normal results of a health history correspond to the appearance and normal functioning of the body. Abnormal results of a health history include any findings that indicate the presence of a disorder, disease, or underlying condition.

Morbidity and mortality rates

Disease and disability are identified during the course of obtaining a health history. There are virtually no risks associated with the verbal exchange of information.

Alternatives

There are no alternatives that are as effective as obtaining a complete health history. The only real alternative is to skip the history. This allows disease

QUESTIONS TO ASK THE DOCTOR

- What are your interpretations of my history, both normal and abnormal?
- What has changed since the last health history was obtained?
- What do you recommend as a result of your interpretation of the information obtained in this health history?
- When do you want to repeat the health history?

and other pathologic or degenerative processes to go undetected. In the long run, this is not conducive to optimal health.

Resources

BOOKS

Bickley, L. S., and P. G. Szilagyi. *Bates' Guide to Physical Examination and History Taking*, 9th ed. Philadelphia: Lippincott Williams and Wilkins, 2007.

Jarvis, C. *Physical Examination and Health Assessment*, 5th ed. Philadelphia: Saunders, 2007.

Seidel, H. M., J. Ball, J. Dains, and W. Bennedict. *Mosby's Physical Examination Handbook*, 6th ed. St. Louis: Mosby, 2006.

Swartz, M. H. *Textbook of Physical Diagnosis: History and Examination*, 5th ed. Philadelphia: Saunders, 2005.

PERIODICALS

Dalley, A, K. Lynch, P. Feltham, J. Fulcher, and D. Bomba. "The use of smart tokens to permit the secure, remote access of electronic health records." *International Journal of Electronics in Healthcare* 2, no. 1 (2006): 1–11.

Hendricks, M. M. "Documentation for mammographers." *Radiological Technology* 78, no. 5 (2007): 396M–412M.

Recupero, P. R. "Ethics of medical records and professional communications." *Child and Adolescent Psychiatric Clinics of North America* 17, no. 1 (2008): 37–51.

Schulte, D. J. "Completing and updating health history forms." *Journal of the Michigan Dental Association* 88, no. 7 (2006): 14–21.

Vogel, K. J., V. S. Murthy, B. Dudley, R. E. Grubs, E. Gettig, A. Ford, and S. B. Thomas. "The use of family health histories to address health disparities in an African American community." *Health Promotion Practice* 8, no. 4 (2007): 350–357.

OTHER

"Checkups and Prevention: Recording Your Health History." American Association of Retired Persons. http://www.aarp.org/health/staying_healthy/prevention/a2004-03-01-healthhistory.html (January 4, 2008).

"Family Health History." Genetic Alliance. http://www.geneticalliance.org/ws_display.asp?filter=fhh (January 4, 2008).

"Health History Form." Covenant Health Care. http://www.covenanthealthcare.com/body.cfm?id=574 (January 4, 2008).

Heidekrueger, L. "Measuring Your Family Health History." Genealogy Today. 1999. http://www.genealogytoday.com/articles/genogram.html (January 4, 2008).

"Medical history: How to Compile Your Medical Family Tree." MayoClinic.com. November 1, 2007. http://www.mayoclinic.com/health/medical-history/HQ01707 (January 4, 2008).

"Personal Health History Form." Huntington's Disease Helpful Forms. http://huntingtondisease.tripod.com/hdhelpfulforms/id9.html (January 4, 2008).

"Welcome to My Family Health Portrait." U.S. Department of Health and Human Services. https://familyhistory.hhs.gov/ (January 4, 2008).

ORGANIZATIONS

American Academy of Family Physicians, 11400 Tomahawk Creek Parkway, Leawood, KS, 66211-2672, (913) 906-6000, http://www.aafp.org.

American Academy of Pediatrics, 141 Northwest Point Boulevard, Elk Grove Village, IL, 60007-1098, (847) 434-4000, (847) 434-8000, kidsdocs@aap.org, http://www.aap.org.

American College of Physicians, 190 N. Independence Mall West, Philadelphia, PA, 19106-1572, (215) 351-2400, (800) 523-1546, http://www.acponline.org.

American Medical Association, 515 N. State Street, Chicago, IL, 60610, (800) 621-8335, http://www.ama-assn.org.

L. Fleming Fallon, Jr., M.D., Dr.P.H.

Health Maintenance Organization (HMO)

Definition

A Health Maintenance Organization provides health care coverage to individuals who are enrolled in it. Individuals enroll in an HMO through hospitals, physicians, and other healthcare providers, or through laboratories who have a contract with the HMO.

Purpose

The purpose of an HMO is provide health care coverage at lower costs to the HMO, to the patient, and to the employers or government who offer the HMO as an insurance option. HMOs have advantages and disadvantages, but can be a very important option for many individuals.

Advantages

The advantage to the patient of an HMO over other types of health care insurance are lower costs. For example, a patient may pay a co-pay of $10 for each visit to their primary care physician with HMO coverage, as opposed to 20% with traditional indemnity health care insurance. Frequently, the laboratory fees are covered completely if they are performed at a laboratory that has a contract with the HMO. The HMO monthly premium is usually lower than traditional indemnity insurance plans as well, because the health care providers contract with an HMO to receive a greater number of patients, but in doing so, usually agree to provide care at discounted fees. Another way that most HMOs keep costs down is by setting up a system of care based on specific care plans that are overseen by the patient's primary care physician; the patient cannot make an appointment with a specialist, and be covered by insurance, without prior authorization or referral by their primary care physician. Some HMOs do not have these restrictions, but they tend to have higher premiums. HMOs also focus on preventive healthcare programs to help prevent members from developing chronic conditions that could significantly increase their medical costs.

Disadvantages

A major disadvantage to the patient of an HMO is that his or her preferred health care provider may not have a contract with that HMO and therefore, if the patient wants to see that particular provider, he or she would have to pay for the visits out of pocket. Another disadvantage of HMOs can be that providers may end up being at a financial disadvantage because of the reduced fees required to contract with the HMO. In some areas this has led to very few healthcare providers contracting with certain HMOs and thus the members of the HMO have very little choice in whom to see. For these same reasons, some healthcare providers will not re-sign a contract with an HMO and a patient who has been seeing that healthcare provider for years may end up not being able to choose that healthcare provider for the future.

Resources

ORGANIZATIONS

National Association of Insurance Commissioners, 2301 McGee Street, Suite 800, Kansas City, MO 64108. (816)842-3600.http://www.naic.org/.

OTHER

Medline Plus a service of the National Library of Medicine and the National Institutes of Health, 8600 Rockville Pike, Bethesda, MD 20894.http://www.nlm.nih.gov/medlineplus/ managedcare.html

Renee Laux, M.S.

Heart-lung machines

Definition

The heart-lung machine, sometimes called a pump oxygenator, is medical equipment that provides cardiopulmonary bypass, or mechanical circulatory support of the heart and lungs. The machine may consist of venous and arterial cannula (tubes), polyvinyl chloride (PVC) or silicone tubing, a reservoir (to hold blood), bubbler or membrane oxygenator, cardiotomy (a filtered reservoir), heat exchanger(s), arterial line filter, pump(s), flow meter, inline blood gas and electrolyte analyzer, and pressure-monitoring devices. Treatment provides removal of carbon dioxide from the blood, oxygen delivery to the blood, blood flow to the body, and/or temperature maintenance. Pediatric and adult patients both benefit from this technology.

Purpose

In the **operating room**, the heart-lung machine is used primarily to provide blood flow and respiration for the patient while the heart is stopped. It allows surgeons to perform **heart transplantation**, coronary artery bypass grafting (CABG), open-heart surgery for valve repair or repair of cardiac anomalies, and aortic aneurysm repairs, along with treatment of other cardiac-related diseases.

The heart-lung machine provides the benefit of a motionless heart in an almost bloodless surgical field. Cardioplegia solution is delivered to the heart, resulting in cardiac arrest (heart stoppage). The heart-lung machine is invaluable during this time since the patient is unable to maintain blood flow to the lungs or the body.

In critical care units and **cardiac catheterization** laboratories, the heart-lung machine is used to support and maintain blood flow and respiration. The diseased heart or lung(s) is replaced by this technology, providing time for the organ(s) to heal. The heart-lung machine can be used with venoarterial extracorporeal membrane oxygenation (ECMO), which is used primarily in the treatment of lung disease. Cardiopulmonary support is useful during percutaneous transluminal coronary **angioplasty** (PTCA) and stent procedures performed with cardiac catheterization. Both treatments can be instituted in the critical care unit when severe heart or lung disease is no longer treatable by less-invasive conventional treatments such as pharmaceuticals, intra-aortic balloon pump (IABP), and **mechanical ventilation** with a respirator.

Use of this treatment in the emergency room is not limited to patients suffering heart or lung failure. In severe cases of hypothermia, a patient's **body temperature** can be corrected by extracorporeal circulation with the heart-lung machine. Blood is warmed as it passes over the heat exchanger. The warmed blood returns to the body, gradually increasing the patient's body temperature to normal.

Tertiary care facilities are able to support the staffing required to operate and maintain this technology. Level I trauma centers have access to this specialized treatment and equipment. Being that this technology serves both adult and pediatric patients, specialized children's hospitals may provide treatment with the heart-lung machine for venoarterial ECMO.

Description

The pump oxygenator had its first success on May 6, 1953. Continued research and design have allowed the heart-lung machine to become a standard of care in the treatment of heart and lung disease, while supporting other non-conventional treatments.

Foreign surfaces of the heart-lung machine activate blood coagulation factors, proteins, and platelets, which lead to clot formation. In the heart-lung machine, clot formation would block the flow of blood. As venous and arterial cannulas are inserted, medications are administered to prevent clotting of the blood. This allows blood to flow freely through the heart-lung machine.

Large vessels (veins and arteries) are required for cannulation, to insert the tubes (cannulas) that will carry the blood away from the patient to the heart-lung machine and to return the blood from the heart-lung machine to the patient. Cannulation sites for venous access can include the inferior and superior vena cava, the right atrium (upper chamber of the heart), the femoral vein (in the groin), or internal jugular vein. Oxygen-rich blood can be returned to the aorta, femoral artery, or carotid artery (in the neck). By removing oxygen-poor blood from the right side of the heart and returning oxygen-rich blood to the left side, heart-lung bypass is achieved.

The standard heart-lung machine typically includes up to five pump assemblies. A centrifugal or roller head pump can be used in the arterial position for extracorporeal circulation of the blood. The four remaining pumps are roller pump in design to provide fluid, gas, and liquid for delivery or removal to the heart chambers and surgical field. Left ventricular blood return is accomplished by roller pump, drawing blood away from the heart. Surgical suction created by the roller pump removes accumulated fluid from the general surgical field. The cardioplegia delivery pump is used to deliver a high potassium solution to the coronary vessels. The potassium arrests the heart so that the surgical field is motionless during surgical procedures. An additional pump is available for emergency backup of the arterial pump in case of mechanical failure.

A pump is required to produce blood flow. As of 2007, roller and centrifugal pump designs were the standard of care. Modern heart lung machines can provide pulsatile (pulsed, as from a heartbeat) or non-pulsatile (continuous) blood flow to the systemic circulation.

The roller assembly rotates and engages the tubing, PVC or silicone, which is then compressed against the pump's housing, propelling blood ahead of the roller head. Rotational frequency and inner diameter of the tubing determine blood flow. Because of its occlusive nature, the pump can be used to remove blood from the surgical field by creating negative pressure on the inflow side of the pump head.

The centrifugal pump also has a negative inlet pressure. As a safety feature, this pump disengages when air bubbles are introduced. The centrifugal force draws blood into the center of the device. Blood is propelled and released to the outflow tract tangential to the pump housing. Rotational speed determines the amount of blood flow, which is measured by a flowmeter placed adjacent to the pump housing. If rotational frequency is too low, blood may flow in the wrong direction since the system is non-occlusive in nature. Magnetic coupling links the centrifugal pump to the control unit.

A reservoir collects blood drained from the venous circulation. Tubing connects the venous cannulas to the reservoir. Reservoir designs include open or closed systems. The open system displays graduated demarcations corresponding to blood volume in the container. The design is open to atmosphere, allowing blood to interface with atmospheric gasses. The pliable bag of the closed system eliminates the air-blood interface, while still being exposed to atmospheric pressure. Volume is measured by weight or by change in radius of the container. The closed reservoir collapses when emptied, as an additional safety feature.

Bubble oxygenators use the reservoir for ventilation. When the reservoir is examined from the exterior, the blood is already oxygen rich and appears bright red. As blood enters the reservoir, gaseous emboli are mixed directly with the blood. Oxygen and carbon dioxide are exchanged across the boundary layer of the blood and gas bubbles. The blood will then pass through a filter that is coated with an antifoam solution, which helps to remove fine bubbles. As blood pools in the reservoir, it has already exchanged carbon dioxide and oxygen. From here, tubing carries the blood to the rest of the heart-lung machine.

In opposition to this technique is the membrane oxygenator. Tubing carries the oxygen-poor blood from the reservoir through the pump to the membrane oxygenator. Oxygen and carbon dioxide cross a membrane that separates the blood from the ventilation gasses. As blood leaves the oxygenator, it is oxygen rich and bright red in color.

When blood is ready to be returned from the heart-lung machine to the patient, the arterial line filter will be encountered. This device is used to filter small air bubbles that may have entered, or been generated by, the heart-lung machine. Following this, filter tubing completes the blood path as it returns the blood to the arterial cannula to enter the body.

Fluid being returned from the left ventricle and surgical suction require filtration before the blood is reintroduced to the heart-lung machine. Blood enters a filtered reservoir, called a cardiotomy, which is connected with tubing to the venous reservoir. Other fluids such as blood products and medications are also added into the cardiotomy for filtration of particulate.

Heat exchangers allow body and organ temperatures to be adjusted. The simplest heat exchange design is a bucket of water. As the blood passes through the tubing placed in the bath, the blood temperature will change. A more sophisticated system separates the blood and water interface with a metallic barrier. As the water temperature is changed, so is the blood temperature, which enters the body or organ circulation, which changes the tissue temperature. Once the tissue temperature reaches the desired level, the water temperature is maintained. Being able to cool the blood helps to preserve the organ and body by metabolizing fewer energy stores.

Because respiration is being controlled, and a machine is meeting metabolic demand, it is necessary to monitor the patient's blood chemical makeup. Chemical sensors placed in the blood path are able to detect the amount of oxygen bound to hemoglobin. Other, more elaborate sensors can constantly trend the blood pH, partial pressure of oxygen and carbon dioxide, and electrolytes. This constant trending can quickly analyze the metabolic demands of the body.

Sensors that communicate system pressures are also a necessity. These transducers are placed in areas where pressure is high, after the pump. Readings outside of normal ranges often alert the operator to obstructions in the blood-flow path. The alert of high pressure must be corrected quickly as the heart-lung machine equipment may disengage under the stress of abnormally elevated pressures. Low-pressure readings can be just as serious, alerting the user to faulty connections or equipment. Constant monitoring and proper alarms help to protect the integrity of the system.

Constant scanning of all components and monitoring devices is required. Normal values can quickly change due to device failure or sudden mechanical constrictions. The diagnosis of a problem and quick troubleshooting techniques will prevent additional complications.

Normal results

Continuous scanning of all patient monitors is necessary for proper treatment and troubleshooting. Documentation of patient status is obtained every 15–30 minutes. This information allows the physician and nursing staff to follow trends that will help better manage the patient once treatment is discontinued. At the termination of device support, the perfusionist or ECMO specialist must communicate clearly to the physician all changes in support status. This allows the entire team to assess changes in patient parameters that are consistent with the patient becoming less dependent on the device, while the patient's heart and lungs meet the metabolic demands of the body.

It is the responsibility of the perfusionist or ECMO specialist to be at the device controls at all times.

Resources

BOOKS

Van Meurs, Krisa, Kevin P. Lally, Giles Peek, and Joseph P. Zwischenberger. *Ecmo: Extracorporeal Cardiopulmonary Support in Critical Care*. Ann Arbor, MI: Extracorporeal Life Support Organization, 2005.

OTHER

"Heart Lung Machine." *Your Total Health*. January 19, 2007. http://yourtotalhealth.ivillage.com/heart-lung-machine.html (February 5, 2008).

"Heart Surgery Overview." *Texas Heart Institute*. July 2007. http://www.texasheart.org/HIC/Topics/Proced/index.cfm (February 1, 2008).

Levinson, Mark M. "The Heart-lung Machine." *The Heart Surgery Forum*. 2008. http://www.hsforum.com/stories/storyReader$1486 (February 5, 2008).

ORGANIZATIONS

American Heart Association, 7272 Greenville Avenue, Dallas, TX, 75231, (800) 242-8721, http://www.americanheart.org.

Extracorporeal Life Support Organization, 1327 Jones Drive, Suite 101, Ann Arbor, MI, 48105, (734) 998-6601, http://www.elso.med.umich.edu.

Allison J. Spiwak, M.S.B.M.E.
Tish Davidson, A.M.

Heart-lung transplantation

Definition

Heart-lung transplantation is the surgical replacement of a person's severely diseased or dysfunctional heart and lungs with a healthy human donor heart and lungs.

Purpose

Heart-lung transplantation is an uncommon operation. It is performed when the person has both end-stage lung disease and end-stage heart disease that

Heart-lung transplantation

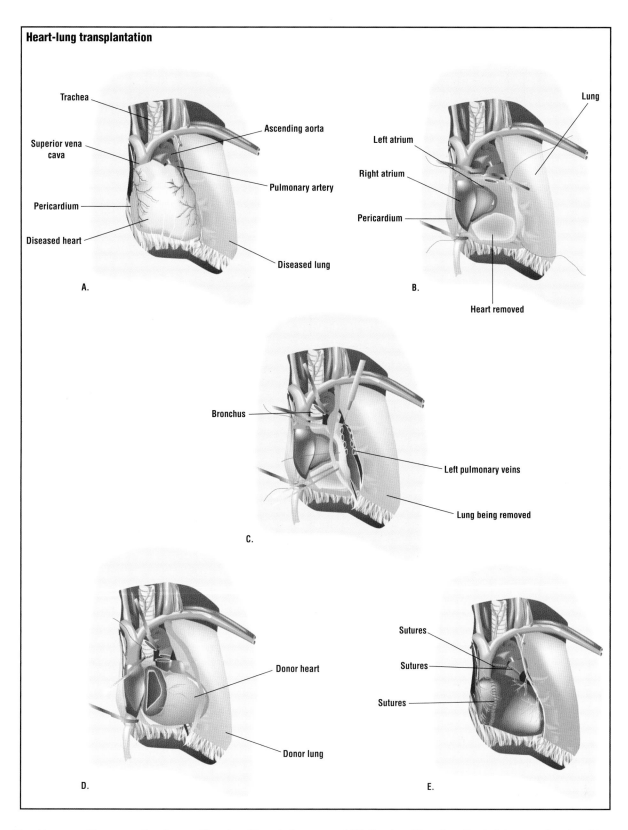

Trachea

Superior vena cava

Pericardium

Diseased heart

Ascending aorta

Pulmonary artery

Diseased lung

A.

Left atrium

Right atrium

Pericardium

Lung

Heart removed

B.

Bronchus

Left pulmonary veins

Lung being removed

C.

Donor heart

Donor lung

D.

Sutures

Sutures

Sutures

E.

Chest is opened to expose the diseased heart and lung to be removed (A). Heart and lung function is taken over by a heart-lung machine. Major blood vessels are severed, and the heart is removed (B). Bronchus and blood vessels leading to the lung are severed, and the lung is removed (C). Donor heart and lung are placed in the patient's the chest cavity (D). They are sutured to their appropriate connections, and the heart is restarted before the patient is taken off the heart-lung machine (E). *(Illustration by GGS Information Services. Cengage Learning, Gale.)*

do nor respond to any other medical treatments. It is also sometimes performed on children with severe congenital heart defects. The purpose of **heart transplantation** is to extend and improve the life of a person who would otherwise die.

Demographics

Heart-lung transplant recipients are not limited by sex, race, or ethnicity. Patients who are severely limited in daily activity, as defined by their doctors, and have a very limited life expectancy, may be candidates for heart-lung transplantation. Healthy donor hearts and lungs are in short supply, therefore, strict rules dictate criteria for transplant recipients. Patients who may be too sick to survive the surgery or the side effects of immunosuppressive therapy are not considered transplant candidates. Other factors that absolutely contraindicate (rule out) heart-lung transplantation include multiple organ system dysfunction, current substance abuse, bone marrow failure, active malignancy (cancer), and HIV infection. Other relative contraindications include age greater than 60, anorexia, obesity, peripheral and coronary vascular disease, ventilator support, steroid dependency, chest wall deformity, resistant bacterial or fungal infections, and certain psychiatric conditions.

According to the Organ Procurement and Transplantation Network, in the United States 961 heart-lung transplants were performed between 1988 and November 2007. Overall, slightly more women than men have received heart-lung transplants in the United States, and more than 800 of the recipients were white. Internationally 800–1,000 heart-lung transplants are performed each year.

Description

Patients with end-stage heart and lung disease unresponsive to medical treatment must have a complete medical examination before they can be put on the transplant waiting list. Many types of tests are done, including blood tests, X-rays, and tests of heart, lung, and other organ function. The results of these tests indicate to doctors how serious the heart disease is and whether the patient is healthy enough to survive the **transplant surgery**.

Patient-donor matching

All patients placed on the waiting list are registered with the United Network for Organ Sharing (UNOS). UNOS has organ transplant specialists who run a national computer network that connects all the transplant centers and organ-donation organizations. Patients

---

KEY TERMS

Aorta—The main artery that carries blood from the heart to the rest of the body. The aorta is the largest artery in the body.

Cardiopulmonary bypass—Mechanically circulating the blood with a heart-lung machine that bypasses the heart and lungs.

Congenital defect—A defect present at birth that occurs during the growth and development of the fetus in the womb.

Coronary vascular disease—Or cardiovascular disease; disease of the heart or blood vessels, such as atherosclerosis (hardening of the arteries).

End-stage heart or lung failure—Severe heart or lung disease that does not respond adequately to medical or surgical treatment.

Nephrotoxicity—A building up of poisons in the kidneys.

Osteoporosis—Loss of bone mass, causing bones to break easily.

Pulmonary hypertension—Increased blood pressure in the blood vessels of the lungs.

Resistant infections—Infections that are not cured by standard antibiotic treatment.

---

are grouped in terms of priority based on how long they can live without a transplant. The list is national and independent of the heart transplant center where the surgery will take place.

Established criteria for donor organ matching include the following:

- anatomic compatibility between the donor and recipient;
- immunologic compatibility between the donor and recipient;
- medical urgency; and
- location of the patient and donor.

The heart and lungs must be transplanted as quickly as possible, therefore, after anatomic and blood group compatibility have been determined, a list of local patients is checked first for a suitable match. After that, a regional list and then a national list are checked. The patient's transplant team of heart and lung transplant specialists makes the final decision as to whether a donor organs are suitable for the patient.

The transplant procedure

Under **general anesthesia**, an incision is made in the patient's chest to access the heart and lungs. Anticoagulation (anti-clotting) and antibiotic medications are provided, and cardiopulmonary bypass to a heart-lung machine is established. Blood flow through the heart is stopped by application of a clamp across the aorta. The surgeon removes the diseased organs. In the heart, the back parts of the patient's own right and left atriums are often left intact, along with the aorta beyond the coronary arteries. This provides large suture lines that allow decreased surgical time and result in fewer bleeding complications.

The donor heart is dissected to match the remaining native heart and aorta. The sutures are made to join the structures. Once completed, the cardiac chambers is filled with the patient's blood that is diverted away from the heart and lung machine. **Mechanical ventilation** of the donor lungs helps inflate the lung tissue.

Diagnosis/Preparation

History, examination, and laboratory studies are performed before referral to a transplant center. These records are reviewed on-site for qualification to be placed on the United Network for Organ Sharing (UNOS) national waiting list. Procedures necessary for evaluation include a chest X-ray, arterial blood samples, air flow studies, ventilation and perfusion scanning (studies the exchange of oxygen with carbon dioxide in the lungs), and **cardiac catheterization** of both the right and left sides of the heart.

Aftercare

The patient will be treated in the **intensive care unit** upon completion of the surgery, and cardiac monitoring will be continued. Medications for cardiac support will be continued until cardiac function stabilizes. Mechanical circulatory support may be continued until cardiac and respiratory functions improve. Ventilator support will be continued until the patient is able to breathe independently. After leaving the intensive care unit, the patient will spend a week or more in a special transplant unit. Medications to prevent organ rejection will be continued indefinitely, as will medications to prevent infection. The patient will be evaluated before discharge and provided with specific instructions to recognize infection and organ rejection. The patient will be given directions to contact the physician after discharge along with criteria for emergency room care.

Risks

General anesthesia and cardiopulmonary bypass carry certain risks unassociated with the heart-lung transplant procedure. Graft rejection and technical failure are often a result of lung injury sustained during the stoppage and restarting of the organ. Infection by cytomegalovirus (CMV) often occurs in the first year, but is usually treatable. Immunosuppressive drugs to prevent rejection have side effects associated with malignancies, lymphomas or tumors of the skin and lips being most common. Osteoporosis and nephrotoxicity are also associated with the immunosuppressive therapies.

Normal results

Lung and cardiac function are drastically improved after transplantation. Strenuous **exercise** may still be limited, but quality of life is greatly improved. The patient will continue with medical visits frequently throughout the first year, including required tissue biopsies to test for rejection and cardiac catheterizations. The frequency of medical visits will decrease after the first year, but invasive medical procedures will still be necessary. Medications to suppress rejection of the organs and prevent infection are continued.

Morbidity and mortality rates

Death within the first 30 days is usually associated with technical and graft failure of the transplanted organ. Causes of death after 30 days often include immune system rejection of the transplant, infection of the airways or other infection, and the development of coronary artery disease. The one-year survival rate is 65%. The five-year survival rate is 40%.

Systemic hypertension (high blood pressure) is common at one year after surgery and can be relieved with medical treatment. Chronic bronchiolitis (infection of the airways) is expected in one-third of patients

QUESTIONS TO ASK THE DOCTOR

- How many of these procedures have been performed at this center in the last year and last five years?
- How many of these procedures has the surgeon performed in the last year and last five years?
- What is the length of time spent on the waiting list for a patient with the pathology of the patient?
- What are the complications associated with this procedure?
- What are the complications associated with the duration of the transplantation?
- What type of limitations will be faced if the transplant is successful?
- How frequent will future medical visits be after the procedure during the first year and after that?

at five years. Hyperlipidemia (high lipid concentration in blood), diabetes mellitus, and kidney dysfunction are also seen in some patients within the first year of transplantation and continue to affect an increasing number of patients each year. Malignancies that include lymphoma and lip and skin tumors are seen at a higher rate than in general populations.

Alternatives

There are no good alternatives when both heart and lungs are seriously diseased. Individuals with only end-stage heart disease sometimes do well with a ventricular-assist device that helps the heart pump. Individuals with end-stage lung disease but a healthy heart often do well with a lung transplant. When both organs are seriously diseased, there are few alternatives to a heart-lung transplant if a suitable donor can be found.

Resources

OTHER

"Heart and Lung Transplant." *eMedicineHealth*. August 18, 2005. http://www.emedicinehealth.com/heart_and_lung_transplant/article_em.htm (February 5, 2008).

Mancini, Mary C. "Heart-Lung Transplantation" *eMedicine*. March 1, 2006. http://www.emedicine.com/med/topic2603.htm (February 5, 2008).

ORGANIZATIONS

American Heart Association, 7272 Greenville Avenue, Dallas, TX, 75231, (800) 242-8721, http://www.americanheart.org.

American Society of Transplantation, 15000 Commerce Parkway, Suite C, Mount Laurel, NJ, 08054, (856) 439-9986, http://www.a-s-t.org.

National Heart, Lung and Blood Institute, National Institutes of Health, P.O. Box 30105, Bethesda, MD, 20824-0105, NHLBIinfo@nhlbi.nih.gov, http://www.nhlbi.nih.gov.

United Network for Organ Sharing, P.O. Box 2484, Richmond, VA, 23218, (804) 782-4800, http://www.unos.org.

Allison Joan Spiwak, M.S.B.M.E.
Tish Davidson, A. M.

Heart catheterization *see* **Cardiac catheterization**

Heart defect surgery *see* **Heart surgery for congenital defects**

Heart resection *see* **Myocardial resection**

Heart sonogram *see* **Echocardiography**

Heart surgery for congenital defects

Definition

Heart surgery for congenital defects consists of a variety of surgical procedures that are performed to repair the many types of heart defects that may be present at birth and can go undiagnosed into adulthood.

Purpose

Heart surgery for congenital defects is performed to repair a defect, providing improved blood flow to the pulmonary and systemic circulations and better oxygen delivery to the body. Congenital heart defects that are symptomatic at birth must be treated with palliative or complete surgical repair. Defects that are not symptomatic at birth may be discovered later in life, and will be treated to relieve symptoms by palliative or complete surgical repair. Surgery is recommended for congenital heart defects that result in a lack of oxygen, a poor quality of life, or when a patient fails to thrive. Even lesions that are asymptomatic may be treated surgically to avoid additional complications later in life.

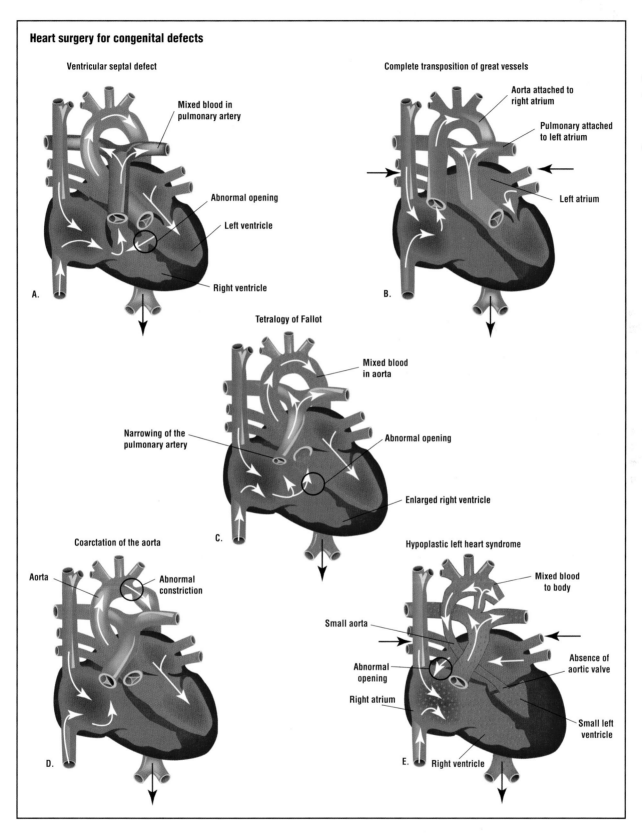

Heart surgery for congenital defects

Ventricular septal defect

Mixed blood in pulmonary artery

Abnormal opening

Left ventricle

Right ventricle

A.

Complete transposition of great vessels

Aorta attached to right atrium

Pulmonary attached to left atrium

Left atrium

B.

Tetralogy of Fallot

Mixed blood in aorta

Narrowing of the pulmonary artery

Abnormal opening

Enlarged right ventricle

C.

Coarctation of the aorta

Aorta

Abnormal constriction

D.

Hypoplastic left heart syndrome

Mixed blood to body

Small aorta

Absence of aortic valve

Abnormal opening

Right atrium

Small left ventricle

E.   Right ventricle

The most common types of congenital heart defects are ventricular septal defect (A), complete transposition of the great vessels (B), tetralogy of Fallot (C), coarctation of the aorta (D), and hypoplastic left heart syndrome (E). *(Illustration by GGS Information Services. Cengage Learning, Gale.)*

Atresia—Lack of development. In tricuspid atresia, the triscupid valve has not developed. In pulmonary atresia, the pulmonary valve has not developed.

Coarctation of the aorta—A congenital defect in which severe narrowing or constriction of the aorta obstructs the flow of blood.

Congenital heart defects—Congenital (conditions that are present at birth) heart disease includes a variety of defects that occur during fetal development.

Cyanotic—Inadequate oxygen in the systemic arterial circulation.

Mitral valve—The heart valve connecting the left atrium and the left ventricle.

Patent ductus arteriosus—A congenital defect in which the temporary blood vessel connecting the left pulmonary artery to the aorta in the fetus fails to close in the newborn.

Pulmonary valve—The heart valve connecting the left atrium and the pulmonary arteries.

Septal defects—Openings in the septum, the muscular wall separating the right and left sides of the heart. Atrial septal defects are openings between the two upper heart chambers and ventricular septal defects are openings between the two lower heart chambers.

Stenosis—A narrowing of the heart's valves.

Tetralogy of Fallot—A cyanotic defect in which the blood pumped through the body has too little oxygen. Tetralogy of Fallot includes four defects: a ventricular septal defect, narrowing at or beneath the pulmonary valve, infundibular pulmonary stenosis (obstruction of blood flow out of the right ventricle through the pulmonary valve), and overriding aorta (the aorta crosses the ventricular septal defect into the right ventricle).

Transposition of the great vessels—A cyanotic defect in which the blood pumped through the body has too little oxygen because the pulmonary artery receives its blood incorrectly from the left ventricle and the aorta incorrectly receives blood flow from the right ventricle.

Tricuspid valve—The heart valve connecting the right atrium and right ventricle.

Demographics

Congenital heart disease is estimated to involve less than 1% of all live births. As some defects are not found until later in life, or may never be diagnosed, this number may actually be higher. Many congenital defects are often incompatible with life leading to miscarriage and stillbirths. During a child's first year of life, the most common defects that are symptomatic include ventricular septal defect (VSD), transposition of the great vessels (TGV), tetralogy of Fallot, coarctation of the aorta, and hypoplastic left heart syndrome. Premature infants have an increased presentation of VSD and patent ductus arteriosus. Diabetic mothers have infants with a higher incidence of congenital heart defects than non-diabetic mothers. Abnormal chromosomes increase the incidence of congenital heart defects. Specific to trisomy 21 (Down syndrome), 23–56% of infants have a congenital heart defect.

Description

Congenital heart defects can be named by a number of specific lesions, but may have additional lesions. Classification best describes lesions by the amount of pulmonary blood flow (increased or decreased pulmonary blood flow) or the presence of an obstruction to blood flow. The dynamic circulation of the newborn as well as the size of the defect will determine the symptoms. Recommended ages for surgery for the most common congenital heart defects are:

- atrial septal defects: during the preschool years
- patent ductus arteriosus: between ages one and two
- coarctation of the aorta: in infancy, if it is symptomatic, at age four otherwise
- tetralogy of Fallot: age varies, depending on the patient's symptoms
- transposition of the great arteries: often in the first weeks after birth, but before the patient is 12 months old

Surgical procedures seek to repair the defect and restore normal pulmonary and systemic circulation. Sometimes, multiple, serial surgical procedures are necessary.

Many congenital defects are often associated so that the surgical procedures described may be combined for complete repair of a specific congenital defect.

Repair for simple cardiac lesions can be performed in the **cardiac catheterization** lab. Catheterization procedures include balloon atrial septostomy and **balloon valvuloplasty**. Surgical procedures include arterial switch, Damus-Kaye-Stansel procedure, Fontan procedure, Ross procedure, shunt procedure, and venous switch or intra-atrial baffle.

Catheterization procedures

Balloon atrial septostomy and balloon valvuloplasty are cardiac catheterization procedures. Cardiac catheterization procedures can save the lives of critically ill neonates and, in some cases, eliminate or delay more invasive surgical procedures. It is expected that catheterization procedures will continue to replace more types of surgery for congenital heart defects in the future. A thin tube called a catheter is inserted into an artery or vein in the leg, groin, or arm and threaded into the area of the heart that needs repair. The patient receives a local anesthetic at the insertion site. General anesthetic or sedation may be used.

BALLOON ATRIAL SEPTOSTOMY. Balloon atrial septostomy is the standard procedure for correcting transposition of the great arteries; it is sometimes used in patients with mitral, pulmonary, or tricuspid atresia. (Atresia is lack of or poor development of a structure.) Balloon atrial septostomy enlarges the atrial septal opening, which normally closes in the days following birth. A special balloon-tipped catheter is inserted into the right atrium and passed into the left atrium. The balloon is inflated in the left atrium and pulled back across the septum to create a larger opening in the atrial septum.

BALLOON VALVULOPLASTY. Balloon valvuloplasty uses a balloon-tipped catheter to open a stenotic (narrowed) heart valve, improving the flow of blood through the valve. It is the procedure of choice in pulmonary stenosis and is sometimes used in aortic and mitral stenosis. A balloon is placed beyond the valve, inflated, and pulled backward across the valve.

Surgical procedures

These procedures are performed under **general anesthesia**. Some require the use of a heart-lung machine, which takes over for the heart and lungs during the procedure, providing cardiopulmonary bypass. The heart-lung machine can cool the body to reduce the need for oxygen, allowing deep hypothermic circulatory arrest (DHCA) to be performed. DHCA benefits the surgeon by creating a bloodless surgical field.

ARTERIAL SWITCH. Arterial switch is performed to correct transposition of the great vessels, where the position of the pulmonary artery and the aorta are reversed. The procedure involves connecting the aorta to the left ventricle and the pulmonary artery to the right ventricle.

DAMUS-KAYE-STANSEL PROCEDURE. Transposition of the great vessels can also be corrected by the Damus-Kaye-Stansel procedure, in which the pulmonary artery is cut in two and connected to the ascending aorta and right ventricle.

VENOUS SWITCH. For transposition of the great vessels, venous switch creates a tunnel inside the atria to redirect oxygen-rich blood to the right ventricle and aorta and venous blood to the left ventricle and pulmonary artery. This procedure differs from the arterial switch and Damus-Kaye-Stansel procedures in that blood flow is redirected through the heart.

FONTAN PROCEDURE. For tricuspid atresia and pulmonary atresia, the Fontan procedure connects the right atrium to the pulmonary artery directly or with a conduit, and the atrial septal defect is closed.

PULMONARY ARTERY BANDING. Pulmonary artery banding is narrowing the pulmonary artery with a band to reduce blood flow and pressure in the lungs. It is used for temporary repair of ventricular septal defect, atrio-ventricular canal defect, and tricuspid atresia. Later, the band can be removed and the defect corrected with a complete repair once the patient has grown.

ROSS PROCEDURE. To correct aortic stenosis, the Ross procedure grafts the pulmonary artery to the aorta.

SHUNT PROCEDURE. For tetralogy of Fallot, tricuspid atresia, or pulmonary atresia, the shunt procedure creates a passage between blood vessels, directing blood flow into the pulmonary or systemic circulations.

OTHER TYPES OF SURGERY. Surgical procedures are also used to treat common congenital heart defects. To close a medium to large ventricular or atrial septal defect, it is recommended that it be sutured or covered with a Dacron patch. For patent ductus arteriosus, surgery consists of dividing the ductus into two and tying off the ends. If performed within the child's first few years, there is practically no risk associated with this operation. Surgery for coarctation of the aorta involves opening the chest wall, removing the defect, and reconnecting the ends of the aorta. If the defect is too long to be reconnected, a Dacron graft is used to replace the missing piece.

Diagnosis/Preparation

Before surgery for congenital heart defects, the patient will receive a complete evaluation, which includes a physical exam, a detailed family history, a **chest x ray**, an **electrocardiogram**, an echocardiogram, and usually, cardiac catheterization. Blood tests will be performed to measure formed blood elements, electrolytes, and blood glucose. Additional tests for sickle cell and digoxin levels may be performed, if applicable. For six to eight hours before the surgery, the patient cannot eat or drink anything.

Aftercare

After heart surgery for congenital defects, the patient goes to an **intensive care unit** for continued cardiac monitoring. The patient may also require continued ventilator support. Chest tubes allow blood to be drained from inside the chest as the surgical site heals. Pain medications will be continued, and the patient may remain under general anesthetic. Within 24 hours, the chest tubes and ventilation may be discontinued. Any cardiac drugs used to help the heart perform better will be adjusted appropriate with the patient's condition.

For temporary procedures, additional follow-up with the physician will be required to judge timing for complete repair. In the meantime, the patient should continue to grow and thrive normally. Complete repair requires follow-up with the physician initially to judge the adequacy of repair, but thereafter will be infrequent with good prognosis. The child should be made aware of any procedure to be communicated for future medical care in adulthood.

Risks

Depending on the institution and the type of congenital defect repair, many risks can be identified, including shock, congestive heart failure, lack of oxygen or too much carbon dioxide in the blood, irregular heartbeat, stroke, infection, kidney damage, lung blood clot, low blood pressure, hemorrhage, cardiac arrest, and **death**. These risks should not impede the surgical procedure, as death is certain without surgical treatment. Neurological dysfunction in the postoperative period occurs in as much as 25% of surgical patients. Seizures are expected in 20% of cases, but are usually limited with no long-

term effects. Additional risks include blood **transfusion** reactions and blood-borne pathogens.

Morbidity and mortality rates

Use of cardiopulmonary bypass has associated risks not related to the congenital defect repair. Procedures performed in association with cardiac catheterization have excellent long-term results, with an associated mortality of 2–4% of procedures. The Fontan procedure carries a survival rate of over 90%. Surgical procedures to repair coarctation of the aorta, in uncomplicated cases, has a risk of operative mortality from 1–2%.

Alternatives

Alternatives are limited for this patient population. Cardiac transplant is an option, but a limited number of organ donors restrict this treatment. Ventricular-assist devices and total artificial heart technology are not yet a suitable option. Temporary procedures do allow additional growth of the patient prior to corrective surgery, allowing them to gain strength and size before treatment.

Resources

BOOKS

"Congenital Heart Disease." In *Current Medical Diagnosis and Treatment*, 37th edition, edited by Stephen McPhee, et al. Stamford: Appleton & Lange, 1997.

Davies, Laurie K., and Daniel G. Knauf. "Anesthetic Management for Patients with Congenital Heart Disease." In *A Practical Approach to Cardiac Anesthesia*, 3rd edition, edited by Frederick A. Hensley, Jr., Donal E. Martin, and Glenn P. Gravlee. Philadelphia, PA: Lippincott Williams & Wilkins, 2000.

DeBakey, Michael E., and Antonio M. Gotto Jr. "Congenital Abnormalities of the Heart." In *The New Living Heart*. Holbrook, MA: Adams Media Corporation, 1997.

Park, Myung K. *Pediatric Cardiology for Practitioners*, 3rd edition. St. Louis: Mosby, 1996.

Texas Heart Institute. "Congenital Heart Disease." In *Texas Heart Institute Heart Owners Handbook*. New York: John Wiley & Sons, 1996.

PERIODICALS

Hicks, George L. "Cardiac Surgery." *Journal of the American College of Surgeons*, 186, no. 2 (February 1998): 129–132.

Rao, P. S. "Interventional Pediatric Cardiology: State of the Art and Future Directions." *Pediatric Cardiology*, 19 (1998): 107–124.

ORGANIZATIONS

American Heart Association. 7320 Greenville Ave., Dallas, TX 75231. (214) 373-6300. http://www.americanheart.org.

Children's Health Information Network. 1561 Clark Drive, Yardley, PA 19067. (215) 493-3068. http://www.tchin.org.

Congenital Heart Anomalies Support, Education & Resources, Inc. 2112 North Wilkins Road, Swanton, OH 43558. (419) 825-5575. http://www.csun.edu/~hfmth006/chaser.

Texas Heart Institute. Heart Information Service. P.O. Box 20345, Houston, TX 77225-0345. http://www.tmc.edu/thi.

Lori De Milto
Allison J. Spiwak, MSBME

Heart transplantation

Definition

Heart transplantation, also called cardiac transplantation, is the replacement of a patient's diseased or injured heart with a healthy donor heart.

Purpose

Heart transplantation is performed on patients with end-stage heart failure or some other life-threatening heart disease. Before a doctor recommends heart transplantation for a patient, all other possible treatments for his or her disease must have been attempted. The purpose of heart transplantation is to extend and improve the life of a person who would otherwise die from heart failure. Most patients who receive a new heart are so sick before transplantation that they cannot live a normal life. Replacing a patient's diseased heart with a healthy, functioning donor heart often allows the recipient to return to normal daily activities.

Demographics

Heart transplant recipients are not limited by sex, race, or ethnicity. Nevertheless, because healthy donor hearts are in short supply, strict rules dictate criteria for heart transplant recipients. Patients who may be too sick to survive the surgery or the side effects of immunosuppressive therapy would not be good transplant candidates.

In 2008, according to the Organ Procurement and Transplantation Network, 2,030 heart transplants were performed in the United States, bringing the total performed since 1988 to 49,132. Of these, people between the ages of 50 and 64 were most likely to receive a heart transplant, while children ages 6–10 were least likely to have heart transplantation surgery. In 2007, men received almost three times more heart transplants than women, and whites had more than twice as many heart transplants as all other races/ethnicities combined. The primary diagnoses of adult patients receiving heart transplantation include coronary artery disease, cardiomyopathy, congenital heart diseases, and retransplantation associated with organ rejection.

These conditions are contraindications for heart transplantation:

- active infection;
- pulmonary hypertension;
- chronic lung disease with loss of more than 40% of lung function;
- untreatable liver or kidney disease;
- diabetes that has caused serious damage to vital organs;
- disease of the blood vessels in the brain, such as a stroke;
- serious disease of the arteries;

Heart transplantation

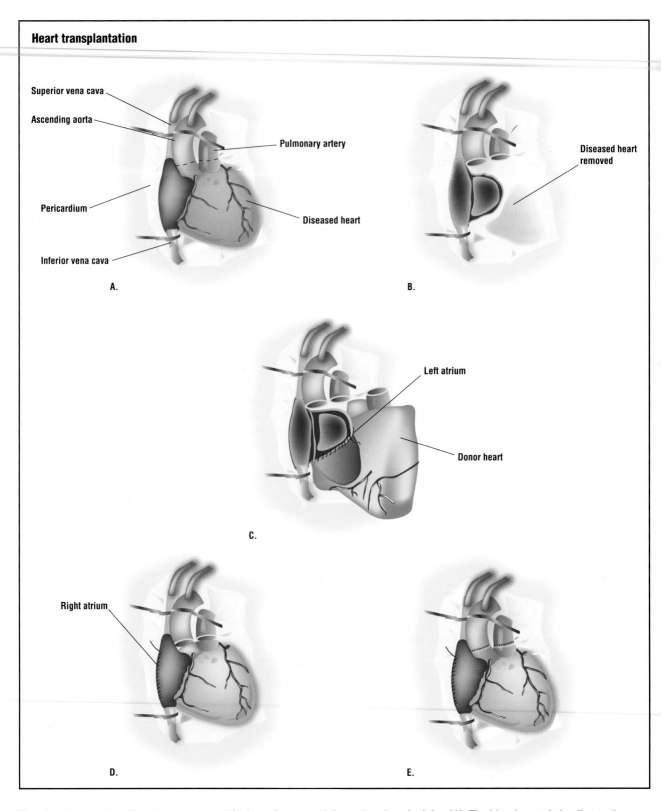

A.

Superior vena cava

Ascending aorta

Pulmonary artery

Pericardium

Diseased heart

Inferior vena cava

B.

Diseased heart removed

C.

Left atrium

Donor heart

D.

Right atrium

E.

For a heart transplantation, the area around the heart is exposed through a chest incision (A). The blood vessels leading to the heart are clamped, and the heart function is replaced by a heart-lung machine. The diseased heart is removed (B). The donor heart is placed in the chest, and the left atrium is attached (C). The right atrium is connected (D), and the aorta and pulmonary artery are finally attached (E). *(Illustration by GGS Information Services. Cengage Learning, Gale.)*

KEY TERMS

Angina—Also called angina pectoris, chest pain or discomfort that occurs when diseased blood vessels restrict blood flow to the heart.

Cardiopulmonary bypass—Mechanically circulating the blood with a heart-lung machine that bypasses the heart and lungs.

Complete blood count (CBC)—A blood test to check the numbers of red blood cells, white blood cells, and platelets in the blood.

Coronary artery disease—Also called atherosclerosis, it is a build-up of fatty matter and debris in the coronary artery wall that causes narrowing of the artery.

Cross-match—A test to determine if patient and donor tissues are compatible.

Echocardiogram—An imaging procedure used to create a picture of the heart's movement, valves, and chambers.

Electrocardiogram (ECG)—A test that measures electrical impulses in the heart.

End-stage heart failure—Severe heart disease that does not respond adequately to medical or surgical treatment.

Endomyocardial biopsy—Removal of a small sample of heart tissue to check it for signs of damage caused by organ rejection.

Graft—To implant living tissue surgically. Graft also refers to the tissue that is transplanted.

Pulmonary hypertension—An increase in the pressure in the blood vessels of the lungs.

• mental illness or any condition that would make a patient unable to take the necessary drugs and treatments on schedule; or

• continuing alcohol or drug abuse.

Description

Patients with end-stage heart disease unresponsive to medical treatment may be considered for heart transplantation. Potential candidates must have a complete medical examination before they can be put on the transplant waiting list. Many types of tests are done, including blood tests, x rays, and tests of heart, lung, and other organ function. The results of these tests indicate to doctors how serious the heart disease is

and whether the patient is healthy enough to survive the **transplant surgery**.

Organ waiting list

A person approved for heart transplantation is placed on the heart transplant waiting list. Patients requesting a heart transplant must be under age 69 at the time they join the list; once on the list they may remain on past that age. All patients on the waiting list are registered with the United Network for Organ Sharing (UNOS). UNOS has organ transplant specialists who run a national computer network that connects all the transplant centers and organ-donation organizations. Patients are grouped in terms of priority based on how long they can live without a transplant. The list is national and independent of the heart transplant center where the surgery will take place. As of 2008, there were 141 UNOS-approved heart transplant programs.

The need for donated hearts outweighs the supply. At any given time, about 3,000 people are waiting for hearts, while only about 2,200 hearts are available each year. When a donor heart becomes available, information about the donor heart is entered into the UNOS computer and compared to information about patients on the waiting list. The computer program produces a list of patients ranked according to blood type, size of the heart, and how urgently they need a heart. Because the heart must be transplanted as quickly as possible, a list of local patients is checked first for a good match. After that, a regional list and then a national list are checked. The patient's transplant team of heart and transplant specialists makes the final decision as to whether a donor heart is suitable for the patient.

The transplant procedure

When a heart becomes available and is approved for a patient, it is packed in a sterile cold solution and rushed to the hospital where the recipient is waiting. The heart can safely remain outside the body for only about four hours, so speed is critical. The recipient will be contacted to return immediately to the hospital if chronic care occurs outside of the hospital.

A general description of the transplant procedure follows. If the operation goes well, the actual surgery takes about three hours.

• The patient undergoes final pre-operative blood work and testing.

• General anesthesia is provided by an anesthesiologist experienced with cardiac patients.

- Intravenous antibiotics are given to prevent bacterial wound infections.
- The patient is put on a heart/lung machine, which performs the functions of the heart and lungs by pumping the blood to the rest of the body during surgery. This procedure is called cardiopulmonary bypass.
- Once the donor heart has arrived to the operating room, the patient's diseased heart is removed.
- The donor heart is attached to the patient's blood vessels, including the atria, pulmonary artery, and aorta.
- After the blood vessels are connected, the new heart is perfused with the patient's blood and begins beating. If the heart does not begin to beat immediately, the surgeon may use defibrillation (electric shock) to gain a productive rhythm.
- The patient is taken off the heart-lung machine.
- The new heart is stimulated to maintain a regular beat with medications and/or a pacemaker for two to five days after surgery, until the new heart functions normally on its own.

Heart transplant recipients are given immunosuppressive drugs to prevent the body from rejecting the new heart. These drugs are usually started before or during the heart transplant surgery. Immunosuppressive drugs keep the body's immune system from recognizing and attacking the new heart as foreign tissue. Normally, immune system cells recognize and attack foreign or abnormal cells such as bacteria, cancer cells, and cells from a transplanted organ. The drugs suppress the immune cells and allow the new heart to function properly; however, they can also allow infections and other adverse effects to occur to the patient because the patient's natural resistance to infections is suppressed.

The chance of rejection is highest during the first few months after the transplantation, therefore, recipients are usually given a combination of three or four immunosuppressive drugs in high doses during this time. Afterwards, they must take maintenance doses of immunosuppressive drugs for the rest of their lives.

Cost and insurance coverage

The total cost for heart transplantation varies considerably, depending on where it is performed, whether transportation and lodging are needed, and whether there are any complications. The National Foundation for Transplants estimates that the cost for uncomplicated heart transplantation surgery in 2007 was about $350,000. This does not include preoperative care and post-operative follow-up visits.

Insurance coverage for heart transplantation varies, depending on the policy. Most commercial insurance companies pay a fixed percentage of heart transplant costs. **Medicare** pays for heart transplants if the surgery is performed at Medicare-approved centers. **Medicaid** pays for heart transplants in some states. Social workers at the transplant center can help patients and their families figure out their insurance coverage and put them in touch with non-profit organizations that help transplant recipients when insurance is inadequate.

Diagnosis/Preparation

Before patients are put on the transplant waiting list, their blood type is determined so a compatible donor heart can be found. The heart must come from a person with the same blood type as the patient, unless it is blood type O negative. A blood type O negative heart is a universal donor and is suitable for any patient regardless of blood type.

A panel reactive antibodies (PRA) test is also done before heart transplantation. This test tells doctors whether the patient is at high risk for having a hyperacute reaction against a donor heart. A hyperacute reaction is a strong immune response against the new heart that happens within minutes to hours after the new heart is transplanted. If the PRA shows that a patient has a high risk for this kind of reaction, then a cross-match is done between a patient and a donor heart before transplant surgery. A cross-match checks how close the match is between the patient's tissue type and the tissue type of the donor heart. Most people are not high risk, and a cross-match usually is not done before the transplant because the surgery must be done as quickly as possible after a donor heart is found.

While waiting for heart transplantation, patients are given treatment to keep the heart as healthy as possible. They are regularly checked to make sure the heart is pumping enough blood. Intravenous medications may be used to improve cardiac output. If these drugs are not effective, a ventricular-assist device can maintain cardiac output until a donor heart becomes available.

Aftercare

Immediately following surgery, patients are monitored closely in the **intensive care unit** (ICU) of the hospital for 24–72 hours. Most patients need to receive oxygen for four to 24 hours following surgery. Continuous cardiac monitoring is used to diagnose and treat donor heart function. Renal, liver, brain, and pulmonary functions are carefully monitored during this time. Patients are then moved to a transplant unit where they remain a week or more.

Heart transplant patients start taking immunosuppressive drugs before or during surgery to prevent immune rejection of the heart. High doses of immunosuppressive drugs are given at this time because rejection is most likely to happen within the first few months after the surgery. A few months after surgery, lower doses of immunosuppressive drugs usually are given, and then must be taken for the rest of the patient's life.

For about three months after the transplant surgery, patients usually come back to the transplant center twice a week for physical examinations and medical tests. These check for signs of infection, rejection of the new heart, or other complications.

In addition to **physical examination**, the following tests may be done during these visits:

- laboratory tests to check for infection;
- **chest x ray** to check for early signs of lung infection;
- electrocardiogram (ECG) to check heart function;
- echocardiogram to check the function of the ventricles in the heart;
- blood tests to check liver and kidney function;
- complete blood counts (CBC) to check the numbers of blood cells; and
- taking of a small tissue sample from the donor heart (endomyocardial biopsy) to check for signs of rejection.

During the physical examination, blood pressure is checked and heart sounds are monitored with a **stethoscope** to determine if the heart is beating properly and pumping enough blood. Kidney and liver functions are checked because these organs may lose function if the heart is being rejected.

An endomyocardial biopsy is the removal of a small sample of the heart muscle. This is done by **cardiac catheterization**. The heart muscle tissue is examined under a microscope for signs that the heart is being rejected. Endomyocardial biopsy is usually done weekly for the first four to eight weeks after transplant surgery, and then at longer intervals after that.

Risks

The most common and dangerous complications of heart transplant surgery are organ rejection and infection. Immunosuppressive drugs are given to prevent rejection of the heart. Most heart transplant patients have a rejection episode soon after transplantation. Rapid diagnosis ensures quick treatment, and when the response is quick, drug therapy is most successful. Rejection is treated with combinations of immunosuppressive drugs given in higher doses than immunosuppressive maintenance. Most of these rejection situations are successfully treated.

Infection can result from the surgery, but most infections are a side effect of the immunosuppressive drugs. Immunosuppressive drugs keep the immune system from attacking the foreign cells of the donor heart; however, the suppressed immune cells are then unable to adequately fight bacteria, viruses, and other microorganisms. Microorganisms that normally do not affect persons with healthy immune systems can cause dangerous infections in transplant patients taking immunosuppressive drugs.

Patients are given **antibiotics** during surgery to prevent bacterial infection. They may also be given an antiviral drug to prevent virus infections. Patients who develop infections may need to have their immunosuppressive drugs changed or the dose adjusted. Infections are treated with antibiotics or other drugs, depending on the type of infection.

Other complications that can happen immediately after surgery are:

- bleeding;
- pressure on the heart caused by fluid in the space surrounding the heart (pericardial tamponade);
- irregular heart beats;
- reduced cardiac output;
- increased amount of blood in the circulatory system; and
- decreased amount of blood in the circulatory system.

Up to half of all heart transplant patients develop coronary artery disease one to five years after the transplant. The coronary arteries supply blood to the heart. Patients with this problem develop chest pains called angina. Other names for this complication are coronary allograft vascular disease and chronic rejection.

Normal results

Heart transplantation is an appropriate treatment for many patients with end-stage heart failure. The outcomes of heart transplantation depend on the

- Is the transplant center listed with UNOS?
- How many transplants have been performed at this center in the last year, and what is the one-year survival rate?
- May I be introduced to the transplant coordinator and any other physicians who may be involved in patient care?
- What precautions are in place to guarantee that the donor heart will be a correct match?
- If the donor heart is rejected, what is the likelihood of another donor heart becoming available?
- Given my situation, how long do you think the wait on the transplant list will be?
- What type of medical treatment will be supplied while awaiting cardiac transplantation?
- What alternative therapies are available?

patient's age, health, and other factors. According to a year 2004 data collected by the Organ Procurement and Transplantation Network, 88% of transplant recipients survive one year. During the first year, infection and acute rejection are the leading causes of **death**. The three-year survival rate is 82% and the five-year survival rate is 79%.

After transplant, most patients regain normal heart function, meaning the heart pumps a normal amount of blood. A transplanted heart usually beats slightly faster than normal because the heart nerves are cut during surgery. The new heart also does not increase its rate as quickly during **exercise**. Even so, most patients feel much better and their capacity for exercise is dramatically improved from before they received the new heart. About 90% of survivors at five years will have no symptoms of heart failure. Patients return to work and other daily activities. Many are able to participate in sports.

Alternatives

End-stage heart disease is associated with a high mortality rate even with associated medical treatment. A ventricular-assist device can be a viable alternative for patients not eligible for cardiac transplant or who are awaiting a donor heart. Such therapies as the total artificial heart may provide other alternatives for the transplant candidate in the future.

Resources

OTHER

DeMarco, Teresa, et al. "Getting a New Heart." *American Society of Transplantation*. December 2006 http://www.a-s-t.org/files/pdf/patient_education/english/AST-EdBroNEWHEART-ENG.pdf (February 5, 2008).

"Heart Transplantation." *Medline Plus*. April 15, 2008. http://www.nlm.nih.gov/medlineplus/hearttransplantation.html (April 20, 2008).

"Heart Transplantation." *Texas Heart Institute*. July 2007. http://www.texasheartinstitute.org/HIC/Topics/Proced/hearttx.cfm (February 5, 2008).

ORGANIZATIONS

American Heart Association, 7272 Greenville Avenue, Dallas, TX, 75231, (800) 242-8721, http://www.americanheart.org.

American Society of Transplantation, 15000 Commerce Parkway, Suite C, Mount Laurel, NJ, 08054, (856) 439-9986, http://www.a-s-t.org.

National Heart, Lung and Blood Institute, National Institutes of Health, P.O. Box 30105, Bethesda, MD, 20824-0105, NHLBIinfo@nhlbi.nih.gov, http://www.nhlbi.nih.gov.

United Network for Organ Sharing, P.O. Box 2484, Richmond, VA, 23218, (804) 782-4800, http://www.unos.org.

Toni Rizzo
Allison J. Spiwak, M.S.B.M.E.
Tish Davidson, A. M.

Heart valve repair *see* **Mitral valve repair**

Heart valve replacement *see* **Mitral valve replacement; Aortic valve replacement**

Heller myotomy

Definition

A Heller myotomy, also called esophagomyotomy, is a surgical procedure during which the muscles of the lower part of the esophagus are cut. This operation is used to treat a condition called "achalasia," in which spasms of the esophagus prevent the normal passage of liquids and food into the stomach.

Purpose

The esophagus is a muscular tube leading from the throat into the stomach. The upper zone of the esophagus is attached to the throat. It is a muscular ring referred to as the "upper esophageal sphincter," or UES, and is responsible for preventing swallowed food and liquid from passing upward from the esophagus and back into the throat. The lowest area of the esophagus is referred to as the "lower esophageal sphincter," or LES. This area joins with the upper part of the stomach, the cardia. A swallowing disorder is the result of the LES's inability to relax. Cutting the LES can relieve this problem, allowing normal eating and drinking to take place.

Achalasia can be either primary or secondary. Primary achalasia occurs on its own, and is a disorder of the LES itself; no other underlying disorder accounts for the condition. Secondary achalasia occurs when there is another disease that has affected LES functioning. The two most common underlying conditions that can result in achalasia are esophageal cancer and Chagas disease. Symptoms of achalasia include difficulty swallowing, regurgitation, and weight loss.

Men are three to four times more likely to develop esophageal cancer than are women, and African-Americans are about 50% more likely to develop the condition. According to the American Cancer Society, about 16,470 new cases of esophageal cancer will be diagnosed in the United States in 2008, and the disease will be responsible for about 14,280 deaths. The disease is much more common in other countries, such as Iran, northern China, India, and southern Africa, where rates are between ten and 100 times as high as they are in the United States. Still, esophageal cancer rates among white men in Western countries are increasing steadily, at a rate of about 2% per year; the rate has held steady among white women. Among patients diagnosed at all stages of esophageal cancer, five-year survival rates are about 18% in white patients and 11% in African-American patients.

Chagas disease is a parasitic disease found primarily in South America. This protozoan infection is passed to humans during the bite of a bug colloquially referred to as an "assassin bug." It can also be acquired during infected blood transfusions, when food is infected with the protozoa, and by a fetus if its mother is infected. Chagas disease has two phases, acute and chronic. It is during the chronic phase that the lower esophageal sphincter may be affected, causing achalasia.

Achalasia often requires treatment because it can cause a number of complications. Patients with achalasia often suffer from the discomfort of heartburn or gastroesophageal reflux disease. Additionally, the constant exposure of the vulnerable lining of the esophagus to a backwash of stomach acid may result in a condition called Barrett's esophagus. This occurs when the lining cells begin to take on pre-malignant characteristics, and patients have a high risk of eventually developing esophageal cancer. When foods and liquids cannot be fully swallowed, they may also be sucked into the lungs, putting the individual at risk for aspiration pneumonia.

Precautions

Patients who are taking blood thinners, aspirin, or nonsteroidal anti-inflammatory medications may need to discontinue their use in advance of the test, to avoid increasing the risk of bleeding.

Description

Patients undergoing Heller myotomy require general anesthesia. This will be administered in the form of intravenous medications as well as anesthetic gasses that are inhaled. The patient will be intubated and on a ventilator for the duration of the surgery.

A Heller myotomy can be achived through a traditional upper abdominal incision, or through multiple very small laparoscopic incision. These days, the laparasopic approach is most common. Laparoscopic Heller myotomy involves the introduction of a videoscope through one of the keyhole incisions, and the use of other tiny incisions for introducing the miniature surgical instruments necessary for the operation. Once the esophagus is accessed, a lengthwise incision through the outer muscular layer is made. Sometimes, a bit of the stomach is wrapped around the lower part of the esophagus and secured, to try to avoid further gastric reflux. This is referred to as a fundoplication.

Preparations

Patients will need to stop eating and drinking for about 12–16 hours prior to their operation. The evening before the operation, a series of enemas and/or laxatives are used to empty the GI tract of feces. An intravenous line will be placed in order to provide the patient with fluids, general anesthesia agents, sedatives, and pain medicines during the operation. A urinary catheter will be placed in the patient's bladder. The patient will be attached to a variety of monitors to keep track of blood pressure, heart rate, and blood oxygen level throughout the procedure.

Aftercare

The hospital stay after Heller myotomy is usually 2–3 days. Clear liquids are introduced on the same day as the surgery, and within a few days the patient will be allowed to begin taking soft foods. Over time, the patient's diet will slowly be reinstated, progressing gradually from liquids to soft foods to solids. If swallowing remains problematic, a therapist specializing in re-teaching swallowing may be needed to help design a rehabilitative program.

Risks

During the course of a Heller myotomy, there is some risk that the esophagus will become perforated by one of the surgical instruments. Patients who have had a Heller myotomy have a continued high risk of gastric esophageal reflux. Many patients require re-treatment, either another myotomy or removal of a section of esophagus (esophagectomy).

The risk of perforation during Heller myotomy is about 1%. The risk of death is about 0.2%. In general, studies have shown that hospital and surgeon experience with esophagogastrectomy reduces the risk of morbidity and mortality for patients.

Normal results

Normal results occur when the overly tight LES is released, allowing the normal passage of food and liquids through the esophagus and into the stomach.

Abnormal results

Abnormal results include a continued inability to swallow or inadvertent perforation of the esophagus during surgery.

Resources

BOOKS

Abeloff, M. D., et al. *Clinical Oncology,* 3rd ed. Philadelphia: Elsevier, 2004.

Feldman, M., et al. *Sleisenger & Fordtran's Gastrointestinal and Liver Disease.* 8th ed. St. Louis: Mosby, 2005.

Goldman, L., D. Ausiello, eds.*Cecil Textbook of Internal Medicine,* 23rd ed. Philadelphia: Saunders, 2008.

Khatri, V. P., and J. A. Asensio. *Operative Surgery Manual,* 1st ed. Philadelphia: Saunders, 2003.

Townsend, C. M., et al. *Sabiston Textbook of Surgery,* 17th ed. Philadelphia: Saunders, 2004.

Rosalyn Carson-DeWitt, MD

Hemangioma excision

Definition

Hemangioma excision is the use of surgical techniques to remove benign tumors made up of blood vessels that are often located within the skin. Strawberry hemangiomas are often called strawberry birthmarks.

Hemangioma surgery involves the removal of the abnormal growth in a way that minimizes both physical and psychological scarring of the patient.

Purpose

Almost all hemangiomas will undergo a long, slow regression, known as involution, without treatment. The end result of involution is potentially worse than the scarring that would occur with surgery. Thus, surgical intervention is commonly indicated only if the growth of the tumor is life threatening or highly problematic from a medical or psychosocial point of view. For example, tumor growths that affect the ability of the eye to see, the ear to hear, or the passage of air in and out of the lungs are frequently candidates for surgical treatment. Tumors that have ulcerated are also common candidates for surgical treatment. Surgery after involution can be used to remove remaining scar tissue.

Although controversial, some surgeons also recommend surgery before or during the involution process, in an attempt to minimize the final cosmetic deformity. Small lesions that are in areas that can be excised without cosmetic or functional risk are particularly well-suited to early surgical treatment.

Demographics

Hemangiomas are the most common tumor of infancy, occurring in approximately 10–12% of all white children and are nearly twice as common in premature infants. For unknown reasons, the occurrence in children of black or Asian background is much lower, approximately 0.8–1.4%. The tumors have been reported to be from two to six times more common in females than in males. The great majority of these tumors are located in the head and neck, with the remaining appearing throughout the body, including internally.

At present, an estimated 60% of patients with hemangiomas require some form of corrective surgery sometime during recovery from the tumor surgery. The remaining 40% rely on the spontaneous involution process to resolve the lesion, although complete return to normalcy is extremely rare.

Description

Hemangiomas undergo a characteristic set of stages during the tumor development. Approximately 30% are present at birth, with the remainder appearing within the first few weeks of life, often beginning as

KEY TERMS

Angiography—An x ray of the blood vessels after introduction of a medium that increases the contrast between the vessel path and the surrounding tissues.

Benign—Describes a tumor that is not malignant, that is unlikely to recur or spread to other areas of the body.

Embolization—The purposeful introduction of a substance into a blood vessel to stop blood flow.

Involution—The slow healing and resolution stage of a hemangioma.

Lenticular—Lens-shaped; describes a shape of a surgical excision sometimes used to remove hemangiomas.

Proliferation—The rapid growth stage of a hemangioma.

Purse-string closure—A technique used to close circular or irregularly shaped wounds that involves threading the suture through the edges of the wound and pulling it taut, bringing the edges together.

Radial—Star-shaped or radiating out from a central point; used to describe the scar-folds that results from a purse-string closure.

a well-demarcated pale spot that becomes more noticeable when the child cries. The tumors are highly variable in presentation and range from flat, reddish areas known as superficial hemangiomas, to those that are bluish in color and located further under the skin, and are known as deep hemangiomas.

During the first six to 18 months of life, hemangiomas undergo a stage where they grow at an excessive rate in size due to abnormal cell division. The final size of the tumors can range from tiny, hardly noticeable red areas to large, disfiguring growths. In almost all hemangiomas, a long, slow involution process that follows the proliferation stage can take years to complete. Among the first signs of the involution process is a deepening of the red color of the tumor, a graying of the surface, and the appearance of white spots. In general, 50% of all hemangiomas are completely involuted by age five, and 75–90% have completed the process by age seven.

Once a decision to treat a hemangionma with surgery is made, the exact technique to be utilized must also be determined. The most commonly used technique for small lesions is very straightforward and involves removing the abnormal vascular tissue with a lenticular, or lens-shaped excision, that results in a linear scar. Recently, some surgeons have been advocating the use of an elliptical, circular, or irregular incision shapes, followed by a purse-string-type closure. This technique does result in a scar having radial (star-shaped) ridges that can take several weeks to flatten. However, the overall result is a shorter scar that can be followed up by removal, using the lenticular excision technique.

Larger, more extensive lesions may require **angiography**, a process that maps the path of the vessels feeding the lesion, and embolization, the deliberate blocking of these blood vessels using small particles of inert material. This process is followed by complete removal of the abnormal tissue.

Depending on the size and nature of the tumor, the excision surgery can be done on an outpatient or inpatient basis. For very small lesions, local anesthetic may be sufficient, but for the great majority, **general anesthesia** is necessary to keep the patient comfortable.

Diagnosis/Preparation

Initial correct diagnosis of the hemangioma is necessary for effective treatment. Generally, hemangiomas are not present at birth; they proliferate during the first year of the patient's life, and then commonly begin an involution process. These clinical characteristics distinguish hemangiomas from another type of congenital vascular lesion called a vascular malformation. Vascular malformations are always present at birth, do not proliferate, and do not involute. Vascular malformations are developmental abnormalities and can involve veins, arteries, or lymphatic tissue. Because of the lack of rapid proliferation, the expectation for vascular malformations differs from those with a hemangioma, and so the precise type of lesion has a significant impact on treatment decisions.

Aftercare

Aftercare for a hemangioma excision involves **wound care** and maintenance such as changing of **bandages**.

Risks

The greatest risk of hemangioma excision is bleeding during the operation, as these tumors are comprised of abnormal blood vessels. Surgeons often utilize special surgical tools to reduce this risk, including thermoscalpels (an electrically heated scapel) and electrocauteries (a tool that stops bleeding using an electrical charge).

A second risk of the surgery is recurrence of the tumor, that is, an incomplete excision of the abnormally growing tissue. Surgery may also result in scarring that is at least as noticeable as what would remain after involution, if not more so. Patients and their caregivers should carefully consider this possibility when deciding to undergo surgical treatment for hemangiomas.

Other risks of the surgery are very low, and include those that accompany any surgical procedure, such as reactions to anesthesia and possible infections of the incision.

Normal results

Completely normal appearance after surgery is very rare. However, for significantly disfiguring tumors or those that impact physical function, the surgical scar may be preferable to the presence of the tumor.

Morbidity and mortality rates

Morbidity and mortality resulting from this surgery is close to zero, particularly because of the new surgical techniques and tools that prevent intra-operative bleeding of the tumor.

Alternatives

Several alternatives to surgical excision include observation ("watchful waiting"), treatment with steroids during the proliferation stage to shrink the tumor and speed the involution process, and **laser surgery** techniques to alter the appearance of the tumor. Commonly, a combination of these treatment methods, including surgery, will be used to tailor a therapeutic approach for a patient's particular tumor.

Resources

BOOKS

DuFresne, Craig R. "The Management of Hemangiomas and Vascular Malformations of the Head and Neck." In *Plastic Surgery: Indications, Operations, and Outcomes,* Volume 2, edited by Craig A. Vander Kolk, et al. St. Louis, MO: Mosby, 2000.

Waner, Milton, and James Y. Suen. *Hemangiomas and Vascular Malformations of the Head and Neck.* New York: Wiley-Liss, 1999.

PERIODICALS

Mulliken, John B., Gary F. Rogers, and Jennifer J. Marler. "Circular Excision of Hemangioma and Purse-String Closure: The Smallest Possible Scar." *Plastic and Reconstructive Surgery* 109 (April 15, 2002): 1544.

ORGANIZATIONS

American Society of Plastic Surgeons. 444 E. Algonquin Rd. Arlington Heights, IL 60005. (800) 475-2784.www. plasticsurgery.org.

Vascular Birthmark Foundation. P.O. Box 106, Latham, NY 12110. (877) VBF-LOOK (daytime) and (877) VBF-4646 (evenings and weekends). www.birthmark.org.

OTHER

Sargent, Larry A. "Hemangiomas." In *Tennessee Craniofacial Center Monographs,* 2000 [cited March 23, 2003] www.erlanger.org/craniofacial/book.

Michelle Johnson, MS, JD

Hematocrit

Definition

The hematocrit is a test that measures the percentage of blood that is comprised of red blood cells.

Purpose

The hematocrit is used to screen for anemia, or is measured on a person to determine the extent of anemia. An anemic person has fewer or smaller than normal red blood cells. A low hematocrit, combined with other abnormal blood tests, confirms the diagnosis. The hematocrit is decreased in a variety of common conditions including chronic and recent acute blood loss, some cancers, kidney and liver diseases, malnutrition, vitamin B_{12} and folic acid deficiencies, iron deficiency, pregnancy, systemic lupus erythematosus, rheumatoid arthritis and peptic ulcer disease. An elevated hematocrit is most often associated with severe burns, diarrhea, shock, Addison's disease, and dehydration, which is a decreased amount of water in the tissues. These conditions reduce the volume of plasma water causing a relative increase in RBCs, which concentrates the RBCs, called hemoconcentration. An elevated hematocrit may also be caused by an absolute increase in blood cells, called polycythemia. This may be secondary to a decreased amount of oxygen, called hypoxia, or the result of a proliferation of blood forming cells in the bone marrow (polycythemia vera).

Critically high or low levels should be immediately called to the attention of the patient's nurse or doctor. **Transfusion** decisions are based on the results of laboratory tests, including the hematocrit. Generally, transfusion is not considered necessary if the hematocrit is above 21%. The hematocrit is also used as a guide to how many transfusions are needed. Each unit of packed red blood cells administered to an adult is expected to increase the hematocrit by approximately 3% to 4%.

Precautions

Fluid volume in the blood affects hematocrit values. Accordingly, the blood sample should not be taken from an arm receiving IV fluid or during hemodialysis. It should be noted that pregnant women have extra fluid, which dilutes the blood, decreasing the hematocrit. Dehydration concentrates the blood, which increases the hematocrit.

In addition, certain drugs such as penicillin and chloramphenicol may decrease the hematocrit, while glucose levels above 400 mg/dL are known to elevate results. Blood for hematocrit may be collected either by finger puncture, or sticking a needle into a vein, called venipuncture. When performing a finger puncture, the first drop of blood should be wiped away because it dilutes the sample with tissue fluid. A nurse or phlebotomist usually collects the sample following cleaning and disinfecting the skin at the site of the needle stick.

KEY TERMS

Anemia—A lack of oxygen carrying capacity commonly caused by a decrease in red blood cell number, size, or function.

Dehydration—A decreased amount of water in the tissues.

Hematocrit—The volume of blood occupied by the red blood cells, and expressed in percent.

Hypoxia—A decreased amount of oxygen in the tissues.

Polycythemia—A condition in which the amount of RBCs are increased in the blood.

Description

Blood is made up of red blood cells, white blood cells (WBCs), platelets, and plasma. A decrease in the number or size of red cells also decreases the amount of space they occupy, resulting in a lower hematocrit. Conversely, an increase in the number or size of red cells increases the amount of space they occupy, resulting in a higher hematocrit. Thalassemia minor is an exception in that it usually causes an increase in the number of red blood cells, but because they are small, it results in a decreased hematocrit.

The hematocrit may be measured manually by centrifugation. A thin capillary tube called a microhematocrit tube is filled with blood and sealed at the bottom. The tube is centrifuged at 10,000 RPM (revolutions per minute) for five minutes. The RBCs have the greatest weight and are forced to the bottom of the tube. The WBCs and platelets form a thin layer, called the buffy coat, between the RBCs and the plasma, and the liquid plasma rises to the top. The height of the red cell column is measured as a percent of the total blood column. The higher the column of red cells, the higher the hematocrit. Most commonly, the hematocrit is measured indirectly by an automated blood cell counter. It is important to recognize that different results may be obtained when different measurement principles are used. For example, the microhematocrit tube method will give slightly higher results than the electronic methods when RBCs of abnormal shape are present because more plasma is trapped between the cells.

Aftercare

Discomfort or bruising may occur at the puncture site. Pressure to the puncture site until the bleeding stops reduces bruising; warm packs relieve discomfort.

Some people feel dizzy or faint after blood has been drawn, and lying down and relaxing for awhile is helpful for these people.

Risks

Other than potential bruising at the puncture site, and/or dizziness, there are no complications associated with this test.

Normal results

Normal values vary with age and sex. Some representative ranges are:

- at birth: 42-60%
- six to 12 months: 33-40%
- adult males: 42-52%
- adult females: 35-47%

Resources

BOOKS

Chernecky, Cynthia C. and Barbara J. Berger. *Laboratory Tests and Diagnostic Procedures.* 3rd ed. Philadelphia: W. B. Saunders Company, 2001.

Kee, Joyce LeFever. *Handbook of Laboratory and Diagnostic Tests.* 4th ed. Upper Saddle River, NJ: Prentice Hall, 2001.

Kjeldsberg, Carl R. *Practical Diagnosis of Hematologic Disorders.* 3rd ed. Chicago: ASCP Press, 2000.

ORGANIZATIONS

American Association of Blood Banks. 8101 Glenbrook Road, Bethesda, Maryland 20814. (301) 907-6977. Fax: (301) 907-6895. http://www.aabb.org.

Victoria E. DeMoranville
Mark A. Best

Hemispherectomy

Definition

Hemispherectomy is a surgical treatment for epilepsy in which one of the two cerebral hemispheres, which together make up the majority of the brain, is removed.

Purpose

Hemispherectomy is used to treat epilepsy when it cannot be sufficiently controlled by medications.

The cerebral cortex is the wrinkled outer portion of the brain. It is divided into left and right hemispheres, which communicate with each other through a bundle of nerve fibers called the corpus callosum, located at the base of the hemispheres.

The seizures of epilepsy are due to unregulated electrical activity in the brain. This activity often begins in a discrete brain region called the focus of the seizure, and then spreads to other regions. Removing or disconnecting the focus from the rest of the brain can reduce seizure frequency and intensity.

In some people with epilepsy, there is no single focus. If there are multiple focal points within one hemisphere, or if the focus is undefined but restricted to one hemisphere, hemispherectomy may be indicated for treatment.

Removing an entire hemisphere of the brain is an effective treatment. The hemisphere that is removed is usually quite damaged by the effects of multiple seizures, and the other side of the brain has already assumed many of the functions of the damaged side. In addition, the brain has many "redundant systems," which allow healthy regions to make up for the loss of the damaged side.

Children who are candidates for hemispherectomy usually have significant impairments due to their epilepsy, including partial or complete paralysis and partial or complete loss of sensation on the side of the body opposite to the affected brain region.

Demographics

Epilepsy affects up to 1% of all people. Approximately 40% of patients are inadequately treated by medications, and so may be surgery candidates. Hemispherectomy is a relatively rare type of epilepsy surgery. The number performed per year in the United States is likely less than 100. Hemispherectomy is most often considered in children, whose brains are better able to adapt to the loss of brain matter than adults.

Description

Hemispherectomy may be "anatomic" or "functional." In an anatomic hemispherectomy, a hemisphere is removed, while in a functional hemispherectomy, some tissue is left in place, but its connections to other brain centers are cut so that it no longer functions.

Several variations of the anatomic hemispherectomy exist, which are designed to minimize complications. Lower portions of the brain may be left relatively intact, or muscle tissue may be transplanted in order to protect the brain's ventricles (fluid-filled cavities) and prevent leakage of cerebrospinal fluid from them.

Most surgical centers perform functional hemispherectomy. In this procedure, the temporal lobe (that region closest to the temple) and the part of the central portion of the cortex are removed. Additionally, numerous connecting fibers within the remaining brain are severed, as is the corpus callosum, which connects the two hemispheres.

During either procedure, the patient is under **general anesthesia**, lying on the back. The head is shaved and a portion of the skull is removed for access to the brain. After all tissue has been cut and removed and all bleeding is stopped, the underlying tissues are sutured and the skull and scalp are replaced and sutured.

Diagnosis/Preparation

The candidate for hemispherectomy has epilepsy untreatable by medications, with seizure focal points that are numerous or ill defined, but localized to one hemisphere. Such patients may have one of a wide variety of disorders that have caused seizures, including:

- neonatal brain injury
- Rasmussen disease
- hemimegalencephaly
- Sturge-Weber syndrome

The candidate for any type of epilepsy surgery will have had a wide range of tests prior to surgery. These include **electroencephalography** (EEG), in which electrodes are placed on the scalp, on the brain surface, or within the brain to record electrical activity. EEG is used to attempt to locate the focal point(s) of the seizure activity.

Several neuroimaging procedures are used to obtain images of the brain. These may reveal structural abnormalities that the neurosurgeon must be aware of. These procedures will include **magnetic resonance imaging** (MRI), x rays, computed tomography (**CT**) **scans**, or **positron emission tomography** (**PET**) imaging.

Neuropsychological tests may be done to provide a baseline against which the results of the surgery are measured. A Wada test may also be performed, in which a drug is injected into the artery leading to one half of the brain, putting it to sleep. This allows the neurologist to determine where in the brain language and other functions are localized, and may also be useful for predicting the result of the surgery.

Aftercare

Immediately after the operation, the patient may be on a mechanical ventilator for up to 24 hours. Patients remain in the hospital for at least one week.

> ## WHO PERFORMS THE PROCEDURE AND WHERE IS IT PERFORMED?
>
> Hemispherectomy is performed by a neurosurgical team in a hospital. It is also performed by a relatively small number of specialized centers.

Physical and occupational therapy are part of the rehabilitation program to improve strength and motor function.

Risks

Hemorrhage during or after surgery is a risk for hemispherectomy. Disseminated intravascular coagulation, or blood clotting within the circulatory system, is a risk that may be managed with **anticoagulant drugs**. "Aseptic meningitis," an inflammation of the brain's covering without infection, may occur. Hydrocephalus, or increased fluid pressure within the remaining brain, may occur in 20–30% of patients. **Death** from surgery is a risk that has decreased as surgical techniques have improved, but it still occurs in approximately 2% of patients.

The patient will lose any remaining sensation or muscle control in the extremities on the side opposite the removed hemisphere. However, upper arm and thigh movements may be retained, allowing adapted function with these parts of the body.

Normal results

Seizures are eliminated in 70–85% of patients, and reduced by 80% in another 10–20% of patients. Patients with Rasmussen disease, which is progressive, will not benefit as much. Medications may be reduced, and some improvement in intellectual function may occur.

Morbidity and mortality rates

Death may occur in 1–2% of patients undergoing hemispherectomy. Serious but treatable complications may occur in 10–20% of patients.

Alternatives

Corpus callosotomy may be an alternative for some patients, although its ability to eliminate seizures completely is much less. Multiple subpial transection, in which several bundles of nerve fibers are cut, is also an alternative for some patients.

Resources

BOOKS

Devinsky, O. *A Guide to Understanding and Living with Epilepsy.* Philadelphia: EA Davis, 1994.

ORGANIZATIONS

Epilepsy Foundation. http://www.epilepsyfoundation.org.

Richard Robinson

Hemodialysis *see* **Kidney dialysis**

Hemodialysis fistula *see* **Arteriovenous fistula**

Hemoglobin test

Definition

Hemoglobin is a protein inside red blood cells that carries oxygen. A hemoglobin test reveals how much hemoglobin is in a person's blood. This information can be used to help physician's diagnose and monitor anemia (a low hemoglobin level) and polycythemia vera (a high hemoglobin level).

Purpose

A hemoglobin test is performed to determine the amount of hemoglobin in a person's red blood cells (RBCs). This is important because the amount of oxygen available to tissues depends upon how much oxygen is in the RBCs, and local perfusion of the tissues. Without sufficient hemoglobin, the tissues lack oxygen and the heart and lungs must work harder to compensate.

A low hemoglobin measurement usually means the person has anemia. Anemia results from a decrease in the number, size, or function of RBCs. Common causes include excessive bleeding, a deficiency of iron, vitamin B$_{12}$, or folic acid, destruction of red cells by antibodies or mechanical trauma, and structurally

abnormal hemoglobin. Hemoglobin levels are also decreased due to cancer, kidney diseases, other chronic diseases, and excessive IV fluids. An elevated hemoglobin may be caused by dehydration (decreased water), hypoxia (decreased oxygen), or polycythemia vera. Hypoxia may result from high altitudes, smoking, chronic obstructive lung diseases (such as emphysema), and congestive heart failure. Hemoglobin levels are also used to determine if a person needs a blood **transfusion**. Usually a person's hemoglobin must be below 7–8 g/dL before a transfusion is considered, or higher if the person has heart or lung disease. The hemoglobin concentration is also used to determine how many units of packed red blood cells should be transfused. A common rule of thumb is that each unit of red cells should increase the hemoglobin by approximately 1.0–1.5 g/dL.

Precautions

Fluid volume in the blood affects hemoglobin values. Accordingly, the blood sample should not be taken from an arm receiving IV fluid. It should also be noted that pregnant women and people with cirrhosis, a type of permanent liver disease, have extra fluid, which dilutes the blood, decreasing the hemoglobin. Dehydration, a decreased amount of water in the body, concentrates the blood, which may cause an increased hemoglobin result.

Certain drugs such as **antibiotics**, **aspirin**, antineoplastic drugs, doxapram, indomethacin, **sulfonamides**, primaquine, rifampin, and trimethadione, may also decrease the hemoglobin level.

A nurse or phlebotomist usually collects the sample by inserting a needle into a vein, or venipuncture, after cleaning the skin, which helps prevent infections.

Description

Hemoglobin is a complex protein composed of four subunits. Each subunit consists of a protein, or polypeptide chain, that enfolds a heme group. Each heme contains iron (Fe^{2+}) that can bind a molecule of oxygen. The iron gives blood its red color. After the first year of life, 95–97% of the hemoglobin molecules contain two pairs of polypeptide chains designated alpha and beta. This form of hemoglobin is called hemoglobin A.

Hemoglobin is most commonly measured in whole blood. Hemoglobin measurement is most often performed as part of a **complete blood count** (CBC), a test that includes counts of the red blood cells, white blood cells, and platelets (thrombocytes).

Some people inherit hemoglobin with an abnormal structure. The abnormal hemoglobin results from a point mutation in one or both genes that code for the alpha or beta polypeptide chains. Examples of hemoglobin abnormalities resulting from a single amino acid substitution in the beta chain are sickle cell and hemoglobin C disease. Most abnormal hemoglobin molecules can be detected by hemoglobin electrophoresis, which separates hemoglobin molecules that have different electrical charges.

Preparation

No special preparation is required other than cleaning and disinfecting the skin at the puncture site. Blood is collected in a tube by venipuncture. The tube has an anticoagulant in it so that the blood does not clot in the tube, and so that the blood will remain a liquid.

Aftercare

Discomfort or bruising may occur at the puncture site. Pressure to the puncture site until the bleeding stops reduces bruising; warm packs relieve discomfort. Some people feel dizzy or faint after blood has been drawn, and lying down and relaxing for awhile is helpful for these people.

Risks

Other than potential bruising at the puncture site, and/or dizziness, there are usually no complications associated with this test.

Normal results

Normal values vary with age and sex, with women generally having lower hemoglobin values than men.

Normal results for men range from 13–18 g/dL. For women the normal range is 12–16 g/dL. Critical limits (panic values) for both males and females are below 5.0 g/dL or above 20.0 g/dL.

A low hemoglobin value usually indicates the person has anemia. Different tests are done to discover the cause and type of anemia. Dangerously low hemoglobin levels put a person at risk of a heart attack, congestive heart failure, or stroke. A high hemoglobin value indicates the body may be making too many red blood cells. Other tests are performed to differentiate the cause of the abnormal hemoblogin level. Laboratory scientists perform hemoglobin tests using automated laboratory equipment. Critically high or low levels should be immediately called to the attention of the patient's doctor.

Resources

BOOKS

Chernecky, Cynthia C. and Barbara J. Berger. *Laboratory Tests and Diagnostic Procedures*. 3rd ed. Philadelphia: W. B. Saunders Company, 2001.

Kee, Joyce LeFever. *Handbook of Laboratory and Diagnostic Tests*. 4th ed. Upper Saddle River, NJ: Prentice Hall, 2001.

Kjeldsberg, Carl R. *Practical Diagnosis of Hematologic Disorders*. 3rd ed. Chicago: ASCP Press, 2000.

ORGANIZATIONS

American Association of Blood Banks. 8101 Glenbrook Road, Bethesda, Maryland 20814. (301) 907-6977. Fax: (301) 907-6895. http://www.aabb.org.

OTHER

Uthman, Ed. *Blood Cells and the CBC*. 2000. [cited February 17, 2003]. http://web2.iadfw.net/uthman/blood_cells.html (accessed june 12, 2008).

Victoria E. DeMoranville
Mark A. Best, M.D.

Hemoperfusion

Definition

Hemoperfusion is a treatment technique in which large volumes of the patient's blood are passed over an adsorbent substance in order to remove toxic substances from the blood. Adsorption is a process in which molecules or particles of one substance are attracted to the surface of a solid material and held there. These solid materials are called sorbents. Hemoperfusion is sometimes described as an extracorporeal form of treatment because the blood is pumped through a device outside the patient's body.

The sorbents most commonly used in hemoperfusion are resins and various forms of activated carbon or charcoal. Resin sorbents are presently used in Europe but not in the United States; since 1999, all hemoperfusion systems manufactured in the United States use cartridges or columns containing carbon sorbents. A newer type of cartridge containing an adsorbent polymer has been undergoing clinical tests in the United States since the summer of 2002.

Purpose

Hemoperfusion has three major uses:

- to remove nephrotoxic drugs or poisons from the blood in emergency situations (a nephrotoxic substance is one that is harmful to the kidneys);
- to remove waste products from the blood in patients with kidney disease; and
- to provide supportive treatment before and after transplantation for patients in liver failure.

Hemoperfusion is more effective than other methods of treatment for removing certain specific poisons from the blood, particularly those that bind to proteins in the body or are difficult to dissolve in water. It is used to treat overdoses of **barbiturates**, meprobamate, glutethimide, theophylline, digitalis, carbamazepine, methotrexate, ethchlorvynol, and **acetaminophen**, as well as treating paraquat poisoning. Paraquat is a highly toxic weed killer that is sometimes used by people in developing countries to commit suicide.

Description

A hemoperfusion system can be used with or without a hemodialysis machine. After the patient has been made comfortable, two catheters are placed in the arm, one in an artery and one in a nearby vein. After the catheters have been checked for accurate placement, the catheter in the artery is connected to tubing leading into the hemoperfusion system, and the catheter in the vein is connected to tubing leading from the system through a pressure monitor. The patient is given heparin at the beginning of the procedure and at 15–20-minute intervals throughout the hemoperfusion in order to prevent the blood from clotting. The patient's blood pressure is also taken regularly. A typical hemoperfusion treatment takes about three hours.

Hemoperfusion works by pumping the blood drawn through the arterial catheter into a column or cartridge containing the sorbent material. As the blood passes over the carbon or resin particles in the column,

the toxic molecules or particles are drawn to the surfaces of the sorbent particles and trapped within the column. The blood flows out the other end of the column and is returned to the patient through the tubing attached to the venous catheter. Hemoperfusion is able to clear toxins from a larger volume of blood than hemodialysis or other filtration methods; it can process over 300 mL of blood per minute.

Preparation

In emergency situations, preparation of the patient may be limited to cleansing the skin on the inside of the arm with an antiseptic solution and giving a local anesthetic to minimize pain caused by the needles used to insert the catheters.

The hemoperfusion system is prepared by sterilizing the cartridge containing the sorbent and rinsing it with heparinized saline solution. The system is then pressure-tested before the tubing is connected to the catheters in the patient's arm.

Normal results

Normal results include satisfactory clearance of the toxic substance or waste products from the patient's blood. The success of hemoperfusion depends in part, however, on the nature of the drug or poison to be cleared from the blood. Some drugs, such as the tricyclic antidepressants, enter the tissues of the patient's body as well as the bloodstream. As a result, even though hemoperfusion may remove as much as 80% of the drug found in the blood plasma, that may be only a small fraction of the total amount of the drug in the patient's body.

Risks

The risks associated with hemoperfusion are similar to those for hemodialysis, including infection, bleeding, blood clotting, destruction of blood platelets, an abnormal drop in blood pressure, and equipment failure. When hemoperfusion is performed by a qualified health professional, the risks are minor compared to the effects of poisoning or organ failure.

Resources

BOOKS

"Dialysis." In *The Merck Manual of Diagnosis and Therapy,* 18th ed. Edited by Mark H. Beers, Robert S. Porter, Thomas V. Jones, Justin L. Kaplan, and Michael Berkwits. Whitehouse Station, NJ: Merck Research Laboratories, 2006.

"Elimination of Poisons." In *The Merck Manual of Diagnosis and Therapy,* 18th ed. Edited by Mark H. Beers, Robert S. Porter, Thomas V. Jones, Justin L. Kaplan, and Michael Berkwits. Whitehouse Station, NJ: Merck Research Laboratories, 2006.

Nissenson, Allen R., and Richard N. Fine. *Clinical Dialysis,* 4th ed. New York: McGraw-Hill Professional, 2005.

PERIODICALS

Borra, M., et al. "Advanced Technology for Extracorporeal Liver Support System Devices." *International Journal of Artificial Organs* 25 (October 2002): 939–949.

Cameron, R. J., P. Hungerford, and A. H. Dawson. "Efficacy of Charcoal Hemoperfusion in Massive Carbamazepine Poisoning." *Journal of Toxicology: Clinical Toxicology* 40 (2002): 507–512.

Hsu, H. H., C. T. Chang, and J. L. Lin. "Intravenous Paraquat Poisoning-Induced Multiple Organ Failure and Fatality: A Report of Two Cases." *Journal of Toxicology: Clinical Toxicology* 41 (2003): 87–90.

Reiter, K., et al. "In Vitro Removal of Therapeutic Drugs with a Novel Adsorbent System." *Blood Purification* 20 (2002): 380–388.

OTHER

Deshpande, Girish G. "Toxicity. Carbamazepine." *eMedicine.* February 13, 2008. http://www.emedicine.com/ped/topic2732.htm (April 21, 2008).

Kirkland, Lisa, and Alan W. Horn. "Toxicity, Theophylline." *eMedicine.* January 11, 2007. http://www.emedicine.com/med/topic2261.htm (April 21, 2008).

ORGANIZATIONS

American Academy of Emergency Medicine, 555 East Wells Street, Suite 1100, Milwaukee, WI, 53202-3823, (800) 884-2236, http://www.aaem.org.

Center for Emergency Medicine of Western Pennsylvania, 230 McKee Place, Suite 500, Pittsburgh, PA, 15213, (412) 647-5300, http://www.centerem.org.

National Kidney Foundation, 30 East 33rd Street, New York, NY, 10016, (212) 889-2210, (800) 622-9010, http://www.kidney.org.

Society of Toxicology, 1821 Michael Faraday Drive, Suite 300, Reston, VA, 20190, (703) 438-3115, http://www.toxicology.org.

Rebecca Frey, Ph.D.
Laura Jean Cataldo, R.N., Ed.D.

∎ Hemorrhoidectomy

Definition

A hemorrhoidectomy is the surgical removal of a hemorrhoid, which is an enlarged, swollen, inflamed cluster of vascular tissue combined with smooth muscle and connective tissue located in the lower part of the rectum or around the anus. A hemorrhoid is not a varicose vein in the strictest sense. Hemorrhoids are also known as piles.

Purpose

The primary purpose of a hemorrhoidectomy is to relieve the symptoms associated with hemorrhoids that have not responded to more conservative treatments. These symptoms commonly include bleeding and pain. In some cases the hemorrhoid may protrude from the patient's anus. Less commonly, the patient may notice a discharge of mucus or have the feeling that they have not completely emptied the bowel after defecating. Hemorrhoids are usually treated with dietary and medical measures before surgery is recommended because they are not dangerous, and are only rarely a medical emergency. Many people have hemorrhoids that do not produce any symptoms at all.

As of 2003, inpatient hemorrhoidectomies are performed significantly less frequently than they were as recently as the 1970s. In 1974, there were 117 hospital hemorrhoidectomies performed per 100,000 people in the general United States population; this figure declined to 37 per 100,000 by 1987.

Hemorrhoidectomy

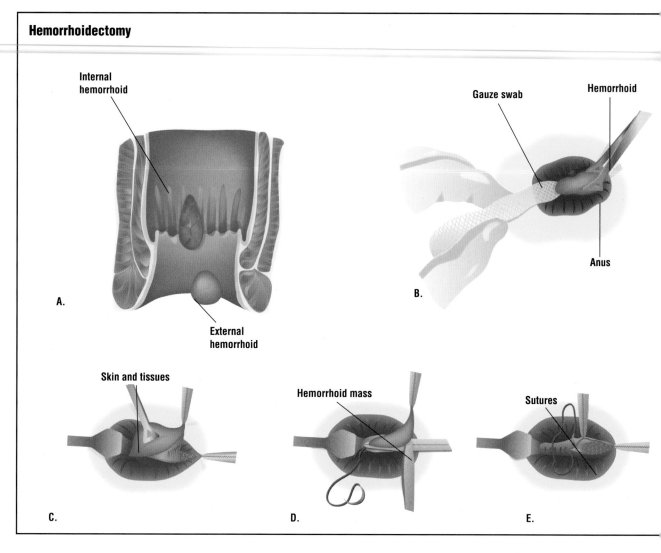

Hemorrhoids can occur inside the rectum, or at its opening (A). To remove them, the surgeon feeds a gauze swab into the anus and removes it slowly. A hemorrhoid will adhere to the gauze, allowing its exposure (B). The outer layers of skin and tissue are removed (C), and then the hemorrhoid itself (D). The tissues and skin are then repaired (E). *(Illustration by GGS Information Services. Cengage Learning, Gale.)*

Demographics

Hemorrhoids are a fairly common problem among adults in the United States and Canada; it is estimated that ten million people in North America, or about 4% of the adult population, have hemorrhoids. About a third of these people seek medical treatment in an average year; nearly 1.5 million prescriptions are filled annually for medications to relieve the discomfort of hemorrhoids. Most patients with symptomatic hemorrhoids are between the ages of 45 and 65.

Risk factors for the development of symptomatic hemorrhoids include the following:

- hormonal changes associated with pregnancy and childbirth
- normal aging
- not getting enough fiber in the diet
- chronic diarrhea
- anal intercourse
- constipation resulting from medications, dehydration, or other causes
- sitting too long on the toilet

Hemorrhoids are categorized as either external or internal hemorrhoids. External hemorrhoids develop under the skin surrounding the anus; they may cause

KEY TERMS

Defecation—The act of passing a bowel movement.

Fistula (plural, fistulae)—An abnormal passageway or opening between the rectum and the skin near the anus.

Ligation—Tying off a blood vessel or other structure with cotton, silk, or some other material. Rubber band ligation is one approach to treating internal hemorrhoids.

Piles—Another name for hemorrhoids.

Prolapse—The falling down or sinking of an internal organ or part of the body. Internal hemorrhoids may prolapse and cause a spasm of the anal sphincter muscle.

Psyllium—The seeds of the fleawort plant, taken with water to produce a bland, jelly-like bulk which helps to move waste products through the digestive tract and prevent constipation.

Resection—Surgical removal of part or all of a hemorrhoid, organ, or other structure.

Sclerotherapy—A technique for shrinking hemorrhoids by injecting an irritating chemical into the blood vessels.

Sphincter—A circular band of muscle fibers that constricts or closes a passageway in the body.

Thrombosed—Affected by the formation of a blood clot, or thrombus, along the wall of a blood vessel. Some external hemorrhoids become thrombosed.

pain and bleeding when the vein in the hemorrhoid forms a clot. This is known as a thrombosed hemorrhoid. In addition, the piece of skin, known as a skin tag, that is left behind when a thrombosed hemorrhoid heals often causes problems for the patient's hygiene. Internal hemorrhoids develop inside the anus. They can cause pain when they prolapse (fall down toward the outside of the body) and cause the anal sphincter to go into spasm. They may bleed or release mucus that can cause irritation of the skin surrounding the anus. Lastly, internal hemorrhoids may become incarcerated or strangulated.

Description

There are several types of surgical procedures that can reduce hemorrhoids. Most surgical procedures in current use can be performed on an outpatient level or office visit under **local anesthesia**.

Rubber band ligation is a technique that works well with internal hemorrhoids that protrude outward with bowel movements. A small rubber band is tied over the hemorrhoid, which cuts off the blood supply. The hemorrhoid and the rubber band will fall off within a few days and the wound will usually heal in a period of one to two weeks. The procedure causes mild discomfort and bleeding. Another procedure, sclerotherapy, utilizes a chemical solution that is injected around the blood vessel to shrink the hemorrhoid. A third effective method is infrared coagulation, which uses a special device to shrink hemorrhoidal tissue by heating. Both injection and coagulation techniques can be effectively used to treat bleeding hemorrhoids that do not protrude. Some surgeons use a combination of rubber band ligation, sclerotherapy, and infrared coagulation; this combination has been reported to have a success rate of 90.5%.

Surgical resection (removal) of hemorrhoids is reserved for patients who do not respond to more conservative therapies and who have severe problems with external hemorrhoids or skin tags. Hemorrhoidectomies done with a laser do not appear to yield better results than those done with a scalpel. Both types of surgical resection can be performed with the patient under local anesthesia.

Diagnosis/Preparation

Diagnosis

Most patients with hemorrhoids are diagnosed because they notice blood on their toilet paper or in the toilet bowl after a bowel movement and consult their doctor. It is important for patients to visit the doctor whenever they notice bleeding from the rectum, because it may be a symptom of colorectal cancer or other serious disease of the digestive tract. In addition, such other symptoms in the anorectal region as itching, irritation, and pain may be caused by abscesses, fissures in the skin, bacterial infections, fistulae, and other disorders as well as hemorrhoids. The doctor will perform a digital examination of the patient's rectum in order to rule out these other possible causes.

Following the digital examination, the doctor will use an anoscope or sigmoidoscope in order to view the inside of the rectum and the lower part of the large intestine to check for internal hemorrhoids. The patient may be given a **barium enema** if the doctor suspects cancer of the colon; otherwise, imaging studies are not routinely performed in diagnosing hemorrhoids. In some cases, a laboratory test called a stool guaiac may be used to detect the presence of blood in stools.

A board certified general surgeon who has completed one additional year of advanced training in colon and rectal surgery performs the procedure. Specialists typically pass a board certification examination in the diagnosis and surgical treatment of diseases in the colon and rectum, and are certified by the American Board of Colon and Rectal Surgeons. Most hemorrhoidectomies can be performed in the surgeon's office, an outpatient clinic, or an ambulatory surgery center.

Preparation

Patients who are scheduled for a surgical hemorrhoidectomy are given a sedative intravenously before the procedure. They are also given small-volume saline enemas to cleanse the rectal area and lower part of the large intestine. This preparation provides the surgeon with a clean operating field.

Aftercare

Patients may experience pain after surgery as the anus tightens and relaxes. The doctor may prescribe narcotics to relieve the pain. The patient should take stool softeners and attempt to avoid straining during both defecation and urination. Soaking in a warm bath can be comforting and may provide symptomatic relief. The total recovery period following a surgical hemorrhoidectomy is about two weeks.

Risks

As with other surgeries involving the use of a local anesthetic, risks associated with a hemorrhoidectomy include infection, bleeding, and an allergic reaction to the anesthetic. Risks that are specific to a hemorroidectomy include stenosis (narrowing) of the anus; recurrence of the hemorrhoid; fistula formation; and nonhealing wounds.

Normal results

Hemorrhoidectomies have a high rate of success; most patients have an uncomplicated recovery with no recurrence of the hemorrhoids. Complete recovery is typically expected with a maximum period of two weeks.

- How many of your patients recover from hemorrhoids without undergoing surgery?
- How many hemorrhoidectomies have you performed?
- How many of your patients have reported complications from surgical resection of their hemorrhoids?
- What are the chances that the hemorrhoids will recur?

Morbidity and mortality rates

Rubber band ligation has a 30–50% recurrence rate within five to 10 years of the procedure whereas surgical resection of hemorrhoids has only a 5% recurrence rate. Well-trained surgeons report complications in fewer than 5% of their patients; these complications may include anal stenosis, recurrence of the hemorrhoid, fistula formation, bleeding, infection, and urinary retention.

Alternatives

Doctors recommend conservative therapies as the first line of treatment for either internal or external hemorrhoids. A nonsurgical treatment protocol generally includes drinking plenty of liquids; eating foods that are rich in fiber; sitting in a plain warm water bath for five to 10 minutes; applying anesthetic creams or witch hazel compresses; and using psyllium or other stool bulking agents. In patients with mild symptoms, these measures will usually decrease swelling and pain in about two to seven days. The amount of fiber in the diet can be increased by eating five servings of fruit and vegetables each day; replacing white bread with whole-grain bread and cereals; and eating raw rather than cooked vegetables.

Resources

BOOKS

"Hemorrhoids." Section 3, Chapter 35 in *The Merck Manual of Diagnosis and Therapy*, edited by Mark H. Beers, MD, and Robert Berkow, MD. Whitehouse Station, NJ: Merck Research Laboratories, 1999.

PERIODICALS

Accarpio, G., F. Ballari, R. Puglisi, et al. "Outpatient Treatment of Hemorrhoids with a Combined Technique: Results in 7850 Cases." *Techniques in Coloproctology* 6 (December 2002): 195-196.

Peng, B. C., D. G. Jayne, and Y. H. Ho. "Randomized Trial of Rubber Band Ligation Vs. Stapled Hemorrhoidectomy for Prolapsed Piles." *Diseases of the Colon and Rectum* 46 (March 2003): 291-297.

Thornton, Scott, MD. "Hemorrhoids." *eMedicine*, July 16, 2002 [June 29, 2003]. www.emedicine.com/med/topic2821.htm.

ORGANIZATIONS

American Gastroenterological Association. 4930 Del Ray Avenue, Bethesda, MD 20814. (301) 654-2055; Fax: (301) 652-3890. www.gastro.org.

American Society of Colon and Rectal Surgeons. 85 W. Algonquin Road, Suite 550, Arlington Heights, IL 60005. www.fascrs.org.

National Digestive Diseases Information Clearinghouse (NIDDC). 2 Information Way, Bethesda, MD 20892-3570. www.niddk.nih.gov.

OTHER

National Digestive Diseases Information Clearinghouse (NDDIC). *Hemorrhoids*. Bethesda, MD: NDDIC, 2002. NIH Publication No. 02-3021. www.niddk.nih.gov/health/digest/pubs/hems/hemords.htm.

Laith Farid Gulli, M.D., M.S.
Bilal Nasser, M.D., M.S.
Nicole Mallory, M.S., PA-C

Hepatectomy

Definition

A hepatectomy is the surgical removal of the liver.

Purpose

Hepatectomies are performed to surgically remove tumors from the liver. Most liver cancers start in liver cells called "hepatocytes." The resulting cancer is called hepatocellular carcinoma or malignant hepatoma.

The type of cancer that can be removed by hepatectomy is called a localized resectable (removable) liver cancer. It is diagnosed as such when there is no evidence that it has spread to the nearby lymph nodes or to any other parts of the body. Laboratory tests also show that the liver is working well. As part of a multidisciplinary approach, the procedure can offer a chance of long-term remission to patients otherwise guaranteed of having a poor outcome.

Demographics

According to the National Cancer Institute (NCI), liver cancer is relatively uncommon in the United States, although its incidence is rising, mostly as a result of the spread of hepatitis C. However, it is the most common cancer in Africa and Asia, with more than one million new cases diagnosed each year. In the United States, liver cancer and cancer of the bile ducts only account for about 1.5% of all cancer cases. Liver cancer is also associated with cirrhosis in 50–80% of patients.

Description

The extent of the hepatectomy will depend on the size, number, and location of the cancer. It also depends on whether liver function is still adequate. The surgeon may remove a part of the liver that contains the tumor, an entire lobe, or an even larger portion of the liver. In a partial hepatectomy, the surgeon leaves a margin of healthy liver tissue to maintain the functions of the liver. For some patients, **liver transplantation** may be indicated. In this case, the transplant surgeon performs a total hepatectomy, meaning that the patient's entire liver is removed, and it is replaced with a healthy liver from a donor. A liver transplant is an option only if the cancer has not spread outside the liver and only if a suitable donor liver can be found that matches the patient. While waiting for an adequate donor, the health care team monitors the patient's health while providing other therapy.

The surgical procedure is performed under **general anesthesia** and is quite lengthy, requiring three to four hours. The anesthetized patient is face-up and both arms are drawn away from the body. Surgeons often use a heating pad and wrappings around the arms and legs to reduce losses in **body temperature** during the surgery. The patient's abdomen is opened by an incision across the upper abdomen and a midline-extension incision up to the xiphoid (the cartilage located at the bottom middle of the rib cage). The main steps of a partial hepatectomy then proceed as follows:

- Freeing the liver. The first task of the surgeon is to free the liver by cutting the long fibers that wrap it.
- Removal of segments. Once the surgeon has freed the liver, the removal of segments can start. The surgeon must avoid rupturing important blood vessels to avoid a hemorrhage. Two different techniques can be used. The first has the surgeon make a superficial burn with an electric lancet on the surface of the liver to mark the junction between the sections marked for removal and the rest of the liver. He or she cuts out the section, and then tears towards the hepatic parenchyma. It is the difference in resistance between the parenchyma and the vessels that allows the surgeon to identify the presence of a vessel. At this point, he/she isolates the vessel by removing the surrounding connective tissue, and then clamps it. The surgeon can then cut the vessel, without any danger to the

Hepatectomy

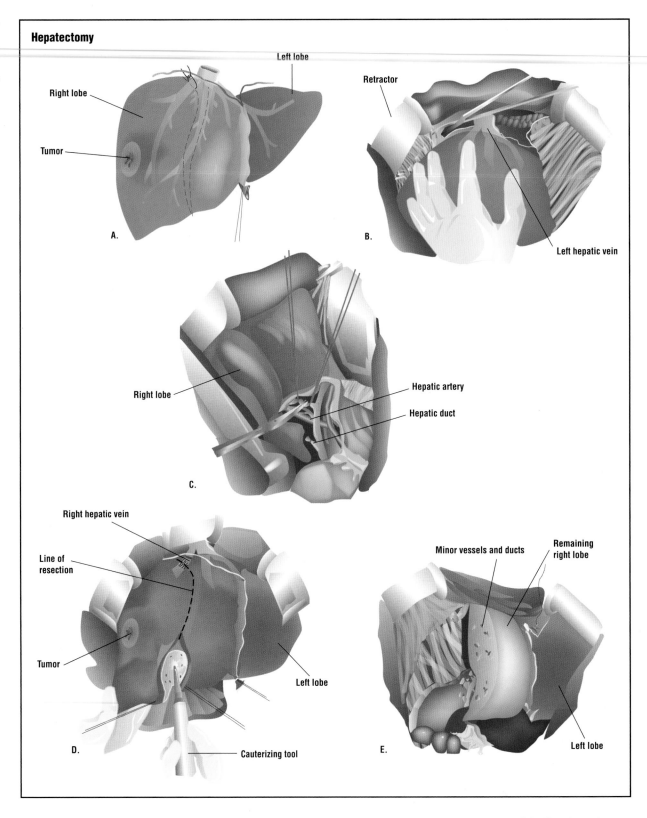

To remove a portion of the liver, the surgeon enters the patient's abdomen, and frees the affected part of the liver from the connecting tissues (B). The artery to the liver and hepatic duct are disconnected from the liver (C). The diseased part of the liver is cut away, and a cauterizing tool is used to stop the bleeding as the surgeon progresses (D). *(Illustration by GGS Information Services. Cengage Learning, Gale.)*

KEY TERMS

Biopsy—The removal of cells or tissues for examination under a microscope.

Cirrhosis—A type of chronic, progressive liver disease in which liver cells are replaced by scar tissue.

Computed tomagraphy (CT) scan—A series of detailed images of areas inside the body taken at various angles; the images are created on a computer linked to an X-ray machine.

Hepatitis—Disease of the liver causing inflammation. Symptoms include an enlarged liver, fever, nausea, vomiting, abdominal pain, and dark urine.

Hepatocellular carcinoma—The most common type of liver tumor.

Hepatocytes—Liver cells.

Hepatoma—A liver tumor.

Magnetic resonance imaging (MRI)—An imaging technique in which a magnet linked to a computer produces images of areas inside the body.

Parenchyma—The essential elements of an organ, used in anatomical nomenclature as a general term to designate the functional elements of an organ, as distinguished from its framework.

Resectable—Part or all of an organ that can be removed by surgery.

patient. The second technique involves identifying the large vessels feeding the segments to be removed. The surgeon operates first at the level of the veins to free and then clamp the vessels required. Finally, the surgeon can make incisions without worrying about cutting little vessels.

Diagnosis/Preparation

A diagnosis of liver cancer requiring an hepatectomy is obtained with the following procedures:

- physical examination;
- blood tests;
- computed tomagraphy (CT) scan;
- ultrasound test;
- magnetic resonance imaging (MRI);
- angiograms; and
- biopsy.

To prepare a patient for a hepatectomy, clean towels are laid across the patient's face, along the sides, and across the knees. The anterior portion of

the chest, the abdomen, and the lower extremities down to the knees are scrubbed with betadine for 10 minutes. In the event of a patient being allergic to iodine, hibiscrub may be used as an alternative. On completion of the scrub, two sterile towels are used to pat the area dry. The area is then painted with iodine in alcohol, and draping proceeds with side drapes, arm board drapes, top and bottom drapes, and a large steridrape. Three suction devices, one diathermy pencil, and a pair of forceps are placed conveniently around the field.

Aftercare

After an hepatectomy, the healing process takes time; the amount of time required to recover varies from patient to patient. Patients are often uncomfortable for the first few days following surgery and they are usually prescribed pain medication. The treating physician or nurse is available to discuss **pain management**. Patients usually feel very tired or weak for a while. Also, patients may have diarrhea and a feeling of fullness in the abdomen. The health care team closely monitors the patient for bleeding, infection, liver failure, or other problems requiring immediate medical attention.

After a total hepatectomy followed by a liver transplant, the patient usually stays in the hospital for several weeks. During that time, the health care team constantly monitors how well the patient is accepting the donated liver. The patient is prescribed drugs to prevent the body from rejecting the transplant, which may cause puffiness in the face, high blood pressure, or an increase in body hair.

Risks

Patients with chronic hepatitis and cirrhosis are at high risk when an hepatectomy is performed.

There are always risks with any surgery, but a hepatectomy that removes 25–60% of the liver carries more than the average risk. Pain, bleeding, infection, and/or injury to other areas in the abdomen, as well as **death**, are potential risks. Other risks include postoperative fevers, pneumonia, and urinary tract infection. Patients who undergo any type of abdominal surgery are also at risk to form blood clots in their legs. These blood clots can break free and move through the heart to the lungs. In the lungs, the blood clot may cause a serious problem called pulmonary embolism, a condition usually treated with blood-thinning medication. In some cases, embolisms can cause death. There are special devices used to keep blood flowing through the legs during surgery to try to prevent clot formation.

There are also risks that are specific only to liver surgery. During the preoperative evaluation, the treatment team tries to evaluate the patient's liver so that they can decide what piece can safely be removed. Removal of a portion of the liver may cause the remaining liver to work poorly for a short period of time. The remaining part of the liver will begin to grow back within a few weeks and will improve; however, a patient may develop liver failure.

Normal results

The results of a hepatectomy are considered normal when liver function resumes following a partial hepatectomy, or when the transplant liver starts functioning in the case of a total hepatectomy.

Morbidity and mortality rates

Liver cancer may be cured by hepatectomy, although surgery is the treatment of choice for only a small fraction of patients with localized disease. Prognosis depends on the extent of the cancer and of liver function impairment. According to the NCI, five-year survival rates are very low in the United States, usually less than 10%. Non-Hispanic white men and women have the lowest incidence of and mortality rates for primary liver cancer. Rates in the black and Hispanic populations are roughly twice as high as the rates in whites. The highest incidence rate is in Vietnamese men (41.8 per 100,000), probably reflecting risks associated with the high prevalence of viral hepatitis infections in their homeland. Other Asian-American groups also have liver cancer incidence and mortality rates several times higher than the white population.

Alternatives

There are no alternatives because hepatectomies are performed when liver cancer does not respond to other treatments.

Resources

BOOKS

Blumgart, L. H., and Y. Fong. *Surgery of the Liver and Biliary Tract,* 3rd ed. Philadelphia: Saunders, 2000.

Carr, B. I. *Hepatocellular Cancer: Diagnosis and Treatment (Current Clinical Oncology).* Totowa, NJ: Humana Press, 2008.

Dionigi, R., and J. Madariaga. *New Technologies for Liver Resections.* Basel, Switzerland: S. Karger Publishing, 1997.

Martin, P. *Liver Transplantation, An Issue of Clinics in Liver Disease.* St. Louis, MO: Elsevier Saunders, 2007.

Okita, K. *Progress in Hepatocellular Carcinoma Treatment.* New York: Springer Verlag, 2000.

PERIODICALS

Ganti, A. L., A. Sardi, and J. Gordon. "Laparoscopic Treatment of Large True Cysts of the Liver and Spleen Is Ineffective." *American Surgeon* 68 (November 2002): 1012–1017.

Hemming, A. W., M. S. Cattral, A. I. Reed, et al. "Liver Transplantation for Hepatocellular Carcinoma." *Annals of Surgery* 233 (May 2001): 652–659.

Joshi, R. M., P. K. Wagle, A. Darbari, D. G. Chhabra, P. S. Patnaik, and M. P. Katrak. "Hepatic Resection for Benign Liver Pathology—Report of Two Cases." *Indian Journal of Gastroenterology* 21 (2002): 157–159.

Kammula, U. S., J. F. Buell, D. M. Labow, S. Rosen, J. M. Millis, and M. C. Posner. "Surgical Management of Benign Tumors of the Liver." *International Journal of Gastrointestinal Cancer* 30 (2001): 141–146.

Matot, I., O. Scheinin, A. Eid, and O. Jurim. "Epidural Anesthesia and Analgesia in Liver Resection." *Anesthesia and Analgesia* 95 (November 2002): 1179–1181.

Zhou, G., W. Cai, H. Li, Y. Zhu, and J. J. Fung. "Experiences Relating to Management of Biliary Tract Complications Following Liver Transplantation in 96 Cases." *Chinese Medical Journal* 115 (October 2002): 1533–1537.

OTHER

Cancer Information Service. National Cancer Institute. http://cis.nci.nih.gov (April 21, 2008).

"Liver Cancer." National Cancer Institute. http://www.nci.nih.gov/cancerinfo/types/liver (April 21, 2008).

ORGANIZATIONS

American College of Surgeons, 633 N. Saint Clair St., Chicago, IL, 60611-3211, (312) 202-5000, (800) 621-4111, (312) 202-5001, postmaster@facs.org, http://www.facs.org.

National Cancer Institute, 6116 Executive Boulevard, Room 3036A, Bethesda, MD, 20892-8322, (800) 422-6237, http://www.cancer.gov.

Society of Toxicology, 1821 Michael Faraday Drive, Suite 300, Reston, VA, 20190, (703) 438-3115, http://www.toxicology.org.

Monique Laberge, Ph.D.
Laura Jean Cataldo, R.N., Ed.D.

Hernia repair, femoral *see* **Femoral hernia repair**

Hernia repair, incisional *see* **Incisional hernia repair**

Hernia repair, inguinal *see* **Inguinal hernia repair**

Hernia repair, umbilical *see* **Umbilical hernia repair**

Heterotopic transplant *see* **Liver transplantation**

Hiatal hernia

Definition

A hiatal hernia is a condition in which a weakness or actual gap or tear in the large muscle of the diaphragm serves as an opening through which the stomach can enter the chest. Hiatal hernias can exist at birth (congenital hiatal hernia) or can develop later in life.

The diaphragm is a large dome-shaped sheet of muscle tissue that spans from the left to the right ribcage. It divides the chest area (thoracic cavity) from the abdominal cavity. The esophageal hiatus is the area of the diagphragm where the esophagus penetrates, joining the stomach below.

Along with other muscles of the abdomen and thoracic cavity, the diaphragm plays an important role in the process of respiration (breathing). During inspiration (breathing in), the muscle of the diaphragm contracts. This increases the volume of the thoracic cavity, and suction allows air to enter the lungs. During expiration, the diaphragm relaxes, and air is expelled from the lungs. The esophagus passes through an area of the diaphragm (the hiatus) on the way to the stomach, which helps prevent the backflow of stomach acid up the esophagus. The diaphragm plays a role in other functions, by virtue of its ability to increase pressure within the abdomen (intra-abdominal pressure)—in this capacity, it is crucial to the acts of vomiting, defecation, and urination.

Demographics

A hiatal hernia can occur due to an injury, or can develop over time due to some inherent weakness in the muscle fibers. Greatly increased intra-abdominal pressure, as may occur during pregnancy, can also induce a hiatal hernia. The following factors may contribute to the development of a hiatal hernia:

- Obesity
- Family history of hiatal hernia
- Repeated straining due to constipation
- Smoking
- Heavy lifting
- Chronic cough
- Extreme bouts of violent vomiting
- Age (about 60% of people develop some degree of hiatal hernia by the time they reach the age of 60)

Description

A hiatal hernia occurs when the stomach enters the chest cavity through a weakness or tear in the area of the diaphragm where the esophagus passes through. The most common form of hiatal hernia occurs when the gastroesophageal junction (the area where the esophagus enters the stomach) slides upward through the hernia opening. This is referred to as a sliding hiatal hernia. A rolling or paraesophageal hiatal hernia is much more rare. In this instance, the gastroesophageal junction doesn't protrude up into the thoracic cavity; instead, a portion of the stomach slides up alongside the esophagus, and protrudes into the chest cavity through the hiatal opening. This type of hiatal hernia is more dangerous, since there is a risk that the narrow confines through which the stomach protrudes will prevent proper blood circulation into this area of the stomach, causing its tissue to become oxygen deprived (strangulated).

While some people can have a hiatal hernia without any recognizable symptoms, other people have clear-cut discomfort related to the condition. Symptoms of a hiatal hernia are very similar to symptoms of gastric acid reflux, and include

- Heartburn
- Chest pain
- Nausea
- Frequent belching

Symptoms often get worse based on position (lying down, leaning forward) and activity (lifting heavy objects, straining for any reason). Over time, symptoms can worsen and cause coughing and asthma-like symptoms, sore throat, and swallowing problems (dysphagia). Anemia can develop when chronic acid reflux causes esophagitis with erosions of the esophagus or upper stomach.

Diagnosis/Preparations

Hiatal hernia is sometimes diagnosed when a **chest x ray** is performed for some other reason. In other instances, tests such as a barium swallow (upper GI series) or upper endoscopy may be performed specifically to look for the presence of a hiatal hernia.

Treatment

Treatment of a hiatal hernia often starts with treatment of the symptoms of gastroesophageal reflux that it induces, including medications such as antacids, H-2 blockers, and proton pump inhibitors. Practical recommendations include weight loss, stopping smoking, elevating the head of the bed at night, so that gravity discourages acid reflux, adjusting the diet to avoid constipation (and therefore straining at stool), and avoiding activities that cause straining (such as heavy lifting).

In some cases, surgical interventions will be required, particularly with very large hiatal hernias or with the rolling or paraesophageal form of hiatal hernia. Several surgical approaches may be utilized, all with the purpose of pulling the stomach back down into the abdomen, and decreasing the size of the hiatal opening. The surgery may be performed through an incision in the chest (thoracic access), abdomen (abdominal access), or using minimally invasive, laparoscopic techniques. Some of the surgeries used include Nissen fundoplication, Belsey (Mark IV) fundoplication, and Hill repair.

Resources

BOOKS

Feldman, M., et al. *Sleisenger & Fordtran's Gastrointestinal and Liver Disease*. 8th ed. St. Louis: Mosby, 2005.
Khatri, V. P., and J. A. Asensio. *Operative Surgery Manual*. 1st ed. Philadelphia: Saunders, 2003.
Townsend, C. M., et al. *Sabiston Textbook of Surgery*. 17th ed. Philadelphia: Saunders, 2004.

Rosalyn Carson-DeWitt, MD

HIDA Scan

Definition

A HIDA scan (hepatobiliary iminodiacetic acid scan), also called cholescintigraphy, is performed in order to assess the patency and functioning of the gallbladder and the bile ducts. A radioactive tracer chemical, called iminodiacetic acid, is injected into a vein. Over time, the radioactive chemical goes to the liver and is excreted into the bile ducts. A special scanner that picks up radioactive signals (similar to a Geiger counter) allows the generation of images of the liver, gallbladder, and bile ducts to be recorded. Although the contrast material utilized is radioactive, the scan itself does not involve any radiation exposure to the patient.

Purpose

HIDA scans are usually done when patients have signs of gallbladder disease, including chronic indigestion, fever, white or clay colored bowel movements, colicky right upper quadrant pain, jaundice, nausea, vomiting.

The gallbladder is an organ that is located behind the liver. It is a muscular pouch that contains fluid called bile which is crucial to the digestion of fats. When crystals form in the bile, the crystals can clump together and create gallstones. Gallstones can irritate the inside of the gallbladder, causing it to become swollen and painful. This condition is called cholecystitis. Gallstones can also block the ducts that lead from the gallbladder, the liver, or the pancreas to the upper part of the small intestine, the duodenum. When this happens, pain in the right upper quadrant of the abdomen can be quite severe. Under very rare circumstances, the obstruction may be caused not by a gallstone, but by the presence of a parasite, blood clot, or tumor. Blockages may also result in jaundice, an increase in bilirubin in the blood which can cause the whites of the eyes and the skin to turn yellow. Sometimes, obstruction of the biliary system leads to bacterial infection, a condition called cholangitis.

KEY TERMS

Bile—A fluid produced by the liver and stored in the gallbladder. Bile is important for the appropriate digestion of fats in the intestine.

Biliary system—The term used to describe the system of ducts that carries the bile flow through the liver and the gallbladder, and ultimately empties into the duodenum.

Cholangitis—A bacterial infection of the biliary system.

Cholecystitis—Swelling and inflammation of the gall bladder.

Duodenum—The first part of the small intestine. The duodenum receives stomach contents, as well as digestive juices from the gallbladder, liver, and pancreas.

Jaundice— A condition in which elevated bilirubin in the bloodstream causes the whites of the eyes and the skin to turn yellow.

Demographics

95% of the time, gallbladder inflammation or cholecystitis is due to the presence of gallstones. Gallstones strike about 0.6% of the general population. Some ethnic groups are more prone to gallstones than others (for example, more than 75% of Native Americans over the age of 60 have gallstones). Between the ages of 20 and 60, women are thre times as likley as men to develop gallstones.

Description

During a HIDA scan, a radioactive dye or tracer is injected into a vein in the arm. As the tracer proceeds through the liver, gallbladder, and small intestine, a scanner positioned over the abdomen records a series of images. Scans are preformed at set intervals (usually about every 5–10 minutes) over the course of the 90-minute examination. If the tracer is moving very slowly through the patient's system, the patient may be asked to return as late as the next day in order to repeat a scan to see whether tracer is still present.

Another chemical, called cholecystokinin or CCK, may also be used during the course of a HIDA scan. CCK stimulates the gallbladder to contract, and images taken following CCK injection can give important information about how well the gallbladder is functioning.

Preparation

Bismuth (found in certain heartburn medicines) and barium (used to perform x-ray studies such as upper and lower GI series) can both interfere with the scanning results. Therefore, patients should be advised to delay undergoing a HIDA scan by at least four days after the use of bismuth or barium. Patients are also asked to stop eating and drinking during the four to twelve hours prior to the HIDA scan. Women who are breastfeeding and who undergo a HIDA scan should feed their baby with formula for two days following the procedure, and should pump and discard their breast milk, since it will be contaminated with the radioactive dye.

Patients are often asked to eat a fatty meal the night before having a HIDA scan.

Aftercare

There is no aftercare necessary following a HIDA scan. The patient can return to a normal diet and normal activities.

Risks

HIDA scans pose very little risk to the patient, although some patients do experience pain during the course of the exam, due to contraction of the inflamed gall bladder. Under rare circumstances, patients may exhibit signs of allergy to the tracer.

Normal results

Normal results of a HIDA scan show the gallbladder in the appropriate anatomical location, with normal measurements and shape. Scanning over time reveals that the tracer progresses in an appropriate and timely fashion through the liver, into the gallbladder, and then into the duodenum.

Abnormal results

A HIDA scan is abnormal when the gallbladder is not normal size, or if a blockage (from either a gallstone or inflammation) prevents the gallbladder or duodenum from being visualized because the tracer cannot flow freely through the normal route. Liver disease may be present if the liver does not take up the tracer from the bloodstream. If tracer is evident outside of the usually path of the biliary system, there may be some kind of a leak from the bile ducts or the gallbladder. If cholecystokinin has been administered, swelling or scarring of the gallbladder wall may be indicated by the continued presence of radioactive tracer in the gallbladder, which cannot perform its normally activity of contracting to empty bile into the duodenum.

Resources

BOOKS

Feldman, M., et al.*Sleisenger & Fordtran's Gastrointestinal and Liver Disease.* 8th ed. St. Louis: Mosby, 2005.

Grainger, R. G., et al. *Grainger & Allison's Diagnostic Radiology: A Textbook of Medical Imaging.* 4th ed. Philadelphia: Saunders, 2001.

Mettler, F. A. *Essentials of Radiology,* 2nd ed. Philadelphia: Saunders, 2005.

Rosalyn Carson-DeWitt, MD

Hip osteotomy

Definition

A hip osteotomy is a surgical procedure in which the bones of the hip joint are cut, reoriented, and fixed in a new position. Healthy cartilage is placed in the weight-bearing area of the joint, followed by reconstruction of the joint in a more normal position.

Purpose

To understand hip surgery, it is helpful to have a brief description of the structure of the human hip. The femur, or thigh bone, is connected to the knee at its lower end and forms part of the hip joint at its upper end. The femur ends in a ball-shaped piece of bone called the femoral head. The short, slanted segment of the femur that lies between the femoral head and the long vertical femoral shaft is called the neck of the femur. In a normal hip, the femoral head fits snugly into a socket called the acetabulum. The hip joint thus consists of two parts, the pelvic socket or acetabulum, and the femoral head.

The hip is susceptible to damage from a number of diseases and disorders, including arthritis, traumatic injury, avascular necrosis, cerebral palsy, or Legg-Calve-Perthes (LCP) disease in young patients. The hip socket may be too shallow, too large, or too small, or the femoral head may lose its proper round contour. Problems related to the shape of the bones in the hip joint are usually referred to as hip dysplasia. **Hip replacement** surgery is often the preferred treatment for disorders of the hip in older patients. Adolescents and young adults, however, are rarely considered for this type of surgery due to their active lifestyle; they have few good options for alleviating their pain and improving joint function if they are stricken by a hip disorder. Osteotomies are performed in these patients, using the patient's own tissue in order to restore joint function in the hip and eliminate pain. An osteotomy corrects a hip deformity by cutting and repositioning the bone, most commonly in patients with misalignment of certain joints or mild osteoarthritis. The procedure is also useful for people with osteoarthritis in only one hip who are too young for a total joint replacement.

Demographics

The incidence of hip dysplasia is four per 1000 live births in the general world population, although it occurs much more frequently in Lapps and Native Americans. In addition, the condition tends to run in families and is more common among girls and first-borns. Acetabular dysplasia patients are usually in their late teens to early thirties, with the female-male ratio in the United States being five to one.

Description

A hip osteotomy is performed under **general anesthesia**. Once the patient has been anesthetized, the surgeon makes an incision to expose the hip joint. The surgeon then proceeds to cut away portions of damaged bone and tissue to change the way they fit together in the hip joint. This part of the procedure may involve removing bone from the femoral head or from the acetabulum, allowing the bone to be moved slightly within the joint. By changing the position of these bones, the surgeon tries to shift the brunt of the patient's weight from damaged joint surfaces to healthier cartilage. He or she then inserts a metal plate or pin to keep the bone in its new place and closes the incision.

There are different hip osteotomy procedures, depending on the type of bone correction required. Two common procedures are:

- Varus rotational osteotomy (VRO), also called a varus derotational osteotomy (VDO). In some patients, the femoral neck is too straight and is not angled far enough toward the acetabulum. This condition is called femoral neck valgus or just plain valgus. The VRO procedure corrects the shape of the femoral neck. In other patients, the femoral neck is not straight enough, in which case the condition is referred to as a femoral neck varus.

- Pelvic osteotomy. Many hip disorders are caused by a deformed acetabulum that cannot accommodate the femoral head. In this procedure, the surgeon redirects the acetabular cartilage or augments a deficient acetabulum with bone taken from outside the joint.

KEY TERMS

Acetabular dysplasia—A type of arthritis resulting in a shallow hip socket.

Acetabulum—The hollow, cuplike portion of the pelvis into which the femoral head is fitted to make the hip joint.

Arthrodesis—Surgical fusion of the femoral head to the acetabulum.

Avascular necrosis—Destruction of cartilage tissue due to impaired blood supply.

Femoral head—The upper end of the femur.

Hip dysplasia—Abnormal development of the hip joint.

Legg-Calve-Perthes disease (LCP)—A disorder in which the femoral head deteriorates within the hip joint as a result of insufficient blood supply.

Osteotomy—The surgical cutting of any bone.

Valgus—A deformity in which a body part is angled away from the midline of the body.

Varus—A deformity in which a body part is angled toward the midline of the body.

Diagnosis/Preparation

A **physical examination** performed by a pediatrician or an orthopaedic surgeon is the best method for diagnosing developmental dysplasia of the hip. Other aids to diagnosis include **ultrasound** examination of the hips during the first six months of life. An ultrasound study is better than an x ray for evaluating hip dysplasia in an infant because much of the hip is made of cartilage at this age and does not show up clearly on x rays. Ultrasound imaging can accurately determine the location of the femoral head in the acetabulum, as well as the depth of the baby's hip socket. An x-ray examination of the pelvis can be performed after six months of age when the child's bones are better developed. Diagnosis in adults also relies on x-ray studies.

To prepare for a hip osteotomy, the patient should come to the clinic or hospital one to seven days prior to surgery. The physician will review the proposed surgery with the patient and answer any questions. He or she will also review the patient's medical evaluation, laboratory test results, and x-ray findings, and schedule any other tests that are required. Patients are instructed not to eat or drink anything after midnight the night before surgery to prevent nausea and vomiting during the operation.

WHO PERFORMS THE PROCEDURE AND WHERE IS IT PERFORMED?

A hip osteotomy is performed in a hospital by surgeons who specialize in the treatment of hip disorders, such as reconstructive orthopedic surgeons, pediatric orthopedic surgeons, and physiatrists.

Aftercare

Immediately following a hip osteotomy, patients are taken to the **recovery room** where they are kept for one to two hours. The patient's blood pressure, circulation, respiration, temperature, and wound drainage are carefully monitored. **Antibiotics** and fluids are given through the IV line that was placed in the arm vein during surgery. After a few days the IV is disconnected; if antibiotics are still needed, they are given by mouth for a few more days. If the patient feels some discomfort, pain medication is given every three to four hours as needed.

Patients usually remain in the hospital for several days after a hip osteotomy. Most VRO patients also require a body cast that includes the legs, which is known as a spica cast. Because of the extent of the surgery that must be done and healing that must occur to restore the pelvis to full strength, the patient's hip may be kept from bearing the full weight of the upper body for about eight to 10 weeks. A second operation may be performed after the patient's pelvis has healed to remove some of the hardware that the surgeon had inserted. Full recovery following an osteotomy usually takes longer than with a total hip replacement; it may be about four to six months before the patient can walk without assistive devices.

Risks

Although complications following hip osteotomy are rare, there is a small chance of infection or blood clot formation. There is also a very low risk of the bone not healing properly, surgical damage to a nerve or artery, or poor skin healing.

Normal results

Full recovery from an osteotomy takes six to 12 months. Most patients, however, have good outcomes following the procedure.

Alternatives

One alternative is to postpone surgery, if the patient's pain can be sufficiently controlled with medication to allow reasonable comfort, and if the patient is willing to accept a lower range of motion in the affected hip.

Surgical alternatives to a hip osteotomy include:

- Total hip replacement. Total hip replacement is an operation designed to replace the entire damaged hip joint. Various prosthetic designs and types of procedures are available. The procedure involves surgical removal of the damaged parts of the hip joint and replacing them with artificial components made from ceramic or metal alloys. The bearing surface is usually made from a durable type of polyethylene, but other materials including ceramics, newer plastics, or metals may be used.
- Arthrodesis. This procedure is rarely performed as of 2003, but is considered particularly effective for younger patients who are short in stature and otherwise healthy. Arthrodesis relieves pain by fusing the femoral head to the acetabulum. It has none of the limitations that a joint replacement or other procedure imposes on the patient's activity level. An arthrodesis is especially suited for patients with strong backs and no other symptoms. The procedure generally requires internal fixation with a plate and screws. The patient may be immobilized in a cast while healing takes place. An arthrodesis can be converted to a total hip replacement at a later date.
- Pseudarthrosis. This procedure is also called a Girdlestone operation. A pseudarthrosis involves removing the femoral head without replacing it with an artificial part. It is performed in patients with hip infections and those whose bones cannot tolerate a reconstructive procedure. Pseudarthrosis leaves the patient with one leg shorter and usually less stable than the other. After this procedure, the patient almost always needs at least one crutch, especially for long-distance walking.

Resources

BOOKS

Browner, B., J. Jupiter, A. Levine, and P. Trafton. *Skeletal Trauma: Fractures, Dislocations, Ligamentous Injuries,* 3rd ed. Philadelphia: Saunders, 2002.

Callaghan, J. J., A. G. Rosenberg, and H. E. Rubash, eds. *The Adult Hip,* 2nd ed. Philadelphia: Lippincott Williams & Wilkins, 2006.

Canale, S. T. *Campbell's Operative Orthopedics,* 10th ed. St. Louis, MO: Mosby, 2002.

Dutton, Mark. *Orthopaedic Examination, Evaluation, and Intervention.* New York: McGraw-Hill, 2004.

Klapper, R., and L. Huey. *Heal Your Hips: How to Prevent Hip Surgery—and What to Do If You Need It.* New York: John Wiley & Sons, 1999.

MacNicol, M. F., ed.*Color Atlas and Text of Osteotomy of the Hip.* St. Louis, MO: Mosby, 1996.

Skinner, Harry. *Current Diagnosis & Treatment in Orthopedics.* New York: McGraw-Hill, 2006.

Staheli, L. T. *Fundamentals of Pediatric Orthopedics,* 4th ed. Philadelphia: Lippincott Williams & Wilkins, 2007.

PERIODICALS

Devane, P. A., R. Coup, and J. G. Horne. "Proximal Femoral Osteotomy for the Treatment of Hip Arthritis in Young Adults." *ANZ Journal of Surgery* 72 (March 2002): 196–199.

Ganz, R., and M. Leunig. "Osteotomy and the Dysplastic Hip: The Bernese Experience." *Orthopedics* 25 (September 2002): 945–946.

Ito, H., A. Minami, H. Tanino, and T. Matsuno. "Fixation with Poly-L-Lactic Acid Screws in Hip Osteotomy: 68 Hips Followed for 18–46 Months." *Acta Orthopaedica Scandinavica* 73 (January 2002): 60–64.

Millis, M. B., and Y. J. Kim. "Rationale of Osteotomy and Related Procedures for Hip Preservation: A Review." *Clinical Orthopaedics and Related Research* 405 (December 2002): 108–121.

OTHER

"Developmental Dysplasia of the Hip." Medical Encyclopedia, MedlinePlus. September 28, 2007. www.nlm.nih.gov/medlineplus/ency/article/000971.htm (April 21, 2008).

"Perthes Disease." American Academy of Orthopaedic Surgeons. October 2007. http://orthoinfo.aaos.org/topic.cfm?topic = A00070&return_link = 0 (April 21, 2008).

"Types of Surgery." Arthritis Foundation. June 6, 2007. http://www.arthritis.org/types-surgery.php (April 21, 2008).

ORGANIZATIONS

American Academy of Orthopaedic Surgeons, 6300 N. River Road, Rosemont, IL, 60018-4262, (847) 823-7186, (800) 346-AAOS, (847) 823-8125, http://www.aaos.org.

American College of Surgeons, 633 N. Saint Clair St., Chicago, IL, 60611-3211, (312) 202-5000, (800) 621-4111, (312) 202-5001, postmaster@facs.org, http://www.facs.org.

American Society for Bone and Mineral Research, 2025 M Street, NW, Suite 800, Washington, DC, 20036-3309, (202) 367-1161, http://www.asbmr.org.

Arthritis Foundation, P.O. Box 7669, Atlanta, GA, 30357-0669, (800) 283-7800, http://www.arthritis.org.

Orthopedic Trauma Association, 6300 N. River Road, Suite 727, Rosemont, IL, 60018-4226, (847) 698-1631, http://www.ota.org/links.htm.

Monique Laberge, Ph.D.
Laura Jean Cataldo, R.N., Ed.D.

Hip prosthesis surgery *see* **Hip revision surgery**

Hip replacement

Definition

Hip replacement is a procedure in which the surgeon removes damaged or diseased parts of the patient's hip joint and replaces them with new artificial parts. The operation itself is called hip **arthroplasty**. Arthroplasty comes from two Greek words, *arthros*, or joint, and *plassein*, "to form or shape." It is a type of surgery done to replace or reconstruct a joint. The artificial joint itself is called a prosthesis. Hip prostheses may be made of metal, ceramic, plastic, or various combinations of these materials.

Purpose

Hip arthroplasty has two primary purposes: pain relief and improved functioning of the hip joint.

Pain relief

Because total hip replacement (THR) is considered major surgery, with all the usual risks involved, it is usually not considered as a treatment option until the patient's pain cannot be managed any longer by more conservative nonsurgical treatment.

Joint pain interferes with a person's quality of life in many ways. If the pain in the hip area is chronic, affecting the person even when he or she is resting, it can lead to depression and other emotional disturbances. Severe chronic pain also strains a person's relationships with family members, employer, and workplace colleagues; it is now recognized to be the most common underlying cause of suicide in the United States.

In most cases, however, pain in the hip joint is a gradual development. Typically, the patient finds that their hip begins to ache when they are exercising vigorously, walking, or standing for a long time. They may cut back on athletic activities only to find that they are starting to limp when they walk and that sitting down is also becoming uncomfortable. Many patients then begin to have trouble driving, sitting through a concert or movie, or working at a desk without pain. It is usually at this point, when a person's ability to live independently is threatened, that he or she considers hip replacement surgery.

Joint function

Restoration of joint function is the other major purpose of hip replacement surgery. The hip joint is one of the most active joints in the human body, designed for many different types of movement. It consists of the head (top) of the femur (thighbone), which is shaped like a ball, and a part of the pelvic bone called the acetabulum, which looks like a hollow or socket. In a healthy hip joint, a layer of cartilage lies between the head of the femur and the acetabulum. The cartilage keeps the bony surfaces from grinding against each other, and allows the head of the femur to rotate or swivel in different directions inside the socket formed by the acetabulum. It is this range of motion, as well as the hip's ability to support the weight of the upper body, that is gradually lost when the hip joint deteriorates. The prostheses that are used in hip replacement surgery are intended to restore as much of the functioning of to the hip joint as possible. The level of function in the hip after the surgery depends in part on the reason for the damage to the joint.

Disorders and conditions that may lead to the need for hip replacement surgery include:

- Osteoarthritis (OA). Osteoarthritis is a disorder in which the cartilage in the joints of the body gradually breaks down, allowing the surfaces of the bones to rub directly and wear against each other. Eventually the patient experiences swelling, pain, inflammation, and increasing loss of mobility. OA most often affects adults over age 45, and is thought to result from a combination of wear and tear on the joint, lifestyle, and genetic factors. OA is the most common cause of joint damage requiring hip replacement.

Acetabulum—The socket-shaped part of the pelvis that forms part of the hip joint.

Analgesic—A medication given to relieve pain.

Ankylosing spondylitis—A form of inflammatory arthritis in which the bones in the spine and pelvis gradually fuse when inflamed connective tissue is replaced by bone.

Arthrodesis—A surgical procedure sometimes used to treat younger patients with hip problems, in which the head of the femur is fused directly to the acetabulum.

Arthroplasty—The medical term for surgical replacement of a joint. Arthroplasty can refer to knee as well as hip replacement.

Autologous blood—The patient's own blood is drawn and set aside for use during surgery in case a transfusion is needed.

Avascular necrosis—A disorder in which bone tissue dies and collapses following the temporary or permanent loss of its blood supply; it is also known as osteonecrosis.

Cartilage—A whitish elastic connective tissue that allows the bones forming the hip joint to move smoothly against each other.

Cortisone—A steroid compound used to treat autoimmune diseases and inflammatory conditions. It is sometimes injected into a joint to relieve the pain of arthritis.

Deep venous thrombosis (DVT)—The formation of a blood clot in the deep vein of the leg. It is considered a serious complication of hip replacement surgery.

Epidural—A method of administering anesthesia by injecting it into the lower spine in the space around the spinal cord. Epidural anesthesia blocks sensation in the parts of the body below the level of the injection.

Femur—The medical name for the thighbone.

Heterotopic bone—Bone that develops as an excess growth around the hip joint following surgery.

Nonsteroidal anti-inflammatory drugs (NSAIDs)—A term used for a group of analgesics that also reduce inflammation when used over a period of time. NSAIDs are often given to patients with osteoarthritis.

Orthopaedics—The branch of surgery that treats deformities or disorders affecting the musculoskeletal system.

Osteolysis—Dissolution and loss of bone resulting from inflammation caused by particles of debris from a prosthesis.

Osteotomy—A surgical alternative to a hip prosthesis, in which the surgeon cuts through the pelvis or femur in order to realign the hip.

Prosthesis (plural, prostheses)—An artificial device that substitutes for or supplements a missing or damaged body part. Prostheses may be either external or implanted inside the body.

Tourniquet—A tube or pressure cuff that is tightened around a limb in order to compress a vein to stop bleeding.

- Rheumatoid arthritis (RA). Rheumatoid arthritis is a disease that begins earlier in life than OA and affects the whole body. Women are three times as likely as men to develop RA. Its symptoms are caused by the immune system's attacks on the body's own cells and tissues. Patients with RA often suffer intense pain even when they are not putting weight on the affected joints.

- Trauma. Damage to the hip joint from a fall, automobile accident, or workplace or athletic injury may trigger the process of cartilage breakdown in the hip joint.

- Avascular necrosis. Avascular necrosis, which is also called osteonecrosis, is a disorder caused by the loss of blood supply to bone tissue. Bone starved for blood supply becomes weak and eventually collapses. The most common reasons for loss of blood supply include trauma, the use of steroid medications, certain blood

disorders, and alcoholism. Avascular necrosis often affects the top of the femur that forms part of the hip joint. It develops most frequently in adults between the ages of 30 and 50.

- Ankylosing spondylitis (AS). Ankylosing spondylitis is a less common form of arthritis that primarily affects the bones in the spine and pelvis. These bones gradually fuse together when the body replaces inflamed tendons or ligaments with new bone instead of elastic connective tissue. AS typically develops in the patient's late teens or early twenties, with three times as many men affected as women.

Demographics

Between 200,000 and 300,000 hip replacement operations are performed in the United States each year, most of them in patients over the age of 60. According to the American Academy of Orthopaedic Surgeons (AAOS), only 5–10% of total hip replacements were in patients younger than 50. There are two reasons for this concentration in older adults. Arthritis and other degenerative joint disorders are the most common health problems requiring hip replacement, and they become more severe as people grow older. The second reason is the limited life expectancy of the prostheses used in hip replacements. Because THR is a complex procedure and requires a long period of recovery after surgery, doctors generally advise patients to put off the operation as long as possible so that they will not need to undergo a second operation later to insert a new prosthesis.

This demographic picture is changing rapidly, however, because of advances in designing hip prostheses, as well as changes in older Americans' rising expectations of quality of life. Many people are less willing to tolerate years of pain or limited activity in order to postpone surgery. In addition, hip prostheses are lasting longer than those used in the 1960s; one study found that 65% of the prostheses in patients who had had THR before the age of 50 were still intact and functioning well 25 years after the surgery. A larger number of hip replacements are now being done in younger patients, and the operation itself is being performed more often. One expert estimates that the annual number of hip replacements in the United States will rise to 600,000 by 2015.

Description

Hip replacement surgery is a relatively recent procedure that had to wait for the invention of plastics and other synthetic materials to make reliable prostheses that could withstand years of wear. The first successful total hip replacement was performed in 1962 by Sir John Charnley (1911–1982), a British orthopedic surgeon who designed a device that is still known as a Charnley prosthesis. Charnley used a stainless steel ball mounted on a stem that was inserted into the patient's thighbone to replace the femoral head. A high-density polyethylene socket was fitted into the acetabular side of the joint. Both parts of the Charnley prosthesis were secured to their respective sides of the joint with acrylic polymer cement. More recent developments include the use of cobalt chrome alloys or ceramic materials in place of stainless steel, as well as methods for holding the prosthesis in place without cement.

There are three major types of hip replacement surgery performed in the United States: a standard procedure for hip replacement; a newer technique known as minimally invasive surgery (MIS), pioneered in Chicago in February 2001; and revision surgery, which is done to replace a loosened or damaged prosthesis.

Standard hip replacement surgery

A standard hip replacement operation takes between one and a half and three hours. The patient may be given a choice of general, spinal, or epidural anesthesia. An epidural anesthesia, which is injected into the space around the spinal cord to block sensation in the lower body, causes less blood loss and also lowers the risk of blood clots or breathing problems after surgery. After the patient is anesthetized, the surgeon makes an incision 8–12 in (20–30 cm) long down the side of the patient's upper thigh. The surgeon may then choose to enter the joint itself from the side, back, or front. The back approach is the most common. The ligaments and muscles under the skin are then separated.

Once inside the joint, the surgeon separates the head of the femur from the acetabulum and removes the head with a saw. The surgeon uses a power drill and a special reamer to remove the cartilage from the acetabulum and shape it to accept the acetabular part of the prosthesis. This part of the new prosthesis is a curved piece of metal lined with plastic or ceramic.

After selecting the correct size for the patient, the surgeon inserts the acetabular component. If the new joint is to be cemented, the surgeon will attach the component to the bone with a type of epoxy. Otherwise, the metal plate will be held in place by screws or by the tightness of the fit itself.

To replace the femoral head, the surgeon first drills a hole inside the thighbone to accept a stem for the femoral component. The stem may be cemented in place or held in place by the tightness of the fit. A metal or ceramic ball to replace the head of the femur is then attached to the stem.

After the prosthesis is in place, an x ray is taken to verify that it is correctly positioned. The incision is then washed with saline solution as a safeguard against infection. The sutures used to close the deeper layers of tissue are made of a material that the body eventually absorbs, while the uppermost layer of skin is closed with metal surgical **staples**. The staples are removed 10–14 days after surgery.

Finally, a large triangular pillow known as a Charnley pillow is placed between the patient's ankles to prevent dislocation of the hip during the first few days after surgery.

Minimally invasive hip replacement surgery

Minimally invasive surgery (MIS) is a new technique of hip replacement introduced in 2001. Instead of making one long incision, the surgeon uses two 2-in (5 cm) incisions or one 3.5-in (9 cm) incision. Using newly designed smaller implements, the surgeon removes the damaged bone and inserts the parts of the new prosthesis. MIS hip replacement takes only an hour and a half. As there is less bleeding, the patient can leave the hospital the next day. However, obese patients or those with very weak bones are not considered for MIS.

Revision surgery

Revision surgery is most commonly performed to replace a prosthesis that no longer fits or functions well because the bone in which it is implanted has deteriorated with age or disease. Revision surgery is a much more complicated process than first-time hip replacement; it sometimes requires a specialized prosthesis, as well as bone grafts from the patient's pelvis, and its results are not usually as good. On the other hand, some patients have had as many as three revision operations with satisfactory results.

Diagnosis/Preparation

Because pain in the hip joint is usually a gradual development, its cause has been diagnosed in most cases by the time the patient is ready to consider hip replacement surgery. The doctor will have taken a careful medical and employment history in order to determine the most likely cause of the pain and whether the patient's job may be a factor. The doctor will also ask about a family history of osteoarthritis as well as other disorders known to run in families. The patient will be asked about injuries, falls, or other accidents that may have affected the hip joint, and about his or her use of alcohol and prescription medications—particularly steroids, which can cause avascular necrosis.

The patient will then be given a complete **physical examination** to evaluate his or her fitness for surgery. Certain disorders, including Parkinson's disease, dementia and other conditions of altered mental status, kidney disease, advanced osteoporosis, disorders associated with muscle weakness, diabetes, and an unstable cardiovascular system are generally considered contraindications to hip replacement surgery. People with weakened immune systems may also be advised against surgery. In the case of obesity, the operation may be postponed until the patient loses weight. The stress placed on the hip joint during normal walking can be as high as three times the patient's body weight; thus, each pound in weight reduction equals three pounds in stress reduction. Consequently, weight reduction lowers an obese patient's risk of complications after the operation.

The doctor will also order an x ray of the affected hip. The results will show the location and extent of damage to the hip joint.

Diagnostic tests

The doctor may also order one or more specialized tests, depending on the known or suspected causes of the pain:

- Aspiration. Aspiration is a procedure in which fluid is withdrawn from the joint by a needle and sent to a laboratory for analysis. It is done to check for infection in the joint.

- Arthrogram. An arthrogram is a special type of x ray in which a contrast dye is injected into the hip to outline the cavity surrounding the joint.

- Magnetic resonance imaging (MRI). An MRI uses a large magnet, radio waves, and a computer to generate images of the head and back. It is helpful in diagnosing avascular necrosis.

- Computed axial tomography (CAT) scan. A CAT scan is another specialized type of x ray that uses computers to generate three-dimensional images of the hip joint. It is most often used to evaluate the severity of avascular necrosis and to obtain a more accurate picture of malformed or unusually shaped joints.

- Bone densitometry test. This test measures the density or strength of the patient's bones. It does not require injections; the patient lies flat on a padded table while an imager passes overhead. This test is most often given to patients at risk for osteoporosis or other disorders that affect bone density.

Preoperative preparation

Hip replacement surgery requires extensive and detailed preparation on the patient's part because it affects so many aspects of life.

LEGAL AND FINANCIAL CONSIDERATIONS. In the United States, physicians and hospitals are required to verify the patient's insurance benefits before surgery and to obtain pre-certification from the patient's insurer or from **Medicare**. Without health insurance, the total cost of a hip replacement can run tens of thousands of dollars. In addition to insurance documentation, patients are legally required to sign an **informed consent** form prior to surgery to signify that the patient is a knowledgeable participant in making healthcare decisions. The doctor will discuss all of the following with the patient before he or she signs the form: the nature of the surgery; reasonable alternatives to the surgery; and the risks, benefits, and uncertainties of each option. Informed consent also requires the doctor to make sure that the patient understands the information that has been given.

MEDICAL CONSIDERATIONS. Patients are asked to do the following in preparation for hip replacement surgery:

- Get in shape physically by doing exercises for strengthening the heart and lungs, building up the muscles around the hip, and increasing the range of motion of the hip joint. Many clinics and hospitals distribute illustrated pamphlets of pre-operation exercises.
- Lose weight if the surgeon recommends it.
- Quit smoking as smoking weakens the cardiovascular system and increases the risks that the patient will have breathing difficulties under anesthesia.
- Make donations of one's own blood for storage in case a transfusion is necessary during surgery. This procedure is known as autologous blood donation; it has the advantage of avoiding the risk of transfusion reactions or transmission of diseases from infected blood donors.
- Have necessary dental work completed before the operation. This precaution is necessary because small numbers of bacteria enter the bloodstream whenever a dentist performs any procedure that causes the gums to bleed. Bacteria from the mouth can be carried to the site of the hip replacement and cause an infection.
- Discontinue taking birth control pills and any anti-inflammatory medications (aspirin or NSAIDs) two weeks before surgery. Most doctors also recommend discontinuing any alternative herbal preparations at this time, as some of them interact with anesthetics and pain medications.

LIFESTYLE CHANGES. Hip replacement surgery requires a long period of **recovery at home** after leaving the hospital. Since the patient's physical mobility will be limited, he or she should do the following before the operation:

- Arrange for leave from work, help at home, help with driving, and similar tasks and commitments.
- Obtain a handicapped parking permit.
- Check the living quarters thoroughly for needed adjustments to furniture, appliances, lighting, and personal conveniences. People recovering from hip replacement surgery must minimize bending, stooping, and any risk of falling.
- Stock up on nonperishable groceries, cleaning supplies, and similar items in order to minimize the need for shopping.
- Have a supply of easy-care clothing with elastic waistbands and simple fasteners in front rather than complicated ties or buttons in the back. Shoes should be slip-ons or fastened with Velcro.

Many hospitals and clinics now have classes for patients scheduled for hip replacement surgery. These classes answer questions regarding preparation for the operation and what to expect during recovery, but in addition they provide opportunities for patients to share concerns and experiences. Studies indicate that patients who have attended these pre-operation classes are less anxious before surgery and generally recover more rapidly.

Aftercare

Aftercare following hip replacement surgery begins while the patient is still in the hospital. Most patients will remain there for five to 10 days after the operation. During this period, the patient will be given fluids and antibiotic medications intravenously to prevent infection. Medications for pain will be given every three to four hours, or through a device known as a PCA (patient-controlled anesthesia), which is a small pump that delivers a dose of medication into the IV when the patient pushes a button. To get the lungs back to normal functioning, a respiratory therapist will ask the patient to cough several times a day or breathe into blow bottles.

Aftercare during the hospital stay is also intended to lower the risk of a venous thromboembolism (VTE), or blood clot in the deep veins of the leg. Prevention of VTE involves medications to thin the blood; exercises for the feet and ankles while lying in bed; and wearing thromboembolic deterrent (TED) or deep vein thrombosis (DVT) stockings. TED stockings are made of nylon (usually white) and may be knee-length or thigh-length; they help to reduce the risk of a blood clot forming in the leg vein by putting mild pressure on the veins. TED stockings are worn for two to six weeks after surgery.

Physical therapy is also begun during the patient's hospital stay, often on the second day after the operation. The physical therapist will introduce the patient to using a walker or crutches and explain how to manage such activities as getting out of bed or showering without dislocating the new prosthesis. In addition to increasing the patient's level of physical activity each day, the physical therapist will help the patient select special equipment for recovery at home. Commonly recommended devices include a reacher for picking up objects without bending too far, a sock cone and special shoehorn, and bathing equipment.

Following **discharge from the hospital**, the patient may go to a skilled nursing facility, rehabilitation center, or directly home. Ongoing physical therapy is the most important part of recovery for the first four to five months following surgery. Most insurance companies in the United States allow home visits by a home health aide, visiting nurse, and physical therapist for three to four weeks after surgery. The physical therapist will monitor the patient's progress, as well as suggest specific exercises to improve strength and range of motion. After the home visits, the patient is encouraged to take up other forms of physical activity in addition to the exercises; swimming, walking, and pedaling a stationary bicycle are all good ways to speed recovery. The patient may take a mild medication for pain (usually **aspirin** or ibuprofen) 30–45 minutes before an **exercise** session, if needed.

Most patients can start driving six to eight weeks after the operation and return to work full time after eight to 10 weeks, depending on the amount and type of physical exertion their jobs requires. Some patients arrange to work on a part-time basis until their normal level of energy returns.

Risks

Hip replacement surgery involves both short- and long-term risks.

Short-term risks

The most common risks associated with hip replacement are as follows:

- Dislocation of the new prosthesis. Dislocation is most likely to occur in the first 10–12 weeks after surgery. It is a risk because the ball and socket in the prosthesis are smaller than the parts of the natural joint, and can move out of place if the patient places the hip in certain positions. The three major rules for avoiding dislocation are: do not cross the legs when lying, sitting, or standing; never lean forward past a 90° angle at the waist; and do not roll the legs inward toward each other—keep the feet pointed forward or turned slightly outward.
- Deep vein thrombosis (DVT). There is some risk (about 1.5% in the United States) of a clot developing in the deep vein of the leg after hip replacement surgery because the blood supply to the leg is cut off by a tourniquet during the operation. The blood-

thinning medications and TED stockings used after surgery are intended to minimize the risk of DVT.
- Infection. The risk of infection is minimized by storing autologous blood for transfusion and administering intravenous antibiotics after surgery. Infections occur in fewer than 1% of hip replacement operations.
- Injury to the nerves that govern sensation in the leg. This problem usually resolves over time.

Long-term risks

The long-term risks of hip replacement surgery include:

- Inflammation related to wear and tear on the prosthesis. Tiny particles of debris from the prosthesis can cause inflammation in the hip joint and lead eventually to dissolution and loss of bone. This condition is known as osteolysis.
- Heterotopic bone. Heterotopic bone is bone that develops in the space between the femur and the pelvis after hip replacement surgery. It can cause stiffness and pain, and may have to be removed surgically. The cause is not completely understood, but is thought to be a reaction to the trauma of the operation. In the United States, patients are usually given indomethacin (Indocin) to prevent this process; in Germany, surgeons are using postoperative radiation treatments together with Indocin.
- Changed length of leg. Some patients find that the operated leg remains slightly longer than the other leg even after recovery. This problem does not interfere with mobility and can usually be helped by an orthotic shoe insert.
- Loosening or damage to the prosthesis itself. This development is treated with revision surgery.

Normal results

Normal results are relief of chronic pain, greater ease of movement, and much improved quality of life. Specific areas of improvement depend on a number of factors, including the patient's age, weight, and previous level of activity; the disease or disorder that caused the pain; the type of prosthesis; and the patient's attitude toward recovery. In general, total hip replacement is considered one of the most successful procedures in modern surgery.

It is difficult to estimate the "normal" lifespan of a hip prosthesis. The figure quoted by many surgeons— between 10 and 15 years—is based on statistics from the early 1990s. It is too soon to tell how much longer the newer prostheses will last. In addition, as hip replacements become more common, the increased size of the worldwide patient database will allow for more accurate predictions. It is known that younger patients and obese patients wear out hip prostheses more rapidly.

Morbidity and mortality rates

Information about mortality and complication rates following THR is limited because the procedure is considered elective. The most important factor affecting morbidity and mortality rates in the United States, according to a Harvard study, is the volume of THRs performed at a given hospital or by a specific surgeon: the higher the volume, the better the outcomes.

Alternatives

Nonsurgical alternatives

The most common conservative alternatives to hip replacement surgery are assistive devices (canes or walkers) to reduce stress on the affected hip; exercise regimens to maintain joint flexibility; dietary changes, particularly if the patient is overweight; and **analgesics**, or painkilling medications. Most patients who try medication begin with an over-the-counter NSAID such as ibuprofen (Advil). If the pain cannot be controlled by nonprescription analgesics, the doctor may give the patient cortisone injections, which relieve the pain of arthritis by reducing inflammation. Unfortunately, the relief provided by cortisone tends to diminish with each injection; moreover, the drug can produce serious side effects.

Complementary and alternative (CAM) approaches

Complementary and alternative forms of therapy cannot be used as substitutes for hip replacement surgery, but they are helpful in managing pain before and after the operation, and in speeding physical recovery. Many patients also find that CAM therapies help them maintain a positive mental attitude in coping with the emotional stress of surgery and physical therapy. CAM therapies that have been shown to relieve the pain of rheumatoid and osteoarthritis include acupuncture, music therapy, naturopathic treatment, homeopathy, Ayurvedic medicine, and certain herbal preparations. Chronic pain from other disorders affecting the hip has been successfully treated with **biofeedback**, relaxation techniques, chiropractic manipulation, and mindfulness meditation.

Some types of movement therapy are recommended in order to postpone the need for hip surgery. Yoga, tai chi, qigong, and dance therapy help to

> ## WHO PERFORMS THE PROCEDURE AND WHERE IS IT PERFORMED?
>
> Hip replacement surgery is performed by an orthopedic surgeon, who has received advanced training in surgical treatment of disorders of the musculoskeletal system. Qualification for this specialty in the United States requires a minimum of five years of training after medical school. Most orthopedic surgeons who perform joint replacements have had additional specialized training in these specific procedures. If surgery is being considered, it is a good idea to find out how many hip replacements the surgeon performs each year; those who perform 200 or more have had more opportunities to refine their technique.
>
> Hip replacement surgery can be performed in a hospital with a department of orthopedic surgery, but is also performed in specialized clinics or institutes for joint disorders. MIS is performed in a small number of specialized facilities and teaching hospitals attached to major university medical schools.

maintain strength and flexibility in the hip joint, and to slow down the deterioration of cartilage and muscle tissue. Exercise in general has been shown to reduce a person's risk of developing osteoporosis.

Alternative surgical procedures

Other surgical options include:

- Osteotomy. An osteotomy is a procedure in which the surgeon cuts the thigh bone or pelvis in order to realign the hip. It is done more frequently in Europe than in the United States, but it has the advantage of not requiring artificial materials.

- Arthrodesis. This type of operation is rarely performed except in younger patients with injury to one hip. In this procedure, the head of the femur is fused to the acetabulum with a plate and screws. The major advantage of arthrodesis is that it places fewer restrictions on the patient's activity level than a hip replacement.

- Pseudarthrosis. In this procedure, the head of the femur is removed without any replacement, resulting in a shorter leg on the affected side. It is usually performed when the patient's bones are too weak for implanting a prosthesis or when the hip joint is badly infected. This procedure is sometimes called a

Girdlestone operation, after the surgeon who first used it in the 1940s.

Resources

BOOKS

Canale, S. T., ed. *Campbell's Operative Orthopaedics*, 10th ed. St. Louis: Mosby, 2003.

DeLee, J. C., and D. Drez. *DeLee and Drez's Orthopaedic Sports Medicine*, 2nd ed. Philadelphia: Saunders, 2005.

Khatri, V. P., and J. A. Asensio. *Operative Surgery Manual*, 1st ed. Philadelphia: Saunders, 2003.

Townsend, C. M., et al. *Sabiston Textbook of Surgery*, 17th ed. Philadelphia: Saunders, 2004.

PERIODICALS

"Arthritis—Hip Replacement." *Harvard Health Letter* 27 (February 2002): i4.

Daitz, Ben. "In Pain Clinic, Fruit, Candy and Relief." *New York Times*, December 3, 2002.

Drake, C., M. Ace, and G. E. Maale. "Revision Total Hip Arthroplasty." *AORN Journal* 76 (September 2002): 414–417, 419–427.

"Hip Replacement Surgery Viable Option for Younger Patients, Thanks to New Prostheses." *Immunotherapy Weekly* (March 13, 2002): 10.

Hungerford, D. S. "Osteonecrosis: Avoiding Total Hip Arthroplasty." *Journal of Arthroplasty* 17 (June 2002) (4 Supplement 1): 121–124.

Laupacis, A., R. Bourne, C. Rorabeck, et al. "Comparison of Total Hip Arthroplasty Performed With and Without Cement: A Randomized Trial." *Journal of Bone and Joint Surgery, American Volume* 84-A (October 2002): 1823–1828.

Lie, S. A., L. B. Engesaeter, L. I. Havelin, et al. "Early Postoperative Mortality After 67,548 Total Hip Replacements: Causes of Death and Thromboprophylaxis in 68 Hospitals in Norway from 1987 to 1999." *Acta Orthopaedica Scandinavica* 73 (August 2002): 392–399.

Mantilla, C. B., T. T. Horlocker, D. R. Schroeder, et al. "Frequency of Myocardial Infarction, Pulmonary Embolism, Deep Venous Thrombosis, and Death Following Primary Hip or Knee Arthroplasty." *Anesthesiology* 96 (May 2002): 1140–1146.

Solomon, D. H., E. Losina, J. A. Baron, et al. "Contribution of Hospital Characteristics to the Volume-Outcome Relationship: Dislocation and Infection Following Total Hip Replacement Surgery." *Arthritis and Rheumatism* 46 (September 2002): 2436–2444.

White, R. H. and M. C. Henderson. "Risk Factors for Venous Thromboembolism After Total Hip and Knee Replacement Surgery." *Current Opinion in Pulmonary Medicine* 8 (September 2002): 365–371.

ORGANIZATIONS

American Academy of Orthopaedic Surgeons (AAOS). 6300 North River Road, Rosemont, IL 60018. (847) 823-7186 or (800) 346-AAOS. http://www.aaos.org (accessed April 1, 2008).

American Physical Therapy Association (APTA). 1111 North Fairfax Street, Alexandria, VA 22314. (703)684-APTA or (800) 999-2782. http://www.apta.org (accessed April 1, 2008).

National Center for Complementary and Alternative Medicine (NCCAM) Clearinghouse. P.O. Box 7923, Gaithersburg, MD 20898. (888) 644-6226. TTY: (866) 464-3615. Fax: (866) 464-3616. http://www.nccam.nih.gov (accessed April 1, 2008).

National Institute of Arthritis and Musculoskeletal and Skin Diseases (NIAMS) Information Clearinghouse. National Institutes of Health, 1 AMS Circle, Bethesda, MD 20892. (301) 495-4484. TTY: (301) 565-2966. http://www.niams.nih.gov (accessed April 1, 2008).

Rush Arthritis and Orthopedics Institute. 1725 West Harrison Street, Suite 1055, Chicago, IL 60612. (312) 563-2420. http://www.rush.edu (accessed April 1, 2008).

OTHER

Hip Universe. http://www.hipuniverse.homestead.com (accessed April 1, 2008).

Questions and Answers About Hip Replacement. Bethesda, MD: National Institutes of Health, 2001. NIH Publication No. 01-4907.

Rebecca Frey, PhD
Rosalyn Carson-DeWitt, MD

Hip revision surgery

Definition

Hip revision surgery, which is also known as revision total hip **arthroplasty**, is a procedure in which the surgeon removes a previously implanted artificial hip joint, or prosthesis, and replaces it with a new prosthesis. Hip revision surgery may also involve

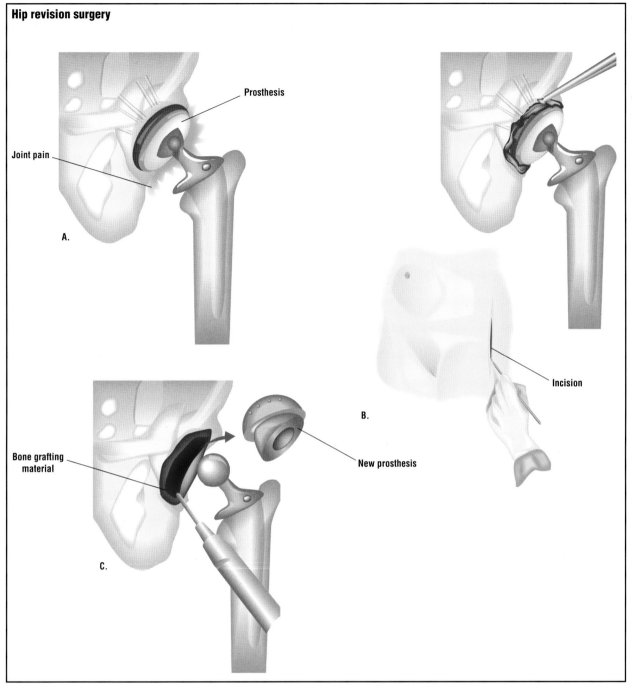

Hip revision surgery

Degeneration of the joint around the prosthesis causes pain for some patients who have undergone hip replacement (A). To repair it, an incision is made in the hip and the old prosthesis is removed (B). Bone grafts may be planted in the hip, and a new prosthesis is attached (C). *(Illustration by GGS Information Services. Cengage Learning, Gale.)*

the use of bone grafts. The bone graft may be an autograft, which means that the bone is taken from another site in the patient's own body; or an allograft, which means that the bone tissue comes from another donor.

Purpose

Hip revision surgery has three major purposes: relieving pain in the affected hip; restoring the patient's mobility; and removing a loose or damaged

Acetabulum—The socket-shaped part of the pelvis that forms part of the hip joint.

Allograft—A graft of bone or other tissue taken from a donor.

Analgesic—A medication given to relieve pain.

Arthroscope—An instrument that contains a miniature camera and light source mounted on a flexible tube. It allows a surgeon to see the inside of a joint or bone during surgery.

Autograft—A graft of bone or other tissue taken from the body of the patient undergoing surgery.

Femur—The medical name for the thighbone. The femur is the largest bone in the human body.

Impaction grafting—The use of crushed bone from a donor to fill in the central canal of the femur during hip revision surgery.

Metaphysis—The widened end of the shaft of a long tubular bone such as the femur.

Orthopedics (sometimes spelled orthopaedics)—The branch of surgery that treats deformities or disorders affecting the musculoskeletal system.

Osteolysis—Dissolution and loss of bone resulting from inflammation caused by particles of polyethylene debris from a prosthesis.

Osteotomy—The cutting apart of a bone or removal of bone by cutting. An osteotomy is often necessary during hip revision surgery in order to remove the femoral part of the old prosthesis from the femur.

Prosthesis (plural, prostheses)—An artificial device that substitutes for or supplements a missing or damaged body part. Prostheses may be either external or implanted inside the body.

Quadriceps muscles—A set of four muscles on each leg located at the front of the thigh. The quadriceps straighten the knee and are used every time a person takes a step.

Templating—A term that refers to the surgeon's use of x-ray images of an old prosthesis as a template or pattern guide for a new implant.

prosthesis before irreversible harm is done to the joint. Hip prostheses that contain parts made of polyethylene typically become loose because wear and tear on the prosthesis gradually produces tiny particles from the plastic that irritate the soft tissue around the prosthesis. The inflamed tissue begins to dissolve the underlying bone in a process known as osteolysis. Eventually, the soft tissue expands around the prosthesis to the point at which the prosthesis loses contact with the bone.

In general, a surgeon will consider revision surgery for pain relief only when more conservative measures, such as medication and changes in the patient's lifestyle, have not helped. In some cases, revision surgery is performed when x-ray studies show loosening of the prosthesis, wearing of the surfaces of the hip joint, or loss of bone tissue even though the patient may not have experienced any discomfort. In most cases, however, increasing pain in the affected hip is one of the first indications that revision surgery is necessary.

Other less common reasons for hip revision surgery include fracture of the hip, the presence of infection, or dislocation of the prosthesis. In these cases, the prosthesis must be removed in order to prevent long-term damage to the hip itself.

Demographics

The demographics of hip revision surgery are likely to change significantly over the next few decades as the proportion of people over 65 in the world's population continues to increase. However, demographic information about this procedure is difficult to evaluate. This difficulty is due in part to the fact that total **hip replacement** (THR) itself is a relatively new procedure dating back only to the early 1960s. Since the design of hip prostheses and the materials used in their manufacture have changed over the last 40 years, it is difficult to predict whether prostheses implanted in the early 2000s will last longer than those used in the past and, if so, whether improved durability will affect the need for revision surgery. On the other hand, more THRs are being performed in younger patients who are more likely to wear out their hip prostheses relatively quickly because they are more active and living longer than the previous generation of THR recipients. In addition, recent improvements in surgical technique as well as in prosthesis design have made hip revision surgery a less risky procedure than it was even a decade ago. One Scottish surgeon has reported performing as many as four hip revisions on selected patients, with highly successful outcomes.

While information on the epidemiology of both THR and hip revision surgery is limited, one study found that three to six times as many THRs were performed as revision surgeries. Women had higher rates of both procedures than men, and Caucasians had higher rates than African Americans. Other researchers have reported that one reason for the lower rate of hip replacement and revision procedures among African Americans is the difference in social networks. African Americans are less likely than Caucasians to know someone who has had hip surgery, and they are therefore less likely to consider it as a treatment option.

Description

Hip revision surgery is hard to describe in general terms because the procedure depends on a set of factors unique to each patient. These factors include the condition of the patient's hip and leg bones; the type of prosthesis originally used; whether the original prosthesis was cemented or held in place without cement; and the patient's age and overall health. Unlike standard THR, however, hip revision surgery is a much longer and more complicated procedure. It is not unusual for a hip revision operation to take from five to eight hours.

The most critical factor affecting the length of the operation and some of the specific steps in hip revision surgery is the condition of the bone tissue in the femur. Defects in the bone are classified in four stages, including:

- Type I. Minimal bone defects.
- Type II. Most of the damage lies at the metaphysis (the flared end of the femur), with minimal damage to the shaft of the bone.
- Type III. All of the damage lies at the metaphysis.
- Type IV. There is extensive bone loss in the femoral shaft as well as at the metaphysis.

The first stage in all hip revision surgery is the removal of the old prosthesis. The part attached to the acetabulum is removed first. The hip socket is cleaned and filled with morselized bone, which is bone in particle form. The new shell and liner are then pressed into the acetabulum.

Revision of the femoral component is the most complicated part of hip revision surgery. If the first prosthesis was held in place by pressure rather than cement, the surgeon usually cuts the top of the femur into several pieces to remove the implant. This cutting apart of the bone is known as osteotomy. The segments of bone are cleaned and the new femoral implant is pressed or cemented in place. If the patient's bone has been classified as Type IV, bone grafts may be added to strengthen the femur. These grafts consist of morselized bone from a donor (allograft bone) that is packed into the empty canal inside the femur. This technique is called impaction grafting. The segments of the femur are then reassembled around the new implant and bone grafts, and held in place with surgical wire.

A newer technique that was originally designed to help surgeons remove old cement from prostheses that were cemented in place can sometimes be used instead of osteotomy. This method involves the use of a ballistic chisel powered by controlled bursts of pressurized nitrogen. The ballistic chisel is used most often to break up pieces of cement from a cemented prosthesis, but it can also be used to loosen a prosthesis that was held in place only by tightness of fit. In addition to avoiding the need for an osteotomy, the ballistic chisel takes much less time. The surgeon uses an arthroscope in order to view the progress of the chisel while he or she is working inside the femur itself.

After all the cement has been removed from the inner canal of the femur, the surgeon washes out the canal with saline solution, inserts morselized bone if necessary, and implants the new femoral component of the prosthesis. After both parts of the prosthesis have been checked for correct positioning, the head of the femoral component is fitted into the new acetabular component and the incision is closed.

Diagnosis/Preparation

Diagnosis

In most cases, increasing pain, greater difficulty in placing weight on the hip, and loss of mobility in the hip joint are early indications that revision surgery is necessary. The location of the pain may point to the part of the prosthesis that has been affected by osteolysis. The pain is felt in both the hip area and the thigh when both parts of the prosthesis have become loose; if only the femoral component has been affected, the patient usually feels pain only in the thigh. However, some patients do not experience any discomfort even though their prosthesis is loosening or wearing against surrounding structures. In addition, a minority of patients who have had THR have always had pain from their artificial joints, and these patients may not consider their discomfort new or significant.

In general, diagnostic imaging that shows bone loss, loosening of the prosthesis, or wearing away of the joint tissues is an essential aspect of hip revision surgery—many orthopedic surgeons will not consider the procedure unless the x-ray studies reveal one or more of these signs. X-ray studies are also used to diagnose fractures of the hip or dislocated prostheses. In some cases, the doctor may order a computed tomography (CT) scan to confirm the extent and location of suspected osteolysis; recent research indicates that **CT scans** can detect bone loss around a hip prosthesis at earlier stages than radiography.

Infections related to a hip prosthesis are a potentially serious matter. Estimated rates of infection following THR range between one in 300 operations and one in 100. Infections can develop at any time following THR, ranging from the immediate postoperative period to 10 or more years later. The symptoms of superficial infections include swelling, pain, and redness in the skin around the incision, but are usually treatable with **antibiotics**. With deep infections, antibiotics may not work and the new joint is likely to require revision surgery.

Preoperative preparation

Certain health conditions or disorders are considered contraindications for hip revision surgery, including:

- a current hip infection
- dementia or other severe mental disorder
- severe vascular disease
- poor condition of the skin covering the hip
- extreme obesity
- paralysis of the quadriceps muscles
- terminal illness

Patients who are considered appropriate candidates for hip revision surgery are asked to come to the hospital about a week before the operation. X rays and other diagnostic images of the hip are reviewed in order to select the new prosthesis. This review is called templating because the diagnostic images serve as a template for the new implant. The surgeon will also decide whether special procedures or instruments will be needed to remove the old prosthesis.

Aftercare

Aftercare for hip revision surgery is essentially the same as for hip replacement surgery. The major difference is that some patients with very weak bones are asked to use canes or walkers all the time following revision surgery rather than trying to walk without assistive devices.

Risks

Risk factors

Factors that lower a patient's chances for a good outcome from hip revision surgery include the following:

- Sex. Men are more likely to have poor outcomes from revision surgery than women.
- Age. Older patients, particularly those over 75, are more likely to have complications following revision surgery.
- Race. African Americans have a higher rate of complications than Caucasian or Asian Americans.
- Socioeconomic status (SES). Patients with lower incomes do not do as well as patients in higher income brackets.
- Presence of other chronic diseases or disorders.
- Obesity. Many surgeons will not perform hip revision surgery on patients weighing 300 pounds or more.
- Genetic factors. Recent British research indicates that patients who carry an inflammation control gene known as TNF-238A are twice as likely to require replacement of a hip prosthesis as those who lack this gene.

Specific risks of hip revision surgery

Risks following hip revision surgery are similar to those following hip replacement surgery, including deep venous thrombosis and infection. The length of the patient's leg, however, is more likely to be affected following revision surgery. Dislocation is considerably more common because the tissues surrounding the bone are weaker as well as the bone itself usually being more fragile. One group of researchers found that the long-term rate of dislocation following revision surgery may be as high as 7.4%.

Normal results

In general, hip revision surgery has less favorable outcomes than first-time replacement surgery. The greater length and complexity of the procedure often require a longer hospital stay as well as a longer period of **recovery at home**. The range of motion in the new joint is usually smaller than in the first prosthesis, and the patient may experience greater long-term discomfort. In addition, the new prosthesis is not expected to last as long. The life expectancy of implants used in first-time hip replacement surgery is usually given as 10–15 years, whereas revision implants may need to be removed after between eight and 10 years.

WHO PERFORMS THE PROCEDURE AND WHERE IS IT PERFORMED?

Hip revision surgery is performed by an orthopedic surgeon, who has received advanced training in surgical treatment of disorders of the musculoskeletal system. Qualification for this specialty in the United States requires a minimum of five years of training after medical school. Most orthopedic surgeons who perform joint replacements and revision surgery have had additional specialized training in these specific procedures. It is a good idea to find out how many hip revisions the surgeon performs each year; those who perform 200 or more have had more opportunities to refine their technique.

In many cases, hip revision surgery is done by the surgeon who performed the first replacement operation. Some surgeons, however, refer patients to colleagues who specialize in hip revision procedures.

Hip revision surgery can be performed in a hospital with a department of orthopedic surgery, but is also performed in specialized clinics or institutes for joint disorders.

Morbidity and mortality rates

There are relatively few analyses of mortality and morbidity following hip revision surgery in comparison to studies of complications following THR.

Alternatives

Nonsurgical alternatives

In some cases, medications can be used to control the patient's pain, or the patient may prefer to use assistive devices rather than undergo revision surgery. If infection is present, however, surgery is necessary in order to remove the old prosthesis and any areas of surrounding bone that may be infected.

Alternative and complementary treatments

Alternative and complementary approaches that have been shown to control discomfort after hip revision surgery include mindfulness meditation, **biofeedback**, acupuncture, and relaxation techniques. Music therapy, humor therapy, and aromatherapy are helpful

to some patients in maintaining a positive mental attitude and relieving emotional stress before surgery or during recovery at home.

Resources

BOOKS

Canale, S. T., ed. *Campbell's Operative Orthopaedics*, 10th ed. St. Louis: Mosby, 2003.

DeLee, J. C., and D. Drez. *DeLee and Drez's Orthopaedic Sports Medicine*, 2nd ed. Philadelphia: Saunders, 2005.

Khatri, V. P., and J. A. Asensio. *Operative Surgery Manual*, 1st ed. Philadelphia: Saunders, 2003.

Townsend, C. M., et al. *Sabiston Textbook of Surgery*, 17th ed. Philadelphia: Saunders, 2004.

PERIODICALS

Alberton, G. M., W. A. High, and B. F. Morrey. "Dislocation After Revision Total Hip Arthroplasty: An Analysis of Risk Factors and Treatment Options." *Journal of Bone and Joint Surgery, American Volume* 84-A (October 2002): 1788–1792.

Blake, V. A., J. P. Allegrante, L. Robbins, et al. "Racial Differences in Social Network Experience and Perceptions of Benefit of Arthritis Treatments Among New York City Medicare Beneficiaries with Self-Reported Hip and Knee Pain." *Arthritis and Rheumatism* 47 (August 15, 2002): 366–371.

Drake, C., M. Ace, and G. E. Maale. "Revision Total Hip Arthroplasty." *AORN Journal* 76 (September 2002): 414–417, 419–427.

Mahomed, N. N., J. A. Barrett, J. N. Katz, et al. "Rates and Outcomes of Primary and Revision Total Hip Replacement in the United States Medicare Population." *Journal of Bone and Joint Surgery, American Volume* 85-A (January 2003): 27–32.

Nelissen, R. G., E. R. Valstar, R. G. Poll, et al. "Factors Associated with Excessive Migration in Bone Impaction Hip Revision Surgery: A Radiostereometric Analysis Study." *Journal of Arthroplasty* 17 (October 2002): 826–833.

Puri, L., R. L. Wixson, S. H. Stern, et al. "Use of Helical Computed Tomography for the Assessment of Acetabular Osteolysis After Total Hip Arthroplasty."

Journal of Bone and Joint Surgery, American Volume 84-A (April 2002): 609–614.

ORGANIZATIONS

American Academy of Orthopaedic Surgeons (AAOS). 6300 North River Road, Rosemont, IL 60018. (847) 823-7186 or (800) 346-AAOS. http://www.aaos.org (accessed April 1, 2008).

American Physical Therapy Association (APTA). 1111 North Fairfax Street, Alexandria, VA 22314. (703)684-APTA or (800) 999-2782. http://www.apta.org (accessed April 1, 2008).

National Center for Complementary and Alternative Medicine (NCCAM) Clearinghouse. P.O. Box 7923, Gaithersburg, MD 20898. (888) 644-6226. TTY: (866) 464-3615. Fax: (866) 464-3616. http://www.nccam.nih.gov (accessed April 1, 2008).

National Institute of Arthritis and Musculoskeletal and Skin Diseases (NIAMS) Information Clearinghouse. National Institutes of Health, 1 AMS Circle, Bethesda, MD 20892. (301) 495-4484. TTY: (301) 565-2966. http://www.niams.nih.gov (accessed April 1, 2008).

Rush Arthritis and Orthopedics Institute. 1725 West Harrison Street, Suite 1055, Chicago, IL 60612. (312) 563-2420. http://www.rush.edu (accessed April 1, 2008).

OTHER

Hip Universe. June 15, 2003 [cited July 1, 2003]. http://www.hipuniverse.homestead.com (accessed April 1, 2008).

Questions and Answers About Hip Replacement. Bethesda, MD: National Institutes of Health, 2001. NIH Publication No. 01-4907.

Rebecca Frey, PhD
Rosalyn Carson-DeWitt, MD

Histocompatibility testing *see* **Human leukocyte antigen test**

HLA test *see* **Human leukocyte antigen test**

HMOs *see* **Managed care plans**

Home care

Definition

Home care is a form of skilled health care service provided where a patient lives. It is sometimes called domiciliary care. Patients can receive home care services whether they live in their own homes, with or without family members, or in an assisted living facility. According to the National Center for Health Statistics (NCHS), about 1.3 million persons in the United States receive home care.

Description

The goal of home care is to allow the patient to remain living at home, regardless of age or disability. After surgery, a patient may require home care services that may range from such homemaking services as cooking or cleaning to skilled medical care. In the United States, most home care (about 80%) is still provided by members of patients' families; however, some patients also require home health aides or personal care attendants to help them with activities of daily living (ADLs), which are usually defined as activities necessary for adequate self-care, such as bathing, dressing, going to the toilet, and the like. A second category, instrumental activities of daily living (IADLs), refers to tasks that a person must be capable of carrying out in order to live independently. IADLs include being able to perform light housework, prepare meals, take medications, go shopping for groceries or clothes, use the telephone, and manage money.

Medical, dental, and nursing care may all be delivered in patients' homes, which allows them to feel more comfortable and less anxious. The professionals most often involved in home care in the United States are nurses, followed by physical therapists and home health aides. Therapists from speech-language pathology, physical therapy, and respiratory therapy departments often make regular home visits, depending on a patient's specific needs. General nursing care is provided by both registered and licensed practical nurses; however, there are also nurses who are clinical specialists in psychiatry, obstetrics, and cardiology who may provide care when necessary. Home health aides provide what is called custodial care in domestic settings; their duties are similar to those of nurses' aides in the hospital. Professionals who deliver care to patients in their homes are employed either by independent for-profit home-care agencies, hospital agencies, or hospital departments. Personal care attendants can also be hired privately by patients; however, not only is it more difficult to evaluate an employee's specific background and credentials when he or she is not associated with a certified agency or hospital, but medical insurance may not cover the expense of an employee who does not come from an approved source.

Home care nurses provide care for patients of every age, economic class, and level of disability. Some nurses provide specialized **hospice**, mental health, or pediatric care. Home care nursing often involves more than biomedical-based care, depending on a patient's religious or spiritual background.

The NCHS reported that 76% of the 1.3 million persons receiving home care in the United States lived with a primary caregiver, usually a spouse, adult son or daughter, another relative, or a parent (in that order). Of adults aged 65, 6–7% needed assistance with ADLs, compared to 20.6% of persons over 85. Women were more likely to need assistance with ADLs than men. With regard to payment, 710,000 persons paid through **Medicare** and 277,000 through **Medicaid**.

Viewpoints

Most patients are more comfortable in their own homes, rather than in a hospital setting. Depending on the patient's living status and relationships with others in the home, however, the home is not always the best place for caregiving. Consequently, home care continues to grow in popularity. Hospital stays have been shortened considerably, starting in the 1980s with the advent of the diagnosis-related group (DRG) reimbursement system as part of a continuing effort to reduce healthcare costs. But as a result, many patients come home "quicker and sicker," and in need of some form of care or help that family or friends may not be able to offer. Community-based healthcare services are expanding, giving patients more options for assistance at home.

History

It is helpful to have some basic information about the evolution of home care in order to understand the public's demand for quality healthcare, cost containment, and the benefits of advances in both medical and communication technologies. Members of Roman Catholic religious orders in Europe first delivered home care in the late seventeenth century. Today, there are many home care agencies and visiting nurse associations (VNAs) that continue to deliver a wide range of home care services to meet the specific needs of patients throughout the United States and Canada.

Social factors have historically influenced home care delivery, and continue to do so today. Before the 1960s, home care was a community-based delivery system that provided care to patients whether they could pay for the services or not. Agencies relied on charitable contributions from private citizens or charitable organizations, as well as some limited government funding. Life expectancy of the United States population began to rise as advances in medical science saved patients who might have died in years past. As a result, more and more elderly or disabled people required medical care in their homes, as well as in institutions. In response, the federal government put Medicare and Medicaid programs into place in 1965 to help fund and regulate healthcare delivery for this population.

Funding and regulation

Government involvement resulted in regulations that changed the focus of home care from a nursing care delivery service to care delivery under the direction of a physician. Home care delivery is paid for either by the government through Medicare and/or Medicaid; by private insurance or health maintenance organizations (HMOs); by patients themselves; or by certain non-profit community, charitable disease advocacy organizations (e.g., ACS), or faith-based organizations.

Home care delivery services provided by Medicare-certified agencies are tightly regulated. For example, a patient must be homebound in order to receive Medicare-reimbursed home care services. The homebound requirement—one of many—means that the patient must be physically unable to leave home (other than for infrequent trips to the doctor or hospital), thereby restricting the number of persons eligible for home care services. Private insurance companies and HMOs also have certain criteria for the number of visits that will be covered for specific conditions and services. Restrictions on the payment source, the physician's orders, and the patient's specific needs determine the length and scope of services.

Assessment and implementation

Since home care nursing services are provided on a part-time basis, patients, family members, or other caregivers are encouraged and taught to do as much of the care as possible. This approach goes beyond payment boundaries; it extends to the amount of responsibility the patient and his or her family or caregivers are willing or able to assume in order to reach expected outcomes. Nurses who have received special training as case managers visit the patient's home and draw up a plan of care based on assessing the patient, listing the diagnoses, planning the care delivery, implementing specific interventions, and evaluating outcomes or the efficacy of the implementation phase. Planning the care delivery includes assessing the care resources within the circle of the patient's caregivers.

At the time of the initial assessment, the visiting nurse, who is working under a physician's orders, enlists professionals in other disciplines who might be involved in achieving expected outcomes, whether those outcomes include helping the patient return to a certain level of health and independence or maintaining the existing level of health and mobility. The nurse provides instruction to the patient and caregiver(s) regarding the patient's particular disease(s) or condition(s) in order to help the patient achieve an agreed-upon level of independence. Home care nurses are committed to helping patients make good decisions about their care by providing them with reliable information about their conditions. Since home care relies heavily on a holistic approach, care delivery includes teaching coping mechanisms and promoting a positive

attitude to motivate patients to help themselves to the extent that they are able. Unless the patient is paying for home care services out-of-pocket and has unlimited resources or a specific private **long-term care insurance** policy, home care services are scheduled to end at some point. Therefore, the goal of most home care delivery is to move both the patient and the caregivers toward becoming as independent as possible during that time.

Professional implications

Home care delivery is influenced by a number of variables. Political, social, and economic factors place significant constraints on care delivery. Differences among nurses, including their level of education, years of work experience, type of work experience, and level of cultural competence (cross-cultural sensitivity) all influence care delivery to some extent.

Some of the professional issues confronting home care nurses include:

- legal issues
- ethical concerns
- safety issues
- nursing skills and professional education

Legal issues

The legal considerations connected with delivering care in a patient's private residence are similar to those of care delivered in healthcare facilities, but have additional aspects. For example, what would a home care nurse do if she or he had heard the patient repeatedly express the desire not to be resuscitated in case of a heart attack or other catastrophic event, and, during a home visit, the nurse finds the patient unresponsive and cannot find the orders not to resuscitate in the patient's chart? What happens if the patient falls during home care delivery? While processes, protocols, and standards of practice cannot be written to address every situation that may arise in a domestic setting, timely communication and strong policy are essential to keep both patients and home care staff free of legal liability.

Ethical concerns

Ethical implications are closely tied to legal implications in home care—as in the case of missing do-not-resuscitate (DNR) orders. For example, what measures are appropriate if a home care nurse finds a severe diabetic and recovered alcoholic washing down a candy bar with a glass of bourbon? The patient is in his or her own residence and has the legal right to do as he or she chooses. Or, what about the family member who has a bad fall while the nurse is in the home providing care? Should the nurse care for that family member as well? What is the nurse's responsibility to the patient when he or she notices that a family member is taking money from an unsuspecting patient? Complex ethical issues are not always addressed in policy statements. Ongoing communication between the home care agency and the nurse in the field is essential to address problematic situations.

Safety issues

Safety issues in home care require attention and vigilance. The home care nurse does not have security officers readily available if a family member becomes violent either toward the healthcare worker or the patient. Sometimes, home care staff is required to visit patients in high-crime areas or after dark. All agencies should have some type of supervisory personnel available 24 hours a day, seven days a week, so that field staff can reach them with any concerns. Also, clear policy statements that cover issues of personal safety must be documented and communicated regularly and effectively.

Technological advances

With advances in technology and the increased effort to control cost, home care delivery services are using "telecare," which uses communications technology to transmit medical information between the patient and the healthcare provider. Providing care to patients without being in their immediate presence is a relatively new form of home nursing, and is not without its problems. While some uncertainty exists regarding legal responsibilities and the potential for liability, much has been done to make telecare an effective way to hold costs down for some patients. Home care nurses who are required to make telecare visits should know what regulations exist in the particular state before providing care. The chief problem lies in diagnosing and prescribing over the phone. Technological advances have enabled patients to access telecare through the Internet using personal computers or using televisions. With the most recent advances in telecare, the following services may now be offered:

- instant access to patient records

- prescriptions for treatment

- assessment of possible dangers to the patient

- evaluation of the patient's treatment and medication

- follow-up care

Resources

BOOKS

Abrams, William B., Mark H Beers, and Robert Berkow, eds. *The Merck Manual of Geriatrics*, 3rd edition. Whitehouse Station, NJ: Merck & Co., Inc., 2000–2006.

Anderson, Patsy, and Deolinda Mignor. *Home Care Nursing: Using an Accreditation Approach*. Clifton Park, NY: Thomson Delmar Learning, 2008.

Bradshaw, Ann. *Caring for the Older Person: Practical Care in Hospital, Care Home, or At Home*. Hoboken, NJ: John Wiley and Sons, 2007.

Rice, Robyn. *Home Care Nursing Practice: Concepts and Application*, 3rd edition. Philadelphia: Mosby, 2001.

PERIODICALS

Blouin, G., and B. Fowler. "Improving Medication Management in Home Care: Issues and Solutions." *Journal of Palliative Medicine* 10 (December 2007): 1423–1424.

Buhler-Wilkerson, K. "Care of the Chronically Ill at Home: An Unresolved Dilemma in Health Policy for the United States." *Milbank Quarterly* 85, no. 4 (2007): 611–639.

Goulet, C., et al. "A Randomized Clinical Trial of Care for Women with Preterm Labor: Home Management Versus Hospital Management." *CMAJ* 164, no. 7 (April 3, 2001): 985–991.

Hoenig, Helen, Donald H. Taylor, Jr, and Frank A. Sloan. "Does Assistive Technology Substitute for Personal Assistance among the Disabled Elderly?" *American Journal of Public Health* 93, no. 2 (February 2003): 330–337.

Reuben, D. B. "Better Care for Older People with Chronic Diseases: An Emerging Vision." *Journal of the American Medical Association* 298 (December 12, 2007): 2673–2674.

Spratt, G., and Petty, T.L. "Partnering for Optimal Respiratory Home Care: Physicians Working with Respiratory Therapists to Optimally Meet Respiratory Home Care Needs." *Respiratory Care*, 46, no. 5 (May 2001): 475–488.

ORGANIZATIONS

Centers for Medicare & Medicaid Services (CMS). 7500 Security Boulevard, Baltimore, MD 21244-1850. (800) 633-4227. http://www.cms.hhs.gov/ (accessed April 1, 2008).

Hospice Foundation of America. 2001 S. Street NW, Suite 300, Washington, DC 20009. (800) 854-3402. (202) 638-5419l. Fax: (202) 638-5312; E-mail: jon@hospicefoundation.org. http://www.hospicefoundation.org (accessed April 1, 2008).

Joint Commission. One Renaissance Blvd., Oakbrook Terrace, IL 60181. (630) 792-5000. http://www.jointcommission.org (accessed April 1, 2008).

National Association for Home Care & Hospice. 228 7th Street, SE, Washington, DC 20003. (202) 547-7424. Fax: (202) 547-3540.

National Center for Health Statistics (NCHS). 3311 Toledo Road, Hyattsville, MD 20782. (800) 232-4636. http://www.cdc.gov/nchs/ (accessed April 1, 2008).

U.S. Department of Health and Human Services. 200 Independence Avenue, S.W., Washington, DC 20201. (202) 619-0257. (877) 696-6775. http://www.dhhs.gov/ (accessed April 1, 2008).

Visiting Nurse Associations of America (VNAA). 900 19th St, NW, Suite 200, Washington, DC 20006. (202) 384-1420. vnaa@vnaa.org. http://www.vnaa.org (accessed April 1, 2008).

Susan Joanne Cadwallader
Crystal H. Kaczkowski, MSc
Rebecca Frey, PhD

Homocysteine test *see* **Cardiac marker tests**

Hospice

Definition

The term hospice refers to an approach to end-of-life care as well as to a type of facility for supportive care of terminally ill patients. Hospice programs provide palliative (care that relieves discomfort but does not improve the patient's condition or cure the disease) patient-centered care, and other services. The goal of hospice care, whether delivered in the patient's home or in a healthcare facility, is the provision of humane and compassionate medical, emotional, and spiritual care to the **dying**.

Description

Early history

The English word "hospice" is derived from the Latin *hospitium*, which originally referred to the guesthouse of a monastery or convent. The first hospices date back to the Middle Ages, when members of religious orders frequently took in dying people and nursed them during their last illness. Other hospices were built along the routes to major pilgrimage shrines in medieval Europe, such as Rome, Compostela, and Canterbury. Pilgrims who died during their journey were cared for in these hospices. The modern hospice movement, however, may be said to have begun in the United Kingdom during the middle of the nineteenth century. In Dublin, the Roman Catholic Sisters of Charity undertook to provide a clean, supportive environment for care for the terminally ill. Their approach spread throughout England and as far as Asia, Australia, and

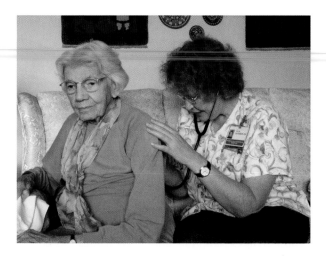

A nurse cares for a 95-year-old woman in a hospice. *(Jim West/Alamy)*

Africa; but until the early 1970s, it had not been accepted on any large scale in the United States.

Two physicians, Drs. Cicely Saunders and Elisabeth Kübler-Ross, are credited with introducing the hospice concept in the United States. Dame Saunders had originally trained as a nurse in England and afterward attended medical school. She founded St. Christopher's Hospice just outside London in 1962. St. Christopher's pioneered an interdisciplinary team approach to the care of the dying. This approach made great strides in **pain management** and symptom control. Dr. Saunders also developed the basic tenets of hospice philosophy, including:

- acceptance of death as the natural conclusion of life
- delivery of care by a highly trained, interdisciplinary team of health professionals who communicate among themselves regularly
- an emphasis on effective pain management and comprehensive home care services
- counseling for the patient and bereavement counseling for the family after the patient's death
- ongoing research and education as essential features of hospice programs

During this same period, Dr. Kübler-Ross, a psychiatrist working in Illinois, published results from her groundbreaking studies of dying patients. Her books about the psychological stages of response to catastrophe and her lectures to health professionals helped to pave the way for the development and acceptance of hospice programs in the United States. The merit of the five stages of acceptance that Dr. Kübler-Ross outlines is that they are not limited to use in counseling the dying. Many patients who become disabled—especially those whose disability and physical impairment are

KEY TERMS

Analgesic—A type of medication given to relieve pain.

Hospice—An approach for providing compassionate, palliative care to terminally ill patients and counseling or assistance for their families. The term may also refer to a hospital unit or freestanding facility devoted to the care of terminally ill patients.

Palliative—A type of care that is intended to relieve pain and suffering, but not to cure.

Patient-controlled analgesia (PCA)—An approach to pain management that allows the patient to control the timing of intravenous doses of analgesic drugs.

sudden occurrences—go through the same stages of "grieving" for the loss of their previous physical health or quality of life. Paraplegics, quadriplegics, amputees, and patients with brain-stem injuries all progress through these same stages of acceptance—and they are not dying.

The first hospice programs in North America opened during the 1970s. In New Haven, Connecticut, the Yale University School of Medicine started a hospice **home care** program in 1974, adding inpatient facilities in 1979. In 1976, another hospice/home-care program, the Hospice of Marin, began in northern California. After a slow start, interest in and enthusiasm for the hospice concept grew. Health professionals as well as the public at large embraced the idea of **death** with dignity. The notion of quality care at the end of life combined with grief counseling and bereavement care (counseling and support for families and friends of dying persons) gained widespread acceptance. The hospice movement also benefited from government efforts to contain healthcare costs when reimbursement for inpatient **hospital services** was sharply reduced. Home-based hospice care is a cost-effective alternative to end-of-life care in a hospital or skilled nursing facility.

Acceptance by mainstream medical professionals

The hospice approach emphasizes caring instead of curing, and some health professionals initially found that this orientation was inconsistent with their previous education, experiences, beliefs, and traditions. Moreover, the involvement of complementary and alternative medicine practitioners was sometimes

unsettling for health professionals unaccustomed to interacting with these persons. As a result of this early period of tension, the Academy of Hospice Physicians was established in 1988 to bring together doctors from a variety of specialties to awaken interest in hospice care among their colleagues and answer their concerns.

In the 1990s, the Academy changed its name to the American Academy of Hospice and Palliative Medicine (AAHPM). Its present purposes include the recognition of palliative care and the management of terminal illness as a distinctive medical discipline; the accreditation of training programs in hospice care; and the support of further research in the field. Most members of the AAHPM believe that more work needs to be done to encourage primary care practitioners and other physicians to refer patients to hospices. A study found that a significant minority of family practitioners and internists have problems interacting with hospices and hospice staff. In the late 1990s, however, the American Board of Medical Specialties (ABMS) recognized hospice and palliative medicine as a board-certified subspecialty. As of 2006, there were 2,883 physicians in the United States who were certified in this subspecialty.

Models of hospice care

HOSPITAL- AND HOME-BASED HOSPICE CARE. According to the National Hospice and Palliative Care Organization (NHPCO), there were 3,650 hospice programs operating in the United States in 2004, including Puerto Rico and Guam. In 1999, hospice programs in the United States cared for over 600,000 people, or 29% of those who died that year. By 2004, this number had increased to 1,060,000 patients.

There are several successful hospice models. As of 2007, over 95% of hospice care is delivered in patients' homes, although the hospice programs that direct the care may be based in medical facilities. Home health agency programs care for patients at home, while hospital-based programs may devote a special wing, unit, or floor to hospice patients. Freestanding independent for-profit hospices devoted exclusively to care of the terminally ill also exist. Most hospice programs offer a combination of services, both inpatient and home-care programs, allowing patients and families to make use of either or both as needed.

One limitation of present hospice models is that most require physicians to estimate that the patient is not likely to live longer than six months. This requirement is related to criteria for **Medicare** eligibility, which has covered hospice care since 1982. Unfortunately,

Medicare eligibility means that terminal patients with uncertain prognoses are often excluded from hospice care, as well as homeless and isolated patients. In addition, pressures to contain healthcare costs have continued to shorten the length of patients' stays in hospices. The shortened time span in turn has made it more difficult for pastoral and psychological counselors to help patients and their families deal effectively with the complex issues of terminal illness.

Another present issue for hospice care in the United States and Western Europe is the need for greater understanding of concepts of death in Eastern cultures. For example, the Chinese notion of a "good death" differs from Western perspectives in several significant ways. As more people from non-Western cultures emigrate to North America and eventually seek hospice care, their concepts of **death and dying** will need to be incorporated in hospice care programs.

One challenge that confronts the hospice movement in the United States as of the early 2000s is the need to accommodate the rapid increase in the size of the elderly population (defined as people over the age of 65), which is expected to double between 2000 and 2030. The group of those over 85 is expected to increase from 4.2 million in 2000 to 8.9 million by 2030. In addition to the sheer number of elderly patients who will need hospice care, hospices must also care for people with a wider range of terminal conditions. In the 1970s, most hospice patients were people diagnosed with end-stage cancer. In 2002, however, people with cancer accounted for only 51% of hospice patients; the others were diagnosed with end-stage heart, kidney, or liver disorders; dementia; lung disease; or AIDS.

The demographics of hospice patients has also changed since the 1970s. In the early years of the hospice movement, almost all patients were middle-class Caucasians. In the early 2000s, 9.2% of hospice patients were African American, 4.3% were Hispanic, 8% were Asian, and 3.7% were multiracial. African Americans, however, appear to be more reluctant than members of other racial groups to consider hospice at the end of life even when their doctor strongly recommends it.

SPECIALIZED HOSPICES. The first hospices in the United States and the United Kingdom were established to meet the needs of adult patients; in the early 1970s, only four hospice programs in the United States accepted children. In 1977, a dying eight-year-old boy was denied admission to a hospice because of his age. This incident prompted the foundation of hospices just for children beginning in 1983, as well as the admission of children to other hospices. As of 2007, almost all hospices in the United States and Canada will accept children as patients.

In 1995, the National Prison Hospice Association (NPHA) was founded to meet the needs of prison inmates with terminal illness. Prisoners are much more resistant than most people to accept the fact that they are dying because death in prison feels like the ultimate defeat. Many are also very suspicious of medical care given within the prison, and are afraid to appear weak and vulnerable in the eyes of other inmates. A surprisingly high number refuse to take pain medications for this reason. The NPHA trains medical professionals and volunteers to understand the special needs of terminally ill prison inmates and their families.

Hospices in the United States and Canada accept patients from all religious backgrounds and faith traditions. Hospices that are related to a specific religion or spiritual tradition, however, often offer special facilities or programs to meet the needs of patients from that tradition. For example, there are Jewish hospices that observe the dietary regulations, Sabbath rituals, and other parts of *Halakhah* (Jewish religious law). The National Institute for Jewish Hospice (NIJH), founded in 1985, has accredited 40 hospice programs for Jewish patients as of 2007. Hospices related to the various branches of Christianity have a priest or pastor on call for prayer, administration of the sacraments, and similar Christian religious observances. The Zen Hospice Project, founded in 1987, sponsors programs reflecting the Buddhist tradition of compassionate service and maintains a 25-bed unit within the Laguna Honda Hospice in San Francisco, California.

Aspects of hospice care

GENERAL ENVIRONMENT. The goal of freestanding hospices and even hospital-based programs is the creation and maintenance of warm, comfortable, home-like environments. Rather than the direct overhead lights found in hospitals, these hospices use floor and table lamps along with natural light to convey a sense of brightness and uplift. Some hospices offer music or art programs and fill patient rooms with original artwork and fresh flowers.

PAIN MANAGEMENT AND PSYCHOSPIRITUAL SUPPORT. Along with acceptance of death as a natural part of the life cycle, health professionals who refer patients to or work in hospice programs must become especially well informed about pain management and symptom control. This knowledge is necessary because about 80% of hospice patients are dying of end-stage cancer. In traditional medical settings, pain medication is often administered when the patient requests it. Hospice care approaches pain control quite differently. By administering pain medication regularly, before it is needed, hospice caregivers hope to prevent pain from recurring. Since addiction and other long-term consequences of narcotic **analgesics** are not a concern for the terminally ill, hospice caregivers focus on relieving pain as completely and effectively as possible. Hospice patients often have **patient-controlled analgesia** (PCA) pumps that allow them to control their pain medication.

Symptom relief often requires more than simply using narcotic analgesia. Hospices consider the patient and family as the unit of care; family is broadly defined as embracing all persons who are close to the patient, not just blood relatives. Seeking to relieve physical, psychological, emotional, and spiritual discomfort, hospice teams rely on members of the clergy, pastoral counselors, social workers, psychiatrists, massage therapists, and trained volunteers to comfort patients and family members, in addition to the solace offered by nurses and physicians. A study published in early 2008 reported that patients and family members who received spiritual care while they were in a hospice setting thought that they received better overall care than those who did not. The single most important spiritual need mentioned by patients was individual devotional activities.

Since the patient and his or her family members are considered the unit of care, hospice programs continue to support families and loved ones after the patient's death. Grief and bereavement counseling as well as support groups offer opportunities to express and resolve emotional concerns and share them with others.

COMPLEMENTARY AND ALTERNATIVE THERAPIES. In addition to mainstream medicine, many hospices offer patients and families the opportunity to use complementary and alternative approaches to control symptoms and improve well being. Acupuncture, music therapy, pet therapy, bodywork, massage therapy, aromatherapy, Reiki (energy healing), Native American ceremonies, herbal treatments, and other non-Western practices may be used to calm and soothe patients and their families. A study of complementary and alternative therapies within hospice programs found that patients who received these treatments reported greater overall satisfaction with hospice care than those who did not.

Resources

BOOKS

Hospice and Palliative Nurses Association. *Hospice and Palliative Nursing: Scope and Standards of Practice.* Silver Spring, MD: American Nurses Association, 2007.

Jacob, Bob. *Perspective: Hospice Poems.* Simsbury, CT: Antrim House, 2007.

Kübler-Ross, Elisabeth. *On Death and Dying.* New York: Macmillan, 1969.

Pelletier, Kenneth R., MD. *The Best Alternative Medicine,* Part I, Chapter 11, "Spirituality and Healing." New York: Simon & Schuster, 2002.

Russo, Richard, ed. *A Healing Touch: True Stories of Life, Death, and Hospice.* Camden, ME: Down East Books, 2008.

Saunders, Cicely M. *Cicely Saunders: Selected Writings 1958–2004.* New York: Oxford University Press, 2006.

PERIODICALS

Daaleman, T. P., et al. "Spiritual Care at the End of Life in Long-Term Care." *Medical Care* 46 (January 2008): 85–91.

Demmer, C. and J. Sauer. "Assessing Complementary Therapy Services in a Hospice Program." *American Journal of Hospice and Palliative Care* 19 (September–October 2002): 306–314.

Friedrichsdorf, S. J., S. Remke, B. Symalla, et al. "Developing a Pain and Palliative Care Programme at a US Children's Hospital." *International Journal of Palliative Nursing* 13 (November 2007): 534–542.

Ludke, R. L., and D. R. Smucker. "Racial Differences in the Willingness to Use Hospice Services." *Journal of Palliative Medicine* 10 (December 2007): 1329–1337.

Mak, M. H. "Awareness of Dying: An Experience of Chinese Patients with Terminal Cancer." *Omega (Westport)* 43 (2001): 259–279.

Ogle, K., B. Mavis, and T. Wang. "Hospice and Primary Care Physicians: Attitudes, Knowledge, and Barriers." *American Journal of Hospice and Palliative Care* 20 (January–February 2003): 41–51.

ORGANIZATIONS

American Academy of Hospice and Palliative Medicine (AAHPM). 4700 West Lake Avenue, Glenview, IL 60025-1485. (847) 375-4712. http://www.aahpm.org (accessed April 1, 2008).

Children's Hospice International (CHI). 1101 King Street, Suite 360, Alexandria, VA 22314. (703) 684-0330 or (800) 2-4-CHILD. http://www.chionline.org (accessed April 1, 2008).

Hospice Foundation of America. 2001 S Street NW, Suite 300, Washington, DC 20009. (800) 854-3402. http://www.hospicefoundation.org (accessed April 1, 2008).

National Hospice and Palliative Care Organization (NHPCO). 1700 Diagonal Road, Suite 625, Alexandria, VA 22314. (703) 837-1500 or (800) 658-8898 (Helpline). http://www.nhpco.org (accessed April 1, 2008).

National Institute for Jewish Hospice (NIJH). 732 University Street, North Woodmere, NY 11581. (800) 446-4448. http://www.nijh.org/ (accessed April 1, 2008).

National Prison Hospice Association (NPHA). P. O. Box 4623, Boulder, CO 80306. (303) 447-8051. http://www.npha.org (accessed April 1, 2008).

Zen Hospice Project. 273 Page Street, San Francisco, CA 94102. (415) 863-2910. http://www.zenhospice.org (accessed April 1, 2008).

Barbara Wexler
Rebecca Frey, PhD

Hospital-acquired infections

Definition

A hospital-acquired infection, also called a nosocomial infection, is an infection that first appears between 48 hours and four days after a patient is admitted to a hospital or other healthcare facility.

Description

About 10% of patients admitted to acute care hospitals and long-term care facilities in the United States develop a hospital-acquired, or nosocomial, infection, with an annual total of 1.7 million infections and 99,000 deaths as of 2007. The annual cost of treating these infections is estimated to run between $4.5 billion and $11 billion. Hospital-acquired infections are usually related to a device, procedure, or treatment used to diagnose or treat the patient's initial illness or injury. The Centers for Disease Control (CDC) of the U.S. Department of Health and Human Services has shown that many of these infections are preventable through the adherence to strict guidelines by healthcare workers when caring for patients. What can make these infections so troublesome is that they occur in people whose health is already compromised by the condition for which they were first hospitalized.

Hospital-acquired infections may be caused by bacteria, viruses, fungi, or parasites. These microorganisms may already be present in the patient's body or may come from the environment, contaminated hospital equipment, healthcare workers, or other patients. There are three basic routes of infection transmission: direct contact (diseases are spread by touching infected objects or persons); droplet (diseases are spread by coughing and sneezing); and airborne (diseases are spread by microorganisms that remain suspended in the air for long periods of time).

Depending on the causal agents involved, an infection may start in any part of the body. A localized infection is limited to a specific part of the body and has local symptoms. For example, if a surgical wound in the abdomen becomes infected, the area around the wound becomes red, hot, and painful. A generalized infection is one that enters the bloodstream and causes systemic symptoms such as fever, chills, low blood pressure, or mental confusion. This can lead to sepsis, a serious, rapidly progressive multi-organ infection, sometimes called blood poisoning, that can result in **death**.

Hospital-acquired infections may develop from the performance of surgical procedures; from the insertion of catheters (tubes) into the urinary tract, nose, mouth, or blood vessels; or from material from the nose or mouth that is aspirated (inhaled) into the lungs. According to the CDC, the most common types of hospital-acquired infections are urinary tract infections (UTIs) (32%), surgical wound infections (22%), pneumonia (15%), and bloodstream infections (14%). The University of Michigan Health System reports that the most common sources of infection in their hospital are urinary catheters, central venous (in the vein) catheters, and endotracheal tubes (tubes going through the mouth into the stomach). Catheters going into the body allow bacteria to move along the outside of the tube into the body where they find their way into the bloodstream. A study in the journal *Infection Control and Hospital Epidemiology* shows that about 24% of patients with catheters will develop catheter-related infections, of which 5.2% will become bloodstream infections. Death has been shown to occur in 4–20% of catheter-related infections.

Hospital-acquired infections in the United States are monitored by the National Healthcare Safety Network (NHSN), formed in 2005 by a merger of three health surveillance systems previously established by the CDC. The NHSN monitors healthcare personnel safety as well as patient safety.

Causes

All hospitalized patients are at risk of acquiring an infection from their treatment or surgery. Some patients are at greater risk than others, especially young children, the elderly, and persons with compromised immune systems. The surveillance database compiled by the CDC shows that the overall infection rate among children in intensive care is 6.1%, with the primary causes being venous catheters and ventilator-associated pneumonia. The risk factors for hospital-acquired infections in children include parenteral nutrition (tube or intravenous feeding), the use of **antibiotics** for more than 10 days, use of invasive devices, poor postoperative status, and immune system dysfunction. Other risk factors that increase the opportunity for hospitalized adults and children to acquire infections are:

KEY TERMS

Abscess—A localized pocket of pus at a site of infection.

Aseptic—Sterile conditions with no harmful microorganisms present.

Catheter—A thin, hollow tube inserted into the body at specific points in order to infuse medications, blood components, or nutritional fluids into the body, or to withdraw fluids from the body such as gastric fluid or urine.

Culture—A swab of blood, sputum, pus, urine, or other body fluid planted in a special medium, incubated, and allowed to grow for identification of infection-causing organisms.

Generalized infection—An infection that has entered the bloodstream and has general systemic symptoms such as fever, chills, and low blood pressure.

Localized infection—An infection that is limited to a specific part of the body and has local symptoms.

Nosocomial infection—An infection acquired in the hospital.

Sepsis—A rapidly spreading state of poisoning in the body, usually involving the whole body.

• a prolonged hospital stay

• severity of underlying illness

• compromised nutritional or immune status

• use of indwelling catheters

• failure of health care workers to wash their hands between patients or before procedures

• prevalence of antibiotic-resistant bacteria from the overuse of antibiotics

Any type of invasive (enters the body) procedure can expose a patient to the possibility of infection. Some common procedures that increase the risk of hospital-acquired infections include:

• urinary bladder catheterization

• respiratory procedures such as intubation or mechanical ventilation

• surgery and the dressing or drainage of surgical wounds

• gastric drainage tubes into the stomach through the nose or mouth

• intravenous (IV) procedures for delivery of medication, transfusion, or nutrition

Urinary tract infection (UTI) is the most common type of hospital-acquired infection and has been shown to occur after urinary catheterization. Catheterization is the placement of a catheter through the urethra into the urinary bladder to empty urine from the bladder; or to deliver medication, relieve pressure, or measure urine in the bladder; or for other medical reasons. Normally, a healthy urinary bladder is sterile, with no harmful bacteria or other microorganisms present. Although bacteria may be in or around the urethra, they normally cannot enter the bladder. A catheter, however, can pick up bacteria from the urethra and give them an easy route into the bladder, causing infection. Bacteria from the intestinal tract are the most common type to cause UTIs. Patients with poorly functioning immune systems or who are taking antibiotics are also at increased risk for UTI caused by a fungus called *Candida*. The prolonged use of antibiotics, which may reduce the effectiveness of the patient's own immune system, has been shown to create favorable conditions for the growth of this fungal organism.

Invasive surgical procedures, the second most common cause of nosocomial infections, increase a patient's risk of getting an infection by giving bacteria a route into normally sterile areas of the body. An infection can be acquired from contaminated surgical equipment or from the hands of healthcare workers. Following surgery, the surgical wound can become infected from contaminated **dressings** or the hands of healthcare workers who change the dressing. Other wounds can also become easily infected, such as those caused by trauma, burns, or pressure sores that result from prolonged bed rest or wheel chair use.

Pneumonia is the third most common type of hospital-acquired infection. Bacteria and other microorganisms are easily introduced into the throat by treatment procedures performed to treat respiratory illnesses. Patients with chronic obstructive lung disease, for example, are especially susceptible to infection because of frequent and prolonged antibiotic therapy and long-term **mechanical ventilation** used in their treatment. The infecting microorganisms can come from contaminated equipment or the hands of healthcare workers as procedures are conducted such as respiratory intubation, suctioning of material from the throat and mouth, and mechanical ventilation. Once introduced through the nose and mouth, microorganisms quickly colonize the throat area. This means that they grow and form a colony, but have not yet caused an infection. Once the throat is colonized, it is easy for a patient to aspirate the microorganisms into the lungs, where infection develops that leads to pneumonia.

Bloodstream infections are the fourth most common type of hospital-acquired infections. Many hospitalized patients need continuous medications, transfusions, or nutrients delivered into their bloodstream. An intravenous (IV) catheter is placed in a vein and the medications, blood components, or liquid nutritional components are infused into the vein. Bacteria from the surroundings, contaminated equipment, or healthcare workers' hands can enter the body at the site of catheter insertion. A local infection may develop in the skin around the catheter. The bacteria can also enter the blood through the vein and cause a generalized infection. The longer a catheter is in place, the greater the risk of infection.

Other hospital procedures that may put patients at risk for nosocomial infection are gastrointestinal procedures, obstetric procedures, and **kidney dialysis**.

Symptoms

Fever is often the first sign of infection. Other symptoms and signs of infection are rapid breathing, mental confusion, low blood pressure, reduced urine output, and a high **white blood cell count**. Patients with a UTI may have pain when urinating and blood in the urine. Symptoms of pneumonia may include difficulty breathing and inability to cough. A localized infection begins with swelling, redness, and tenderness on the skin or around a surgical wound or other open wound, which can progress rapidly to the destruction of deeper layers of muscle tissue, and eventually sepsis.

Diagnosis

An infection is suspected any time a hospitalized patient develops a fever that cannot be explained by the underlying illness. Some patients, especially the elderly, may not develop a fever. In these patients, the first signs of infection may be rapid breathing or mental confusion.

Diagnosis of a hospital-acquired infection is determined by any of the following:

- evaluation of symptoms and signs of infection
- examination of wounds and catheter entry sites for redness, swelling, or the presence of pus or an abscess
- a complete physical examination and review of underlying illness
- laboratory tests, including complete blood count (CBC), especially to look for an increase in infection-fighting white cells; urinalysis, looking for white cells or evidence of blood in the urinary tract; cultures of the infected area, blood, sputum, urine, or other body fluids or tissue to find the causative organism
- chest x ray may be done when pneumonia is suspected to look for the presence of white blood cells and other inflammatory substances in lung tissue
- review of all procedures performed that might have led to infection

Treatment

Cultures of blood, urine, sputum, other body fluids, or tissue are especially important in order to identify the bacteria, fungi, virus, or other microorganism causing the infection. Once the organism has been identified, it will be tested again for sensitivity to a range of antibiotics so that the patient can be treated quickly and effectively with an appropriate medicine to which the causative organism will respond. While waiting for these test results, treatment may begin with common broad-spectrum antibiotics such as penicillin, **cephalosporins**, **tetracyclines**, or erythromycin.

More and more often, however, some types of bacteria are becoming resistant to these standard antibiotic treatments, especially when patients with chronic illnesses are frequently given antibiotic therapy for long periods of time. When resistance develops, a different, more powerful, and more specific antibiotic must be used to which the specific organism has been shown to respond. Two strong antibiotics that have been effective against resistant bacteria are vancomycin and imipenem, although some bacteria are developing resistance to these antibiotics as well. A newer generation of tetracycline antibiotics known as glycylcyclines was introduced in 2005; the first of these, tigecycline, was developed specifically to target drug-resistant microorganisms. The prolonged use of antibiotics is also known to reduce the effectiveness of the patient's own immune system, sometimes becoming a factor in the development of infection.

Fungal infections are treated with antifungal medications. Examples of these are amphotericin B, nystatin, ketoconazole, itraconazole, and fluconazole.

Viruses do not respond to antibiotics. A number of antiviral drugs have been developed that slow the growth or reproduction of viruses, such as acyclovir, ganciclovir, foscarnet, and amantadine.

Prevention

Hospitals take a variety of steps to prevent nosocomial infections, including:

- Adoption of an infection control program such as the one sponsored by the Centers for Disease Control

(CDC), which includes quality control of procedures known to lead to infection, and a monitoring program to track infection rates to see if they go up or down.

- Employment of an infection control practitioner for every 200 beds.
- Identification of high-risk procedures and other possible sources of infection.
- Strict adherence to hand-washing rules by healthcare workers and visitors to avoid passing infectious microorganisms to or between hospitalized patients.
- Strict attention to aseptic (sterile) technique in the performance of procedures, including use of sterile gowns, gloves, masks, and barriers.
- Sterilization of all reusable equipment such as ventilators, humidifiers, and any devices that come in contact with the respiratory tract.
- Frequent changing of dressings for wounds and use of antibacterial ointments under dressings.
- Removal of nasogastric (nose to stomach) and endotracheal (mouth to stomach) tubes as soon as possible.
- Use of an antibacterial-coated venous catheter that destroys bacteria before they can get into the bloodstream.
- Preventing contact between respiratory secretions and health care providers by using barriers and masks as needed.
- Use of silver alloy-coated urinary catheters that destroy bacteria before they can migrate up into the bladder.
- Limitations on the use and duration of high-risk procedures such as urinary catheterization.
- Isolation of patients with known infections.
- Sterilization of medical instruments and equipment to prevent contamination.
- Reductions in the general use of antibiotics to encourage better immune response in patients and reduce the cultivation of resistant bacteria.

Resources

BOOKS

Ayliffe, Graham, and Mary English. *Hospital Infection: From Miasmas to MRSA*. New York: Cambridge University Press, 2003.

Mayhall, C. Glen, ed. *Hospital Epidemiology and Infection Control*, 3rd ed. Philadelphia: Lippincott Williams and Wilkins, 2004.

PERIODICALS

Crane, S. J., D. Z. Uzlan, and L. M. Baddour. "Bloodstream Infections in a Geriatric Cohort: A Population-Based Study." *American Journal of Medicine* 120 (December 2007): 1078–1083.

Edwards, Jonathan R., et al. "National Healthcare Safety Network (NHSN) Report, Data Summary for 2006, Issued June 2007." *American Journal of Infection Control* 35 (June 2007): 290–301.

Kilgore, M. L., K. Ghosh, C. M. Beavers, et al. "The Costs of Nosocomial Infections." *Medical Care* 46 (January 2008): 101–104.

Rose, W. E., and M. J. Rybak. "Tigecycline: First of a New Class of Antimicrobial Agents." *Pharmacotherapy* 26 (August 2006): 1099–1110.

Wang, L., and J. F. Barrett. "Control and Prevention of MRSA Infections." *Methods in Molecular Biology* 391 (2007): 209–225.

ORGANIZATIONS

Centers for Disease Control and Prevention (CDC). 1600 Clifton Road, Atlanta, GA 30333. 404-639-3311. http://www.cdc.gov/health/ (accessed April 1, 2008).

National Healthcare Safety Network (NHSN). Division of Healthcare Quality Promotion, MS-A24, Centers for Disease Control and Prevention,1600 Clifton Road, NE, Atlanta, GA 30333. (800) 893-0485. http://www.cdc.gov/ncidod/dhqp/nhsn_members.html (accessed April 1, 2008).

OTHER

Centers for Disease Control and Prevention (CDC). *Questions and Answers about Healthcare-Associated Infections*. Atlanta, GA: CDC, 2007.

Siegel, J. D., et al. *Guideline for Isolation Precautions: Preventing Transmission of Infectious Agents in Healthcare Settings, June 2007*. Atlanta, GA: CDC, 2007.

Toni Rizzo
L. Lee Culvert
Rebecca Frey, PhD

Hospital services

Definition

Hospital services is a term that refers to medical and surgical services and the supporting laboratories, equipment and personnel that make up the medical and surgical mission of a hospital or hospital system.

Purpose

Hospital services make up the core of a hospital's offerings. They are often shaped by the needs or wishes of its major users to make the hospital a one-stop or core institution of its local community or medical network. Hospitals are institutions comprising basic services and personnel—usually departments of medicine and surgery—that administer clinical and other services for specific diseases and conditions, as well as emergency services. Hospital services cover a range of medical offerings from basic health care necessities or training and research for major medical school centers to services designed by an industry-owned network of such institutions as health maintenance organizations (HMOs). The mix of services that a hospital may offer depends almost entirely upon its basic mission(s) or objective(s).

There are three basic types of hospitals in the United States: proprietary (for-profit) hospitals; nonprofit hospitals; and charity- or government-supported hospitals. The services within these institutions vary considerably, but are usually organized around the basic mission(s) or objective (s) of the institution:

- Proprietary hospitals. For-profit hospitals include both general and specialized hospitals, usually as part of a healthcare network like Humana or HCA, which may be corporately owned. The main objective of proprietary hospitals is to make a profit from the services provided.

- Teaching or community hospitals. These are hospitals that serve several purposes: they provide patients for the training or research of interns and residents; they also offer services to patients who are unable to pay for services, while attempting to maintain profitability. Nonprofit centers like the University of California at San Francisco (UCSF) or the Mayo Clinics combine service, teaching, and profitability without being owned by a corporation or private owner.

- Government-supported hospitals. This group includes tax-supported hospitals for counties, communities and cities with voluntary hospitals (community or charity hospitals) run by a board of citizen administrators who serve without pay. The main objective of this type of hospital is to provide health care for a community or geographic region.

Demographics

As of 2006, the total number of hospitals in the United States, including military and prison hospitals, is over 7,569. Of this total, approximately 3,000 are non-government-related nonprofit hospitals; almost 800 are investor-owned; and 1,156 are government (state, county, or local) hospitals.

Description

Over the past two decades, hospital services in the United States have declined markedly as a percentage of health care costs, from 43.5% in 1980 to about 31% in 2005. This decline was due to shortened lengths of

---

KEY TERMS

Auxiliary hospital services—A term used broadly to designate such nonmedical services as financial services, birthing classes, support groups, etc. that are instituted in response to consumer demand.

Health maintenance organization (HMO)—A broad term that covers a variety of prepaid systems providing health care within a certain geographic area to all persons covered by the HMO's contract.

Intensivist—A physician who specializes in caring for patients in intensive care units.

Nonprofit hospitals—Hospitals that combine a teaching function with providing for uninsured within large, complex networks technically designated as nonprofit institutions. While the institution may be nonprofit, however, its services are allowed to make a profit.

Proprietary hospitals—Hospitals owned by private entities, mostly corporations, that are intended to make a profit as well as provide medical services. Most hospitals in health maintenance organizations and health networks are proprietary institutions.

Teaching hospitals—Hospitals whose primary mission is training medical personnel in collaboration with (or ownership by) a medical school or research center.

---

hospital stay, the move from inpatient to outpatient facilities for surgery, and a wave of hospital mergers in the 1990s that consolidated services and staff. Since 2001, however, spending on hospital care in the United States has been growing faster than other sectors of the economy as a result of increasing demand for hospital services. Forty percent of the rise in spending on hospital care is due to escalating costs for hospital services attributed to population growth, the aging of the general population, and growing discontent with the limitations imposed by managed care. In addition, new medical technologies have allowed hospitals to provide life-saving diagnostic and therapeutic alternatives that were unavailable in the 1990s.

At the same time that the use of hospital services is increasing nationwide, government support of hospital services with **Medicaid** and **Medicare** has been decreasing, putting pressure upon hospitals to treat the uninsured and make up for $21.6 billion in uncompensated care (year 2002). This trend has put pressure on for-profit, not-for-profit and teaching hospitals to provide a broader range of community services or such "low-end" services as mental health care, preventive health services, and general pediatric care. In addition, very recent changes in Federal laws governing the entry of hospitals into new markets—Certificate of Need laws—allow health care providers to offer new hospital services, resulting in the growth of ambulatory surgical centers, special tertiary surgery centers and specialty hospitals that treat a single major disease category. These legislative changes encourage the offering of "high-end" services that are increasingly demanded by consumers.

Hospital services define the core features of a hospital's organization. The range of services may be limited in such specialty hospitals as cardiovascular centers or cancer treatment centers, or very broad to meet the needs of the community or patient base, as in full service health maintenance organizations (HMOs), rural charity centers, urban health centers, or medical research centers. Hospital services are usually the most general in large urban areas or underserved rural areas, broadly encompassing many services ordinarily offered by other medical providers. The basic services that hospitals offer include:

- short-term hospitalization
- emergency room services
- general and specialty surgical services
- x ray/radiology services
- laboratory services
- blood services

HMO hospitals add a number of special and auxiliary services to the basic list, including:

- pediatric specialty care
- greater access to surgical specialists
- physical therapy and rehabilitation services
- prescription services
- home nursing services
- nutritional counseling
- mental health care
- family support services
- genetic counseling and testing
- social work or case management services
- financial services

Hospitals funded by state, regional, or local government, as well as charity hospitals and hospitals within research and teaching centers, are pressed by community needs to provide for the uninsured or underinsured with more basic services:

- primary care services
- mental health and drug treatment
- infectious disease clinics
- hospice care
- dental services
- translation and interpreter services

Diagnosis/Preparation

Most hospitals have extensive surgical services that include preoperative testing, which may include x rays, **CT scans**, ultrasonography, blood tests, **urinalysis**, and/or an EKG. Medication counseling is offered for current patient prescriptions and how they should be taken during and after surgery. **Informed consent** forms are made available to patients, as well as patient advocate services for questions and assistance in understanding the consent form and similar documents. An anesthesiologist or an assistant discuss with the patient the patient's history of allergies, previous reactions to anesthesia and special precautions that will be taken. Intravenous medications are usually begun in the patient's room before surgery to relax the patient, with **general anesthesia** administered in the **operating room**.

Aftercare

According to the National Center for Health Statistics of the Centers for Disease Control and Prevention (CDC), 44.9 million inpatient surgical procedures were performed in the United States in 2005, followed closely by 31.5 million outpatient surgeries. The procedures that were performed most frequently included:

- appendectomy
- breast biopsy
- carotid endarterectomy
- cataract surgery
- cesarian section
- gall baldder surgery
- debridement of wound, infection, burn
- dilatation and curettage or d & c
- hemorrhoidectomy
- hysterectomy
- hysteroscopy
- inguinal hernia repair
- lower back surgery
- mastectomy
- colectomy
- revision of peritoneal adhesions
- tonsillectomy

Inpatient aftercare

After inpatient surgery, most patients are taken to a **recovery room** and monitored by nursing staff until they regain full consciousness. If there are complications or if the patient develops respiratory or cardiac problems, he or she is transferred to a surgical **intensive care unit** equipped to deal with acute needs. Intensive care units (ICU) are highly advanced facilities in which patients are monitored by special equipment that measures their heart rate, breathing, blood pressure, and blood oxygen level. Some patients require a respirator to breathe for them and additional intravenous lines to deliver medication and fluids. Once stabilized, patients are transferred to their hospital room.

After returning to the room, the patient is encouraged to sit up, start walking, and do as much as possible to return to a normal level of activity. Special diets may be provided, as well as pain-killing medications and **antibiotics** if needed. A respiratory therapist will usually visit the patient with breathing equipment intended to help the patient's lung function return to normal. A physical therapist may introduce the patient to an **exercise** program or to skills needed to manage with temporary or permanent physical limitations.

Discharge personnel help the patient plan to go home. Some hospitals follow up with an outpatient nurse or social worker service. Pharmaceutical services may be offered to fill take-home prescriptions without the requirement of visiting an outside pharmacy. Medical equipment, like wheelchairs or crutches and other durable equipment, may be provided by the hospital and then purchased by the patient for use at home.

Outpatient aftercare

Outpatient or ambulatory surgery services make up almost half of all surgeries in the United States as a result of advances in surgical equipment and technique that allow for laser treatments and other minimally invasive procedures. Outpatient procedures require comparatively little aftercare for the patient due to both the nature of the surgical procedure and the advantages of being able to use regional or **local anesthesia**. Aftercare in hospital outpatient clinics, **ambulatory surgery centers**, or office-based practices requires that patients recover from anesthetics in the facility. After the anesthetic has worn off, the patient is briefly monitored for complications and released to go home. Many surgical procedures now allow patients to go home after a short recovery period on the same day as the surgery, and benefit from minimal pain and a speedier recovery.

Morbidity and mortality rates

According to a health consumer organization, 195,000 people die each year in America's hospitals as a result of **medical errors**. In recent years, many hospitals have introduced special safeguards to cut down on the number of mistakes in medication and surgical services. Two new practices have been adopted by quality hospitals. Computerized order entries for medications cut down drastically on the number of misread prescriptions. The other innovation reduces the number of medical errors in intensive care units by using specially trained physicians—intensivists—in the unit. Hospitals that have introduced these patient safety features can be found on the Internet at conssumer health sites.

Proprietary hospitals generally offer more services and "high end" care than government or community hospitals, with teaching hospitals offering the most highly developed new procedures and techniques along with services for the poor and special populations. For-profit hospitals, however, do not have lower rates of morbidity or mortality in their delivery of hospital services. One study in 2000 published by General Internal Medicine found that patients at for-profit hospitals suffered two to four times more complications from surgery as well as delays in diagnosing and treating illness than did patients in nonprofit hospitals. Previous research has shown that **death** rates are 25% higher in proprietary hospitals than in teaching hospitals, and 6–7% higher in proprietary hospitals than in nonprofit institutions.

Resources

PERIODICALS

Birkmeyer, J. D., E. V. Finlayson, and C. M. Birkmeyer. "Volume Standards for High-Risk Surgical Procedures: Potential Benefits of the Leapfrog Initiative." *Surgery* 130 (September 2001): 415–422.

Relman, Arnold, MD. "Dr. Business." *The American Prospect* 8 (September 1, 1997).

ORGANIZATIONS

Accreditation Association for Ambulatory Health Care (AAAHC). 3201 Old Glenview Road, Suite 300, Wilmette, IL 60091-2992. (847) 853-6060. www.aahc.org.

American Hospital Association. One North Franklin, Chicago, IL 60606-3421. (312) 422-3000. www.hospitalconnect.com.

Joint Commission on Accreditation of Healthcare Organizations (JCAHO). One Renaissance Blvd., Oakbrook Terrace, IL 60181. (630) 792-5000 or (630) 792-5085. www.jcaho.org/.

OTHER

Employee Benefits Research Institute (EBRI). "The Role of the Health Care Sector in the U.S. Economy." www.ebri.org/press/.

HealthPages.com. "All Hospitals Are Not Created Equal." www.healthpages.com.

HealthScope.com. "Hospitals." www.healthscope.com.

Nancy McKenzie, PhD

Human leukocyte antigen test

Definition

The human leukocyte antigen (HLA) test, also known as HLA typing or tissue typing, identifies antigens on the white blood cells (WBCs) that determine tissue compatibility for organ transplantation (that is, histocompatibility testing). There are six loci on chromosome 6, where the genes that produce HLA antigens are inherited: HLA-A, HLA-B, HLA-C, HLA-DR, HLA-DQ, and HLA-DP.

Unlike most blood group antigens, which are inherited as products of two alleles (types of gene that occupy the same site on a chromosome), many different alleles can be inherited at each of the HLA loci. These are defined by antibodies (antisera) that recognize specific HLA antigens, or by DNA probes that recognize the HLA allele. Using specific antibodies, 26 HLA-A alleles, 59 HLA-B alleles, 10 HLA-C alleles, 26 HLA-D alleles, 22 HLA-DR alleles, nine HLA-DQ alleles, and six HLA-DP alleles can be recognized. This high degree of genetic variability (polymorphism) makes finding compatible organs more difficult than finding compatible blood for **transfusion**.

Purpose

HLA typing, along with ABO (blood type) grouping, is used to provide evidence of tissue compatibility. The HLA antigens expressed on the surface of the lymphocytes of the recipient are matched against those from various donors. Human leukocyte antigen typing is performed for kidney, bone marrow, liver, pancreas, and heart transplants. The probability that a transplant will be successful increases with the number of identical HLA antigens.

Graft rejection occurs when the immune cells (T-lymphocytes) of the recipient recognize specific HLA antigens on the donor's organ as foreign. The T-lymphocytes initiate a cellular immune response that result in graft rejection. Alternatively, T-lymphocytes

KEY TERMS

Allele—Types of genes that occupy the same site on a chromosome.

Ankylosing spondylitis—An inflammatory arthropathy (arthritis-like) of the vertebral column and sacroiliac joints.

Antibody—A protein (immunoglobulin) produced by B-lymphocytes in response to stimulation by a specific antigen.

Antigen—A molecule, usually a protein, that elicits the production of a specific antibody or immune response.

Autoimmune disorders—A disorder caused by a reaction of an individual's immune system against the organs or tissues of one's own body.

B-lymphocyte—A type of blood cell that is active in immune response.

Cornea—The transparent outer layer of the eye. It covers the iris and lens.

Histocompatibility testing—Testing of genotypes of a recipient and potential donor to see if rejection would occur when tissues are transplanted.

Lymphocyte—A class of white blood cell that is responsible for the immune response to antigens.

Macrophage—A type of blood cell derived from monocytes that are stimulated by inflammation and stimulate antibody production.

Monocyte—A type of white blood cell produced in bone marrow.

Phenotype—A trait produced by a gene. For example, the specific HLA antigen(s) inherited for the HLA-A locus is the phenotype for that gene.

present in the grafted tissue may recognize the host tissues as foreign and produce a cell-mediated immune response against the recipient. This is called graft versus host disease (GVHD), and it can lead to life-threatening systemic damage in the recipient. Human leukocyte antigen testing is performed to reduce the probability of both rejection and GVHD.

Typing is also used along with blood typing and DNA tests to determine the parentage (that is, for paternity testing). The HLA antigens of the mother, child, and alleged father can be compared. When an HLA antigen of the child cannot be attributed to the mother or the alleged father, then the latter is excluded as the father of the child.

A third use of HLA testing called linkage analysis is based on the region where the HLA loci are positioned, the major histocompatibility complex (MHC), which contains many other genes located very close to the HLA loci. The incidence of crossing-over between HLA genes during fertilization of the egg by sperm is generally less than 1%. Consequently, the HLA antigens from all six loci are inherited together and segregate with many other genes located within the same region of chromosome 6. Many of the MHC-region genes are involved in immunological processes. As a result, alleles that are known to increase the chance of developing various autoimmune diseases have remained associated with specific HLA alleles. For example, 2% of people who have the HLA-B27 allele develop an arthritic condition of the vertebrae called ankylosing spondylitis. However, approximately nine out of ten white persons who have ankylosing spondylitis are positive for HLA-B27. Because of this association, the disease and this HLA type are linked. Thus, a person with ankylosing spondylitis who is also HLA-B27 positive would have family with a much higher likelihood of developing ankylosing spondylitis than those who are not. Some notable autoimmune diseases that have a strong association with HLA antigens include Hashimoto's thyroiditis (an autoimmune disorder involving underproduction by the thyroid gland) associated with HLA-DR5; Graves' disease (an autoimmune disorder associated with overproduction by the thyroid gland), associated with HLA-B8 and Dw3; and hereditary hemochromatosis (excess iron stores), associated with HLA-A3, B7, and B14.

Precautions

HLA testing is performed using WBCs. If possible, this test should be postponed if the patient has recently undergone a transfusion, because any WBCs from the transfusion may interfere with the tissue typing of the patient's lymphocytes.

Description

The HLA gene products can be grouped into three classes. Class I consists of the products of the genes located on the HLA-A, HLA-B, and HLA-C loci. These HLA antigens are found on all nucleated cells. Class II molecules consist of antigens inherited as genes from the HLA-DR, HLA-DQ, and HLA-DP loci. These HLA antigens are normally found only on B-lymphocytes, macrophages, monocytes, dendritic cells, endothelial cells, and activated T-lymphocytes. Class III molecules are not evaluated in histocompatibility testing.

Because the HLA loci are closely linked, the HLA antigens are inherited as a group of six antigens is called a haplotype. The probability of siblings having identical haplotypes is one in four. Therefore, siblings provide the opportunity for the best matches. They can donate bone marrow, a kidney, and a section of their livers, but they cannot donate other solid organs. Approximately 85% of transplants are organs from cadavers, and because the HLA antigens are so highly polymorphic, the chance of identical haplotypes decreases quickly.

Histocompatibility testing consists of three tests, HLA antigen typing (tissue typing), screening of the recipient for anti-HLA antibodies (antibody screen), and the lymphocyte crossmatch (compatibility test). HLA antigen typing may be performed by serological (blood fluid) or DNA methods. In either case, HLA typing of HLA-A, HLA-B, HLA-DR, and HLA-DQ antigens is performed for solid organ transplants. HLA typing of HLA-C antigens is also included when tissue typing is performed for bone marrow transplants.

The antibody screen is performed in order to detect antibodies in the recipient's serum that react with HLA antigens. The most commonly used method of HLA antibody screening is the microcytotoxicity test. If an antibody against an HLA antigen is present, it will bind to the cells. The higher the number of different HLA antibodies, the lower the probability of finding a compatible match.

The third component of a histocompatibility study is the crossmatch test. In this test peripheral blood lymphocytes from the donor are separated into B and T lymphocyte populations. In the crossmatch, serum from the recipient is mixed with T-cells or B-cells from the donor. A positive finding indicates the presence of preformed antibodies in the recipient that are reactive against the donor tissues. An incompatible T-cell crossmatch contraindicates transplantation of a tissue from the T-cell donor.

Preparation

The HLA test requires a blood sample. There is no need for the patient to fast before the test.

Aftercare

The patient may feel discomfort when blood is drawn from a vein. Bruising may occur at the puncture site, or the person may feel dizzy or faint. Pressure should be applied to the puncture site until the bleeding stops to reduce bruising. Warm packs can also be placed over the puncture site to relieve discomfort.

Risks

Risks for this test are minimal, but may include slight bleeding from the puncture site, fainting or feeling lightheaded after having blood taken, or hematoma (blood accumulating under the puncture site).

Normal results

HLA typing either by serologic (blood fluid) or DNA methods is reported as the phenotype for each HLA loci tested. The antibody screen test is reported as the percentage of panel reactive antibodies (PRA). The percent PRA is the number of wells reactive with the patient's serum expressed in percent. The cross-match is reported as compatible or incompatible.

Tissue typing results for both donors and recipients and antibody screen results for recipients are submitted to the United Network for Organ Sharing (UNOS) database. The database searches all regional donors that are ABO-compatible for an HLA-identical match. If none is found, the database searches the national database for ABO compatible donors and scores the match. A point system is used based upon several parameters, including the number of matching HLA loci, the length of time the recipient has been waiting, the recipient's age, and the PRA score.

Resources

BOOKS

American Association of Blood Banks Technical Manual.13th ed., Bethesda, MD: American Association of Blood Banks, 1999.

Beutler, E., et al., eds. William's Hematology, 7th ed. New York: McGraw-Hill, Inc. 2005.

Henry, J. B. Clinical Diagnosis and Management by Laboratory Methods, 20th ed. New York: W. B. Saunders Company, 2001.

ORGANIZATIONS

American Association of Blood Banks. 8101 Glenbrook Rd., Bethesda, MD 20814. (301) 907-6977. http://www.aabb.org/content.

United Network for Organ Sharing (UNOS). http://www.unos.org/.

OTHER

National Institutes of Health. http://www.nlm.nih.gov/medlineplus/ency/article/003551.htm.

Advances in HLA Typing. http://www.marrow.org/PHYSICIAN/Adv_in_Auto_Allo_Tx/Adv_in_HLA_Typing/index.html.

Organ Donor.Gov. http://www.organdonor.gov/.

Mark A Best
Laura Jean Cataldo, RN, EdD

Hydrocele repair *see* **Hydrocelectomy**

Hydrocelectomy

Definition

Hydrocelectomy, also known as hydrocele repair, is a surgical procedure performed to correct a hydrocele. A hydrocele is an accumulation of peritoneal fluid in a membrane called the tunica vaginalis, which covers the front and sides of the male testes. Hydroceles occur because of defective absorption of tissue fluid or irritation of the membrane leading to overproduction of fluid. In addition to filling the tunic vaginalis, the fluid may also fill a portion of the spermatic duct (epididymis) in the scrotum.

Purpose

A hydrocelectomy is performed to correct a hydrocele and prevent its recurrence.

Demographics

Hydroceles are found in male children or adult males (usually over 40). They have no known association with a man's ethnic background or lifestyle factors.

Description

A hydrocele usually appears as a soft swelling in the membrane surrounding the testes. It is not usually painful and does not damage the testes. It typically occurs on one side only; only 7–10% occur on both sides of the scrotum. Inflammation is not usually present, although if the hydrocele occurs in conjunction with epididymitis (inflammation of the epididymis), the testes may be inflamed and painful. The main symptom of a hydrocele that occurs without epididymitis is scrotal swelling. As the hydrocele fills with fluid and grows, the scrotum itself gets larger. Some men may have pain or discomfort from the increased size of the scrotal mass. Hydroceles are usually congenital, found in a large percentage (80% or more) of male children and in 1% of adult males over 40.

The most common congenital hydrocele is caused by a failure of a portion of the testicular membrane (processus vaginalis, a membrane that descends with the testicles in the fetus) to close normally. This failure to close allows peritoneal (abdominal) fluid to flow into the scrotum. Although surgery is the usual treatment, it is not performed until the child is at least two years of age, giving the processus vaginalis sufficient time to close by itself. More than 80% of newborn boys are reported to have a patent (open) processus vaginalis, but it closes spontaneously in the majority

Hydrocelectomy

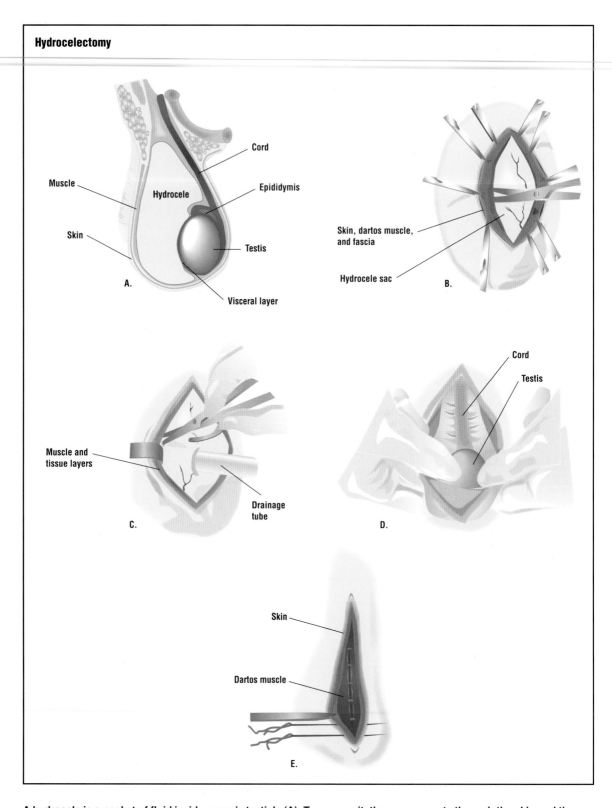

A hydrocele is a pocket of fluid inside a man's testicle (A). To remove it, the surgeon cuts through the skin and tissue layers (B), then drains the hydrocele with a tube (C). The hydrocele is opened completely (D), and skin and tissue layers are stitched (E). *(Illustration by GGS Information Services. Cengage Learning, Gale.)*

KEY TERMS

Aspiration—The process of removing fluids or gases from the body by suction.

Epididymis—A coiled segment of spermatic duct within the scrotum, attached to the back of the testis.

Epididymitis—Inflammation of the epididymis.

Inguinal hernia—An opening, weakness, or bulge in the lining tissue of the abdominal wall in the groin area, with protrusion of the large intestine.

Hydrocele—An accumulation of fluid in the membrane that surrounds the testes.

Scrotum—A pouch of skin containing the testes, epididymis, and portions of the spermatic cords.

Testis (plural, testes)—The male sex gland, held within the scrotum.

Transillumination—A technique in which the doctor shines a strong light through body tissues in order to examine an organ or structure.

Tunica vaginalis—A sac-like membrane covering the outer surface of the testes.

of children before they are 12 months old. The processus is not expected to close spontaneously in children over 18 months.

In adults, hydroceles develop slowly, usually as a result either of a defect in the tunica vaginalis that causes overproduction of fluid, or as a result of blocked lymphatic flow that may be related to an obstruction in the spermatic cord. Hydroceles may also develop as a result of inflammation or infection of the epididymis; trauma to the scrotal area; or in association with cancerous tumors in the groin area. A hydrocele can occur at the same time as an inguinal hernia.

Hydroceles can be treated with aspiration or surgery. To aspirate the collected fluid, the doctor inserts a needle into the scrotum and directs it toward the hydrocele. Suction is applied to remove (aspirate) as much fluid as possible. While aspiration is usually successful, it is a temporary correction with a high potential for recurrence of the hydrocele. Aspiration may have longer-term success when certain medications are injected during the procedure (sclerotherapy). There is a higher risk of infection with aspiration than with surgery.

Generally, surgical repair of a hydrocele will eliminate the hydrocele and prevent recurrence. In adults, surgery is used to remove large or painful hydroceles.

It is the preferred method of treatment for children over two years of age. It is also standard practice to remove hydroceles that reoccur after aspiration.

Patients are given **general anesthesia** for hydrocele repair surgery. A hydrocelectomy is typically performed on an outpatient basis with no special precautions required. The extent of the surgery depends on whether other problems are present. If the hydrocele is uncomplicated, the doctor makes an incision directly into the scrotum. After the canal between the abdominal cavity and the scrotum is repaired, the hydrocele sac is removed, fluid is removed from the scrotum, and the incision is closed with sutures. If there are complications, such as the presence of an inguinal hernia, an incision is made in the groin area. This approach allows the doctor to repair the hernia or other complicating factors at the same time as correcting the hydrocele. Some surgeons use a minimally invasive laparoscopic approach to repair a hydrocele. The operation is performed through a tiny incision using a lighted, camera-tipped, tube-like instrument (laparoscope) that allows the passage of instruments for the repair while displaying images of the procedure on a monitor in the **operating room**.

Diagnosis

Diagnosis will begin with taking a careful history, including sexual history, recent injury, or illnesses, and observing signs and symptoms. Hydroceles can sometimes be diagnosed in the doctor's office by visual examination and palpation (touch). Hydroceles are distinguished from other testicular problems by transillumination (shining a light source through the hydrocele so that the tissue lights up) and **ultrasound** examinations of the area around the groin and scrotum.

Preparation

The patient will be given standard pre-operative blood and urine tests at some time prior to surgery. Before the operation, the physician or nurse will explain the procedure, the type of anesthesia to be used, and, in some cases, the need for a temporary drain to be inserted. The drain will be placed during surgery to reduce the chances of postoperative infection and fluid accumulation.

Aftercare

Immediately following surgery, the patient will be taken to a recovery area and checked for any undue

WHO PERFORMS THE PROCEDURE AND WHERE IS IT PERFORMED?

A hydrocelectomy is performed in a hospital operating room or a one-day surgery center by a general surgeon or urologist.

bleeding from the incision. **Body temperature** and blood pressure will be monitored. Patients will usually go home the same day for a brief recovery period at home. Follow-up appointments are usually scheduled for several weeks after surgery so that the doctor can check the incision for healing and to be sure there is no infection. The patient may notice swelling for several months after the procedure; however, prolonged swelling, fever, or redness in the incision area should be reported to the surgeon immediately.

Risks

Hydrocelectomy is considered a safe surgery, with only a 2% risk of infection or complications. Injury to spermatic vessels can occur, however, and affect the man's fertility. As with all surgical procedures, reactions to anesthesia, bleeding from the surgical incision, and internal bleeding can also occur.

Normal results

Surgery usually corrects the hydrocele and the underlying defect completely; recurrence is rare. The long-term outlook is excellent. There may be swelling of the scrotum for up to a month. The adult patient is able to resume most activities within seven to 10 days, although heavy lifting and sexual activities may be delayed for up to six weeks. Children will be able to resume normal activities in four to seven days.

Morbidity and mortality rates

Chronic infection after surgical repair can increase morbidity. There are no instances reported of **death** following a hydrocele repair.

Alternatives

A hydrocele is most often a congenital defect that is commonly corrected surgically. There are no recommended alternatives and no known measures to prevent the occurrence of congenital hydroceles.

QUESTIONS TO ASK THE DOCTOR

- Why is this surgery necessary?
- How will it improve my condition (my child's condition)?
- Is surgery the only option for correction of this problem?
- How many times have you performed this surgery? What are the usual results?
- How will I (my child) feel after the surgery?
- How soon can I (my child) resume normal activities?

Resources

BOOKS

"Disorders of the Scrotum." Section 17, Chapter 219 in *The Merck Manual of Diagnosis and Therapy*, edited by Mark H. Beers, MD, and Robert Berkow, MD. Whitehouse Station, NJ: Merck Research Laboratories, 1999.

Sabiston, D. C., and H. K. Lyrly. *Essentials of Surgery.* Philadelphia, PA: W. B. Saunders Co., 1994.

Way, Lawrence W., MD. *Current Surgical Diagnosis and Treatment*, 10th ed. Stamford, CT: Appleton & Lange, 1994.

PERIODICALS

Chalasani, V., and H. H. Woo. "Why Not Use a Small Incision to Treat Large Hydroceles?" *ANZ Journal of Surgery* 72 (August 2002): 594-595.

Fearne, C. H., M. Abela, and D. Aquilina. "Scrotal Approach for Inguinal Hernia and Hydrocele Repair in Boys." *European Journal of Pediatric Surgery* 12 (April 2002): 116-117.

ORGANIZATIONS

National Kidney and Urologic Diseases Information Clearinghouse. 31 Center Drive, MSC 2560, Building 31, Room 9A-04, Bethesda, MD 20892-2560. (800) 891-5390. www.niddk.nih.gov.

OTHER

Dolan, James P., MD. *Hydrocele Repair.* www.kernanhospital.com.

Men's Health Topics. *Hydrocele.* www.uro.com/hydrocele.htm.

L. Lee Culvert

Hypophysectomy

Definition

Hypophysectomy, or hypophysis, is the surgical removal of the pituitary gland.

Purpose

The pituitary gland is a small, oval-shaped endocrine gland about the size of a pea located in the center of the brain above the back of the nose. Its major role is to produce hormones that regulate growth and metabolism in the body. Removing this important gland is a drastic step that is usually taken in the case of cancers or tumors that resist other forms of treatment, especially craniopharyngioma tumors. Hypophysectomy may also be performed to treat Cushing's syndrome, a hormonal disorder caused by prolonged exposure of the body's tissues to high levels of the hormone cortisol, in most cases associated with benign tumors called pituitary adenomas. The goal of the surgery is to remove the tumor and try to partially preserve the gland.

Demographics

Craniopharyngiomas account for less than 5% of all brain tumors. Half of all craniopharyngiomas occur in children, with symptoms most often appearing between the ages of five and ten. Cushing's syndrome is relatively

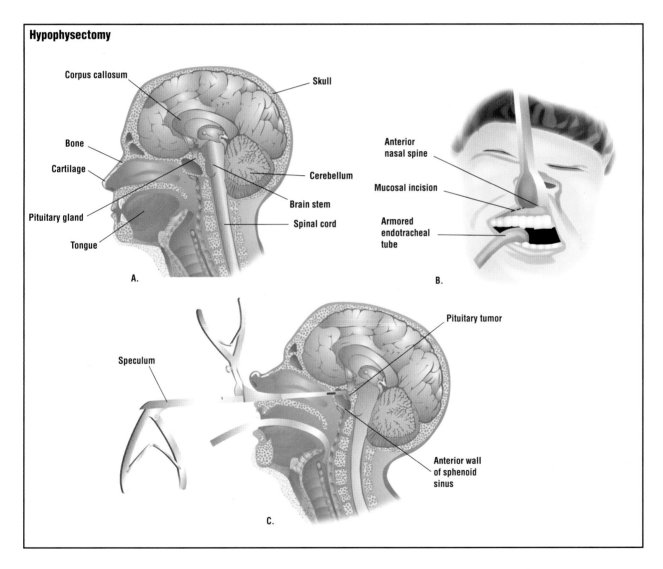

Hypophysectomy

Hypophysectomy is a procedure to access and remove the pituitary gland (A). To access it, an incision is made beneath the patient's upper lip to enter the nasal cavity (B). A speculum is inserted, and special forceps are used to remove the pituitary tumor (C). *(Illustration by GGS Information Services. Cengage Learning, Gale.)*

Adenoma—A benign tumor in which cells form recognizable glandular structures.

Cerebrospinal fluid (CSF)—A clear, colorless fluid that contains small quantities of glucose and protein. CSF fills the ventricles of the brain and the central canal of the spinal cord.

Craniotomy—A surgical incision into the skull.

Cushing's disease—A disease in which too many hormones called glucocorticoids are released into the blood. This causes fat to build up in the face, back, and chest, and the arms and legs to become very thin. Other symptoms include excessive blood sugar levels, weak muscles and bones, a flushed face, and high blood pressure.

Electrocardiogram—A recording of the electrical activity of the heart on a moving strip of paper.

Endocrine system—Group of glands and parts of glands that control metabolic activity. The pituitary, thyroid, adrenals, ovaries, and testes are all part of the endocrine system.

Hormone—A chemical made in one place that has effects in distant places in the body. Hormone production is usually triggered by the pituitary gland.

Hypopituitarism—A medical condition where the pituitary gland produces lower than normal levels of its hormones.

Magnetic resonance imaging (MRI)—A special imaging technique used to visualize internal structures of the body, particularly the soft tissues.

Metabolism—The sum of all the physical and chemical processes required to maintain life and also the transformation by which energy is made available for the uses of the body.

Pituitary gland—A small, oval-shaped endocrine gland situated at the base of the brain in the fossa (depression) of the sphenoid bone. Its overall role is to regulate growth and metabolism. The gland is divided into the posterior and anterior pituitary, each responsible for the production of its own unique hormones.

Pituitary tumors—Tumors found in the pituitary gland. Most pituitary tumors are benign, meaning that they grow very slowly and do not spread to other parts of the body.

rare in the United States, most commonly affecting adults aged 20–50. An estimated 10–15 of every million people are affected each year. However, the Pituitary Network Association reports that one out of every five people worldwide has a pituitary tumor. The earliest study was performed in 1936, by Dr. R. T. Costello of the Mayo Foundation who found pituitary tumors in 22.4% of his studied population with statistics not having changed significantly since that time.

Description

There are several surgical approaches to the pituitary. The surgeon chooses the best one for the specific procedure. The pituitary lies directly behind the nose, and access through the nose or the sinuses is often the best approach. A **craniotomy** (opening the skull) and lifting the frontal lobe of the brain will expose the delicate neck of the pituitary gland. This approach works best if tumors have extended above the pituitary fossa (the cavity in which the gland lies).

Surgical methods using new technology have made other approaches possible. Stereotaxis is a three-dimensional aiming technique using x rays or scans for guidance. Instruments can be placed in the brain with pinpoint accuracy through tiny holes in the skull. These instruments can then manipulate brain tissue, either to destroy it or remove it. Stereotaxis is also used to direct radiation with similar precision using a gamma knife. Access to some brain lesions can be gained through the blood vessels using tiny tubes and wires guided by x rays.

Diagnosis/Preparation

A patient best prepares for a hypophysectomy by keeping as healthy and relaxed as possible. Informed surgical consent is always required.

The patient is first seen for evaluation of pituitary functions by the treatment team. An MRI scan of the pituitary gland is performed and the patient is seen by a neurosurgeon in an outpatient clinic or at the hospital to assess whether hypophysectomy is suitable.

The patient checks into the hospital the day before surgery and undergoes blood tests, chest x rays, or an **electrocardiogram** to assess anesthesia fitness. Four to five sticks are attached on buttons on the forehead and marked for a special MRI scan. These buttons and scan help the neurosurgeon to accurately remove the pituitary tumor using sophisticated visualization computers. The patient is visited by the anesthesiologist (the physician who puts the patient to sleep for the operation) and he is asked to fast (nothing to eat or drink) from midnight before the day of surgery. If the hypophysectomy is performed through the nose, the patient is advised to practice breathing through the mouth as the nose will be packed after the surgery.

Aftercare

The operation takes about one to two hours, following which the patient is taken to the recovery area for about two hours before returning to the neurosurgical ward. The following postoperative measures are the normally taken:

- The patient's nose is packed to stop bleeding.
- There may be a dressing on a site of incision in the abdominal wall or thigh if a graft was necessary.
- A drip is attached to the hand and foot and other lines are attached to monitor the heart and breathing.
- A urinary catheter is placed to monitor fluid output.
- The patient has an oxygen mask.

Once in the ward, the patient is allowed to eat and drink the same night, after he or she has recovered from the anesthesia. If fluid intake and output are in balance, the drip and urinary catheter are removed the next morning. The nurses continue to monitor the amount of fluid taken and the amount of urine passed by the patient for a few days. The blood is usually tested the day following surgery. The nasal pack stays for about four days. Once the nasal pack is removed, patients commonly experience moisture coming through the nose and blood-stained mucus occurs frequently. If all is well, patients are usually discharged the following day. There are no sutures to be removed. The sutures in the nose are degradable and the graft site is usually glued together. Patients are advised not to blow their nose or insert anything in the nose.

Risks

The risks associated with hypophysectomy are numerous. Procedures are painstakingly selected to minimize risk and maximize benefit. A special risk associated with surgery on the pituitary is the risk of destroying the entire gland and leaving the entire endocrine system without regulation. Historically, this was the purpose of hypophysectomy, when the procedure was performed to suppress hormone production. After the procedure, the endocrinologist, a physician specializing in the study and care of the endocrine system, would provide the patient with all

WHO PERFORMS THE PROCEDURE AND WHERE IS IT PERFORMED?

Hypophysectomies are performed by neurosurgeons or surgeons specialized in endocrinology. Endocrinologists are physicians with special education, training, and interest in the practice of clinical endocrinology. These physicians devote a significant part of their career to the evaluation and management of patients with endocrine disease. These physicians are usually members of the American Association of Clinical Endocrinologists and a majority are certified by Boards recognized by the American Board of Medical Specialties.

A hypophysectomy is major surgery and is always performed in a hospital setting.

the hormones needed. Patients with no pituitary function did and still do quite well because of the available hormone replacements.

Other specific risks include;

- Hypopituitarism. Following surgery, if the pituitary gland has normal activity, it may become underactive and the patient may require hormone replacement therapy. Diabetes insipidus (DI) (excessive thirst and excessive urine) is not uncommon in the first few days following surgery. The vast majority of cases clear but a small number of individuals need hormone replacement.
- Cerebrospinal fluid (CSF) leakage. CSF leakage from the nose can occur following hypophysectomy. If it happens during surgery, the surgeon will repair the leak immediately. If it occurs after the nasal pack is removed, it may require diversion of the CSF away from the site of surgery or repair.
- Infection. Infection of the pituitary gland is a serious risk as it may result in abscess formation or meningitis. The risk is very small and the vast majority of cases are treatable by antibiotics. Patients are usually given antibiotics during surgery and until the nasal pack is removed.
- Bleeding. Nasal bleeding or bleeding in the cavity of the tumor after removal may occur. If the latter occurs it may lead to deterioration of vision as the visual nerves are very close to the pituitary region.
- Nasal septal perforation. This may also occur during surgery, although it is very uncommon.
- Visual impairment. A very rare occurrence, but still a risk.

QUESTIONS TO ASK THE DOCTOR

- Should I stop any medications before surgery?
- How long will the surgery last?
- What are the possible risks and complications?
- How long will it be before I can resume normal activities?
- How many hypophysectomies do you perform each year?
- Are there alternatives to surgery?

- Incomplete tumor removal. Tumors may not be completely removed, due to their attachment to vital structures.

Normal results

In the past, complete removal of the pituitary was the goal for cancer treatment. Nowadays, removal of tumors with preservation of the gland is the goal of the surgery.

Morbidity and mortality rates

A follow-up study performed at the Massachusetts General Hospital and involving 349 patients who underwent surgery for pituitary adenomas between 1978 and 1985 documented 39 deaths over the 13 year follow-up. The primary cause of **death** was cardiovascular (27.5%) followed by non-pituitary cancer (20%) and pituitary-related deaths (20%). When compared to the population at large, the primary cause of death was also cardiovascular (40%), followed by cancers (at 24%).

Alternatives

Surgery is a common treatment for pituitary tumors. For patients in whom hypophysectomy has failed or who are not suitable candidates for surgery, radiotherapy is another possible treatment. Radiation therapy uses high-energy x rays to kill cancer cells and shrink tumors. Radiation to the pituitary gland is given over a six-week period, with improvement occurring in 40–50% of adults and up to 80% of children. It may take several months or years before patients feel better from radiation treatment alone. However, the combination of radiation and the drug mitotane (Lysodren) has been shown to help speed recovery. Mitotane suppresses cortisol production and lowers plasma and urine hormone levels. Treatment with mitotane alone can be successful in 30–40% of patients. Other drugs used alone or in combination to control the production of excess cortisol are aminoglutethimide, metyrapone, trilostane, and ketoconazole.

Resources

BOOKS

Biller, Beverly M. K. and Gilbert H. Daniels. "Neuroendocrine Regulation and Diseases of the Anterior Pituitary and Hypothalamus." In *Harrison's Principles of Internal Medicine,* edited by Anthony S. Fauci, et al. New York: McGraw-Hill, 1997.

Jameson, J. Larry. "Anterior Pituitary." In *Cecil Textbook of Medicine,* edited by J. Claude Bennett and Fred Plum. Philadelphia: W. B. Saunders, 1996.

Youmans, Julian R. "Hypophysectomy." In *Neurological Surgery*. Philadelphia: W. B. Saunders, 1990.

PERIODICALS

Buchinsky, F. J., T. A. Gennarelli, S. E. Strome, D. G. Deschler, and R. E. Hayden. "Sphenoid Sinus Mucocele: A Rare Complication of Transsphenoidal Hypophysectomy." *Ear Nose Throat Journal* 80 (December 2001): 886–888.

Davis, K. T., I. McDuffie, L. A. Mawhinney, and S. A. Murray. "Hypophysectomy Results in a Loss of Connexin Gap Junction Protein from the Adrenal Cortex." *Endocrine Research* 26 (November 2000): 561–570.

Dizon, M. N. and D. L. Vesely. "Gonadotropin-secreting Pituitary Tumor Associated with Hypersecretion of Testosterone and Hypogonadism After Hypophysectomy." *Endocrinology Practice* 3 (May-June 2002): 225–231.

Nakagawa, T., M. Asada, T. Takashima, and K. Tomiyama. "Sellar Reconstruction After Endoscopic Transnasal Hypophysectomy." *Laryngoscope* 11 (November 2001): 2077–2081.

Volz, J., U. Heinrich, and S. Volz-Koster. "Conception and Spontaneous Delivery After Total Hypophysectomy." *Fertility and Sterility* 77 (March 2002): 624–625.

ORGANIZATIONS

American Association of Clinical Endocrinologists (AACE). 1000 Riverside Ave., Suite 205, Jacksonville, FL 32204. (904) 353-7878. http://www.aace.com/.

American Association of Endocrine Surgeons (AAES). MetroHealth Medical Center, H920, 2500 MetroHealth Drive, Cleveland, OH 44109-1908. (216) 778-4753. http://www.endocrinesurgeons.org.

OTHER

"Hypophysectomy." University of Dundee. Tayside University Hospitals. 2000 [cited June 24, 2003]. http://www.dundee.ac.uk/medicine/tayendoweb/images/hypophysectomy.htm.

J. Ricker Polsdorfer, MD
Monique Laberge, Ph.D.

Hypospadias repair

Definition

Hypospadias repair refers to a group of surgical approaches used to correct or reconstruct parts of the external genitalia and urinary tract related to a displaced meatus, or opening of the urethra. The urethra is the passageway that carries urine from the bladder to the outside of the body. Hypospadias is the medical term for a birth defect in which the urethra opens on the underside of the penis (in boys) or into the vagina (in girls). The word hypospadias comes from two Greek words that mean underneath and rip or tear, because severe forms of hypospadias in boys look like large tears in the skin of the penis.

Hypospadias is one of the most common congenital abnormalities in males. It was described in the first and second centuries A.D. by Celsus, a Roman historian of medicine, and Galen, a Greek physician. The first attempt to correct hypospadias by surgery was made in 1874 by Duplay, a French surgeon; as of 2003, more than 200 different procedures for the condition have been reported in the medical literature.

Hypospadias repair is, however, controversial because it is genital surgery. Some people regard it as unnecessary interference with a child's body and a traumatic experience with psychological consequences extending into adult life. Others maintain that boys with untreated hypospadias are far more likely than those who have had surgery to develop fears about intimate relationships and sexuality. There is little information about the emotional aftereffects of hypospadias repair on girls.

Purpose

Although there are several different surgical procedures used at present to correct hypospadias depending on its severity, all have the following purposes:

- To permit emptying of the bladder standing up. The abnormal location of the urethral meatus on the underside of the penis forces many boys to void urine sitting down, which leads to anxiety about using public restrooms or otherwise being seen undressed by other males.
- To correct a condition associated with hypospadias known as chordee. Chordee, which comes from the French *cordée*, which means tied or corded, is a condition in which the penis bends downward during an erection. This curving or bending makes it difficult to have normal sexual intercourse as an adult.

- To prevent urinary tract infections (UTIs). It is common in hypospadias for the urethral meatus to be stenotic, or abnormally narrowed. A stenotic urethra increases the risk of frequent UTIs.
- To lower the risk of developing testicular cancer. Hypospadias has been identified as a risk factor for developing testicular cancer after adolescence.
- To confirm the boy's sexual identity by improving the outward appearance of the penis. The external genitals of babies with severe hypospadias may look ambiguous at birth, causing stress for the parents about their child's gender identity.

Demographics

Hypospadias is much more common in males than in females. In Canada and the United States, the incidence of hypospadias in boys is estimated to be 1:250 live births. In girls, the condition is very rare, estimated at 1:500,000 live births. One troubling phenomenon is the reported doubling of cases of hypospadias in both Europe and North America since the 1970s without any obvious explanation. According to a recent press release from the U.S. Centers for Disease Control and Prevention (CDC), data from two surveillance systems monitoring birth defects in the United States show that the rate of hypospadias rose from 36 per 10,000 male births in 1968 to 80 per 10,000 male births in 1993. In addition to the increase in the number of cases reported, the proportion of severe cases has also risen, which means that the numerical increase cannot be explained as the result of better reporting.

The severity of hypospadias is defined according to the distance of the urethral opening from its normal location at the tip of the penis. In mild hypospadias, which is sometimes called coronal/glandular hypospadias, the urethral opening is located on the shaft of the penis just below the glans. In mild to moderate hypospadias, the opening is located further down the shaft of the penis toward the scrotum. In severe hypospadias, which is also called penoscrotal hypospadias, the urethral opening is located on the scrotum. About 80–85% of hypospadias are classified as mild; 10–15% as mild to moderate; and 3–6% as severe.

Although the causes of hypospadias are not yet fully understood, the condition is thought to be the end result of a combination of factors. The following have been associated with an increased risk of hypospadias:

- Genetic inheritance. Hypospadias is known to run in families; a boy with hypospadias has a 28% chance of having a male relative with the condition.

Hypospadias repair

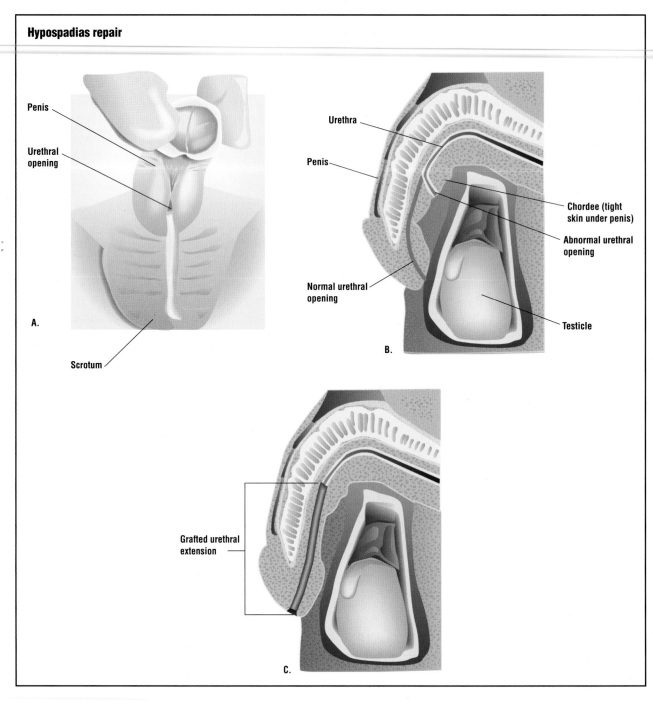

In hypospadias, the urethral opening is at the base of the penis, instead of the tip (A). Tissue grafts are used to create an extension for the urethra (C) and alleviate the tight skin, or chordee, on the underside of the penis. *(Illustration by GGS Information Services. Cengage Learning, Gale.)*

- Genetic disorders. Hypospadias is found in boys with a deletion on human chromosome 4p, also known as Wolf-Hirschhorn syndrome; and in persons with a variety of intersex conditions related to chromosomal abnormalities. Several different genetic mutations responsible for a deficiency in 5-alpha reductase, an enzyme needed to convert testosterone to a stronger androgen needed for urethral development, have been found in boys with hypospadias.

- Low birth weight. Several studies in the United Kingdom as well as in the United States have shown that male infants with hypospadias weigh less and are

Androgen—Any substance that promotes the development of masculine characteristics in a person. Testosterone is one type of androgen; others are produced in the adrenal glands located above the kidneys.

Chordee—A condition associated with hypospadias in which the penis bends downward during erections.

Circumcision—The removal of the foreskin of the penis.

Cryptorchidism—A developmental disorder in which one or both testes fail to descend from the abdomen into the scrotum before birth. It is the most common structural abnormality in the male genital tract.

Degloving—Separating the skin of the penis from the shaft temporarily in order to correct chordee.

Dehiscence—A separation or splitting apart. In hypospadias repair, dehiscence refers to the reopening of the tip of the penis or the coming apart of the entire repair.

Fistula (plural, fistulae)—An abnormal passage between two internal organs or between an internal organ and the surface of the body. The formation of fistulae is one of the possible complications of hypospadias repair.

Glans—The cap-shaped structure at the end of the penis.

Hernia—The protrusion of a loop or piece of tissue through an incision or abnormal opening in other tissues.

Inguinal—Referring to the groin area.

Meatus—The medical term for the opening of the urethra.

Stenotic—Abnormally narrowed. The urethral meatus is often stenotic in patients with uncorrected hypospadias.

Stent—A thin plastic tube inserted temporarily to hold the urethra open following hypospadias repair.

Testosterone—The major male sex hormone, produced in the testes.

Urethra—The canal or passageway that carries urine from the bladder to the outside of the body.

Urology—The branch of medicine that deals with disorders of the urinary tract in both males and females, and with the genital organs in males.

---

smaller at birth than controls. It is thought that these low measurements are markers of fetal androgen dysfunction.

- Drugs taken by the mother during pregnancy. Diethylstilbestrol (DES), a synthetic hormone that was prescribed for many women between 1938 and 1971 to prevent miscarriage, has been associated with an increased risk of stenosis of the urethral meatus as well as hypospadias in the sons of women who took the medication. Boys born to mothers addicted to cocaine also have an abnormally high rate of hypospadias.

- Environmental contamination. One proposal for explaining the rising rate of hypospadias and other birth defects in males is the so-called endocrine disruptor hypothesis. Many pesticides, fungicides, and other environmental pollutants contain estrogenic or anti-androgenic substances that interfere with the normal androgen pathways in embryonic tissue development—in birds and other animals as well as in humans.

- Assisted reproduction. A study done in Baltimore of children who were conceived through in vitro fertilization (IVF) between 1988 and 1992 found that the incidence of hypospadias among the males was five times that of male infants in a control group.

With regard to ethnic and racial differences in the American population, the CDC reports that Caucasians have the highest rates of hypospadias, Hispanics have the lowest, and African Americans have intermediate rates. Other studies have found that hypospadias is more common in males of Jewish or Italian descent than in other ethnic groups.

Description

Correction of hypospadias in boys

The specific surgical procedure used depends on the severity of the hypospadias. The objectives of surgery always include widening the urethral meatus; correcting chordee, if present; reconstructing the missing part of the urethra; and making the external genitalia look as normal as possible. Most repair procedures take between one-and-a-half and three hours, and are performed under **general anesthesia**. Mild hypospadias can be corrected in a one-step procedure known as a meatal advancement and glanduloplasty, or MAGPI. In a MAGPI procedure, the opening of the urethra is moved forward and the head of the penis is reshaped. More severe hypospadias can also be corrected in one operation, which involves degloving the penis (separating the skin from the shaft) in order to cut the bands of tissue that cause chordee, and constructing a new urethra that will reach to the tip of the penis. The specific technique of reconstruction is usually decided in the **operating room**, when the surgeon can determine how much tissue will be needed to make the new urethra. In some cases, tissue must be taken from the inner arm or the lining of the mouth. In a few cases, the repair may require two or three stages spaced several months apart.

There is some remaining disagreement among professionals regarding the best age for hypospadias repair in boys. Most surgeons think the surgery should be done between 12 and 18 months of age, on the ground that gender identity is not fully established prior to toilet training and the child is less likely to remember the operation. Some doctors, however, prefer to wait until the child is about three years old, particularly if the repair involves extensive reconstruction of the urethra.

Recent advances in hypospadias repair include the use of tissue glues and other new surgical adhesives that speed healing and reduce the risk of fistula formation. In addition, various synthetic materials are being tested for their suitability in constructing artificial urethras, which would reduce the risk of complications related to **skin grafting**.

Correction of hypospadias in girls

The most common surgical technique for correcting hypospadias in girls is construction of a new urethra that opens to the outside of the body rather than emptying into the vagina. Tissue is taken from the front wall of the vagina for this purpose.

Diagnosis/Preparation

Diagnosis

The diagnosis of hypospadias in boys is often made at the time of delivery during the newborn examination. The condition may also be diagnosed before birth by **ultrasound**; according to a group of Israeli researchers, ultrasound images of severe hypospadias resemble the outline of a tulip flower. Ultrasound is also used prior to surgical repair to check for other abnormalities, as about 18% of boys with hypospadias also have cryptorchidism (undescended testicles), inguinal hernia, or defects of the upper urinary tract.

Hypospadias in girls may not be discovered for several months after birth because of the difficulty of examining the vagina in newborn females.

Preparation

Male infants with hypospadias should not be circumcised as the foreskin may be needed for tissue grafting during repair of the hypospadias.

Some surgeons prescribe small doses of male hormones to be given to the child in advance to increase the size of the penis and improve blood supply to the area. The child may also be given a mild sedative immediately before surgery to minimize memories of the procedure.

Aftercare

Short-term aftercare

Many anesthesiologists provide a penile nerve block to minimize the child's postoperative discomfort. **Dressings** are left in place for about four days. The surgeon places a stent, which is a short plastic tube held in place with temporary **stitches**, or a catheter to keep the urethra open. The patient is usually given a course of **antibiotics** to reduce the risk of infection until the dressings and the stent or catheter are removed, usually 10–14 days after surgery.

The child should be encouraged to drink plenty of fluids after returning home in order to maintain an adequate urinary output. Periodic follow-up tests of adequate urinary flow are typically scheduled for three weeks, three months, and 12 months after surgery.

Long-term aftercare

Boys who have had any type of hypospadias repair should be followed through adolescence to exclude the possibility of chronic inflammation or scarring of the urethra. In some cases, psychological counseling may also be necessary.

Risks

In addition to the risks of bleeding and infection that are common to all operations under general anesthesia, there are some risks specific to hypospadias repair:

- Wound dehiscence. Dehiscence means that the incision splits apart or reopens. It is treated by a follow-up operation.
- Bladder spasms. These are a reaction to the presence of a urinary catheter, and are treated by giving medications to relax the bladder muscles.
- Fistula formation. A fistula is an abnormal opening that forms between the reconstructed urethra and the skin. Most fistulae that form after hypospadias

Surgery to correct hypospadias is done by a pediatric urologist, a surgeon with advanced training in urology as well as in treating disorders affecting children. According to the Society for Pediatric Urology (SPU), pediatric urologists educated in the United States have completed two years in a general surgery residency after medical school, followed by four years in a urologic surgery residency and an additional two years in a pediatric urology fellowship program.

Surgical procedures to correct mild or mild to moderate hypospadias with little chordee may be done on an outpatient basis. Correction of moderate or severe hypospadias with some chordee, however, involves hospitalizing the child for 1–2 days. Parents can usually arrange to stay overnight with their child.

surgery close by themselves within a few months. The remainder can be closed surgically.

- Recurrent chordee. This complication requires another operation to remove excess fibrous tissue.

- Urethral stenosis. Narrowing of the urethral opening after surgery is treated by dilating the meatus with urethral probes.

Normal results

Hypospadias repair in both boys and girls has a high rate of long-term success. In almost all cases, the affected children are able to have normal sexual intercourse as adults, and almost all are able to have children.

Morbidity and mortality rates

Surgical repair of hypospadias has a fairly high short-term complication rate:

- leakage of urine from the area around the urethral meatus: 3–9%

- formation of a fistula: 0.6–23% for one-stage procedures; 2–37% for two-stage procedures

- urethral stenosis: 8.5%

- persistent chordee: less than 1%

- How often do you perform hypospadias repair, and what is your success rate?

- How severe is my child's hypospadias, and what procedure do you recommend to correct it?

- What do you consider the best age for corrective genital surgery and why?

Alternatives

There are no medical treatments for hypospadias as of 2007. The only alternative to surgery in childhood is postponement until the child is old enough to decide for himself (or herself) about genital surgery.

Resources

BOOKS

Behrman RE, et al. *Nelson Textbook of Pediatrics.* 17th ed. Philadelphia: Saunders, 2004.

Wein, AJ, et al. *Campbell-Walsh Urology.* 9th ed. Philadelphia: Saunders, 2007.

PERIODICALS

Greenfield, S. P. "Two-Stage Repair for Proximal Hypospadias: A Reappraisal." *Current Urology Reports* 4 (April 2003): 151-155.

Hendren, W. H. "Construction of a Female Urethra Using the Vaginal Wall and a Buttock Flap: Experience with 40 Cases." *Journal of Pediatric Surgery* 33 (February 1998): 180–187.

Hughes, I. A., et al. "Reduced Birth Weight in Boys with Hypospadias: An Index of Androgen Dysfunction?" *Archives of Disease in Childhood: Fetal and Neonatal Edition* 87 (September 2002): F150–F151.

Klip, H., et al. "Hypospadias in Sons of Women Exposed to Diethylstilbestrol in Utero: A Cohort Study." *Lancet* 359 (March 30, 2002): 1102–1107.

Meizner, I., et al. "The 'Tulip Sign': A Sonographic Clue for In-Utero Diagnosis of Severe Hypospadias." *Ultrasound in Obstetrics and Gynecology* 19 (March 2002): 250–253.

ORGANIZATIONS

American Academy of Pediatrics (AAP). 141 Northwest Point Boulevard, Elk Grove Village, IL 60007. (847) 434-4000. http://www.aap.org.

American Board of Urology (ABU). 2216 Ivy Road, Suite 210, Charlottesville, VA 22903. (434) 979-0059. http://www.abu.org.

American Urological Association (AUA). 1120 North Charles Street, Baltimore, MD 21201. (410) 727-1100. http://www.auanet.org.

Society for Pediatric Urology (SPU). C/o HealthInfo, 870 East Higgins Road, Suite 142, Schaumburg, IL 60173. http://www.spuonline.org.

OTHER

Centers for Disease Control Press Release. "Hypospadias Trends in Two U.S. Surveillance Systems." http://www.cdc.gov/od/oc/media/pressrel/hypospad.htm.

Gatti, John M., Andrew Kirsch, and Howard M. Snyder III. "Hypospadias." eMedicine. January 31, 2003 [cited April 25, 2003]. http://www.emedicine.com/PED/topic1136.htm.

Santanelli, Fabio and Francesca R. Grippaudo. "Urogenital Reconstruction, Penile Hypospadias." eMedicine. November 6, 2002 [cited April 24, 2003]. http://www.emedicine.com/plastic/topic495.htm.

Silver, Richard I. "Recent Research Topics in Hypospadias." Society for Pediatric Urology Newsletter 1 (October 1999). http://www.kids-urology.com/HypospadiasResearch.html.

Rebecca Frey, Ph.D.

Hysterectomy

Definition

Hysterectomy is the surgical removal of all or part of the uterus. In a total hysterectomy, the uterus and cervix are removed. In some cases, the fallopian tubes and ovaries are removed along with the uterus, which is a hysterectomy with bilateral **salpingo-oophorectomy**. In a subtotal hysterectomy, only the uterus is removed. In a radical hysterectomy, the uterus, cervix, ovaries, oviducts, lymph nodes, and lymph channels are removed. The type of hysterectomy performed depends on the reason for the procedure. In all cases, menstruation permanently stops and a woman loses the ability to bear children.

Purpose

The most frequent reason for hysterectomy in American women is to remove fibroid tumors, accounting for 30% of these surgeries. Fibroid tumors are non-cancerous (benign) growths in the uterus that can cause pelvic, low back pain, and heavy or lengthy menstrual periods. They occur in 30–40% of women over age 40, and are three times more likely to be present in African-American women than in Caucasian women. Fibroids do not need to be removed unless they are causing symptoms that interfere with a woman's normal activities.

Treatment of endometriosis is the reason for 20% of hysterectomies. The endometrium is the lining of the uterus. Endometriosis occurs when the cells from the endometrium begin growing outside the uterus. The outlying endometrial cells respond to the hormones that control the menstrual cycle, bleeding each month the way the lining of the uterus does. This causes irritation of the surrounding tissue, leading to pain and scarring.

Twenty percent of hysterectomies are done because of heavy or abnormal vaginal bleeding that cannot be linked to any specific cause and cannot be controlled by other means. Another 20% are performed to treat prolapsed uterus, pelvic inflammatory disease, or endometrial hyperplasia, a potentially pre-cancerous condition.

About 10% of hysterectomies are performed to treat cancer of the cervix, ovaries, or uterus. Women with cancer in one or more of these organs almost always have the organ(s) removed as part of their cancer treatment.

Demographics

Hysterectomy is the second most common operation performed on women in the United States. About 556,000 of these surgeries are done annually. By age 60, approximately one out of every three American women will have had a hysterectomy. It is estimated that 30% of hysterectomies are unnecessary.

The frequency with which hysterectomies are performed in the United States has been questioned in recent years. It has been suggested that a large number of hysterectomies are performed unnecessarily. The United States has the highest rate of hysterectomies of any country in the world. Also, the frequency of this surgery varies across different regions of the United States. Rates are highest in the South and Midwest, and are higher for African-American women. In recent years, although the number of hysterectomies performed has declined, the number of hysterectomies performed on younger women aged 30s and 40s is increasing, and 55% of all hysterectomies are performed on women ages 35–49.

Description

A hysterectomy is classified according to what structures are removed during the procedure and what method is used to remove them.

Total hysterectomy

A total hysterectomy, sometimes called a simple hysterectomy, removes the entire uterus and the cervix.

Hysterectomy (abdominal)

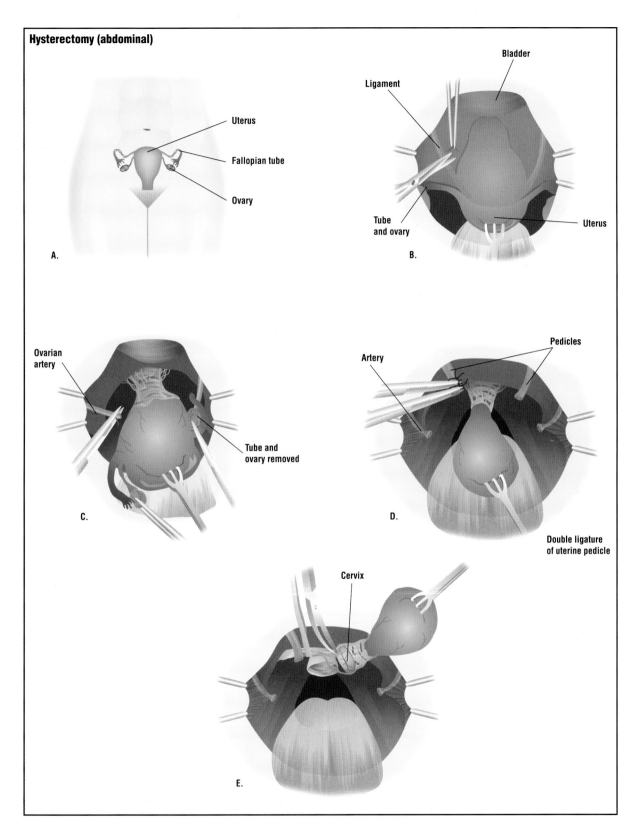

A.

B. Ligament / Bladder / Tube and ovary / Uterus

C. Ovarian artery / Tube and ovary removed

D. Artery / Pedicles / Double ligature of uterine pedicle

E. Cervix

In a hysterectomy, the reproductive organs are accessed through a lower abdominal incision or laparoscopically (A). Ligaments and supporting structures called pedicles connecting the uterus to surrounding organs are severed (B). Arteries to the uterus are severed (C). The uterus, fallopian tubes, and ovaries are removed (D and E). *(Illustration by GGS Information Services. Cengage Learning, Gale.)*

The ovaries are not removed and continue to secrete hormones. Total hysterectomies are usually performed in the case of uterine and cervical cancer. This is the most common kind of hysterectomy.

In addition to a total hysterectomy, a procedure called a bilateral salpingo-oophorectomy is sometimes performed. This surgery removes the ovaries and the fallopian tubes. Removal of the ovaries eliminates the main source of the hormone estrogen, so menopause occurs immediately. Removal of the ovaries and fallopian tubes is performed in about one-third of hysterectomy operations, often to reduce the risk of ovarian cancer.

Subtotal hysterectomy

If the reason for the hysterectomy is to remove uterine fibroids, treat abnormal bleeding, or relieve pelvic pain, it may be possible to remove only the uterus and leave the cervix. This procedure is called a subtotal hysterectomy (or partial hysterectomy), and removes the least amount of tissue. The opening to the cervix is left in place. Some women believe that leaving the cervix intact aids in their achieving sexual satisfaction. This procedure, which used to be rare, is now performed more frequently.

Subtotal hysterectomy is easier to perform than a total hysterectomy, but leaves a woman at risk for cervical cancer. She will still need to get yearly Pap smears.

Radical hysterectomy

Radical hysterectomies are performed on women with cervical cancer or endometrial cancer that has spread to the cervix. A radical hysterectomy removes the uterus, cervix, above part of the vagina, ovaries, fallopian tubes, lymph nodes, lymph channels, and tissue in the pelvic cavity that surrounds the cervix. This type of hysterectomy removes the most tissue and requires the longest hospital stay and a longer recovery period.

Methods of hysterectomy

There are two ways that hysterectomies can be performed. The choice of method depends on the type of hysterectomy, the doctor's experience, and the reason for the hysterectomy.

ABDOMINAL HYSTERECTOMY. About 75% of hysterectomies performed in the United States are abdominal hysterectomies. The surgeon makes a 4–6-in (10–15-cm) incision either horizontally across the pubic hair line from hip bone to hip bone or vertically from navel to pubic bone. Horizontal incisions leave a less noticeable scar, but vertical incisions give the surgeon a better view of the abdominal cavity. The blood vessels, fallopian tubes, and ligaments are cut away from the uterus, which is lifted out.

Abdominal hysterectomies take from one to three hours. The hospital stay is three to five days, and it takes four to eight weeks to return to normal activities.

The advantages of an abdominal hysterectomy are that the uterus can be removed even if a woman has internal scarring (adhesions) from previous surgery or her fibroids are large. The surgeon has a good view of the abdominal cavity and more room to work. Also, surgeons tend to have the most experience with this type of hysterectomy. The abdominal incision is more painful than with vaginal hysterectomy, and the recovery period is longer.

VAGINAL HYSTERECTOMY. With a vaginal hysterectomy, the surgeon makes an incision near the top of the vagina. The surgeon then reaches through this incision to cut and tie off the ligaments, blood vessels, and fallopian tubes. Once the uterus is cut free, it is removed through the vagina. The operation takes one to two hours. The hospital stay is usually one to three days, and the return to normal activities takes about four weeks.

The advantages of this procedure are that it leaves no visible scar and is less painful. The disadvantage is that it is more difficult for the surgeon to see the uterus and surrounding tissue. This makes complications more common. Large fibroids cannot be removed using this technique. It is very difficult to remove the ovaries during a vaginal hysterectomy, so this approach may not be possible if the ovaries are involved.

Vaginal hysterectomy can also be performed using a laparoscopic technique. With this surgery, a tube containing a tiny camera is inserted through an incision in the navel. This allows the surgeon to see the uterus on a video monitor. The surgeon then inserts two slender instruments through small incisions in the abdomen and uses them to cut and tie off the blood vessels, fallopian tubes, and ligaments. When the uterus is detached, it is removed though a small incision at the top of the vagina.

This technique, called laparoscopic-assisted vaginal hysterectomy, allows surgeons to perform a vaginal hysterectomy that might otherwise be too difficult. The hospital stay is usually only one day. Recovery time is about two weeks. The disadvantage is that this operation is relatively new and requires great skill by the surgeon.

Any vaginal hysterectomy may have to be converted to an abdominal hysterectomy during surgery if complications develop.

Diagnosis/Preparation

Before surgery the doctor will order blood and urine tests. The woman may also meet with the anesthesiologist to evaluate any special conditions that might affect the administration of anesthesia. On the evening before the operation, the woman should eat a light dinner and then have nothing to eat or drink after midnight.

Aftercare

After surgery, a woman will feel some degree of discomfort; this is generally greatest in abdominal hysterectomies because of the incision. Hospital stays vary from about two days (laparoscopic-assisted vaginal hysterectomy) to five or six days (abdominal hysterectomy with bilateral salpingo-oophorectomy). During the hospital stay, the doctor will probably order more blood tests.

Return to normal activities such as driving and working takes anywhere from two to eight weeks, again depending on the type of surgery. Some women have emotional changes following a hysterectomy. Women who have had their ovaries removed will probably start hormone replacement therapy.

Risks

Hysterectomy is a relatively safe operation, although like all major surgery it carries risks. These include unanticipated reaction to anesthesia, internal bleeding, blood clots, damage to other organs such as the bladder, and post-surgery infection.

Other complications sometimes reported after a hysterectomy include changes in sex drive, weight gain, constipation, and pelvic pain. Hot flashes and other symptoms of menopause can occur if the ovaries are removed. Women who have both ovaries removed and who do not take estrogen replacement therapy run an increased risk for heart disease and osteoporosis (a condition that causes bones to be brittle). Women with a history of psychological and emotional problems before the hysterectomy are likely to experience psychological difficulties after the operation.

As in all major surgery, the health of the patient affects the risk of the operation. Women who have chronic heart or lung diseases, diabetes, or iron-deficiency anemia may not be good candidates for this operation. Heavy smoking, obesity, use of steroid drugs, and use of illicit drugs add to the **surgical risk**.

Normal results

Although there is some concern that hysterectomies may be performed unnecessarily, there are many conditions for which the operation improves a woman's quality of life. In the Maine Woman's Health Study, 71% of women who had hysterectomies to correct moderate or severe painful symptoms reported feeling better mentally, physically, and sexually after the operation.

Morbidity and mortality rates

The rate of complications differs by the type of hysterectomy performed. Abdominal hysterectomy is associated with a higher rate of complications (9.3%), while the overall complication rate for vaginal hysterectomy is 5.3%, and 3.6% for laparoscopic vaginal hysterectomy. The risk of **death** from hysterectomy is about one in every 1,000 women. The rates of some of the more commonly reported complications are:

- excessive bleeding (hemorrhaging): 1.8–3.4%
- fever or infection: 0.8–4.0%
- accidental injury to another organ or structure: 1.5–1.8%

Alternatives

Women for whom a hysterectomy is recommended should discuss possible alternatives with their doctor and consider getting a **second opinion**, since this is major surgery with life-changing implications. Whether an alternative is appropriate for any

WHO PERFORMS THE PROCEDURE AND WHERE IS IT PERFORMED?

Hysterectomies are usually performed under the strict conditions of a hospital operating room. The procedure is generally performed by a gynecologist, a medical doctor who has specialized in the areas of women's general health, pregnancy, labor and childbirth, prenatal testing, and genetics.

QUESTIONS TO ASK THE DOCTOR

- Why is a hysterectomy recommended for my particular condition?
- What type of hysterectomy will be performed?
- What alternatives to hysterectomy are available to me?
- Will I have to start hormone replacement therapy?

individual woman is a decision she and her doctor should make together. Some alternative procedures to hysterectomy include:

- Embolization. During uterine artery embolization, interventional radiologists put a catheter into the artery that leads to the uterus and inject polyvinyl alcohol particles right where the artery leads to the blood vessels that nourish the fibroids. By killing off those blood vessels, the fibroids have no more blood supply, and they die off. Severe cramping and pain after the procedure is common, but serious complications are less than 5% and the procedure may protect fertility.

- Myomectomy. A myomectomy is a surgery used to remove fibroids, thus avoiding a hysterectomy. Hysteroscopic myomectomy, in which a surgical hysteroscope (telescope) is inserted into the uterus through the vagina, can be done on an outpatient basis. If there are large fibroids, however, an abdominal incision is required. Patients typically are hospitalized for two to three days after the procedure and require up to six weeks recovery. Laparoscopic myomectomies are also being done more often. They only require three small incisions in the abdomen, and have much shorter hospitalization and recovery times. Once the fibroids have been removed, the surgeon must repair the wall of the uterus to eliminate future bleeding or infection.

- Endometrial ablation. In this surgical procedure, recommended for women with small fibroids, the entire lining of the uterus is removed. After undergoing endometrial ablation, patients are no longer fertile. The uterine cavity is filled with fluid and a hysteroscope is inserted to provide a clear view of the uterus. Then, the lining of the uterus is destroyed using a laser beam or electric voltage. The procedure is typically done under anesthesia, although women can go home the same day as the surgery. Another newer procedure involves using a balloon, which is filled with superheated liquid and inflated until it fills

the uterus. The liquid kills the lining, and after eight minutes the balloon is removed.

- Endometrial resection. The uterine lining is destroyed during this procedure using an electrosurgical wire loop (similar to endometrial ablation).

Resources

BOOKS

Katz, VL, et al. *Comprehensive Gynecology*. 5th ed. St. Louis: Mosby, 2007.

Khatri, VP and JA Asensio. *Operative Surgery Manual*. 1st ed. Philadelphia: Saunders, 2003.

Townsend, CM, et al. *Sabiston Textbook of Surgery*. 17th ed. Philadelphia: Saunders, 2004.

PERIODICALS

Kovac, S. Robert. "Hysterectomy Outcomes in Patients with Similar Indications." *Obstetrics & Gynecology* 95, no. 6 (June 2000): 787–93.

ORGANIZATIONS

American Cancer Society. 1599 Clifton Rd., NE, Atlanta, GA 30329-4251. (800) 227-2345. http://www.cancer.org.

American College of Obstetricians and Gynecologists. 409 12th St., SW, P.O. Box 96920, Washington, DC 20090-6920. http://www.acog.org.

National Cancer Institute. Building 31, Room 10A31, 31 Center Drive, MSC 2580, Bethesda, MD 20892-2580. (800) 422-6237. http://www.nci.nih.gov.

OTHER

Bachmann, Gloria. "Hysterectomy." eMedicine. May 3, 2002 [cited March 13, 2003]. http://www.emedicine.com/med/topic3315.htm.

Bren, Linda. "Alternatives to Hysterectomy: New Technologies, More Options." Food and Drug Administration. October 29, 2001 [cited March 13, 2003]. http://www.fda.gov/fdac/features/2001/601_tech.html.

Debra Gordon
Stephanie Dionne Sherk

Hysteroscopy

Definition

Hysteroscopy enables a physician to look through the vagina and neck of the uterus (cervix) to inspect the cavity of the uterus with an instrument called a hysteroscope. Hysteroscopy is used as both a diagnostic and a treatment tool.

Purpose

Diagnostic hysteroscopy can be used to help determine the cause of infertility, dysfunctional uterine bleeding, and repeated miscarriages. It can also help locate polyps and fibroids, as well as intrauterine devices (IUDs).

The procedure is also used to investigate and treat gynecological conditions, often done instead of or in addition to, performing a dilation and curettage (D&C).

A D&C is a surgical procedure that expands the cervical canal (dilation) so that the lining of the uterus can be scraped (curettage). A D&C can be used to take a sample of the lining of the uterus for analysis. However, hysteroscopy has advantages over a D&C because the doctor can take tissue samples of specific areas and view any fibroids, polyps, or structural abnormalities. In addition, small fibroids and polyps may be removed via the hysteroscope (in combination with other instruments that are inserted through canals in the hysteroscope), thus avoiding more invasive and complicated open surgery. This approach is also used to remove IUDs that have become embedded in the wall of the uterus.

Demographics

There is no research available to indicate that hysteroscopy is performed more or less frequently on any subset of the female population.

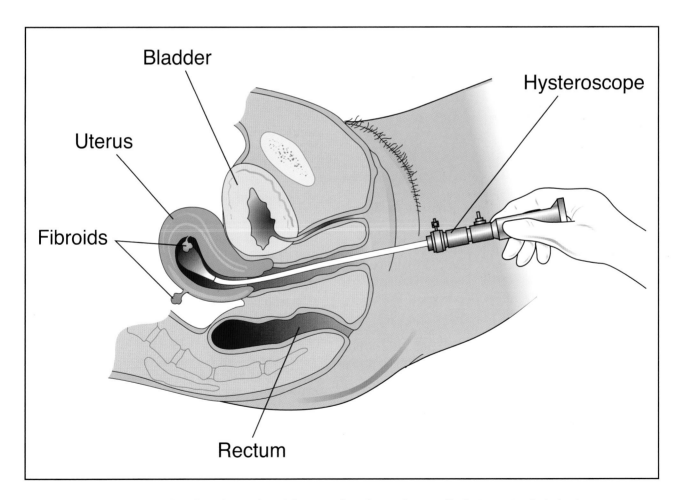

Hysteroscopy is a procedure that allows inspection of the uterus by using a telescope-like instrument called a hysteroscope.
(Illustration by Electronic Illustrators Group. Cengage Learning, Gale.)

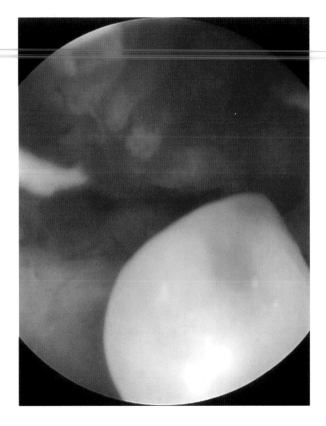

Hysteroscopy of an intrauterine polyp. *(Ism/Phototake. Reproduced by permission.)*

Description

The hysteroscope is an extremely thin telescope-like instrument that looks like a lighted tube. The modern hysteroscope is so thin that it can fit through the cervix with only minimal or no dilation.

Before inserting the hysteroscope, the doctor administers an anesthetic. Once it has taken effect, the doctor dilates the cervix slightly, and then inserts the hysteroscope through the cervix to reveal the inside of the uterus. Ordinarily, the walls of the uterus are touching each other. In order to get a better view, the uterus may be inflated with carbon dioxide gas or fluid. Hysteroscopy takes approximately 30 minutes.

Treatment involving the use of hysteroscopy is usually performed as a short-stay hospital procedure with regional or **general anesthesia**. Tiny **surgical instruments** may be inserted through the hysteroscope to remove polyps or fibroids. A small sample of tissue lining the uterus is often removed for examination, especially if the patient has experienced any abnormal vaginal bleeding.

Diagnosis/Preparation

If the procedure is performed under general anesthesia, the patient should have nothing to eat or drink after midnight the night before the procedure. Routine lab tests may be ordered if the procedure is performed in a hospital. Occasionally, a mild sedative is administered to help the patient relax. The patient is asked to empty her bladder. She is then placed in position (usually in a special chair that tilts back) and the vagina is cleansed. Usually, a local anesthetic is administered around the cervix, although a regional anesthetic that blocks nerves connected to the pelvic region or a general anesthetic may be required for some patients.

Aftercare

It is normal to experience light bleeding for one to two days after surgical hysteroscopy. Mild cramping or pain is common after operative hysteroscopy, but usually diminishes within eight hours. If carbon dioxide gas was used, the resulting discomfort usually subsides within 24 hours.

Risks

Diagnostic hysteroscopy rarely causes complications. The primary risk is infection. Prolonged bleeding may follow a surgical hysteroscopy to remove a growth. Another complication is perforation of the uterus, bowel, or bladder, caused by over-forceful advancement of the hysteroscope. An infrequent but dangerous complication is increased fluid absorption from the uterus into the bloodstream. Keeping track of the amount of fluid used during the procedure can minimize this complication. Surgery under general anesthesia poses the additional risks typically associated with this type of anesthesia.

The procedure is not performed on women with acute pelvic inflammatory disease (PID) due to the potential of exacerbating the condition. Hysteroscopy should be scheduled after menstrual bleeding has ended and before ovulation to avoid a potential interruption of a new pregnancy.

Patients should notify their health care provider if, after the hysteroscopy, they develop any of the following symptoms:

- abnormal discharge
- heavy vaginal bleeding
- fever over 101°F (38.3°C)
- severe lower abdominal pain

Normal results

Normal hysteroscopy reveals a healthy uterus with no fibroids or other growths. Abnormal results include uterine fibroids, polyps, or a septum (an extra fold of tissue down the center of the uterus). Sometimes, precancerous or malignant growths are discovered.

Morbidity and mortality rates

The rate of complications during diagnostic hysteroscopy is very low, about 0.01%. Surgical hysteroscopy is associated with a higher number of complications. Perforation of the uterus occurs in 0.8% of procedures and excess bleeding in 1.2–3.5% of cases. **Death** as a result of hysteroscopy occurs at a rate of 2.4 per 100,000 procedures performed.

Alternatives

A laparoscope (an instrument which is attached to a video camera and a light source, is inserted through

the abdominal wall) may be used to visualize the outside of the uterus or perform a surgical procedure on the pelvic organs. **Laparoscopy** and hysteroscopy are sometimes performed simultaneously to maximize their diagnostic capabilities.

Resources

BOOKS

Baggish, Michael, S., Rafael F. Calle, and Hubert Guedi. *Hysteroscopy: Visual Perspectives of Uterine Anatomy, Physiology, and Pathology*, 3rd ed. Baltimore: Lippincott Williams & Wilkins, 2007.

Pagana, Kathleen D., and Timothy J. Pagana. *Diagnostic Testing and Nursing Implications*, 5th edition. St. Louis: Mosby, 1999.

Valle, Rafael F. *Manual of Clinical Hysteroscopy*, 2nd edition. London: Informa Healthcare, 2004.

PERIODICALS

Murdoch, J. A., and T. J. Gan. "Anesthesia for Hysteroscopy." *Anesthesiology Clinics of North America* 19, no. 1 (March 2001): 125–40.

Neuwirth, R. S. "Special Article: Hysteroscopy and Gynecology: Past, Present, and Future." *Journal of American Association of Gynecology Laparoscopy* 8, no. 2 (May 2001): 193–8.

ORGANIZATIONS

American Association of Gynecologic Laparoscopists. 6757 Katella Avenue. Cypress, CA, 90630-5105. http://www.aagl.org/.

American College of Obstetricians and Gynecologists. 409 12th St., S.W., P.O. Box 96920, Washington, DC 20090-6920. http://www.acog.org/.

OTHER

Gordon, A. G. "Complications of Hysteroscopy." Practical Training and Research in Gynecologic Endoscopy. February 17, 2003. http://www.gfmer.ch/Books/Endoscopy_book/Ch24_Complications_hyster.html.

Maggie Boleyn, RN, BSN
Stephanie Dionne Sherk
Laura Jean Cataldo, RN, EdD

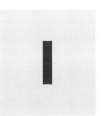

Ibuprophen *see* **Nonsteroidal anti-inflammatory drugs**

ICU *see* **Intensive care unit**

ICU equipment *see* **Intensive care unit equipment**

Ileal conduit surgery

Definition

There are many surgical techniques for urinary diversion surgery. They fall into two categories: continent diversion and conduit diversion. In continent diversion, also known as continent catheterizable stomal reservoir, a separate rectal reservoir for urine is created, which allows evacuation from the body. In conduit diversion, or orthotopic urethral anastomotic procedure, an intestinal stoma or conduit for release of urine is created in the abdominal wall so that a catheter or ostomy can be attached for the release of urine. An ileal conduit is a small urine reservoir that is surgically created from a small segment of bowel. Both techniques are forms of **reconstructive surgery** to replace the bladder or bypass obstructions or disease in the bladder so that urine can pass out of the body. Both procedures have been used for years and should be considered for all appropriate patients. Ileal conduit surgery, the easiest of the reconstructive surgeries, is the gold standard by which other surgical techniques, both continent and conduit, have been compared as the techniques have advanced over the decades.

Purpose

The bladder creates a reservoir for the liquid wastes created by the kidneys as a result of the ability of these organs to filter and retain glucose, salts, and minerals that the body needs. When the bladder must be removed; or becomes diseased, injured, obstructed, or develops leak points; the release of urinary wastes from the kidneys becomes impaired, endangering the kidneys with an overburden of poisons. Reasons for disabling the urinary bladder are: cancer of the bladder; neurogenic sources of bladder dysfunction; bladder sphincter detrusor overactivity that causes continual urge incontinence; chronic inflammatory diseases of the bladder; tuberculosis; and schistosomiasis, which is an infestation of the bladder by parasites, mostly occurring Africa and Asia. Radical **cystectomy**, removal of the bladder, is the predominant treatment for cancer of the bladder, with radiation and chemotherapy as other alternatives. In both cases, urinary diversion is often necessitated, either due to the whole or partial removal of the bladder or to damage done by radiation to the bladder.

Demographics

Urinary diversion has a long history and, over the last two decades, has developed new techniques for urinary tract reconstruction to preserve renal function and to increase the quality of life. A number of difficulties had to be solved for such progress to take place. Clean intermittent catheterization by the patient became possible in the 1980s, and many patients with loss of bladder function were able to continue to have urine release through the use of catheters. However, it soon became clear that catheterization left a residue that cumulatively, and over time, increased the risk of infection, which subsequently decreased kidney function through reflux, or backup, of urine into the kidneys. A new way had to be found. With the advent of surgical anatomosis (the grafting of vascularizing tissue for the repair and expansion of organ function) as well as with the ability to include a flap-type of valve to prevent backup, bladder reconstructive surgery that allowed for protection of the kidneys became possible.

Ileal conduit surgery

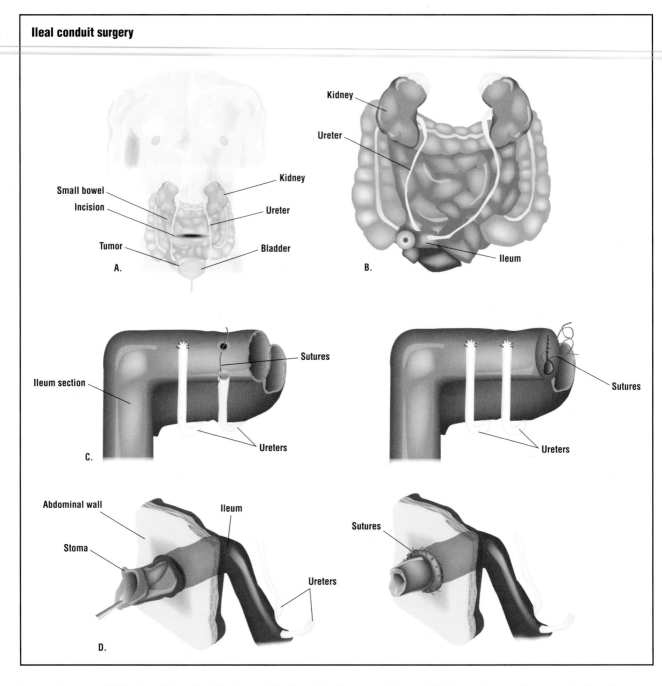

In a cystectomy with ileal conduit, an incision is made in the patient's lower abdomen (A). The ureters are disconnected from the bladder, which is then removed (B). They are then attached to a section of ileum (small intestine) that has been removed and refashioned for that purpose (C). A stoma, or hole in the abdominal wall, is created at the site to allow drainage of the urine (D). *(Illustration by GGS Information Services. Cengage Learning, Gale.)*

Description

Ileal conduit surgery consists of open abdominal surgery that proceeds in the following three stages:

- Isolating the ileum, which is the last section of small bowel. The segment used is about 5.9–7.8 in (15–20 cm) in length.

- The segment is then anastomosed, or grafted, to the ureters with absorbable sutures.

- A stoma, or opening in skin, is created on the right side of the abdomen.

- The other end of the bowel segment is attached to the stoma, which drains into an ostomy bag.

Neo-bladder—A term that refers to the creation of a reservoir for urine made from intestinal tissue that allows for evacuation.

Ostomy—A pouch attached to an outlet through the abdominal wall that allows urine to drain and be collected after the surgical removal of the bladder.

Stoma—A term used for the opening in the abdomen created to reroute urine to an external collection pouch, or ostomy.

Urinary conduit diversion—A type of urinary diversion or rerouting that uses a conduit made from an intestinal segment to channel urine to an outside collection pouch.

Stents are used to bypass the surgical site and divert urine externally, ensuring that the anastomotic site has adequate healing time. Continent surgeries are more extensive than the ileal conduit surgery and are not described here. Both types of surgery require an extensive hospitalization with careful monitoring of the patient for infections, removal of stents placed in the bowel during surgery, and removal of catheters.

Diagnosis/Preparation

Ileal conduit surgery is recommended depending on what conditions are being treated; whether the urinary diversion is immediately necessary; for the relief of pain or discomfort; or for relatively healthy individuals or individuals with terminal illness. Three major decisions that must be made by the physician and patient include:

• The type of surgery to restore bladder function: either by sending urine through the ureters to a new repository fashioned in the rectum, or by creating a conduit for the removal of the urine out through the stomach wall and into a permanent storage pouch or ostomy outside the body.

• The type of material out of which to fashion the reservoir or conduit.

• Where to place the stoma outlet for patient use.

Recent research has shown there is little difference in infection rates or in renal deterioration between the conduit surgical techniques and the continent techniques. The patient's preference becomes important as to which type of surgery and resulting procedures for urination they want. Of course, some patients, unable to conduct catheterization due to debilitating diseases like multiple sclerosis or neurological injuries, should be encouraged to have the reservoir or continent procedures.

Materials for fashioning continent channels have included sections of the appendix, stomach, ileum and cecum of the intestines, and for the reservoir, sigmoid and ureter tissues, usually with an anti-refluxing mechanism to maximize continence. A segment of the ileum is often preferred, unless the tissue has received radiation. In this case, other tissue must be used. Ileum is preferred because the ileal tissue of the intestines accommodates larger urine volume at lower pressure.

Many urinary diversion procedures are performed in conjunction with surgery for recurrent cancer or complications of pelvic radiation. Fistula development and repeated repair as well as ureteral obstruction also are reasons to have the surgery. If the surgery is considered because of cancer, the physician and the patient need to discuss how appropriate the surgery is for cure or for relieving pain. Highly relevant are the patient's age, medical condition, and ability to comprehend both the procedure and the patient's role in the changed state that will result with the surgery. In general, ileal conduit surgery is easier, faster, and has fewer complications than continent reservoir surgery.

In addition to these considerations, great emphasis must be put on preparing the patient psychologically, and physicians must make themselves available for counseling and questions before proceeding with patient evaluation for the procedures. The renal system must be assessed using pylography, which is the visualization of the renal pelvis of the kidneys to determine the health of each renal system. Patients with renal disease or abnormalities are not good candidates for urinary diversion. Bowel preparation and prophylactic **antibiotics** are necessary to avoid infection with the surgery. Bowel preparation includes injecting a clear-liquid diet preoperatively for two days, followed by using a cleansing enema or enemas until the bowel runs clear. The importance of these preparations must be explained to the patient: leaking from the bowel during surgery can be life threatening. For ileal conduits, the placement of the stoma must be decided. This is accomplished after the physician evaluates the patient's abdomen in both a sitting and standing position, to avoid placing the stoma in a fatty fold of the abdomen. The input from a stomal therapist is important for this preparation with the patient.

Aftercare

Ureteral stents are generally removed one week after surgery. A **urine culture** is taken from each stent. Radiologic contrast studies are carried out to ensure against ureteral anastomotic leakage or obstruction. On the seventh postoperative day, a contrast study is performed to ensure pouch integrity. Thereafter, ureteral stents may be removed, again with radiologic control. When it has been determined that the ureteral anastomoses and pouch are intact, the suction drain is removed. The patient is shown how to support the operative site when sleeping and with breathing and coughing. Fluids and electrolytes are infused intravenously until the patient can take liquids by mouth. The patient is usually able to get up in eight to 24 hours and leave the hospital in about a week.

Patients are taught how to care for the ostomy, and family members are educated as well. Appropriate supplies and a schedule of how to change the pouch are discussed, along with skin care techniques for the area surrounding the stoma. Often, a stomal therapist will make a home visit after discharge to help the patient return to normal daily activities.

Risks

This surgery includes the major risks of thrombosis and heart difficulties that can result from abdominal surgery. Many difficulties can occur after urinary diversion surgery, including urinary leakage, problems with a stoma, changes in fluid balance, and infections over time. However, urinary diversion is usually tolerated well by most patients, and reports indicate that patient satisfaction is very high. Common complications are stricture caused by inflammation or scar tissue from surgery, disease, or injury. The incidence of urine leakage for all types of ureterointestinal anastomoses is 3–5% and occurs within the first 10 days after surgery. According to some researchers, this incidence of leakage can be reduced to near zero if stents are used during surgery.

Normal results

Complete healing is expected without complications, with the patient returning to normal activities once they have recovered from surgery.

Morbidity and mortality rates

Possible complications associated with ileal conduit surgery include bowel obstruction, blood clots, urinary tract infection, pneumonia, skin breakdown around the stoma, stenosis of the stoma, and damage to the upper urinary tract by reflux. Pyelonephritis, or bacterial infection of a kidney, occurs both in the early postoperative period and over the long term. Approximately 12% of patients diverted with ileal conduits and 13% in those diverted with anti-refluxing colon conduits have this complication. Pyelonephritis is associated with significant mortality.

Alternatives

An alternative to ileal conduit surgery is continent surgery in which a neo-bladder is fashioned from bowel segments, allowing the patient to evacuate the urine and avoid having an external appliance. The procedures of continent diversion are more complicated, require more hospitalization, and have higher complication rates than conduit surgery. Many patients, unable to manage a stoma, are good candidates for continent diversion.

Resources

BOOKS

Novick, Andrew C., et al. *Operative Urology: At the Cleveland Clinic,* 1st ed. Totowa, NJ: Humana Press, 2006.

Tanagho, Emil A. and Jack W. McAninch. *Smith's General Urology,* 17h ed. New York: McGraw-Hill Professional, 2007.

Walsh, P., et al. *Campbell's Urology,* 8th ed. St. Louis: Elsevier, 2000.

PERIODICALS

Estape, R., L. E. Mendez, R. Angioli, and M. Penalver. "Gynecologic Oncology: Urinary Diversion in Gynecological Oncology." *Surgical Clinics of North America* 81, no. 4 (August 2002).

ORGANIZATIONS

National Digestive Diseases Information Clearinghouse. 2 Information Way, Bethesda, MD 20892-3570. http://www2.niddk.nih.gov.

United Ostomy Association, Inc. (UOA). 19772 MacArthur Blvd., Suite 200, Irvine, CA 92612-2405. (800) 826-0826. http://www.uoa.org.

Wound, Ostomy and Continence Nurses Society. 15000 Commerce Parkway, Suite C. Mt. Laurel, NJ 08054. 888-224-WOCN (9626).http://www.wocn.org/

OTHER

"Urinary Diversion." American Urological Association. http://www.urologyhealth.org.

Nancy McKenzie, PhD
Laura Jean Cataldo, RN, EdD

Ileoanal anastomosis

Definition

Ileoanal anastomosis is a surgical procedure in which the large intestine is bypassed and the lower portion of the small intestine is directly attached to the anal canal. It is also called an ileal pouch-anal anastomosis.

Purpose

An ileoanal anastomosis is an invasive procedure performed in patients who have not responded to more conservative treatments. The small intestine is composed of three major sections: the duodenum, which is the upper portion into which the stomach empties; the jejunum, which is the middle portion; and the ileum. The ileum is the last portion of the small intestine and empties into the large intestine. The large intestine is composed of the colon, where stool is formed, and the rectum, which empties to the outside of the body through the anal canal.

Surgical removal of the bowel is usually a procedure of last resort for a patient who has not responded to less invasive medical therapies. For example, many patients with ulcerative colitis, an inflammatory condition of the colon and rectum, can be treated by medications or dietary changes that control the symptoms of the disease. For patients who fail to respond to these approaches, however, the creation of an ileoanal anastomosis removes most or all of the diseased tissue. Certain types of colon cancer and a condition called familial adenomatous polyposis, or FAP, in which the inner lining of the colon becomes covered with abnormal growths, may also be treated with ileoanal anastomosis.

Demographics

Most patients—more than 85%—who undergo an ileoanal anastomosis are being treated for ulcerative colitis; familial adenomatous polyposis is the next most common condition requiring the surgery. The average age of patients at surgery is 35 years, and the majority of patients are male.

Description

A surgical anastomosis is the connection of two cut or separate tubular structures to make a continuous channel. To perform an ileoanal anastomosis, the surgeon detaches the ileum from the colon and the anal canal from the rectum. He or she then creates a pouch-like structure from ileal tissue to act as a rectum and connects it directly to the anal canal. This procedure offers distinct advantages over a conventional **ileostomy**, a procedure in which the ileum is connected to the abdominal wall. A conventional ileostomy leaves the patient incontinent (i.e., unable to control the emptying of waste from the body) and unable to have normal bowel movements. Instead, the patient's waste is excreted through an opening in the abdominal wall into a bag. An ileoanal anastomosis, however, removes the diseased large intestine while allowing the patient to pass stool normally without the need of a permanent ileostomy.

An ileoanal anastomosis is usually completed in two separate surgeries. During the first operation, the surgeon makes a vertical incision through the patient's abdominal wall and removes the colon. This procedure is called a colectomy. The inner lining of the rectum is also removed in a procedure called a mucosal proctectomy. The muscles of the rectum and anus are left in place so that the patient will not be incontinent. Next, the surgeon makes a pouch by stapling sections of the small intestine together with surgical **staples**. The pouch may be J-, W-, or S-shaped, and acts as reservoir for waste (as the rectum does) to decrease the frequency of the patient's bowel movements. Once the pouch is constructed, it is connected to the anal canal to form the anastomosis. To allow the anastomosis time to heal before stool begins to pass through, the surgeon creates a temporary "loop" ileostomy. The surgeon then makes a small incision through the abdominal wall and brings a loop of the small intestine through the incision and sutures it to the skin. Waste then exits the body through this opening, which is called a stoma, and collects in a bag attached to the

Ileoanal anastomosis

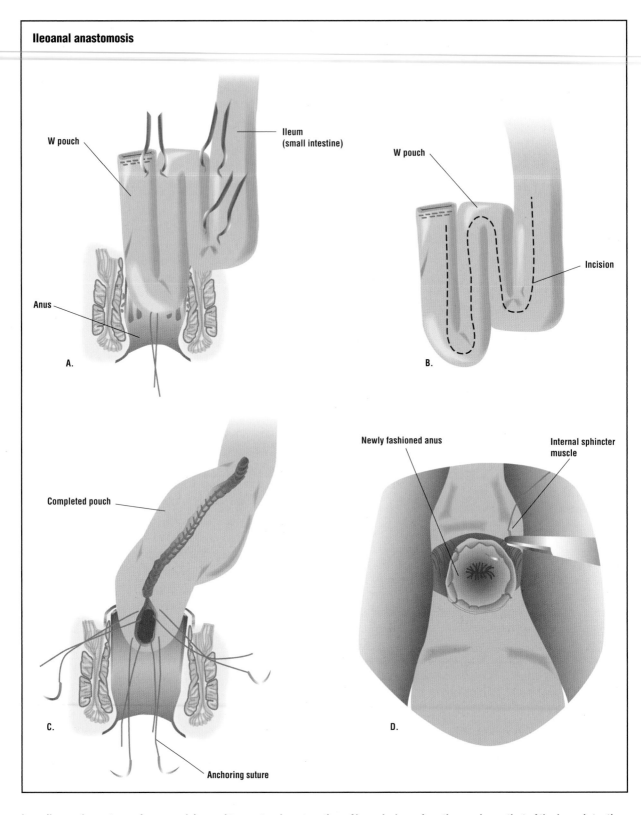

W pouch

Ileum
(small intestine)

W pouch

Incision

Anus

A.

B.

Completed pouch

Newly fashioned anus

Internal sphincter
muscle

C.

D.

Anchoring suture

In an ileoanal anastomosis, a pouch is used to create a large section of bowel whose function replaces that of the large intestine, or colon. In this operation, the ileum (part of the small intestine) is shaped into a W-shaped pouch (A). An incision is made (B) to open up the shape and create the larger pouch, which is left open at one end and brought through the rectal area (C). The bottom of the pouch acts as a new rectum, and a new anus is fashioned (D). *(Illustration by GGS Information Services. Cengage Learning, Gale.)*

KEY TERMS

Anastomosis (plural, anastomoses)—A surgically created joining or opening between two organs or body spaces that are normally separate.

Colon—The portion of the large intestine where stool is formed.

Continent—Able to hold the contents of the bladder or bowel until one can use a bathroom. A continent surgical procedure is one that allows the patient to keep waste products inside the body rather than collecting them in an external bag attached to a stoma.

Enterostomal therapist—A health care provider who specializes in the care of patients with enterostomies (e.g., ileostomies or colostomies).

Ostomy—The surgical creation of an opening from an internal structure to the outside of the body.

Polyp—Any mass of tissue that grows out of a mucous membrane in the digestive tract, uterus, or elsewhere in the body.

Stoma (plural, stomata)—A surgically created opening in the abdominal wall to allow digestive wastes to pass to the outside of the body.

Ileoanal anastomoses are usually performed in hospital operating rooms. They may be performed by a general surgeon, a colorectal surgeon (a medical doctor who focuses on diseases of the colon, rectum, and anus), or a gastrointestinal surgeon (a medical doctor who focuses on diseases of the gastrointestinal system).

outside of the abdomen. In an emergency situation, the surgeon may perform the colectomy and ileostomy during one operation, and create the ileal pouch during another.

In the second operation, the surgeon closes the ileostomy, thus restoring the patient's ability to defecate in the normal manner. This second procedure generally takes place two to three months after the original surgery. The surgeon detaches the ileum from the stoma and attaches it to the newly created pouch. A continuous channel then runs from the small intestine through the ileal pouch and anal canal to the outside of the body. In some instances, the surgeon may decide to combine the two surgeries into one operation without creating a temporary ileostomy.

Diagnosis/Preparation

Because an ileoanal anastomosis is a procedure that is done after a patient has failed to respond to other therapies, the patient's condition has been diagnosed by the time the doctor suggests this surgery.

The patient meets with the operating physician prior to surgery to discuss the details of the surgery and receive instructions on pre- and post-operative care. Immediately before the operation, an intravenous (IV) line is placed in the patient's arm to administer fluid and medications, and the patient is given a bowel preparation to cleanse the bowel for surgery. The location of the stoma is marked on the skin so that it is placed away from bones, abdominal folds, and scars.

Aftercare

Following surgery, the staff will instruct the patient in the care of the stoma, placement of the ileostomy bag, and necessary changes regarding diet and lifestyle. Visits with an enterostomal therapist (ET) or a support group for individuals with ostomies may be recommended to help the patient adjust to living with a stoma. After the anastomosis has healed, which usually takes about two to three months, the ileostomy can then be closed. A dietician may suggest permanent changes in the patient's diet to minimize gas and diarrhea.

Risks

Risks associated with any surgery that involves opening the abdomen include excessive bleeding, infection, and complications due to **general anesthesia**. Specific complications following an ileoanal anastomosis include leakage of stool; anal stenosis (narrowing of the anus); pouchitis (inflammation of the ileal pouch); and pouch failure. Patients who have received a temporary ileostomy may experience obstruction (blockage) of the stoma; stomal prolapse (protrusion of the ileum through the stoma); or a rash or skin irritation around the stoma.

Normal results

After ileoanal anastomosis, patients will usually experience between four and nine bowel movements during the day and one at night; this frequency generally decreases over time. Because of the nature of the surgery, persons with an ileoanal anastomosis retain the ability to control their bowel movements. They can refrain from defecating for extended periods of time, an advantage not afforded by a conventional ileostomy. One study found that 97% of patients were satisfied with the results of the surgery and would recommend it to others with similar disorders.

Morbidity and mortality rates

The overall rate of complications associated with ileoanal anastomosis is approximately 10%. Between 10% and 15% of patients will experience at least one episode of pouchitis, and 10–20% will develop postsurgical pelvic or wound infections. The rate of anastomosis failure requiring the creation of a permanent ileostomy is approximately 5–10%.

Alternatives

An ileostomy is a surgical alternative for patients who are not good candidates for an ileoanal anastomosis. If the patient wishes to retain continence, the surgeon may perform a continent ileostomy. Portions of the small intestine are used to form a pouch and valve; these are then directly attached to the abdominal wall skin to form a stoma. Waste collects inside the internal pouch and is expelled by insertion of a soft, flexible tube through the stoma several times a day.

Resources

BOOKS

Pemberton, John H., and Sidney F. Phillips. "Ileostomy and Its Alternatives." Chapter 105 in *Sleisenger and Fordtran's Gastrointestinal and Liver Disease*, 7th ed. Philadelphia, PA: Elsevier Science, 2002.

Porrett, Theresa and Anthony McGrath. *Stoma Care (Essential Clinical Skills for Nurses)*, 1st ed. Malden, MA: Wiley-Blackwell; 2005.

Rayson, Elizabeth. *Living Well with an Ostomy*, 1st ed. Victoria, Canada: Your Health Press, 2006.

Sklar, Jill and Manuel Sklar. *The First Year: Crohn's Disease and Ulcerative Colitis: An Essential Guide for the Newly Diagnosed*, 2nd ed. New York: Marlowe & Company, 2007.

PERIODICALS

Becker, James M. "Surgical Therapy for Ulcerative Colitis and Crohn's Disease." *Gastroenterology Clinics of North America* 28 (June 1, 1999): 371-90.

ORGANIZATIONS

Crohn's and Colitis Foundation of America. 386 Park Ave. S., 17th Floor, New York, NY 10016. (800) 932-2423. www.ccfa.org.

United Ostomy Association, Inc. (UOA). 19772 MacArthur Blvd., Suite 200, Irvine, CA 92612-2405. (800) 826-0826. http://www.uoa.org.

Wound, Ostomy and Continence Nurses Society. 15000 Commerce Parkway, Suite C. Mt. Laurel, NJ 08054. 888-224-WOCN (9626). http://www.wocn.org/

OTHER

"Surgery for Ulcerative Colitis". Crohn's and Colitis Foundation of America. March, 2006. http://www.ccfa.org/info/surgery/surgeryuc.

Stephanie Dionne Sherk
Laura Jean Cataldo, RN, EdD

Ileoanal reservoir surgery

Definition

Ileoanal reservoir surgery or **ileoanal anastomosis** is a two-stage restorative procedure that removes a part of the colon and uses the ileum (a section of the small intestine) to form a new reservoir for waste that can be expelled through the anus. This surgery is one of several continent surgeries that rely upon a newly created pouch to replace the resected colon and retain the patient's sphincter for natural defecation. Ileoanal reservoir surgery is also called a J-pouch, endorectal pullthrough, or pelvic pouch procedure.

Purpose

A number of diseases require removal of the entire colon or parts of the colon. Proctolectomies (removal of the entire colon) are often performed to treat colon cancer. Another surgical option is the creation of an ileoanal pouch to serve as an internal waste reservoir—an alternative to the use of an external ostomy pouch. An ileoanal reservoir procedure is performed primarily on patients with ulcerative colitis, inflammatory bowel disease (IBD), familial polyposis, or familial adenomatous polyposis (FAP), which is a relatively rare cancer that covers the colon with 100 or more polyps. FAP is caused by a gene mutation on the long arm of human chromosome 5. Ileoanal reservoir surgery is recommended only in those patients who have not previously lost their rectum or anus.

Demographics

The prevalence of familial adenomatous polyposis (FAP) in the United States is two to three cases per 100,000 persons. It develops before age 40 and accounts for about 0.5% of colorectal cancers; this figure is declining, however, as more at-risk families are undergoing detection and prophylactic colon surgery. The annual incidence of ulcerative colitis is 10.4–12 cases per 100,000 people. The prevalence rate is 35–100 cases per 100,000. People of Jewish descent have two to four times the risk of developing ulcerative colitis than people from other ethnic backgrounds. About 20% of ulcerative colitis patients require surgery of the colon.

Description

Conventional ileoanal reservoir surgery is an open procedure that is done in two stages. In the first stage, the surgeon removes the diseased colon and creates a pouch. The second stage is performed three months later, when the temporary drainage conduit is closed and the newly created reservoir allows the patient to defecate in the normal fashion. Both surgeries can also be done together, bypassing the creation of a temporary **ileostomy**.

Some surgeons use a laparoscopic approach to ileoanal surgery. This technique involves the insertion of scaled-down **surgical instruments** and a scope that allows the surgeon to see inside the abdomen through several relatively small incisions (about 3.5 inches [9 cm] compared to 6 inches [16 cm] for an open procedure) in the abdominal wall. Studies indicate that there are few differences in the rates of mortality or complications between laparoscopic surgery and conventional open surgery. Because the incisions are smaller, patients typically require less pain medication with laparoscopic surgery.

Ileoanal surgery includes the following steps:

- The surgeon isolates the ileum or small segment of bowel.
- The segment is then attached to the anus with absorbable sutures.
- A pouch is created out of the small bowel above the anus.

KEY TERMS

Anastomosis—A surgically created joining or opening between two organs or body spaces that are normally separate.

Colon—The portion of the large intestine where stool is formed.

Continent—Able to hold the contents of the bladder or bowel until one can use a bathroom. A continent surgical procedure is one that allows the patient to keep waste products inside the body rather than collecting them in an external bag attached to a stoma.

Ileoanal anastomosis—A reservoir for fecal waste surgically created out of the small intestine. It retains the sphincter function of the anus and allows the patient to defecate in the normal fashion.

Ileum—The third and lowest portion of the small intestine, extending from the jejunum to the beginning of the large intestine.

Polyp—Any mass of tissue that grows out of a mucous membrane in the digestive tract, uterus, or elsewhere in the body.

Sphincter—A circular band of muscle fibers that constricts or closes a passageway in the body.

Stent—A thin rodlike or tubelike device made of wire mesh, inserted into a blood vessel or a section of the digestive tract to keep the structure open.

Stoma (plural, stomata)—A surgically created opening in the abdominal wall to allow digestive wastes to pass to the outside of the body.

- If the surgeon is performing the procedure in two stages, he or she creates a temporary ileostomy. An ileostomy is a tubular bowel segment attached to a stoma at the abdomen that drains into a bag outside the abdomen.
- In the second-stage operation, the surgeon uses an open abdominal procedure to close the temporary pouch.

The surgeon will insert stents to bypass the surgical site and divert urinary and digestive wastes to the outside of the body, thus allowing the new connection between the ileum and the anus to heal properly.

Diagnosis/Preparation

The diagnosis of FAP is usually made after symptoms caused by polyps in the colon, such as rectal bleeding, diarrhea, and abdominal pain, have led to a **physical examination**, the taking of a family history, and in some cases a genetic test. Ulcerative colitis or inflammatory bowel disease patients have usually been treated with medical alternatives before they decide to have surgery. All patients who are candidates for an ileoanal procedure will have an evaluation of the upper gastrointestinal tract, an x ray of the small bowel, and a **colonoscopy** with a pathology review. Most patients will also be given a **sigmoidoscopy** and a digital rectal examination.

The surgeon will need to perform an ileostomy in about 5–10% of cases because the patient's rectal muscles are not strong enough for an anastomosis. This possibility is discussed with the patient, as well as the fact that complications in surgery may lead to an ostomy procedure. The placement of a stoma must be decided in the event that an ileostomy is necessary. The physician evaluates the patient's abdomen while the patient is sitting and then standing, in order to avoid placing the stoma inside a fatty fold of the abdomen. A stomal therapist is often called in to prepare the patient for the possibility that an appliance will be needed. In addition to the medical and surgical considerations of the procedure, the patient requires psychological preparation regarding the changes in function and appearance that accompany this surgery.

Prior to surgery, the patient must undergo a bowel preparation, which includes a clear-liquid diet for two days before the procedure. In addition to drinking nothing but clear fluids, the patient must have a cleansing enema until the bowel runs clear. The importance of a thorough bowel preparation must be explained to the patient, because leakage from the bowel during surgery can be life-threatening.

Aftercare

Open ileaoanal reservoir surgery is a lengthy procedure (as long as five hours) with a slow recovery rate (approximately six weeks) and a relatively long stay in the hospital (about 10 days). The catheters and stents that were used are removed several days after surgery. The patient will be introduced to a special diet in the hospital, and the diet will be altered if needed in response to changes in the chemistry of the colon. The patient's stools are measured, and he or she is monitored for dehydration. In addition, the patient will have the opportunity to discuss his or her concerns about care of the new reservoir and frequency of defecation with staff members before leaving the hospital.

WHO PERFORMS THE PROCEDURE AND WHERE IS IT PERFORMED?

An ileoanal reservoir procedure is performed by a gastrointestinal surgeon specializing in reconstructive bowel or colon surgery. The operation takes place in a general hospital as an inpatient procedure.

Results

For carefully selected patients this procedure, developed over 30 years, is the preferred form of radical colon surgery when the patient's sphincter and rectum are still intact. The advantage of the ileoanal reservoir surgery is that the patient has an internal pouch for the collection of waste material and can pass this waste normally through the anus. Bowel movements may be more fluid, however, and more frequent with the new reservoir. In a small percentage of cases, the surgeon may eventually need to perform an ileostomy due to complications. In one quality of life study for patients who have undergone ileoanal reservoir surgery, researchers found only slight differences in their general health and level of daily activity compared with subjects recruited from the general population.

Morbidity/mortality

Morbidity rates with this procedure have decreased over time due to improvements in technique. The most common complication is inflammation of the pouch, which occurs in as many as 40% of patients. This complication can be treated with medication. Other complications include severe scarring around the incision, and some risk of injury to the nerves that control erection and bladder function. In one major study of 379 patients, researchers at the University of Cincinnati reported that 79 patients had pouch infections (24.3%) and another 20 patients required further surgery for obstructions of the small bowel (6.2%).

Alternatives

The major surgical alternative to an ileoanal reservoir procedure is an ileostomy. In an ileostomy, the patient's fecal matter drains into a plastic bag attached to a stoma on the outside of the patient's abdomen or into a pouch attached to the abdominal wall to be withdrawn through a plastic tube.

Resources

BOOKS

Lange, Vladimir, MD. *Be a Survivor: Colorectal Cancer Treatment Guide*, 1st ed. Los Angeles, CA: Lange Productions, 2006.

Larson, Carol Ann, and Kathleen Ogle. *Positive Options for Colorectal Cancer: Self-Help and Treatment*, 1st ed. Alameda, CA: Hunter House, 2005.

Levin, Bernard, MD , et al. *American Cancer Society's Complete Guide to Colorectal Cancer*, 1st ed. Atlanta: American Cancer Society, 2005.

Pemberton, John H., and Sidney F. Phillips. "Ileostomy and Its Alternatives." In *Sleisenger and Fordtran's Gastrointestinal and Liver Disease*, 7th ed. Philadelphia, PA: Elsevier Science, 2002.

"Tumors of the Gastrointestinal Tract: Large-Bowel Tumors." In *The Merck Manual of Diagnosis and Therapy*, edited by Mark H. Beers, MD, and Robert Berkow, MD. Whitehouse Station, NJ: Merck Research Laboratories, 1999.

PERIODICALS

Allison, Stephen, and Marvin L. Corman. "Intestinal Stomas in Crohn's Disease." *Surgical Clinics of North America* 81, no. 1 (February 1, 2001): 185-95.

Blumberg, D., and D. E. Beck. "Surgery for Ulcerative Colitis." *Gastroenterology Clinics of North America* 31 (March 2002): 219-235.

Pasupathy, S., K. W. Eu, Y. H. Ho, and F. Seow-Choen. "A Comparison Between Open Versus Laparoscopic Assisted Colonic Pouches for Rectal Cancer." *Techniques in Coloproctology* 5 (April 2001): 19-22.

Robb, B., et al. "Quality of Life in Patients Undergoing Ileal Pouch-Anal Anastomosis at the University of Cincinnati." *American Journal of Surgery* 183 (April 2002): 353-360.

ORGANIZATIONS

American Gastroenterological Association, American Digestive Health Foundation. 7910 Woodmont Aveenue, 7th Floor, Bethesda, MD 20814. (301) 654-2055. www.gastro.org.

American Society of Colon and Rectal Surgeons. 85 W. Algonquin Rd., Suite 550, Arlington Heights, IL 60005. www.fascrs.org.

Crohn's and Colitis Foundation of America. 386 Park Ave. S., 17th Floor, New York, NY 10016. (800) 932-2423. www.ccfa.org.

National Digestive Diseases Information Clearinghouse. 2 Information Way, Bethesda, MD 20892-3570. http://www2.niddk.nih.gov.

United Ostomy Association, Inc. (UOA). 19772 MacArthur Blvd., Suite 200, Irvine, CA 92612-2405. (800) 826-0826. www.uoa.org.

OTHER

MDconsult.com. "Inflammatory Bowel Disease (Crohn's Disease and Ulcerative Colitis)." www.MDconsult.com.

"Surgery for Ulcerative Colitis." Crohn's and Colitis Foundation of AmericaMarch, 2006. http://www.ccfa.org/info/surgery/surgeryuc.

Nancy McKenzie, PhD
Laura Jean Cataldo, RN, EdD

Ileorectal anastomosis *see* **Ileoanal anastomosis**

Ileostomy

Definition

An ileostomy is a surgical procedure in which the small intestine is attached to the abdominal wall in order to bypass the large intestine; digestive waste then exits the body through an artificial opening called a stoma (from the Greek word for "mouth").

Purpose

In general, an ostomy is the surgical creation of an opening from an internal structure to the outside of the body. An ileostomy, therefore, creates a temporary or permanent opening between the ileum (the portion of the small intestine that empties to the large intestine) and the abdominal wall. The colon and/or rectum may be removed or bypassed. A temporary ileostomy may be recommended for patients undergoing bowel surgery (e.g., removal of a segment of bowel), to provide the intestines with sufficient time to heal without the stress of normal digestion.

Chronic ulcerative colitis is an example of a medical condition that is treated with the removal of the large intestine. Ulcerative colitis occurs when the body's immune system attacks the cells in the lining of the large intestine, resulting in inflammation and

Ileostomy

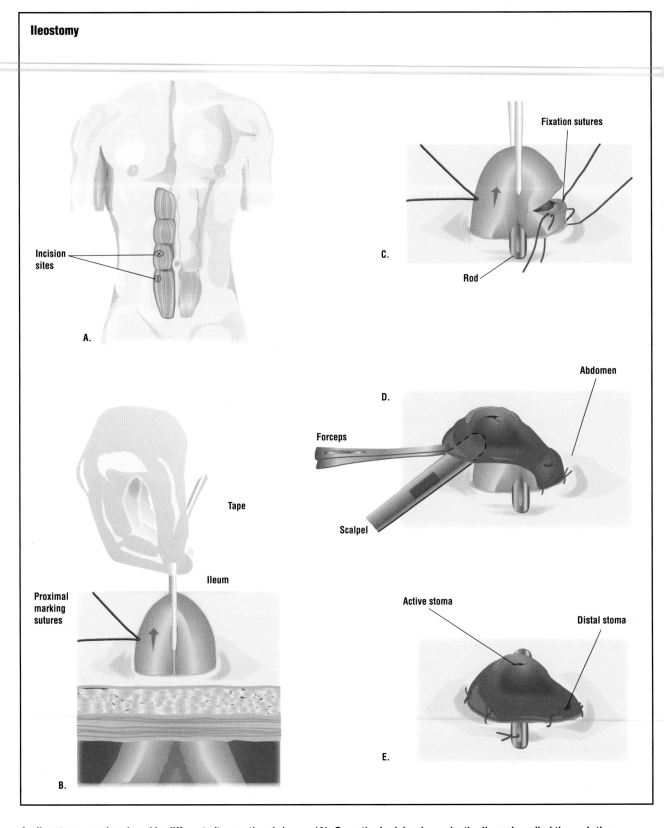

An ileostomy can be placed in different sites on the abdomen (A). Once the incision is made, the ileum is pulled through the incision (B), and a rod is placed under the loop. The loop is cut open, one side is stitched to the abdomen (C). The portion of intestine is flipped open to expose the interior surface (D), and the opposite side is stitched in place (E). *(Illustration by GGS Information Services. Cengage Learning, Gale.)*

KEY TERMS

Anastomosis—A surgically created joining or opening between two organs or body spaces that are normally separate.

Colon—The portion of the large intestine where stool is formed.

Enterostomal therapist—A health care provider who specializes in the care of individuals with enterostomies (e.g. ileostomies or colostomies).

Rectum—The portion of the large intestine where stool is stored until exiting the body through the anal canal.

Stoma (plural, stomata)—A surgically created opening in the abdominal wall to allow digestive wastes to pass to the outside of the body.

tissue damage. Patients with ulcerative colitis often experience pain, frequent bowel movements, bloody stools, and loss of appetite. An ileostomy is a treatment option for patients who do not respond to medical or dietary therapies for ulcerative colitis.

Other conditions that may be treated with an ileostomy include:

- bowel obstructions
- cancer of the colon and/or rectum
- Crohn's disease (chronic inflammation of the intestines)
- congenital bowel defects
- uncontrolled bleeding from the large intestine
- injury to the intestinal tract

Demographics

The United Ostomy Association estimates that approximately 75,000 ostomy surgeries are performed each year in the United States, and that 750,000 Americans have an ostomy. Ulcerative colitis and Crohn's disease affect approximately one million Americans. There is a greater incidence of the diseases among Caucasians under the age of 30 or between the ages of 50 and 70.

Description

For some patients, an ileostomy is preceded by removal of the colon (colonectomy) or the colon and rectum (protocolectomy). After the patient is placed under **general anesthesia**, an incision approximately 8 in (20 cm) long is made down the patient's midline,

through the abdominal skin, muscle, and other subcutaneous tissues. Once the abdominal cavity has been opened, the colon and rectum are isolated and removed. The anal canal is stitched closed. Other patients undergoing ileostomy will have only a temporary bypass of the colon and rectum; examples are patients undergoing **small bowel resection** or the creation of an **ileoanal anastomosis**. An ileoanal anastomosis is a procedure in which the surgeon forms a pouch out of tissue from the ileum and connects it directly to the anal canal.

There are two basic types of permanent ileostomy: conventional and continent. A conventional ileostomy, also called a Brooke ileostomy, involves a separate, smaller incision through the abdominal wall skin (usually on the lower right side) to which the cut end of the ileum is sutured. The ileum may protrude from the skin, often as far as 2 in (5 cm). Patients with this type of stoma are considered fecal-incontinent, meaning they can no longer control the emptying of wastes from the body. After a conventional ileostomy, the patient is fitted with a plastic bag worn over the stoma and attached to the abdominal skin with adhesive. The ileostomy bag collects waste as it exits from the body.

An alternative to conventional ileostomy is the continent ileostomy. Also called a Kock ileostomy, this procedure allows a patient to control when waste exits the stoma. Portions of the small intestine are used to form a pouch and valve; these are directly attached to the abdominal wall skin to form a stoma. Waste collects internally in the pouch and is expelled by insertion of a soft, flexible tube through the stoma several times a day.

Diagnosis/Preparation

The patient meets with the operating physician prior to surgery to discuss the details of the surgery and receive instructions on pre- and **postoperative care**. Directly preceding surgery, an intravenous (IV) line is placed to administer fluid and medications, and the patient is given a bowel prep to cleanse the bowel and prepare it for surgery. The location where the stoma will be placed is marked, away from bones, abdominal folds, and scars.

Aftercare

Following surgery, the patient is instructed in the care of the stoma, placement of the ileostomy bag, and necessary changes to diet and lifestyle. Because the large intestine (a site of fluid absorption) is no longer a part of the patient's digestive system, fecal matter exiting the stoma has a high water content. The patient must therefore be diligent about his or her fluid intake to minimize the risk of dehydration. Visits with an enterostomal therapist (ET) or a support group for individuals with ostomies may be recommended to help the patient adjust to living with a stoma. Once the ileostomy has healed, a normal diet can usually be resumed, and the patient can return to normal activities.

Risks

Risks associated with the ileostomy procedure include excessive bleeding, infection, and complications due to general anesthesia. After surgery, some patients experience stomal obstruction (blockage); inflammation of the ileum; stomal prolapse (protrusion of the ileum through the stoma); or irritation of the skin around the stoma.

Normal results

The physical quality of life of most patients is not affected by an ileostomy, and with proper care most patients can avoid major medical complications. Patients with a permanent ileostomy, however, may suffer emotional aftereffects and benefit from psychotherapy.

Morbidity and mortality rates

Among patients who have undergone a Brooke ileostomy, medical literature reports a 19–70% risk of complications. Small bowel obstruction occurs in 15% of patients; 30% have problems with the stoma; 20–25% require further surgery to repair the stoma; and 30% experience postsurgical infections. The rate of complications is also high among patients who have had a continent ileostomy (15–60%). The most common complications associated with this procedure are small bowel obstruction (7%); wound complications (35%); and failure to restore continence (50%). The mortality rate of both procedures is less than 1%.

Alternatives

Patients with mild to moderate ulcerative colitis may be able to manage their disease with medications. Medications that are given to treat ulcerative colitis include enemas containing hydrocortisone or mesalamine; oral sulfasalazine or olsalazine; oral **corticosteroids**; or cyclosporine and other drugs that affect the immune system.

A surgical alternative to ileostomy is the ileal pouch-anal anastomosis, or ileoanal anastomosis. This procedure, used more frequently than permanent ileostomy in the treatment of ulcerative colitis, is similar to a continent ileostomy in that an ileal pouch is formed. The pouch, however, is not attached to a stoma but to the anal canal. This procedure allows the patient to retain fecal continence. An ileoanal anastomosis usually requires the placement of a temporary ileostomy for 2–3 months to give the connected tissues time to heal.

Resources

BOOKS

Feldman, M, et al. *Sleisenger & Fordtran's Gastrointestinal and Liver Disease*. 8th ed. St. Louis: Mosby, 2005.

Khatri, VP and JA Asensio. *Operative Surgery Manual*. 1st ed. Philadelphia: Saunders, 2003.

Townsend, CM et al. *Sabiston Textbook of Surgery*. 17th ed. Philadelphia: Saunders, 2004.

ORGANIZATIONS

Crohn's and Colitis Foundation of America. 386 Park Ave. S., 17th Floor, New York, NY 10016. (800) 932-2423. www.ccfa.org.

United Ostomy Association, Inc. 19772 MacArthur Blvd., Suite 200, Irvine, CA 92612-2405. (800) 826-0826. www.uoa.org.

OTHER

Hurst, Roger D. "Surgical Treatment of Ulcerative Colitis." [cited May 1, 2003]. www.ccfa.org/medcentral/library/surgery/ucsurg.htm.

Stephanie Dionne Sherk

Immunoassay tests

Definition

Immunoassays are chemical tests used to detect or quantify a specific substance, the analyte, in a blood or body fluid sample, using an immunological reaction. Immunoassays are highly sensitive and specific. Their high specificity results from the use of antibodies and purified antigens as reagents. An antibody is a protein (immunoglobulin) produced by B-lymphocytes (immune cells) in response to stimulation by an antigen. Immunoassays measure the formation of antibody-antigen complexes and detect them via an indicator reaction. High sensitivity is achieved by using an indicator system (e.g., enzyme label) that results in amplification of the measured product.

Immunoassays may be qualitative (positive or negative) or quantitative (amount measured). An example of a qualitative assay is an immunoassay test for pregnancy. Pregnancy tests detect the presence of human chorionic gonadotropin (hCG) in urine or serum. Highly purified antibodies can detect pregnancy within two days of fertilization. Quantitative immunoassays are performed by measuring the signal produced by the indicator reaction. This same test for pregnancy can be made into a quantitative assay of hCG by measuring the concentration of product formed.

Purpose

The purpose of an immunoassay is to measure (or, in a qualitative assay, to detect) an analyte. Immunoassay is the method of choice for measuring analytes normally present at very low concentrations that cannot be determined accurately by other less expensive tests. Common uses include measurement of drugs, hormones, specific proteins, tumor markers, and markers of cardiac injury. Qualitative immunoassays are often used to detect antigens on infectious agents and antibodies that the body produces to fight them. For example, immunoassays are used to detect antigens on *Hemophilus, Cryptococcus*, and *Streptococcus* organisms in the cerebrospinal fluid (CSF) of meningitis patients. They are also used to detect antigens associated with organisms that are difficult to culture, such as hepatitis B virus and *Chlamydia trichomatis*. Immunoassays for antibodies produced in viral hepatitis, HIV, and Lyme disease are commonly used to identify patients with these diseases.

Description

There are several different methods used in immunoassay tests.

- Immunoprecipitation. The simplest immunoassay method measures the quantity of precipitate, which forms after the reagent antibody (precipitin) has incubated with the sample and reacted with its respective antigen to form an insoluble aggregate. Immunoprecipitation reactions may be qualitative or quantitative.
- Particle immunoassays. By linking several antibodies to the particle, the particle is able to bind many antigen molecules simultaneously. This greatly accelerates the speed of the visible reaction. This allows rapid and sensitive detection of antibodies that are markers of such diseases, as infectious mononucleosis and rheumatoid arthritis.
- Immunonephelometry. The immediate union of antibody and antigen forms immune complexes that are too small to precipitate. However, these complexes will scatter incident light and can be measured using an instrument called a nephelometer. The antigen concentration can be determined within minutes of the reaction.
- Radioimmunoassay (RIA) is a method employing radioactive isotopes to label either the antigen or antibody. This isotope emits gamma raysare, which are usually measured following removal of unbound (free) radiolabel. The major advantages of RIA, compared with other immunoassays, are higher sensitivity, easy signal detection, and well-established, rapid assays. The major disadvantages are the health and safety risks posed by the use of radiation and the time and expense associated with maintaining a licensed radiation safety and disposal program. For this reason, RIA has been largely replaced in routine clinical laboratory practice by enzyme immunoassay.
- Enzyme (EIA) immunoassay was developed as an alternative to radioimmunoassay (RIA). These methods use an enzyme to label either the antibody or antigen. The sensitivity of EIA approaches that for RIA, without the danger posed by radioactive isotopes. One of the most widely used EIA methods for detection of infectious diseases is the enzyme-linked immunosorbent assay (ELISA).
- Fluorescent immunoassay (FIA) refers to immunoassays which utilize a fluorescent label or an enzyme label which acts on the substrate to form a fluorescent

product. Fluorescent measurements are inherently more sensitive than colorimetric (spectrophotometric) measurements. Therefore, FIA methods have greater analytical sensitivity than EIA methods, which employ absorbance (optical density) measurement.

- Chemiluminescent immunoassays utilize a chemiluminescent label. Chemiluminescent molecules produce light when they are excited by chemical energy. These emissions are measured by a light detector.

Precautions

Blood samples are collected by vein puncture with a needle. It is not necessary to restrict fluids or food prior to collection. Blood should be collected in tubes containing no additive. Risks of vein puncture include bruising of the skin or bleeding into the skin. Random urine samples are acceptable for drug assays; however, 24-hour urine samples are preferred for hormones and other substances which show diurnal or pulse variation.

Special safety precautions must be observed when performing RIA methods. Radioactive isotopes are used by RIA tests to label antigens or antibodies. Pregnant females should not work in an area where RIA tests are being performed. Personnel handling isotope reagents must wear badges which monitor their exposure to radiation. Special sinks and waste disposal containers are required for disposal of radioactive waste. The amount of radioisotope discarded must be documented for both liquid and solid waste. Leakage or spills of radioactive reagents must be measured for radioactivity; the amount of radiation and containment and disposal processes must be documented.

Normal results

Immunoassays which are qualitative are reported as positive or negative. Quantitative immunoassays are reported in mass units, along with reference intervals (normal ranges) for the test. Normal ranges may be age- and gender-dependent. Positive immunoassay test results for HIV and drugs of abuse generally require confirmatory testing.

Although immunoassays are both highly sensitive and specific, false positive and negative results may occur. False-negative results may be caused by improper sample storage or treatment, reagent deterioration, or improper washing technique. False-positive results are sometimes seen in persons who have certain antibodies, especially to mouse immunoglobulins (immune cells) that may be used in the test. False-positive results have been reported for samples containing small fibrin strands that adhere to the solid phase matrix. False-positives may also be caused by substances in the blood or urine that cross-react or bind to the antibody used in the test.

Preparation

Generally, no special instructions need be given to patients for immunoassay testing. Some assays require a timed specimen collection, while others may have special dietary restrictions.

Aftercare

When blood testing is used for the immunoassay, the vein puncture site will require a bandage or light dressing to accomplish blood clotting.

Risks

Immunoassay is an *in vitro* procedure, and is therefore not associated with complications. When blood is collected, slight bleeding into the skin and subsequent bruising may occur. The patient may become lightheaded or queasy from the sight of blood.

Resources

BOOKS

Cohen, J. et al. *Infectious Diseases.* 2nd ed. St. Louis: Mosby, 2004.

Gershon, A. A. et al. *Infectious Diseases of Children.* 11th ed. St. Louis: Mosby, 2004.

Long, S. S. et al. *Principles and Practice of Pediatric Infectious Diseases.* 2nd ed. London: Churchill Livingstone, 2003.

Mandell, G. L. et al. *Principles and Practice of Infectious Diseases.* 6th ed. London: Churchill Livingstone, 2005.

McPherson, R. A. et al. *Henry's Clinical Diagnosis and Management By Laboratory Methods.* 21st ed. Philadelphia: Saunders, 2007.

Robert Harr
Paul Johnson
Mark A. Best
Rosalyn Carson-DeWitt, MD

Immunologic therapies

Definition

Immunologic therapy is an approach to the treatment of disease that uses medicines for stimulating the body's natural immune response.

Purpose

Immunologic therapy is used to improve the immune system's natural ability to fight such diseases as cancer, hepatitis, and AIDS. These drugs may also be used to help the body recover from immunosuppression resulting from such treatments as chemotherapy or radiation therapy.

Description

Most drugs in this category are synthetic versions of substances produced naturally in the body. In their natural forms, these substances help defend the body against disease. For example, aldesleukin (Proleukin) is an artificial form of interleukin-2, which helps white blood cells work. Aldesleukin is administered to patients with kidney cancers and skin cancers that have spread to other parts of the body. Filgrastim (Neupogen) and sargramostim (Leukine) are versions of natural substances called colony stimulating factors, which encourage the bone marrow to make new white blood cells. Another type of drug, epoetin (Epogen, Procrit), is a synthetic version of human erythropoietin, which stimulates the bone marrow to make new red blood cells. Thrombopoietin stimulates the production of platelets, which are disk-shaped bodies in the blood that are important in clotting. Interferons are substances that the body produces naturally, using cells in the immune system to fight infections and tumors. Synthetic interferons carry such brand names as Alferon, Roferon or Intron A. Some of the interferons that are currently in use as medications are recombinant interferon alfa-2a, recombinant interferon alfa-2b, interferon alfa-n1, and interferon alfa-n3. Alfa interferons are used to treat hairy cell leukemia, malignant melanoma, and Kaposi's

sarcoma, which is a type of cancer associated with HIV infection. In addition, interferons are also used to treat such other conditions as laryngeal papillomatosis, genital warts, and certain types of hepatitis.

Recommended dosage

The recommended dosage depends on the type of immunologic therapy. For some medicines, the physician will decide the dosage for each patient, taking into account a patient's weight and whether he or she is taking other medicines. Some drugs used in immunologic therapy are given only in a hospital under a physician's supervision. Patients who are taking drugs that can be used at home should consult the physician who prescribed the medicine or the pharmacist who filled the prescription for the correct dosage.

Most of these drugs come in an injectable form, which is generally administered by a cancer care provider.

KEY TERMS

Bone marrow—Soft tissue that fills the hollow centers of bones. Blood cells and platelets (disk-shaped bodies in the blood that are important in clotting) are produced in the bone marrow.

Chemotherapy—Treatment of an illness with chemical agents. The term is usually used to describe the treatment of cancer with drugs.

Hepatitis—Inflammation of the liver caused by a virus, chemical, or drug.

Immune response—The body's natural protective reaction against disease and infection.

Immune system—The system that protects the body against disease and infection through immune responses.

Inflammation—Pain, redness, swelling, and heat that usually develop in response to injury or illness.

Seizure—A sudden attack, spasm, or convulsion.

Shingles—A disease caused the Herpes zoster virus—the same virus that causes chickenpox. Symptoms of shingles include pain and blisters along one nerve, usually on the face, chest, stomach, or back.

Sickle cell anemia—An inherited disorder in which red blood cells contain an abnormal form of hemoglobin, a protein that carries oxygen.

Precautions

Aldesleukin

This drug may temporarily increase the patient's risk of getting infections. It may also lower the number of platelets in the blood, and thus interfere with the blood's ability to clot. Taking the following precautions may reduce the chance of such complications:

- Avoiding people with infectious diseases whenever possible.
- Being alert to such signs of infection as fever, chills, sore throat, pain in the lower back or side, cough, hoarseness, or painful or difficult urination. If any of these symptoms occur, the patient should call the physician immediately.
- Being alert to such signs of bleeding problems as black or tarry stools; tiny red spots on the skin; blood in the urine or stools; or any other unusual bleeding or bruising.
- Taking care to avoid cuts or other injuries, particularly when using knives, razors, nail clippers, and other sharp objects. The patient should consult his or her dentist for the best ways to clean the teeth and mouth without injuring the gums. In addition, patients should not have any dental work done without checking with their primary physician.
- Washing hands frequently, and avoiding touching the eyes or inside of the nose unless the hands have just been washed.

Aldesleukin may make some disorders worse, including chickenpox, shingles (herpes zoster), liver disease, lung disease, heart disease, underactive thyroid, psoriasis, immune system problems and mental problems. The medicine may also increase the risk of seizures (convulsions) in people with epilepsy or other seizure disorders. In addition, the drug's effects may be intensified in people with kidney disease, because their kidneys are slow to clear the medicine from their bodies.

Colony stimulating factors

Certain drugs used in treating cancer reduce the body's ability to fight infections. Although colony stimulating factors help restore the body's natural defenses, the process takes time. Getting prompt treatment for infections is important, even while the patient is taking these medications. Patients taking colony stimulating factors should call their physician at the first sign of illness or infection, including a sore throat, fever, or chills.

People with certain medical conditions may have problems if they take colony stimulating factors. Patients with kidney disease, liver disease, or conditions related to inflammation or immune system disorders may find that colony stimulating factors make their disorder worse. People with heart disease may be more likely to experience such side effects as water retention and irregular heart rhythm while taking these drugs. Patients with lung disease may increase their risk of shortness of breath. People with any of these medical conditions should consult their personal physician before using colony stimulating factors.

Epoetin

Epoetin is a medicine that may cause seizures (convulsions), especially in people with epilepsy or other seizure disorders. No one who takes epoetin should drive, operate heavy machinery, or do anything that would be dangerous to themselves or others in the event of a seizure.

Epoetin helps the body make new red blood cells, but it is not effective unless there are adequate stores of iron in the body. The patient's physician may recommend taking iron supplements or certain vitamins that help to maintain the body's iron supply. It is necessary to follow the physician's advice in this instance, as with any dietary supplements that should come only from a physician.

Studies of laboratory animals indicate that epoetin taken during pregnancy causes birth defects in these species, including damage to the bones and spine. The drug, however, has not been reported to cause problems in human babies whose mothers took it during pregnancy. Nevertheless, women who are or may become pregnant should check with their physicians for the most up-to-date information on the safety of taking this medicine during pregnancy.

People with certain medical conditions may have problems if they take epoetin. For example, there appears to be a greater risk of side effects in people with high blood pressure, disorders of the heart or blood vessels, or a history of blood clots. In addition, epoetin may not work properly in people who have bone disorders or sickle cell anemia.

Interferons

Interferons may intensify the effects of alcohol and other drugs that slow down the central nervous system, including antihistamines, over-the-counter cold medicines, allergy medications, sleep aids, anticonvulsants, tranquilizers, some pain relievers, and **muscle relaxants**. Interferons may also intensify the effects of anesthetics, including the local anesthetics used for dental procedures. Patients taking interferons should consult their physicians before taking any of the medications listed above.

Some people experience dizziness, unusual fatigue, or drowsiness while taking these drugs. Because of these possible problems, anyone who takes these drugs should not drive, use heavy machinery, or do anything else that requires full alertness until they have determined how the drugs affect them.

Interferons often cause flu-like symptoms, including fever and chills. The physician who prescribes this medicine may recommend taking **acetaminophen** (Tylenol) before—and sometimes after—each dose to keep the fever from getting too high. If the physician recommends taking acetaminophen, the patient should follow his or her instructions carefully.

Like aldesleukin, interferons may temporarily increase the risk of getting infections and lower the number of platelets in the blood, which may lead to clotting problems. Patients should observe the precautions listed above for reducing the risk of infection and bleeding for aldesleukin.

People who have certain medical conditions may have problems if they take interferons. For example, the drugs may worsen some medical conditions, including heart disease, kidney disease, liver disease, lung disease, diabetes, bleeding problems, and certain psychiatric disorders. In people who have overactive immune systems, these drugs can even increase the activity of the immune system. People who have shingles or chickenpox, or who have recently been exposed to chickenpox, may increase their risk of developing severe problems in other parts of the body if they take interferons. People with a history of seizures or associated mental disorders may be at risk if they take interferon.

Elderly people appear to be at increased risk of side effects from taking interferons.

Interferons may cause changes in the menstrual cycles of teenagers. Young women should discuss this possibility with their physicians. These drugs are not known to cause fetal **death**, birth defects, or other problems in humans when taken during pregnancy. Women who are pregnant or who may become pregnant should ask their physicians for the latest information on the safety of taking these drugs during pregnancy.

Women who are breastfeeding their babies may need to stop while taking this medicine. It is not yet known whether interferons pass into breast milk; however, because of the chance of serious side effects that might affect the baby, women should not breastfeed

while taking interferon. Patients should consult their physician for more specific advice.

General precautions for all types of immunologic therapy

Regular appointments with the doctor are necessary during immunologic therapy treatment. These checkups give the physician a chance to make sure the medicine is working and to monitor the patient for unwanted side effects.

Anyone who has had unusual reactions to the drugs used in immunologic therapy should inform the doctor before resuming the drugs. Any allergies to foods, dyes, preservatives, or other substances should also be reported.

Side effects

Aldesleukin

Aldesleukin may cause serious side effects. It is ordinarily given only in a hospital, where medical professionals can watch for early signs of problems. Medical tests may be performed to check for unwanted side effects. In general, anyone who has breathing problems, fever or chills while being given aldesleukin should consult their doctor at once.

Other side effects should be brought to a physician's attention as soon as possible:

- dizziness
- drowsiness
- confusion
- agitation
- depression
- nausea and vomiting
- diarrhea
- sores in the mouth and on the lips
- tingling of hands or feet
- decrease in urination
- unexplained weight gain of 5 lb (2 kg) or more

Some side effects of aldesleukin are usually temporary and do not need medical attention unless they are bothersome. These include dry skin; itchy or burning rash or redness followed by peeling; loss of appetite; and a general feeling of illness or discomfort.

Colony stimulating factors

Patients sometimes experience mild pain in the lower back or hips in the first few days of treatment with colony stimulating factors. This side effect is not a cause for concern, and usually goes away within a few days. If the pain is intense or causes discomfort, the physician may prescribe a painkiller.

Other possible side effects include headache, joint or muscle pain, and skin rash or itching. These side effects tend to disappear as the body adjusts to the medicine, and do not need medical treatment. If they continue, or if they interfere with normal activities, the patient should consult their physician.

Epoetin

Epoetin may cause such flu-like symptoms as muscle aches, bone pain, fever, chills, shivering, and sweating within a few hours after it is taken. These symptoms usually go away within 12 hours. If they persist or are severe, the patient should call their doctor. Other possible side effects of epoetin that do not need medical attention are diarrhea, nausea or vomiting, and fatigue or weakness.

Other side effects, however, should be brought to a physician's attention as soon as possible. These include headache; vision problems; a rise in blood pressure; fast heartbeat; weight gain; or swelling of the face, fingers, lower legs, ankles, or feet. Anyone who has chest pain or seizures after taking epoetin should seek professional emergency medical attention immediately.

Interferons

Interferons may cause temporary hair loss (alopecia). Although this side effect may be upsetting because it affects the patient's appearance, it is not a sign that something is seriously wrong. The hair should grow back normally after treatment ends.

As the body adjusts to these medications, the patient may experience other side effects that usually go away during treatment. These include flu-like symptoms; alterations in the sense of taste; loss of appetite (anorexia); nausea and vomiting; skin rashes; and unusual fatigue. The patient should consult a doctor if these problems persist or if they interfere with normal life.

Other side effects are more serious and should be brought to a physician's attention as soon as possible:

- confusion
- difficulty thinking or concentrating
- nervousness
- depression
- sleep problems
- numbness or tingling in the fingers, toes, and face

General precautions regarding side effects for all types of immunologic therapy

Other side effects are possible with any type of immunologic therapy. Anyone who has unusual symptoms during or after treatment with these drugs should contact the physician immediately.

Interactions

Anyone who has immunologic therapy should give their physician a list of all other medications that they take, including over-the-counter and herbal preparations. Some combinations of drugs may increase or decrease the effects of one or both drugs, or increase the likelihood of side effects.

Alternatives

Immunoprevention

Immunoprevention is a form of treatment that has been proposed as a form of cancer therapy. There are two types of immunoprevention, active and passive. Treatment that involves such immune molecules as cytokines, which are prepared synthetically, or other immune molecules that are not produced by patients themselves are called passive immunotherapy. By contrast, vaccines are a form of active immune therapy because they elicit an immune response from the patient's body. Cancer vaccines may be made of whole tumor cells or from substances or fragments from the tumor known as antigens.

Adoptive immunotherapy

Adoptive immunotherapy involves stimulating T lymphocytes by exposing them to tumor antigens. These modified cells are grown in the laboratory and then injected into patients. Since the cells taken from a different person for this purpose are often rejected, patients serve both as donor and recipient of their own T cells. Adoptive immunotherapy is particularly effective in patients who have received massive doses of radiation and chemotherapy. In such patients, therapy results in immunosuppression (weakened immune systems), making them vulnerable to viral infections. For example, CMV-specific T cells can reduce the risk of cytomegalovirus (CMV) infection in organ transplant patients.

Resources

BOOKS

"Factors Affecting Drug Response: Drug Interactions." Section 22, Chapter 301 in *The Merck Manual of Diagnosis and Therapy*, edited by Mark H. Beers, MD, and

Robert Berkow, MD. Whitehouse Station, NJ: Merck Research Laboratories, 1999.

Reiger, Paula T. *Biotherapy: A Comprehensive Overview*. Sudbury: Jones and Bartlett, Inc. 2000.

Stern, Peter L., P. C. Beverley, and M. Carroll. *Cancer Vaccines and Immunotherapy*. New York: Cambridge University Press, 2000.

Wilson, Billie Ann, RN, PhD, Carolyn L. Stang, PharmD, and Margaret T. Shannon, RN, PhD. *Nurses Drug Guide 2000*. Stamford, CT: Appleton and Lange, 1999.

PERIODICALS

"Immunoprevention of Cancer: Is the Time Ripe?" *Cancer Research* 60 (May 15, 2000): 2571-2575.

Rosenberg, S. A. "Progress in the Development of Immunotherapy for the Treatment of Patients with Cancer." *Journal of Internal Medicine* 250 (December 2001): 462-475.

Rosenberg, S. A. "Progress in Human Tumor Immunology and Immunotherapy." *Nature* 411 (May 17, 2001): 380-385.

ORGANIZATIONS

American Society of Health-System Pharmacists (ASHP). 7272 Wisconsin Avenue, Bethesda, MD 20814. (301) 657-3000. www.ashp.org.

National Cancer Institute (NCI). NCI Public Inquiries Office, Suite 3036A, 6116 Executive Boulevard, MSC8332, Bethesda, MD 20892-8322. (800) 4-CANCER or (800) 332-8615 (TTY). www.nci.nih.gov.

United States Food and Drug Administration (FDA). 5600 Fishers Lane, Rockville, MD 20857-0001. (888) INFO-FDA. www.fda.gov.

OTHER

National Cancer Institute (NCI). *Treating Cancer with Vaccine Therapy*. www.cancertrials.nci.nih.gov/news/features/vaccine/html/page05.htm.

Nancy Ross-Flanigan
Samuel Uretsky, PharmD
Kausalya Santhanam, Ph.D.
Renee Laux, M.S.

Immunosuppressant drugs

Definition

Immunosuppressant drugs, also called anti-rejection drugs, are used to inhibit or prevent the activity of the body's immune system. They have three major uses as of the early 2000s: to prevent the body from rejecting a transplanted organ; to treat such autoimmune diseases as rheumatoid arthritis (RA), Crohn's disease, ulcerative colitis, and systemic lupus erythematosus (SLE); and to treat a few inflammatory diseases that are not autoimmune disorders, such as long-term allergic asthma.

Purpose

When an organ, such as a liver, heart, or kidney, is transplanted from one person (the donor) into another (the recipient), the immune system of the recipient triggers the same response against the new organ that it would have against any foreign material, setting off a chain of events that can damage the transplanted organ. This process is called rejection. It can occur rapidly (acute rejection), or over a long period of time (chronic rejection). Rejection can occur despite close matching of the donated organ and the transplant patient. Immunosuppressant drugs greatly decrease the risks of rejection, protecting the new organ and preserving its function. These drugs act by blocking the recipient's immune system so that it is less likely to react against the transplanted organ. A wide variety of drugs are available to achieve this aim but work in different ways to reduce the risk of rejection.

In addition to being used to prevent organ rejection, immunosuppressant drugs are also used to treat such severe skin disorders as psoriasis and such other diseases as rheumatoid arthritis, Crohn's disease (chronic inflammation of the digestive tract), and patchy hair loss (alopecia areata). These conditions are termed autoimmune diseases, indicating that the immune system is reacting against the body itself.

Description

Immunosuppressant drugs can be classified according to their specific molecular mode of action. There are four main categories of immunosuppressant drugs currently used in treating patients with transplanted organs:

- Cyclosporins (Neoral, Sandimmune, SangCya). These drugs act by inhibiting T-cell activation, thus preventing T-cells from attacking the transplanted organ.

- Azathioprines (Imuran). These drugs disrupt the synthesis of DNA and RNA as well as the process of cell division. They are sometimes called cytostatic drugs because they inhibit cell division.

- Monoclonal antibodies, including basiliximab (Simulect), daclizumab (Zenpax), and muromonab (Orthoclone OKT3). These drugs act by inhibiting the binding of interleukin-2, which in turn slows down the production of T-cells in the patient's immune system.

- Such corticosteroids as prednisolone (Deltasone, Orasone). These drugs suppress the inflammation associated with transplant rejection.

Most patients are prescribed a combination of drugs—sometimes called a multiple-drug cocktail—after their transplant, one from each of the above main groups; for example, they may be given a combination of

Antibody—A protein produced by the immune system in response to the presence in the body of an antigen.

Antigen—Any substance or organism that is foreign to the body. Examples of antigens include bacteria, bacterial toxins, viruses, or other cells or proteins.

Autoimmune disease—A disease in which the immune system is overactive and produces antibodies that attack the body's own tissues.

Corticosteroids—A class of drugs that are synthetic versions of the cortisone produced by the body. They rank among the most powerful anti-inflammatory agents.

Cortisone—A glucocorticoid compound produced by the adrenal cortex in response to stress. Cortisone is a steroid with anti-inflammatory and immunosuppressive properties.

Cytostatic—A type of drug that inhibits the process of cell division. Azathioprine is an example of a cytostatic drug.

Immune system—The network of organs, cells, and molecules that work together to defend the body from such foreign substances and organisms causing infection and disease as bacteria, viruses, fungi, and parasites.

Immunosuppresive cytotoxic drugs—A class of drugs that function by destroying cells and suppressing the immune response.

Inflammation—A process occurring in body tissues, characterized by increased circulation and the accumulation of white blood cells. Inflammation also occurs in such disorders as arthritis and causes harmful effects.

Lymphocyte—A type of white blood cell involved in the immune response. The two main groups of lymphocytes are the B cells, which carry antibody molecules on their surface; and T cells, which destroy antigens.

Psoriasis—A skin disease characterized by itchy, scaly, red patches on the skin.

T cells—Any of several lymphocytes that have specific antigen receptors, and are involved in cell-mediated immunity and the destruction of antigen-bearing cells.

---

cyclosporin, azathioprine, and prednisolone. Over a period of time, the doses of each drug and the number of drugs taken may be reduced as the risks of rejection decrease. Most transplant patients, however, will need to take at least one immunosuppressive medication for the rest of their lives.

The major limitation of the immunosuppressant drugs in use as of early 2008 is that they cannot target only those cells involved in graft or transplant rejection; they impair the immune responses of other cells as well. In 2007 a major action plan for further research in transplantation noted the importance of developing immunosuppressive drugs with more specific targets.

Immunosuppressants can also be classified according to the specific organ that is transplanted:

- Basiliximab (Simulect) is also used in combination with such other drugs as cyclosporin and corticosteroids in kidney transplants.

- Daclizumab (Zenapax)is also used in combination with such other drugs as cyclosporin and corticosteroids in kidney transplants.

- Muromonab CD3 (Orthoclone OKT3) is used along with cyclosporin in kidney, liver and heart transplants.

- Tacrolimus (Prograf) is used in liver and kidney transplants. It is under study for bone marrow, heart, pancreas, pancreatic island cell, and small bowel transplantation

- Sirolimus (Rapamune, Rapamycin) is used in kidney transplants.

Some immunosuppressants are also used to treat a variety of autoimmune diseases:

- Azathioprine (Imuran) is used not only to prevent organ rejection in kidney transplants, but also in treatment of rheumatoid arthritis. It has been used to treat chronic ulcerative colitis, although it has proved to be of limited value for this use.

- Cyclosporin (Sandimmune, Neoral) is used in heart, liver, kidney, pancreas, bone marrow, and heart/lung transplantation. The Neoral form of cyclosporin has been used to treat psoriasis and rheumatoid arthritis. The drug has also been used to treat many other conditions, including multiple sclerosis, diabetes, and myasthenia gravis.

- Glatiramer acetate (Copaxone) is used in the treatment of relapsing-remitting multiple sclerosis. In one study, glatiramer reduced the frequency of multiple sclerosis attacks by 75% over a two-year period.

- Mycopehnolate (CellCept) is used along with cyclosporin in kidney, liver, and heart transplants. It has also been used to prevent the kidney problems associated with lupus erythematosus.
- Sirolimus (Rapamune, Rapamycin) is used in combination with other drugs, including cyclosporin and corticosteroids, in kidney transplants. The drug is also used to treat patients with psoriasis.

Recommended dosage

Immunosuppressant drugs are available only with a physician's prescription. They come in tablet, capsule, liquid, and injectable forms. The recommended dosage depends on the type and form of immunosuppressant drug and the purpose for which it is being used. Doses may be different for different patients. The prescribing physician or the pharmacist who filled the prescription will advise the patient on the correct dosages.

Patients who are taking immunosuppressant drugs should take them *exactly as directed*. They should never take smaller, larger, or more frequent doses of these medications. In addition, immunosuppressant drugs should never be taken for a longer period of time than directed. The physician will decide exactly how much of the medicine each patient needs. Blood tests are usually necessary to monitor the action of these drugs.

Patients should always consult the prescribing physician before they stop taking an immunosuppressant drug.

Precautions

Patients who are taking immunosuppressant drugs should see their doctor on a regular basis. Periodic checkups will allow the physician to make sure the drug is working as it should and to monitor the patient for unwanted side effects. These drugs are very powerful and can cause such serious side effects as high blood pressure, kidney problems and liver disorders. Some side effects may not show up until years after the medicine was used. Anyone who has been advised to take immunosuppressant drugs should thoroughly discuss the risks and benefits of these medications with the prescribing physician.

Immunosuppressant drugs lower a person's resistance to infection and can make infections harder to treat. The drugs can also increase the chance of uncontrolled bleeding. Anyone who has a serious infection or injury while taking immunosuppressant drugs should get prompt medical attention and should make sure that the treating physician knows that he or she is taking an immunosuppressant medication.

The prescribing physician should be immediately informed if such signs of infection as fever or chills; cough or hoarseness; pain in the lower back or side; painful or difficult urination; bruising or bleeding; blood in the urine; bloody or black, tarry stools occur. Other ways of preventing infection and injury include washing the hands frequently, avoiding sports in which injuries may occur, and being careful when using knives, razors, fingernail clippers, or other sharp objects. Avoiding contact with people who have infections is also important.

In addition, people who are taking or have been taking immunosuppressant drugs should not have such immunizations as smallpox vaccinations without consulting their physician. Because their resistance to infection has been lowered, people taking these drugs might get the disease that the vaccine is designed to prevent. People taking immunosuppressant drugs should avoid contact with anyone who has had a recent dose of oral polio vaccine, as there is a chance that the virus used to make the vaccine could be passed on to them.

Immunosuppressant drugs may cause the gums to become tender and swollen or to bleed. If this happens, a physician or dentist should be notified. Regular brushing, flossing, cleaning, and gum massage may help prevent this problem. A dentist can provide advice on how to clean the teeth and mouth without causing injury.

Special conditions

People who have certain diseases or disorders, or who are taking certain other medicines may have problems if they take immunosuppressant drugs. Before taking these drugs, patients should inform the prescribing physician about any of the following conditions:

ALLERGIES. Anyone who has had unusual reactions to immunosuppressant drugs in the past should let his or her physician know before taking the drugs again. The physician should also be told about any allergies to foods, dyes, preservatives, or other substances.

PREGNANCY. Azathioprine has been considered a cause of birth defects. The British National Formulary, however, states: "Transplant patients immunosuppressed with azathioprine should not discontinue it on becoming pregnant; there is no evidence that azathioprine is teratogenic. There is less experience of ciclosporin in pregnancy but it does not appear to be any more harmful than azathioprine. The use of these drugs during pregnancy needs to be supervised in specialist units. Any risk to the offspring of azathioprine-treated men is small." Nonetheless, patients who are taking any immunosuppressive drug should consult with their physician before conceiving a child, and they should notify the doctor at once when there is any indication of pregnancy.

Basiliximab should not be used during pregnancy. The manufacturer recommends using adequate contraception during use of this drug, and for eight weeks following the final dose.

The manufacturers warn against the use of tacrolimus and mycophenolate during pregnancy, on the basis of findings from animal studies. They recommend using adequate contraception while taking these drugs, and for six weeks after the last dose.

The safety of **corticosteroids** during pregnancy has not been absolutely determined. There is some evidence that use of these drugs during pregnancy may affect the baby's growth; however, this result is not certain, and may vary with the medication used. Patients taking any steroid drug should consult with their physician before starting a family, and should notify the doctor at once if they think they are pregnant.

Most of these medicines have not been studied in humans during pregnancy. Women who are pregnant or who may become pregnant and who need to take immunosuppressants should consult their physicians.

LACTATION. Immunosuppressant drugs pass into breast milk and may cause problems in nursing babies whose mothers take it. Breastfeeding is not recommended for women taking immunosuppressants.

OTHER MEDICAL CONDITIONS. People with any of the following conditions may have problems if they take immunosuppressant drugs:

- People who have shingles (herpes zoster) or chickenpox, or who have recently been exposed to chickenpox, may develop severe disease in other parts of their bodies when they take these medicines.
- Immunosuppressants may produce more intense side effects in people with kidney disease or liver disease, because their bodies are slow to get rid of the medicine.
- Oral forms of immunosuppressants may be less effective in people with intestinal problems, because the medicine cannot be absorbed into the body.

Before using immunosuppressants, people with these or other medical problems should make sure their physicians are aware of their conditions.

Side effects

Increased risk of infection is a common side effect of all immunosuppressant drugs. The immune system protects the body from infections; when the immune system is suppressed, infections are more likely. Taking such **antibiotics** as co-trimoxazole (SXT, TMP-SMX, or TMP-sulfa) prevents some of these infections. Immunosuppressant drugs are also associated with a slightly increased risk of cancer because the immune system plays a role in protecting the body against some forms of cancer. For example, the long-term use of immunosuppressant drugs carries an increased risk of developing skin cancer as a result of the combination of the drugs and exposure to sunlight.

Other side effects of immunosuppressant drugs are minor and usually go away as the body adjusts to the medicine. These include loss of appetite, nausea or vomiting, increased hair growth, and trembling or shaking of the hands. Medical attention is not necessary unless these side effects continue or cause problems.

The treating physician should be notified immediately if any of the following side effects occur:

- unusual tiredness or weakness
- fever or chills
- frequent need to urinate

Interactions

Immunosuppressant drugs may interact with other medicines. When interactions occur, the effects of one or both drugs may change or the risk of side effects may be greater. Other drugs may also have adverse effects on immunosuppressant therapy. It is particularly important for patients taking cyclosporin or tacrolimus to be careful about the possibility of drug interactions. Other examples of problematic interactions are:

- The effects of azathioprine may be greater in people who take allopurinol, a medicine used to treat gout.
- A number of drugs, including female hormones (estrogens), male hormones (androgens), the antifungal drug ketoconazole (Nizoral), the ulcer drug cimetidine (Tagamet), and the erythromycins (used to treat infections), may intensify the effects of cyclosporine. Certain herbs are also reported to interact with cyclosporine.
- When sirolimus is taken at the same time as cyclosporin, the blood levels of sirolimus may be increased to a level that produces severe side effects. Although these two drugs are usually used together, the dose of sirolimus should be taken four hours after the dose of cyclosporin.
- Tacrolimus is eliminated through the kidneys. When this drug is used with other medications that may harm the kidneys, such as cyclosporin, the antibiotics gentamicin and amikacin, or the antifungal drug amphotericin B, the blood levels of tacrolimus may

rise. Careful kidney monitoring is essential when tacrolimus is given with any drug that might cause kidney damage. Tacrolimus is another immunosuppressive drug reported to interact with some over-the-counter herbal preparations.

• The risk of cancer or infection may be greater when immunosuppressant drugs are combined with certain other drugs that also lower the body's ability to fight disease and infection. These drugs include corticosteroids, especially prednisone; the anticancer drugs chlorambucil (Leukeran), cyclophosphamide (Cytoxan) and mercaptopurine (Purinethol); and the monoclonal antibody muromonab-CD3 (Orthoclone), which is also used to prevent transplanted organ rejection.

Not every drug that may interact with immunosuppressant drugs is listed here. Anyone who takes immunosuppressant drugs should give their doctor a list of all other medicines—including herbal formulations—that he or she is taking and should ask whether there are any potential interactions that might interfere with treatment.

Resources

BOOKS

Abbas, A. K., and A. H. Lichtman. *Basic Immunology: Functions and Disorders of the Immune System*, 3rd ed. Philadelphia: Saunders/Elsevier, 2009.

Janeway, Charles A. *Immunobiology: The Immune System in Health and Disease*, 6th ed. New York: Garland Publishers, 2005.

Sompayrac, L. M. *How the Immune System Works*, 3rd ed. Malden, MA: Blackwell, 2008.

PERIODICALS

Allen, D., and J. Bell. "Herbal Medicine and the Transplant Patient." *Nephrology Nursing Journal* 29 (June 2002): 269–274.

Augustine, J. J., and D. F. Hricik. "Minimization of Immunosuppression in Kidney Transplantation." *Current Opinion in Nephrology and Hypertension* 16 (November 2007): 535–541.

Leichtman, A. B. "Balancing Efficacy and Toxicity in Kidney-Transplant Immunosuppression." *New England Journal of Medicine* 357 (December 20, 2007): 2625–2627.

Yang, X.X., et al. "Drug-Herb Interactions: Eliminating Toxicity with Hard Drug Design." *Current Pharmaceutical Design* 12 (2006): 4649–4664.

ORGANIZATIONS

American Association of Immunologists (AAI). 9650 Rockville Pike, Bethesda, MD 20814. (301) 634-7178. www.12.17.12.70/aai/default/asp.

American Society of Health-System Pharmacists (ASHP). 7272 Wisconsin Avenue, Bethesda, MD 20814. (866) 279-0681. www.ashp.org.

National Cancer Institute (NCI). NCI Public Inquiries Office, Room 3036A, 6116 Executive Boulevard, Bethesda, MD 20892-8322. (800) 4-CANCER or (800) 332-8615 (TTY). www.nci.nih.gov.

United States Food and Drug Administration (FDA). 5600 Fishers Lane, Rockville, MD 20857-0001. (888) INFO-FDA. www.fda.gov.

OTHER

British National Formulary. www.bnf.vhn.net/bnf/documents/bnf.2.html#BNFID_35091.

National Cancer Institute (NCI) and the National Institute of Allergy and Infectious Diseases (NIAID). Understanding the Immune System: How It Works. Bethesda, MD: NCI/NIAID, 2003. NIH Publication No. 03-5423.

Prescilla, Randy P., and Tej K. Mattoo. "Immunology of Transplant Rejection." eMedicine, June 14, 2006. http://www.emedicine.com/ped/topic2841.htm [cited January 8, 2008].

U.S. Department of Health and Human Services, National Institutes of Health (NIH). Action Plan for Transplantation Research. Bethesda, MD: NIH, 2007. NIH Publication No. 07-5851. Available online in PDF format at http://www3.niaid.nih.gov/about/overview/planningPriorities/trap2007.pdf. [cited January 8, 2008].

Nancy Ross-Flanigan
Samuel Uretsky, PharmD
Rebecca Frey, Ph.D.

Implantable cardioverter-defibrillator

Definition

The implantable cardioverter-defibrillator (ICD) is a surgically implanted electronic device that directs an electric charge directly into the heart to treat life-threatening arrhythmias.

Purpose

The implantable cardioverter-defibrillator is used to detect and stop life-threatening arrhythmias and restore a productive heartbeat that is able to provide adequate cardiac output to sustain life. The exact indications for the implantation of the device are controversial, but patients suffering from ventricular fibrillation (unproductive heartbeat), ventricular tachycardia (abnormally fast heartbeat), long QT syndrome (an inherited heart disease), or others at risk for sudden cardiac death are potential candidates for this device. A study by the National Institute for Heart, Lung, and Blood of the National Institutes of Health showed a significant increase in survival for patients suffering from ventricular arrhythmias when ICD implant is compared to medication. Several follow-up studies indicate that this may be due to the marked increase in survival for the sickest patients, generally defined as those having a heart weakened to less than 50% of normal, as measured by the ability of the left side of the heart to pump blood. Overall, studies have documented a very low mortality rate of 1–2% annually for persons implanted with the device, compared to approximately 15–25% for patients on drug therapy.

Demographics

ICD implant is limited to patients that face the risk of sudden cardiac death from sustained ventricular arrhythmia, including ventricular tachycardia and ventricular fibrillation. Less than 1% of the more than 100,000 device implants done in the United States are performed on pediatric patients. Reduction in the risk of sudden cardiac death improves to less than 2% for both populations.

Diagnosis

Patients experiencing syncope (fainting) will be monitored with a **cardiac monitor** for arrhythmias. Following unsuccessful medical treatment for sustained ventricular arrhythmias, ICD implant will be indicated.

Description

Similar in structure to a pacemaker, an ICD has three main components: a generator, leads, and an electrode. The generator is encased in a small rectangular container, usually about 2 in (5 cm) wide and around 3 oz (85 g) in weight. Even smaller generators have been developed, measuring 1 in (2.5 cm) in diameter and weighing about 0.5 oz (14 g). The generator is powered by lithium batteries and is responsible for generating the electric shock. The generator is controlled by a computer chip that can be programmed to follow specific steps according to the input gathered from the heart. The programming is initially set and can be changed using a wand programmer, a device that communicates by radio waves through the chest of the patient after implantation. One or two leads, or wires, are attached to the generator. These wires are generally made of platinum with an insulating coating of either silicone or polyurethane. The leads carry the electric shock from the generator. At the tip of each lead is a tiny device called an electrode that delivers the necessary electrical shock to the heart. Thus, the electric shock is created by the generator, carried by the

leads, and delivered by the electrodes to the heart. The decision of where to put the leads depends on the needs of the patient, but they can be located in the left ventricle, the left atrium, or both.

According to the American College of Cardiology, more than 100,000 persons worldwide currently have an ICD. The battery-powered device rescues the patient from a life-threatening arrhythmia by performing a number of functions in order to reestablish normal heart rhythm, which varies with the particular problem of the patient. Specifically, if encountered with ventricular tachycardia, many devices will begin treatment with a pacing regimen. If the tachycardia is not too fast, the ICD can deliver several pacing signals in a row. When those signals stop, the heart may go back to a normal rhythm. If the pacing treatment is not successful, many devices will move onto **cardioversion**. With cardioversion, a mild shock is sent to the heart to stop the fast heartbeat. If the problem detected is ventricular fibrillation, a stronger shock called a **defibrillation** is sent. This stronger shock can stop the fast rhythm and help the heartbeat return to normal. Finally, many ICDs can also detect heartbeats that are too slow; they can act like a pacemaker and bring the heart rate up to normal. ICDs that defibrillate both the ventricles and the atria have also been developed. Such devices not only provide dual-chamber pacing but also can distinguish ventricular from atrial fibrillation. Patients that experience both atrial and ventricle fibrillations, or atrial fibrillation alone, that would not be controlled with a single-chamber device are candidates for this kind of ICD.

Operation

ICD insertion is considered minor surgery, and can be performed in either an **operating room** or an electrophysiology laboratory. The insertion site in the chest will be cleaned, shaved, and numbed with local anesthetic. Generally, left-handed persons have ICDs implanted on the right side, and vice versa, to speed return to normal activities. Two small cuts (incisions) are made, one in the chest wall and one in a vein just under the collarbone. The wires of the ICD are passed through the vein and attached to the inner surface of the heart. The other ends of the wires are connected to the main box of the ICD, which is inserted into the tissue under the collarbone and above the breast. Once the ICD is implanted, the physician will test it several times before the anesthesia wears off by causing the heart to fibrillate and making sure the ICD responds properly. The doctor then closes the incision with sutures (**stitches**), **staples**, or surgical **glue**. The entire procedure takes about an hour.

Immediately following the procedure, a **chest x ray** will be taken to confirm the proper placement of the wires in the heart. The ICD's programming may be adjusted by passing the programming wand over the chest. After the initial operation, the physician may induce ventricular fibrillation or ventricular tachycardia one more time prior to the patient's discharge, although recent studies suggest that this final test is not generally necessary.

A short stay in the hospital is usually required following ICD insertion, but this varies with the patient's age and condition. If there are no complications, complete recovery from the procedure will take about four weeks. During that time, the wires will firmly take hold where they were placed. In the meantime, the patient should avoid heavy lifting or vigorous movements of the arm on the side of the ICD, or else the wires may become dislodged.

After implantation, the cardioverter-defibrillator is programmed to respond to rhythms above the patient's **exercise** heart rate. Once the device is in place, many tests will be conducted to ensure that the device is sensing and defibrillating properly. About 50% of patients with ICDs require a combination of drug therapy and the ICD.

Morbidity and mortality rates

Perioperative mortality demonstrates a 0.4–1.8% risk of death for primary non-thoracotomy implants.

WHO PERFORMS THE PROCEDURE AND WHERE IS IT PERFORMED?

Electrophysiologists are specially trained cardiologists or thoracic surgeons who study and treat problems with the heart conduction system. In a hospital operating room, they often implant the ICD system and oversee the programming or reprogramming of the device. Electrophysiologists receive special continuing medical education to provide successful implantation. Implantation, follow-up, and replacement can be limited at any one institution, therefore an experienced well-trained electrophysiologist should perform these procedures.

The ICD showed improved survival compared to medical therapy, improving by 38% at one year. There is a 96% survival rate at four years for those implanted with ICD. Less then 2% of patients require termination of the device, with a return to only medical therapy.

Normal results

Ventricular tachycardia can be successfully relieved by pacing in 96% of instances with the addition of defibrillation converting 98% of patients to a productive rhythm that is able to sustain cardiac output. Ventricular fibrillation is successfully converted in 98.6–98.8% of all cases. Atrial fibrillation and rapid ventricular response leads to erroneous fibrillation in as many as 11% of patients.

Risks

Environmental conditions that can affect the functioning of the ICD after installation include:

- strong electromagnetic fields such as those used in arc-welding
- contact sports
- shooting a rifle from the shoulder nearest the installation site
- cell phones used on that side of the body
- magnetic mattress pads such as those believed to treat arthritis
- some medical tests such as magnetic resonance imaging (MRI)

storm," in which the machine inappropriately interprets an arrhythmia and gives a series of shocks. Reprogramming can sometimes help alleviate that problem.

QUESTIONS TO ASK THE DOCTOR

- How many of these procedures have been performed by the physician?
- What type of longevity can be expected from the device?
- What will happen during device activation?
- What precautions should be taken in the weeks immediately following implant?
- After implantation how long will it be before normal daily activities can be resumed such as driving, exercise, and work?
- What indications of device malfunction will there be, and when should emergency treatment be sought?
- What precautions should be taken by bystanders when the device activates?
- How will device recalls be communicated?
- Can psychological counseling benefit patient satisfaction and comfort?

Environmental conditions often erroneously thought to affect ICDs include:

- microwave ovens (The waves only affect old, unshielded pacemakers and do not affect ICDs.)
- airport security (Metal detector alarms could be set off, so patients should carry a card stating they have an ICD implanted.)
- anti-theft devices in stores (Patients should avoid standing near the devices for prolonged periods.)

Patients should also be instructed to memorize the manufacturer and make of their ICD. Although manufacturing defects and recalls are rare, they do occur and a patient should be prepared for that possibility.

Aftercare

In general, if the condition of the patient's heart, drug intake, and metabolic condition remain the same, the ICD requires only periodic checking every two months or so for battery strength and function. This is done by placing a special device over the ICD that allows signals to be sent over the telephone to the doctor, a process called trans-telephonic monitoring.

If changes in medications or physical condition occur, the doctor can adjust the ICD settings using a programmer, which involves placing the wand above the pacemaker and remotely changing the internal settings. One relatively common problem is the so-called "ICD

When the periodic testing indicates that the battery is getting low, an elective ICD replacement operation is scheduled. The entire signal generator is replaced because the batteries are sealed within the case. The leads can often be left in place and reattached to the new generator. Batteries usually last from four to eight years.

Alternatives

Patients are treated with medical therapy to reduce the chance of arrhythmia. This alternative has been shown to have a higher rate of sudden death when compared to ICD over the initial three years of treatment, but has not been compared at five years. If the site of ventricular tachycardia generation can be mapped by electrophysiology studies, the aberrant cells can be removed or destroyed. Less then 5% of patients die during this cell removal procedure.

Resources

BOOKS

Libby, P. et al. *Braunwald's Heart Disease*. 8th ed. Philadelphia: Saunders, 2007.

PERIODICALS

Cesario, D.A. "Biventricular Pacing and Defribillator Use in Chronic Heart Failure" *Cardiol Clin* 25 (Nov 2007): 595–603.

Heidbachel, H. "Implantable cardioverter defibrillator therapy in athletes." *Cardiol Clin* 25 (Aug 2007): 467–482.

Leong-Sit, P. "Effect of defibrillation testing on management during implantable cardioverter-defibrillator implantation." *Am Heart J* 152 (December 2006): 1104–1108.

Vorobiof, G. "Effectiveness of the implantable cardioverter defibrillator in blacks versus whites (from MADIT-II)." *Circulation* 98 (Nov 2006): 1383–1386.

Michelle L. Johnson, MS, JD
Allison J. Spiwak, MSBME
Rosalyn Carson-DeWitt, MD

In vitro fertilization

Definition

In vitro fertilization (IVF) is a procedure in which eggs (ova) from a woman's ovary are removed, they are fertilized with sperm in a laboratory procedure, and then the fertilized egg (embryo) is returned to the woman's uterus.

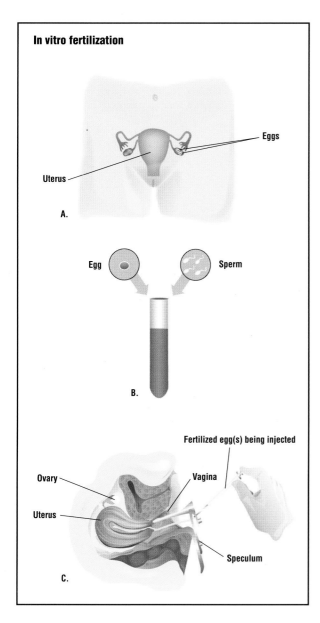

In vitro fertilization

A.

Uterus

Eggs

Egg

Sperm

B.

Fertilized egg(s) being injected

Ovary

Uterus

Vagina

Speculum

C.

For in vitro fertilization, hormones are administered to the patient, and then eggs are harvested from her ovaries (A). The eggs are fertilized by sperm donated by the father (B). Once the cells begin to divide, one or more embryos are placed into the woman's uterus to develop (C). *(Illustration by GGS Information Services. Cengage Learning, Gale.)*

Purpose

IVF is one of several assisted reproductive techniques (ART) used to help infertile couples to conceive a child. If after one year of having sexual intercourse without the use of birth control a woman is unable to get pregnant, infertility is suspected. Some of the reasons for infertility are damaged or blocked fallopian tubes, hormonal imbalance, or endometriosis in the woman. In the man, low sperm count or poor quality sperm can cause infertility.

IVF is one of several possible methods to increase the chances for an infertile couple to become pregnant. Its use depends on the reason for infertility. IVF may be an option if there is a blockage in the fallopian tube or endometriosis in the woman, or low sperm count or poor quality sperm in the man. There are other possible treatments for these conditions, such as surgery for blocked tubes or endometriosis, which may be attempted before IVF.

IVF will not work for a woman who is incapable of ovulating or with a man who is not able to produce at least a few healthy sperm.

Demographics

IVF has been used successfully since 1978, when the first child to be conceived by this method was born in England. Over the past 30 years, thousands of couples have used this method of ART or similar procedures to conceive.

Description

In vitro fertilization is a procedure in which the joining of egg and sperm takes place outside of a woman's body. A woman may be given fertility drugs before this procedure so that several eggs mature in the ovaries at the same time. The mature eggs (ova) are removed from the woman's ovaries using a long, thin needle. The physician has access to the ovaries using one of two possible procedures. One involves inserting the needle

An obstetrician-gynecologist (OB-GYN) with specialized training in IVF supervises the activities of IVF. This specialist performs most of the procedures involving the woman. Most IVF activities are performed in a professional medical office.

Candidates for in-vitro fertilization should consider asking the following questions, including:

- What is the physician's evaluation of IVF and its alternatives for the woman seeking assistance?
- Is the surgeon certified to treat infertility?
- How many procedures has the physician performed?
- What is the physician's overall success rate?
- What is the success rate for women of the same age as the person seeking assistance?

through the vagina (transvaginally); the physician guides the needle to the location in the ovaries with the help of an **ultrasound** machine. In the other procedure, called **laparoscopy**, a small thin tube with a viewing lens is inserted through an incision in the navel. This allows the physician to see on a video monitor inside the uterus to locate the ovaries.

Once the eggs are removed, they are mixed with sperm in a laboratory dish or test tube. (This is the origin of the term "test tube baby.") The eggs are monitored for several days. Once there is evidence that fertilization has occurred and the cells have begun to divide, they are then returned to the woman's uterus.

In the procedure to remove eggs, a sufficient number may be gathered to be frozen and saved (either fertilized or unfertilized) for additional IVF attempts.

Diagnosis/Preparation

Once a woman is determined to be a good candidate for *in vitro* fertilization, she will generally be given fertility drugs to stimulate ovulation and the development of multiple eggs. These drugs may include gonadotropin-releasing hormone agonists (GnRHa), Pergonal, Clomid, or human chorionic gonadotropin (hcg). The maturation of the eggs is then monitored with ultrasound tests and frequent blood tests. If enough eggs mature, a physician will perform the procedure to remove them. The woman may be given a sedative prior to the procedure. A local anesthetic agent may also be used to reduce discomfort during the procedure.

The screening procedures and treatments for infertility can become a long, expensive, and, sometimes, disappointing process. Each IVF attempt takes at least an entire menstrual cycle and can cost $5,000–10,000, which may or may not be covered by health insurance. The anxiety of dealing with infertility can challenge both individuals and their relationship. The added stress and expense of multiple clinic visits, testing, treatments, and surgical procedures can become

overwhelming. Couples may want to receive counseling and support through the process.

Aftercare

After the IVF procedure is performed, the woman can resume normal activities. A pregnancy test can be done approximately 12–14 days after the procedure to determine if it was successful.

Risks

The risks associated with in vitro fertilization include the possibility of multiple pregnancy (since several embryos may be implanted) and ectopic pregnancy (an embryo that implants in the fallopian tube or in the abdominal cavity outside the uterus). There is a slight risk of ovarian rupture, bleeding, infections, and complications of anesthesia. If the procedure is successful and pregnancy is achieved, the pregnancy carries the same risks as any pregnancy achieved without assisted technology.

Normal results

Success rates vary widely among clinics and among physicians performing the procedure. A couple has about a 10% chance of becoming pregnant each time the procedure is performed. Therefore, the procedure may have to be repeated more than once to achieve pregnancy.

Abnormal results include ectopic or multiple pregnancy that may abort spontaneously or that may require termination if the health of the mother is at risk.

Morbidity and mortality rates

The most common cause of morbidity is ectopic pregnancy. Pain is associated with most components of the procedure. Mortality as a result of IVF is extremely rare.

Alternatives

Other types of assisted reproductive technologies might be used to achieve pregnancy. A procedure called intracytoplasmic sperm injection (ICSI) utilizes a manipulation technique that must be performed using a microscope to inject a single sperm into each egg. The fertilized eggs can then be returned to the uterus, as in IVF. In gamete intrafallopian tube transfer (GIFT), the eggs and sperm are mixed in a narrow tube, and then deposited in the fallopian tube, where fertilization normally takes place. Another variation on IVF is zygote intrafallopian tube transfer (ZIFT). As in IVF, the fertilization of the eggs occurs in a laboratory dish. And, similar to GIFT, the embryos are placed in the fallopian tube, rather than in the uterus as with IVF.

Resources

BOOKS

Charlesworth, L. *The Couple's Guide to In Vitro Fertilization: Everything You Need to Know to Maximize Your Chances of Success.* New York: Da Capo Press, 2004.

Olick, D. M. *When Nature's Not Enough: Personal Journeys through In Vitro Fertilization.* Guilford, CT: Lyons Press, 2005.

Sher, G., Davis, V. M., and Stoess, J. *In Vitro Fertilization: The A.R.T. of Making Babies.* 3rd ed. New York: Facts on File, 1999.

Wisot, A. L., and D. R. Meldrum. *Conceptions & Misconceptions: The Informed Consumer's Guide Through the Maze of In Vitro Fertilization & Assisted Reproduction Techniques.* 2nd ed. Vancouver, BC: Hartley and Marks Publishers, 1999.

PERIODICALS

Bourg, C. "Ethical dilemmas in medically assisted procreation: a psychological perspective." *Human Reproduction and Genetic Ethics* 13, no. 2 (2007): 22–31.

Burns, L. H. "Psychiatric aspects of infertility and infertility treatments." *Psychiatric Clinics of North America* 30, no. 4 (2007): 689–716.

Gleicher, N., A. Weghofer, and D. Barad. "Too old for IVF: are we discriminating against older women?" *Journal of Assisted Reproductive Genetics* 24, no. 12 (2007): 639–644.

Munne, S., J. Cohen, and J. L. Simpson. "In vitro fertilization with preimplantation genetic screening." *New England Journal of Medicine* 357, no. 17 (2007): 1769–1770.

Soullier, N., J. Bouver, J. L. Pouly, J. Guilbert, and E. de La Rochebrochard. "Estimating the success of an in vitro fertilization programme using multiple imputation." *Human Reproduction* 23, no. 1 (2008): 187–192.

ORGANIZATIONS

American Board of Obstetrics and Gynecology. 2915 Vine Street, Suite 300, Dallas, TX 75204. (214) 871-1619; Fax: (214) 871-1943. E-mail: info@abog.org. http://www.abog.org.

American College of Obstetricians and Gynecologists. 409 12th St., SW, P.O. Box 96920, Washington, DC 20090-6920. http://www.acog.org.

American Fertility Association. 305 Madison Avenue Suite 449, New York, NY 10165. (888) 917-3777. http://www.afafamilymatters.com/.

American Society for Reproductive Medicine. 1209 Montgomery Highway, Birmingham, AL 35216-2809. (205) 978-5000. http://www.asrm.com.

International Council on Infertility Information Dissemination, Inc. P.O. Box 6836, Arlington, VA 22206. (703) 379-9178. http://www.inciid.org.

OTHER

American Pregnancy Association. Information about In-vitro Fertilization. 2008 [cited January 3, 2008]. http://www.americanpregnancy.org/infertility/ivf.html.

American Society for Reproductive Medicine. Information about In-vitro Fertilization. 2008 [cited January 3, 2008]. http://www.asrm.org/Patients/topics/ivf.html.

American Society for Reproductive Medicine. Information about In-vitro Fertilization. 2008 [cited January 3, 2008]. http://www.asrm.org/Patients/select.html.

National Library of Medicine. Information about In-vitro Fertilization. 2008 [cited January 3, 2008]. http://www.nlm.nih.gov/medlineplus/ency/article/007279.htm.

L. Fleming Fallon, Jr, MD, DrPH

Incision care

Definition

Incision care refers to a series of procedures and precautions related to closing a wound or surgical incision; protecting the cut or injured tissues from contamination or infection; and caring properly for the new skin that forms during the healing process. Incision care begins in the hospital or outpatient clinic and is continued by the patient during **recovery at home**.

Purpose

There are several reasons for caring properly for an incision or wound. These include:

- lowering the risk of postoperative complications, particularly infection
- avoiding unnecessary pain or discomfort
- minimizing scarring
- preventing blood loss

Description

Types of wound or incision closure

Proper care of an incision begins with knowing what material or technique the surgeon used to close the cut. There are four major types of closure used in Canada and the United States as of 2003.

SURGICAL SUTURES. Sutures, or **stitches**, are the oldest method still in use to close an incision. The surgeon uses a sterilized thread, which may be made of natural materials (silk or catgut) or synthetic fibers, to stitch the edges of the cut together with a special curved needle. There are two major types of sutures, absorbable and nonabsorbable. Absorbable sutures are gradually broken down in the body, usually within two months. Absorbable sutures do not have to be removed. They are used most commonly to close the deeper layers of tissue in a large incision or in such areas as the mouth. Nonabsorbable sutures are not broken down in the body and must be removed after the incision has healed. They are used most often to close the outer layers of skin or superficial cuts.

Sutures have several disadvantages. Because they are made of materials that are foreign to the body, they must be carefully sterilized and the skin around the incision cleansed with Betadine or a similar antiseptic to minimize the risk of infection. Suturing also requires more time than newer methods of closure. If the patient is not under **general anesthesia**, the surgeon must first apply or inject a local anesthetic before suturing. Lastly, there is a higher risk of scarring with sutures, particularly if the surgeon puts too much tension on the thread while stitching or selects thread that is too thick for the specific procedure.

SURGICAL STAPLES. Surgical **staples** are a newer method of incision closure. Staples are typically made of stainless steel or titanium. They are used most commonly to close lacerations on the scalp or to close the outer layers of skin in orthopedic procedures. They cannot be used on the face, hand, or other areas of the body where tendons and nerves lie close to

the surface. Staples are usually removed seven to 10 days after surgery.

Staples are less likely to cause infections than sutures, and they also take less time to use. They can, however, leave noticeable scars if the edges of the wound or incision have not been properly aligned. In addition, staples require a special instrument for removal.

STERI-STRIPS. Steri-strips are pieces of adhesive material that can be used in some surgical procedures to help the edges of an incision grow together. They have several advantages, including low rates of infection, speed of application, no need for **local anesthesia**, and no need for special removal. Steri-strips begin to curl and peel away from the body, usually within five to seven days after surgery. They should be pulled off after two weeks if they have not already fallen off. Steri-strips, however, have two disadvantages: they are not as precise as sutures in bringing the edges of an incision into alignment; and they cannot be used on areas of the body that are hairy or that secrete moisture, such as the palms of the hands or the armpits.

LIQUID TISSUE GLUES. Tissue glues are the newest type of incision closure. They are applied to the edges of the incision and form a bond that holds the tissues together until new tissue is formed. The tissue glues most commonly used as of 2003 belong to a group of chemicals known as cyanoacrylates. In addition to speed of use and a low infection rate, tissue glues are gradually absorbed by the body. They are less likely to cause scarring, which makes them a good choice for facial surgery and other cosmetic procedures. They are also often used to close lacerations or incisions in children, who find them less frightening or painful than sutures or staples. Like Steri-strips, however, tissue glues cannot be used on areas of high moisture. They are also ineffective for use on the knee or elbow joints.

Dressings and drainage devices

After the incision is closed, it is covered with a dressing of some sort to keep it dry and clean, and prevent infection. Most **dressings** consist of gauze pads held in place by strips of adhesive tape or ACE **bandages**. An antibiotic ointment may also be applied to the gauze. A newer type of dressing, called OpSite, is a thin transparent membrane made of polyurethane coated with adhesive. It keeps disease organisms out of the wound while holding a layer of moisture close to the skin. This moist environment keeps scabs from forming and speeds up healing of the incision. OpSite can also be used to hold catheters or drainage tubes in place. It cannot, however, be used for severe (third-degree) burns or deep incisions.

Some surgical procedures, such as a **mastectomy** or removal of a ruptured appendix, require the surgeon to insert a drainage device to remove blood, pus, or other tissue fluids from the area of the incision. It is important to prevent these fluids from collecting under the incision because they encourage the growth of disease organisms. The drain may be left in place after the patient leaves the hospital. If so, the patient will need to check and empty the drain daily in addition to general incision care.

Home care of incisions

Guidelines for **home care** of an incision vary somewhat depending on the material that was used for closure, the location and size of the incision, and the nature of the operation. The following section is a general description of the major aspects of incision care.

Patients should ask their doctor for specific information about caring for their incision:

- the type of closure used
- whether another appointment will be needed to remove any sutures or staples

- the length of time that the incision should be kept covered, and the type of dressing that should be used
- whether the incision must be kept dry, and for how long
- any specific signs or symptoms that should be reported to the doctor

Most hospitals and surgery clinics provide patients with written handouts or checklists about incision care; however, it is always helpful to go over the information in the handout with the doctor or nurse, and to ask any further questions that may arise.

BATHING AND SHOWERING. Incisions should be kept dry for several days after surgery, with the exception of incisions closed with tissue **glue**. Incisions closed with nonabsorbable sutures or staples must be kept dry until the doctor removes the sutures or staples, usually about seven to 10 days after surgery. Incisions closed with Steri-strips should be kept dry for about four to five days. If the incision gets wet accidentally, it must be dried at once. Patients with incisions on the face, hands, or arms may be able to take showers or tub baths as long as they are able to hold the affected area outside the water. Patients with incisions in other parts of the body can usually take sponge baths.

It is usually safe to allow incisions closed with tissue glue to get wet during showering or bathing. The patient should, however, dry the area around the incision carefully after washing.

PHYSICAL ACTIVITY AND EXERCISE. Patients should avoid any activity that is likely to pull on the edges of the incision or put pressure on it. Walking and other light activities are encouraged, as they help to restore normal energy levels and digestive functions. Patients should not, however, participate in sports, engage in sexual activity, or lift heavy objects until they have had a postoperative checkup.

MEDICATIONS. Patients are asked to avoid **aspirin** or over-the-counter medications containing aspirin for a week to 10 days after surgery, because aspirin interferes with blood clotting and makes it easier for bruises to form in the skin near the incision. The doctor will usually prescribe codeine or another non-aspirin medication for pain control.

Patients with medications prescribed for other conditions or disorders should ask the doctor before starting to take them again.

SUN EXPOSURE. As an incision heals, the new skin that is formed over the cut is very sensitive to sunlight and will burn more easily than normal skin. Sunburn in turn will lead to worse scarring. Patients should keep the incision area covered for three to nine months from direct sun exposure in order to prevent burning and severe scarring.

SPECIAL CONSIDERATIONS FOR FACIAL INCISIONS. Patients who have had facial surgery are usually given very detailed instructions about incision care because the skin of the face is relatively thin, and incisions in this area can be easily stretched out of alignment. In addition, patients should not apply any cosmetic creams or makeup after surgery without the surgeon's approval because of the risk of infection or allergic reaction.

GENERAL HYGIENE. Infection is the most common complication of surgical procedures. It can be serious; of the 300,000 patients whose incisions become infected each year in the United States, about 10,000 will die. It is important, therefore, to minimize the risk of an infection when caring for an incision at home.

Patients should observe the following precautions about general cleanliness and personal habits:

- Wash hands carefully after using the toilet and after touching or handling trash or garbage; pets and pet equipment; dirty laundry or soiled incision dressings; and anything else that is dirty or has been used outdoors.
- Ask family members, close friends, and others who touch the patient to wash their hands first.
- Avoid contact with family members and others who are sick or recovering from a contagious illness.
- Stop smoking. (Smoking slows down the healing process.)

Normal results

As an incision heals, it is normal to experience some redness, swelling, itching, minor skin irritation or oozing of tissue fluid, or small lumps in the skin near the incision. At first, the skin over the incision will feel thick and hard. After a period of two to six months, the swelling and irritation will go down and the scar tissue will soften and begin to blend into the surrounding tissue.

Risk factors for abnormal results

Some patients are more likely to develop infections or to have their incision split open, which is known as dehiscence. Risk factors for infection or dehiscence include:

- obesity
- diabetes
- malnutrition
- a weakened immune system
- taking corticosteroid medications prescribed for another disorder or condition
- a history of heavy smoking

Warning signs

Patients who notice any of the following signs or symptoms should call their doctor:

- fever of 100.5°F (38°C) or higher
- severe pain in the area of the incision
- intense redness in the area of the incision
- bruising
- bleeding or increased drainage of tissue fluid

Resources

BOOKS

Khatri, VP and JA Asensio. *Operative Surgery Manual.* 1st ed. Philadelphia: Saunders, 2003.

Townsend, CM et al. *Sabiston Textbook of Surgery.* 17th ed. Philadelphia: Saunders, 2004.

PERIODICALS

Farion, K., M. H. Osmond, L. Hartling, et al. "Tissue Adhesives for Traumatic Lacerations in Children and Adults." *Cochrane Database Systems Review* 2002: CD003326.

Mattick, A., G. Clegg, T. Beattie, and T. Ahmad. "A Randomised, Controlled Trial Comparing a Tissue Adhesive (2-octylcyanoacrylate) with Adhesive Strips (Steri-strips) for Paediatric Laceration Repair." *Emergency Medicine Journal* 19 (September 2002): 405–407.

Selo-Ojeme, D. O., and K. B. Lim. "Randomised Clinical Trial of Suture Compared with Adhesive Strip for Skin Closure After HRT Implant." *BJOG: An International Journal of Obstetrics and Gynaecology* 109 (October 2002): 1178–1180.

Takahashi, K., T. Muratani, M. Saito, et al. "Evaluation of the Disinfective Efficacy of Povidone-Iodine with the Use of the Transparent Film Dressing OpSite Wound." *Dermatology* 204 (2002), Supplement 1: 59–62.

OTHER

Higgins, Robert V., Wendel Naumann, and James Hall. "Abdominal Incisions and Sutures in Gynecologic Oncological Surgery." eMedicine, December 21, 2007. http://www.emedicine.com/med/topic3397.htm [accessed April 22, 2008].

Rebecca Frey, Ph.D.

Incisional hernia repair

Definition

Incisional hernia repair is a surgical procedure performed to correct an incisional hernia. An incisional hernia, also called a **ventral hernia**, is a bulge or

Incisional hernia repair

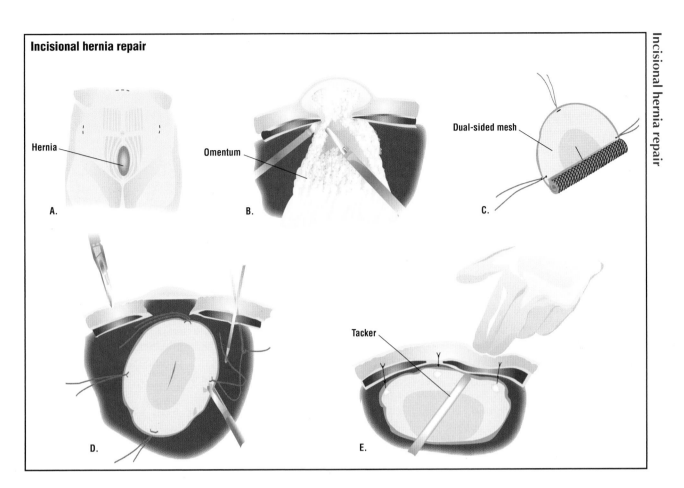

An incisional hernia occurs at the site of a previous incision (A). Intestinal contents break through the abdominal wall and bubble up under the skin. In a laparoscopic repair, the surgeon uses laparoscopic forceps to pull the material, omentum, from the hernia site (B). A mesh pad is inserted into the site to line the hernia site (C and D), and is tacked into place (E). *(Illustration by GGS Information Services. Cengage Learning, Gale.)*

protrusion that occurs near or directly along a prior abdominal surgical incision. The surgical repair procedure is also known as incisional or ventral herniorrhaphy.

Purpose

Incisional hernia repair is performed to correct a weakened area that has developed in the scarred muscle tissue around a prior abdominal surgical incision, occurring as a result of tension (pulling in opposite directions) created when the incision was closed with sutures, or by any other condition that increases abdominal pressure or interferes with proper healing.

Demographics

Because incisional hernias can occur at the site of any type of abdominal surgery previously performed on a wide range of individuals, there is no outstanding profile of an individual most likely to have an incisional hernia. Men, women, and children of all ages and ethnic backgrounds may develop an incisional hernia after abdominal surgery. Incisional hernia occurs more commonly among adults than among children.

Description

An incisional hernia can develop in the scar tissue around any surgery performed in the abdominal area, from the breastbone down to the groin. Depending upon the location of the hernia, internal organs may press through the weakened abdominal wall. The rate of incisional hernia occurrence can be as high as 13% with some abdominal surgeries. These hernias may occur after large surgeries such as intestinal or vascular (heart, arteries, and veins) surgery, or after smaller surgeries such as an **appendectomy** or a **laparoscopy**, which typically requires a small incision at the navel. Incisional hernias themselves can be very small or large and complex, involving growth along the scar tissue of a large incision. They may develop months after the surgery or years after, usually because of inadequate healing or excessive pressure on an abdominal wall scar. The factors that increase the risk of incisional hernia are conditions that increase strain on the abdominal wall, such as obesity, advanced age, malnutrition, poor metabolism (digestion and assimilation of essential nutrients), pregnancy, dialysis, excess fluid retention, and either infection or hematoma (bleeding under the skin) after a prior surgery.

Tension created when sutures are used to close a surgical wound may also be responsible for developing an incisional hernia. Tension is known to influence poor healing conditions because of related swelling and wound separation. Tension and abdominal pressure are greater in people who are overweight, creating greater risk of developing incisional hernias following any abdominal surgery, including surgery for a prior inguinal (groin) hernia. People who have been treated with steroids or chemotherapy are also at greater risk for developing incisional hernias because of the affect these drugs have on the healing process.

The first symptom a person may have with an incisional hernia is pain, with or without a bulge in the abdomen at or near the site of the original surgery.

Incisional hernias can increase in size and gradually produce more noticeable symptoms. Incisional hernias may or may not require surgical treatment.

The effectiveness of surgical repair of an incisional hernia depends in part on reducing or eliminating tension at the surgical wound. The tension-free method used by many medical centers and preferred by surgeons who specialize in hernia repair involves the permanent placement of surgical (prosthetic) steel or polypropylene mesh patches well beyond the edges of the weakened area of the abdominal wall. The mesh is sewn to the area, bridging the hole or weakened area beneath it. As the area heals, the mesh becomes firmly integrated into the inner abdominal wall membrane (peritoneum) that protects the organs of the abdomen. This method creates little or no tension and has a lower rate of hernia recurrence, as well as a faster recovery with less pain. Incisional hernias recur more frequently when **staples** are used rather than sutures to secure mesh to the abdominal wall. Autogenous tissue (skin from the patient's own body) has also been used for this type of repair.

Two surgical approaches are used to treat incisional hernias: either a laparoscopic incisional herniorrhaphy, which uses small incisions and a tube-like instrument with a camera attached to its tip; or a conventional open repair procedure, which accesses the hernia through a larger abdominal incision. Open procedures are necessary if the intestines have become trapped in the hernia (incarceration) or the trapped intestine has become twisted and its blood supply cut off (strangulation). Extremely obese patients may also require an open procedure because deeper layers of fatty tissue will have to be removed from the abdominal wall. Mesh may be used with both types of surgical access.

Minimally invasive laparoscopic surgery has been shown to have advantages over conventional open procedures, including:

- reduced hospital stays
- reduced postoperative pain
- reduced wound complications
- reduced recovery time

Surgical procedure

In both open and laparoscopic procedures, the patient lies on the operating table, either flat on the back or on the side, depending on the location of the hernia. **General anesthesia** is usually given, though some patients may have local or regional anesthesia, depending on the location of the hernia and complexity of the repair. A catheter may be inserted into the bladder to remove urine and decompress the bladder. If the hernia is near the stomach, a gastric (nose or mouth to stomach) tube may be inserted to decompress the stomach.

In an open procedure, an incision is made just large enough to remove fat and scar tissue from the abdominal wall near the hernia. The outside edges of the weakened hernial area are defined and excess tissue removed from within the area. Mesh is then applied so that it overlaps the weakened area by several inches (centimeters) in all directions. Non-absorbable sutures (the kind that must be removed by the doctor) are placed into the full thickness of the abdominal wall. The sutures are tied down and knotted.

In the less-invasive laparoscopic procedure, two or three small incisions will be made to access the hernia site—the laparoscope is inserted in one incision and **surgical instruments** in the others to remove tissue and place the mesh in the same fashion as in an open procedure. Significantly less abdominal wall tissue is removed in laparoscopic repair. The surgeon views the entire procedure on a video monitor to guide the placement and suturing of mesh.

Diagnosis/Preparation

Diagnosis

Reviewing the patient's symptoms and medical history are the first steps in diagnosing an incisional hernia. All prior surgeries will be discussed. The doctor will ask how much pain the patient is experiencing, when it was first noticed, and how it has progressed. The doctor will palpate (touch) the area, looking for any abnormal bulging or mass, and may ask the patient to cough or strain in order to see and feel the hernia more easily. To confirm the presence of the hernia, an **ultrasound** examination or other scan such as computed tomography (CT) may be performed. Scans will allow the doctor to visualize the hernia and to make sure that the bulge is not another type of abdominal mass such as a tumor or enlarged lymph gland. The doctor will be able to determine the size of the defect and whether or not surgery is an appropriate way to treat it. A referral to a surgeon will be made if the doctor believes that medical treatment will not effectively correct the incisional hernia.

Preparation

Many months before the surgery, the patient's doctor may advise weight loss to help reduce the risks of surgery and to improve the surgical results. Control of diabetes and **smoking cessation** are also recommended for a better surgical result. Close to the time

of the scheduled surgery, the patient will have standard preoperative blood and urine tests, an **electrocardiogram**, and a **chest x ray** to make sure that heart and lungs and major organ systems are functioning well. A week or so before surgery, medications may be discontinued, especially **aspirin** or anticoagulant (blood-thinning) drugs. Starting the night before surgery, patients must not eat or drink anything. Once in the hospital, a tube may be placed into a vein in the arm (intravenous line) to deliver fluid and medication during surgery. The patient will be given a preoperative injection of **antibiotics** before the procedure. A sedative may be given to relax the patient.

Aftercare

Immediately after surgery, the patient will be observed in a recovery area for several hours, for monitoring of **body temperature**, pulse, blood pressure, and heart function, as well as observation of the surgical wound for undue bleeding or swelling. Patients will usually be discharged on the day of the surgery; only more complex hernias such as those with incarcerated or strangulated intestines will require overnight hospitalization. Some patients may have prolonged suture-site pain, which may be treated with pain medication or anti-inflammatory drugs. Antibiotics may be prescribed to help prevent postoperative infection.

Once the patient is home, the hernia repair site must be kept clean, and any sign of swelling or redness reported to the surgeon. Patients should also report a fever or any abdominal pain. Outer sutures may have to be removed by the surgeon in a follow-up visit about a week after surgery. Activities may be limited to non-strenuous movement for up to two weeks, depending on the type of surgery performed. To allow proper healing of muscle tissue, hernia repair patients should avoid heavy lifting for at least six to eight weeks after surgery, or longer as advised.

Risks

Long-term complications seldom occur after incisional hernia repair. Short-term risks are greater with obese patients or those who have had multiple earlier operations or the prior placement of mesh patches. The risk of complications has been shown to be about 13%. The risk of recurrence and repeat surgery is as high as 52%, particularly with open procedures or those using staples rather than sutures for wound closure. Some of the factors that cause incisional hernias to occur in the first place, such as obesity and nutritional disorders, will persist in certain patients and encourage the development of a second incisional hernia and repeat

Incisional hernia repair is performed in a hospital operating room or a one-day surgical center by a general surgeon who may specialize in hernia repair procedures.

surgery. Each subsequent time, the surgery will become more difficult and the risk of complications greater. Postoperative infection is higher with open procedures than with laparoscopic procedures.

Postoperative complications may include:

- fluid buildup at the site of mesh placement, sometimes requiring aspiration (draining off)
- postoperative bleeding, though seldom enough to require repeat surgery
- prolonged suture pain, treated with pain medication or anti-inflammatory drugs
- intestinal injury
- nerve injury
- fever, usually related to surgical wound infection
- intra-abdominal (within the abdominal wall) abscess
- urinary retention
- respiratory distress

Normal results

Good outcomes are expected with incisional hernia repair, particularly with the laparoscopic method. Patients will usually go home the day of surgery and can expect a one- to two-week recovery period at home, and then a return to normal activities. The American College of Surgeons reports that recurrence rates after the first repair of an incisional hernia range from 25–52%. Recurrence is more frequent when conventional surgical wound closure with standard sutures (**stitches**) is used. Recurrence after open procedures has been shown to be less likely when mesh is used, although complications, especially infection, have been shown to increase because of the larger abdominal incisions. Laparoscopy with mesh has shown rates of recurrence as low as 3.4%, with fewer complications as well.

Morbidity and mortality rates

Deaths are not reported resulting directly from the performance of herniorrhaphy for incisional hernia.

- What procedure will be performed to correct my hernia?
- What is your experience with this procedure? How often do you perform this procedure?
- Why must I have the surgery?
- What are my options if I do not have the surgery?
- How can I expect to feel after surgery?
- What are the risks involved in having this surgery?
- How quickly will I recover? When can I return to school or work?
- What are my chances of having this type of hernia again?
- What can I do to avoid getting this type of hernia again?

Alternatives

The alternatives to first-time and recurrent incisional hernia repair begin with preventive measures such as:

- Losing weight; maintaining suitable weight for age and height.
- Strengthening abdominal muscles through regular moderate exercise such as walking, tai chi, yoga, or stretching exercises and gentle aerobics.
- Reducing abdominal pressure by avoiding constipation and the buildup of excess body fluids, achieved by adopting a high-fiber, low-salt diet.
- Learning to lift heavy objects in a safe, low-strain way using arm and leg muscles.
- Controlling diabetes and poor metabolism with regular medical care and dietary changes as recommended.
- Eating a healthy, balanced diet of whole foods, high in essential nutrients, including whole grains, fruits and vegetables, limited meat and dairy, and eliminating prepared and refined foods.

Resources

BOOKS

Maddern, Guy J. *Hernia Repair: Open vs. Laparoscopic Approaches.* London: Churchill Livingstone, 1997.

ORGANIZATIONS

American College of Surgeons (ACS), Office of Public Information. 633 North Saint Clair Street, Chicago, IL 60611-3211. (312) 202-5000. http://www.facs.org.

The National Digestive Diseases Information Clearinghouse (NIDDK). 2 Information Way, Bethesda, MD 20892-3570. http://www.niddk.nih.gov/health/digest/nddic.htm.

OTHER

"Hernia." *Focus on Men's Health*. MedicineNet Home. January 2003. http://www.medicinenet.com.

Incisional and Ventral Hernias (Patient Information). Central Montgomery Medical Center, Outpatient Surgery Department. 2100 N. Broad Street, Lansdale, PA 19446. (215) 368-1122.

L. Lee Culvert

Inflatable sphincter *see* Artificial sphincter insertion

▌Informed consent

Definition

Informed consent is a legal document in all 50 states. It is an agreement for a proposed medical treatment or non-treatment, or for a proposed invasive procedure. It requires physicians to disclose the benefits, risks, and alternatives to the proposed treatment, non-treatment, or procedure. It is the method by which fully informed, rational persons may be involved in choices about their health care.

Description

Informed consent stems from the legal and ethical right an individual has to decide what is done to his or her body, and from the physician's ethical duty to make sure that individuals are involved in decisions about their own health care. The process of securing informed consent has three phases, all of which involve information exchange between doctor and patient and are part of patient education. First, in words an individual can understand, the physician must convey the details of a planned procedure or treatment, its potential benefits and serious risks, and any feasible alternatives. The patient should be presented with information on the most likely outcomes of the treatment. Second, the physician must evaluate whether or not the person has understood what has been said, must ascertain that the risks have been accepted, and that the patient is giving consent to proceed with the procedure or treatment with full knowledge and forethought. Finally, the individual must sign the consent form, which documents in generic format the major points of consideration. The

only exception to this is securing informed consent during extreme emergencies.

It is critical that a patient receive enough information on which to base informed consent, and that the consent is wholly voluntary and has not been forced in any way. It is the responsibility of the physician who discusses the particulars with the patient to detail the conversation in the medical record. A physician may, at his or her discretion, appoint another member of the health care team to obtain the patient's signature on the consent form, with the assurance that the physician has satisfied the requirements of informed consent.

The law requires that a reasonable physician/patient standard be applied when determining how much information is considered adequate when discussing a procedure or treatment with the patient. There are three approaches to making this discussion: what the typical physician would say about the intervention (the reasonable physician standard); what an average patient would need to know to be an informed participant in the decision (the reasonable patient standard); and what a patient would need to know and understand to make a decision that is informed (the subjective standard).

There is a theory that the practice of acquiring informed consent is rooted in the post–World War II Nuremberg Trials. At the war crimes tribunal in 1949, 10 standards were put forth regarding physicians' requirements for experimentation on human subjects. This established a new standard of ethical medical behavior for the post–WW II human rights age, and the concept of voluntary informed consent was established. A number of rules accompanied voluntary informed consent. It could only be requested for experimentation for the gain of society, for the potential acquisition of knowledge of the pathology of disease, and for studies performed that avoided physical and mental suffering to the fullest extent possible.

Today, all of the 50 United States have legislation that delineates the required standards for informed consent. For example, the State of Washington employs the second approach outlined as the reasonable patient standard (what an average patient would need to know to be an informed participant in the decision). This approach ensures that a doctor fulfills all professional

Informed consent

responsibilities and provides the best care possible and that patients have choices in decisions about their health care. However, the patient's competence in making a decision is considered. This points to the issue of the patient's mental capacity. Anyone suffering from an illness, anticipating surgery, or undergoing treatment for a disease is under a great deal of stress and anxiety. It may be natural for a patient to be confused or indecisive. When the attending physician has serious doubts about the patient's understanding of the intervention and its risks, the patient may be referred for a psychiatric consultation. This is strictly a precaution to ensure that the patient understands what has been explained; declining to be treated or operated on does not necessarily mean the person is incompetent. It could mean that the person is exercising the right to make his or her own health care decisions.

Although the law requires a formal presentation of the procedure or treatment to the patient, physicians do express doubt as to the wisdom of this. Some believe that informing patients of the risks of treatment might scare them into refusing it, even when the risks of non-treatment are even greater. But patients might have a different view. Without the complete story, for example, a patient might consent to beginning a particular course of chemotherapy. Convinced by the pressures from a pharmaceutical company, it is conceivable that a doctor will use an agent less effective than a newer treatment. By withholding information about treatment alternatives, the physician may be denying the patient a choice and, worse, perhaps a chance of an extended life of greater quality.

Undeniably, physicians in surgery, anesthesia, oncology, infectious disease, and other specialties are faced with issues regarding informed consent. As the federal government takes a more active role in deciding the extent to which patients must be informed of treatments, procedures, and clinical trials in which they voluntarily become enrolled, more and more health care providers must become educated in what must be conveyed to patients. This is emphasized by the report of a case in which a federal court (*Hutchinson v. United States* [91 F2d 560 (9th Cir. 1990)]) ruled in favor of the physician, despite his failure to advise his asthmatic patient, for whom he had prescribed the steroid, prednisone, of the drug's well-known risk of developing aseptic necrosis (bone **death**), which did occur. The practitioner neglected to inform the patient that there were other drugs available with much less serious side effects that could have treated the asthma. However, a higher appellate court reversed the ruling and found the physician guilty. Apparently, the patient had used more conservative drugs in the past with good results. The court believed that if the

physician had merely advised the patient of the more serious side effects of prednisone and offered the patient more conservative treatment, the physician would have avoided liability.

Nursing professionals have a greater role than they might believe in evaluating whether or not consent is informed. When a nurse witnesses the signature of a patient for a procedure, or surgery, he or she is not responsible for providing the details. Rather, the role is to be the patient's advocate, to protect the patient's dignity, to identify any fears, and to determine the patient's degree of comprehension and approval of care to be received. Each patient is an individual, and each one will have a different and unique response depending on his or her personality, level of education, emotions, and cognitive status. If a patient can restate the information that has been imparted, then that will help to confirm that he or she has received enough information and has understood it. The nurse is obligated to report any doubts about the patient's understanding regarding what has been said or any concerns about his or her capacity to make decisions.

Results

The result of informed consent is greater safety and protection for patients, physicians, and society.

Resources

BOOKS

Clarke, S., and J. Oakley. *Informed Consent and Clinician Accountability: The Ethics of Report Cards on Surgeon Performance.* New York: Cambridge University Press, 2007.

Fix, R. M. *Informed Consent.* Florence, KY: Frontline Publishing, 2007.

Getz, K., and D. Boritz. *Informed Consent: The Consumer's Guide to the Risks and Benefits of Volunteering for Clinical Trials.* Boston, MA: CenterWatch, 1999.

Glenn, S. *Informed Consent.* Paris, Ontario, Canada: David C. Cook, 2007.

Manson, N, C., and O. O'Neill. *Rethinking Informed Consent in Bioethics.* New York: Cambridge University Press, 2007.

PERIODICALS

Helmreich, R., J., V. Hundley, A. Norman, J. Ighedosa, and E. Chow. "Research in pregnant women: the challenges of informed consent." *Nursing for Women's Health* 11, no. 6 (2007): 576–585.

Johnson, L. J. "Get informed consent for risky drugs." *Medical Economics* 84, no. 21 (2007): 20–23.

Perez-Carceles, M. D., M. D. Lorenzo, A. Luna, and E. Osuna. "Elderly patients also have rights." *Journal of Medical Ethics* 33, no. 12 (2007): 712–716.

Rossel, M., M. Burnier, and R. Stupp. "Informed consent: true information or institutional review board-approved disinformation?" *Journal of Clinical Oncology* 25, no. 36 (2007): 5835–5836.

Sheach-Leith, V. M. "Consent and nothing but consent? The organ retention scandal." *Sociology of Health and Illness* 29, no. 7 (2007): 1023–1042.

ORGANIZATIONS

American Academy of Family Physicians. 11400 Tomahawk Creek Parkway, Leawood, KS 66211-2672. (913) 906-6000. E-mail: fp@aafp.org. http://www.aafp.org.

American Bar Association. 321 N Clark St., Chicago, IL 60610. 800-285-2221. http://www.abanet.org/home.html.

American College of Physicians. 190 N Independence Mall West, Philadelphia, PA 19106-1572. (800) 523-1546, x2600, or (215) 351-2600. http://www.acponline.org.

American Medical Association. 515 N. State Street, Chicago, IL 60610. 312) 464-5000. http://www.ama-assn.org.

OTHER

American Academy of Pediatrics. Information about Informed Consent. 2007 [cited December 24, 2007]. http://www.aap.org/policy/00662.html.

American Medical Association. Information about Informed Consent. 2007 [cited December 24, 2007]. http://www.ama-assn.org/ama/pub/category/4608.html.

Food and Drug Administration. Information about Informed Consent. 2007 [cited December 24, 2007]. http://google2.fda.gov/search?output = xml_no_dtd&lr = &proxystylesheet = FDA&client = FDA&site = FDA&getfields = *&q = informed + consent.

Office for Human Research Protections. Department of Health and Human Services. Information about Informed Consent. 2007 [cited December 24, 2007]. http://search.hhs.gov/search?q = informed + consent &entqr = 0&ud = 1&sort = date%3AD%3AL%3Ad1 &output = xml_no_dtd&site = HHS&ie = UTF-8&oe = UTF-8&lr = lang_en&client = HHS& proxystylesheet = HHS.

L. Fleming Fallon, Jr, MD, DrPH

Inguinal hernia repair

Definition

Inguinal hernia repair, also known as herniorrhaphy, is the surgical correction of an inguinal hernia. An inguinal hernia is an opening, weakness, or bulge in the lining tissue (peritoneum) of the abdominal wall in the groin area between the abdomen and the thigh. The surgery may be a standard open procedure through an incision large enough to access the hernia or a laparoscopic procedure performed through tiny incisions, using an instrument with a camera attached (laparoscope) and a video monitor to guide the repair. When the surgery involves reinforcing the weakened area with steel mesh, the repair is called hernioplasty.

Purpose

Inguinal hernia repair is performed to close or mend the weakened abdominal wall of an inquinal hernia.

Demographics

The majority of hernias occur in males. Nearly 25% of men and only 2% of women in the United States will develop inguinal hernias. Inguinal hernias occur nearly three times more often in African American adults than in Caucasians. Among children, the risk of groin hernia is greater in premature infants or those of low birth weight. Indirect inguinal hernias will occur in 10–20 children in every 1,000 live births.

Description

About 75% of all hernias are classified as inguinal hernias, which are the most common type of hernia occurring in men and women as a result of the activities of normal living and aging. Because humans stand upright, there is a greater downward force on the lower abdomen, increasing pressure on the less muscled and naturally weaker tissues of the groin area. Inguinal hernias do not include those caused by a cut (incision) in the abdominal wall (incisional hernia). According to the National Center for Health Statistics, about 700,000 inguinal hernias are repaired annually in the United States. The inguinal hernia is usually seen or felt first as a tender and sometimes painful lump in the upper groin where the inguinal canal passes through the abdominal wall. The inguinal canal is the normal route by which testes descend into the scrotum in the male fetus, which is one reason these hernias occur more frequently in men.

Hernias are divided into two categories: congenital (from birth), also called indirect hernias, and acquired, also called direct hernias. Among the 75% of hernias classified as inguinal hernias, 50% are indirect or congenital hernias, occurring when the inguinal canal entrance fails to close normally before birth. The indirect inguinal hernia pushes down from the abdomen and through the inguinal canal. This condition is found in 2% of all adult males and in 1–2% of male children. Indirect inguinal hernias can occur in women, too, when abdominal pressure pushes folds of genital

Inguinal hernia repair

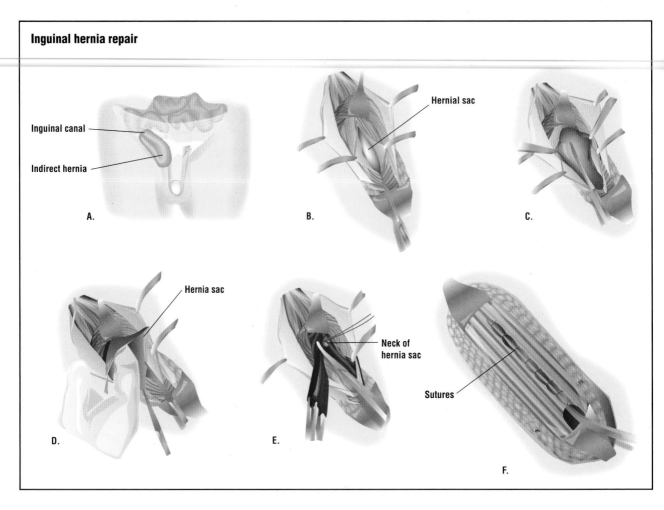

Inguinal canal

Indirect hernia

A.

Hernial sac

B.

C.

Hernia sac

D.

Neck of hernia sac

Sutures

E.

F.

This patient has an indirect inguinal hernia (A). To repair it, the surgeon makes an incision over the area and separates the muscle and tisses to expose the hernia sac (B). The sac is cut open (C), and the contents are replaced into the abdomen (D). The neck of the hernia sac is tied off (E), and the muscles and tissues are sutured (F). *(Illustration by GGS Information Services. Cengage Learning, Gale.)*

tissue into the inquinal canal opening. In fact, women will more likely have an indirect inguinal hernia than direct. Direct or acquired inguinal hernias occur when part of the large intestine protrudes through a weakened area of muscles in the groin. The weakening results from a variety of factors encountered in the wear and tear of life.

Inguinal hernias may occur on one side of the groin or both sides at the same or different times, but occur most often on the right side. About 60% of hernias found in children, for example, will be on the right side, about 30% on the left, and 10% on both sides. The muscular weak spots develop because of pressure on the abdominal muscles in the groin area occurring during normal activities such as lifting, coughing, straining during urination or bowel movements, pregnancy, or excessive weight gain. Internal organs such as the

intestines may then push through this weak spot, causing a bulge of tissue. A congenital indirect inguinal hernia may be diagnosed in infancy, childhood, or later in adulthood, influenced by the same causes as direct hernia. There is evidence that a tendency for inguinal hernia may be inherited.

A direct and an indirect inguinal hernia may occur at the same time; this combined hernia is called a pantaloon hernia.

A femoral hernia is another type of hernia that appears in the groin, occurring when abdominal organs and tissue press through the femoral ring (passageway where the major femoral artery and vein extend from the leg into the abdomen) into the upper thigh. About 3% of all hernias are femoral, and 84% of all femoral hernias occur in women. These are not inquinal hernias, but they can sometimes confuse the

KEY TERMS

Incarcerated hernia—An inguinal hernia that is trapped in place and cannot slip back into the abdominal cavity, often causing intestinal obstruction.

Incisional hernia—Hernia occurring at the site of a prior surgery.

Inguinal hernia—A weak spot in the lower abdominal muscles of the groin through which body organs, usually the large intestines, can push through as a result of abdominal pressure.

Ischemia—The death of tissue that results from lack of blood flow and oxygen.

Laparoscopy—The use of a camera-tipped viewing tube called a laparoscope to perform minimally invasive surgery while viewing the procedure on a video screen.

Strangulated hernia—A twisted piece of herniated intestine that can block blood flow to the intestines.

diagnosis of inguinal hernias because they curve over the inguinal area. They are more often accompanied by intestinal obstruction than inguinal hernias.

Because inguinal hernias do not heal on their own and can become larger or twisted, which may close off the intestines, the prevailing medical opinion is that hernias must be treated surgically when they cause pain or limit activity. Protruding intestines can sometimes be pushed back temporarily into the abdominal cavity, or an external support (truss) may be worn to hold the area in place until surgery can be performed. Sometimes, other medical conditions complicate the presence of a hernia by adding constant abdominal pressure. These conditions, including chronic coughing, constipation, fluid retention, or urinary obstruction, must be treated simultaneously to reduce abdominal pressure and the recurrence of hernias after repair. A relationship between smoking and hernia development has also been shown. Groin hernias occur more frequently in smokers than nonsmokers, especially in women. A hernia may become incarcerated, which means that it is trapped in place and cannot slip back into the abdomen. This causes bowel obstruction, which may require the removal of affected parts of the intestines (**bowel resection**) as well as hernia repair. If the herniated intestine becomes twisted, blood supply to the intestines may be cut off (intestinal ischemia) and the hernia is said to be strangulated, a condition causing severe pain and requiring immediate surgery.

Surgical procedures

In open inguinal hernia repair procedures, the patient is typically given a light **general anesthesia** of short duration. Local or regional anesthetics may be given to some patients. Open surgical repair of an indirect hernia begins with sterilizing and draping the inguinal area of the abdomen just above the thigh. An incision is made in the abdominal wall and fatty tissue removed to expose the inguinal canal and define the outer margins of the hole or weakness in the muscle. The weakened section of tissue is dissected (cut and removed) and the inguinal canal opening is sutured closed (primary closure), making sure that no abdominal organ tissue is within the sutured area. The exposed inguinal canal is examined for any other trouble spots that may need reinforcement. Closing the underlayers of tissue (subcutaneous tissue) with fine sutures and the outer skin with **staples** completes the procedure. A sterile dressing is then applied.

An open repair of a direct hernia begins just as the repair of an indirect hernia, with an incision made in the same location above the thigh, just large enough to allow visualization of the hernia. The surgeon will look for and palpate (touch) the bulging area of the hernia and will reduce it by placing sutures in the fat layer of the abdominal wall. The hernial sac itself will be closed, as in the repair of the indirect hernia, by using a series of sutures from one end of the weakened hernia defect to the other. The repair will be checked for sturdiness and for any tension on the new sutures. The subcutaneous tissue and skin will be closed and a sterile dressing applied.

Laparoscopic procedures are conducted using general anesthesia. The surgeon will make three tiny incisions in the abdominal wall of the groin area and inflate the abdomen with carbon dioxide to expand the surgical area. A laparoscope, which is a tube-like fiberoptic instrument with a small video camera attached to its tip, will be inserted in one incision and **surgical instruments** inserted in the other incisions. The surgeon will view the movement of the instruments on a video monitor, as the hernia is pushed back into place and the hernial sac is repaired with surgical sutures or staples. Laparoscopic surgery is believed to produce less postoperative pain and a quicker recovery time. The risk of infection is also reduced because of the small incisions required in laparoscopic surgery.

The use of surgical (prosthetic) steel mesh or polypropylene mesh in the repair of inguinal hernias has been shown to help prevent recurrent hernias. Instead of the tension that develops between sutures and the skin in a conventionally repaired area, hernioplasty using mesh patches has been shown to virtually eliminate tension. The procedure is often performed in an outpatient facility with **local anesthesia** and patients can walk away the same day, with little restrictions in activity. Tension-free repair is also quick and easy to perform using the laparoscopic method, although general anesthesia is usually used. In either open or laparoscopic procedures, the mesh is placed so that it overlaps the healthy skin around the hernia opening and then is sutured into place with fine silk. Rather than pulling the hole closed as in conventional repair, the mesh makes a bridge over the hole and as normal healing take place, the mesh is incorporated into normal tissue without resulting tension.

Diagnosis/Preparation

Diagnosis

Reviewing the patient's symptoms and medical history are the first steps in diagnosing a hernia. The surgeon will ask when the patient first noticed a lump or bulge in the groin area, whether or not it has grown larger, and how much pain the patient is experiencing. The doctor will palpate the area, looking for any abnormal bulging or mass, and may ask the patient to cough or strain in order to see and feel the hernia more easily. This may be all that is needed to diagnose an inguinal hernia. To confirm the presence of the hernia, an **ultrasound** examination may be performed. The ultrasound scan will allow the doctor to visualize the hernia and to make sure that the bulge is not another type of abdominal mass such as a tumor or enlarged lymph gland. It is not usually possible to determine whether the hernia is direct or indirect until surgery is performed.

Preparation

Patients will have standard preoperative blood and urine tests, an **electrocardiogram**, and a **chest x ray** to make sure that the heart, lungs, and major organ systems are functioning well. A week or so before surgery, medications may be discontinued, especially **aspirin** or anticoagulant (blood-thinning) drugs. Starting the night before surgery, patients must not eat or drink anything. Once in the hospital, a tube may be placed into a vein in the arm (intravenous line) to deliver fluid and medication during surgery. A sedative may be given to relax the patient.

Aftercare

The hernia repair site must be kept clean and any sign of swelling or redness reported to the surgeon. Patients should also report a fever, and men should report any pain or swelling of the testicles. The surgeon may remove the outer sutures in a follow-up visit about a week after surgery. Activities may be limited to non-strenuous movement for up to two weeks, depending on the type of surgery performed and whether or not the surgery is the first hernia repair. To allow proper healing of muscle tissue, hernia repair patients should avoid heavy lifting for six to eight weeks after surgery. The postoperative activities of patients undergoing repeat procedures may be even more restricted.

Prevention of indirect hernias, which are congenital, is not possible. However, preventing direct hernias and reducing the risk of recurrence of direct and indirect hernias can be accomplished by:

- Maintaining body weight suitable for age and height.
- Strengthening abdominal muscles through regular exercise.
- Reducing abdominal pressure by avoiding constipation and the build-up of excess body fluids, achieved by adopting a high-fiber, low-salt diet.
- Lifting heavy objects in a safe, low-stress way, using arm and leg muscles.

Risks

Hernia surgery is considered to be a relatively safe procedure, although complication rates range from 1–26%, most in the 7–12% range. This means that about 10% of the 700,000 inguinal hernia repairs each year will have complications. Certain specialized clinics report markedly fewer complications, often related to whether open or laparoscopic technique is used. One of the greatest risks of inquinal hernia repair is that the hernia will recur. Unfortunately, 10–15% of hernias may develop again at the same site in adults, representing about 100,000 recurrences annually. The risk of recurrence in children is only about 1%. Recurrent hernias can present a serious problem because incarceration and strangulation are more likely and because additional surgical repair is more difficult than the first surgery. When the first hernia repair breaks down, the surgeon must work around scar tissue as well as the recurrent hernia. Incisional hernias, which are hernias that occur at the site of a prior surgery, present the same circumstance of combined scar tissue and hernia and even greater risk of recurrence. Each time a repair is performed, the surgery is less likely to be successful. Recurrence and infection rates for mesh repairs have been shown in some studies to be lower than with conventional surgeries.

Complications that can occur during surgery include injury to the spermatic cord structure; injuries to veins or arteries, causing hemorrhage; severing or entrapping nerves, which can cause paralysis; injuries to the bladder or bowel; reactions to anesthesia; and systemic complications such as cardiac arrythmias, cardiac arrest, or **death**. Postoperative complications include infection of the surgical incision (less in **laparoscopy**); the formation of blood clots at the site that can travel to other parts of the body; pulmonary (lung) problems; and urinary retention or urinary tract infection.

Normal results

Inguinal hernia repair is usually effective, depending on the size of the hernia, how much time has gone by between its first appearance and the corrective surgery, and the underlying condition of the patient. Most first-time hernia repair procedures will be one-day surgeries, in which the patient will go home the same day or in 24 hours. Only the most challenging cases will require an overnight stay. Recovery times will vary, depending on the type of surgery performed. Patients undergoing open surgery will experience little discomfort and will resume normal activities within one to two weeks. Laparoscopy patients will be able to enjoy normal activities within one or two days, returning to a normal work routine and lifestyle within four to seven days, with the exception of heavy lifting and contact sports.

Morbidity and mortality rates

Mortality related to inguinal hernia repair or postoperative complications is unlikely, but with advanced age or severe underlying conditions, deaths do occur. Recurrence is a notable complication and is associated with increased morbidity, with recurrence rates for indirect hernias from less than 1–7% and 4–10% for direct.

Alternatives

If a hernia is not surgically repaired, an incarcerated or strangulated hernia can result, sometimes involving life-threatening bowel obstruction or ischemia.

Resources

BOOKS

Maddern, Guy J. *Hernia Repair: Open vs. Laparoscopic approaches*. London: Churchill Livingstone, 1997.

ORGANIZATIONS

American College of Surgeons (ACS), Office of Public Information. 633 North Saint Clair Street, Chicago, IL 60611-3211. (312) 202-5000. http://www.facs.org.
The National Digestive Diseases Information Clearinghouse (NIDDK). 2 Information Way, Bethesda, MD 20892-3570. http://www.niddk.nih.gov/health/digest/nddic.htm.

OTHER

"Hernia." *Focus on Men's Health*. MedicineNet Home. January 2003. http://www.medicinenet.com.
"Inguinal Hernia." *Laurus Health.com*. February 2001. http://www.laurushealth.com/library.

L. Lee Culvert

Inner ear tube insertion *see* **Endolymphatic shunt**

Intensive care unit

Definition

An intensive care unit, or ICU, is a specialized section of a hospital that provides comprehensive and continuous care for persons who are critically ill and who can benefit from treatment.

Purpose

The purpose of the intensive care unit (ICU) is simple even though the practice is complex. Health-care professionals who work in the ICU or rotate through it during their training provide around-the-clock intensive monitoring and treatment of patients seven days a week. Patients are generally admitted to an ICU if they are likely to benefit from the level of care provided. Intensive care has been shown to benefit patients who are severely ill and medically unstable—that is, they have a potentially life-threatening disease or disorder.

Although the criteria for admission to an ICU are somewhat controversial—excluding patients who are either too well or too sick to benefit from intensive care—there are four recommended priorities that intensivists (specialists in critical care medicine) use to decide this question. These priorities include:

- critically ill patients in a medically unstable state who require an intensive level of care (monitoring and treatment)
- patients requiring intensive monitoring who may also require emergency interventions
- patients who are medically unstable or critically ill and who do not have much chance for recovery due to the severity of their illness or traumatic injury
- patients who are generally not eligible for ICU admission because they are not expected to survive (Patients in this fourth category require the approval of the director of the ICU program before admission.)

ICU care requires a multidisciplinary team that consists of but is not limited to intensivists (clinicians who specialize in critical illness care); pharmacists and nurses; respiratory care therapists; and other medical consultants from a broad range of specialties including surgery, pediatrics, and anesthesiology. The ideal ICU will have a team representing as many as 31 different health care professionals and practitioners who assist in patient evaluation and treatment. The intensivist will provide treatment management, diagnosis, interventions, and individualized care for each patient recovering from severe illness.

Demographics

A large and comprehensive study conducted in 1992 by the Society of Critical Care Medicine in collaboration with the American Hospital Association found that approximately 8% of all licensed hospital beds in the United States were designated for intensive care. The average size of an adult or pediatric ICU averaged 10–12 beds per unit. Small hospitals with

fewer than 100 beds usually had one ICU, whereas larger hospitals with more than 300 beds usually had several ICUs designated for medical, surgical, and coronary patients. Smaller hospitals do not usually have a full-time board-certified specialist in critical care medicine, whereas larger medical centers generally employ certified intensivists—60% of hospitals with more than 500 beds had full-time specialist directors at the time the survey was conducted.

In a 2006 report, the Society of Critical Care Medicine noted that there are approximately 6,000 ICUs in the United States, caring for 55,000 critically ill patients each day. Statistics reveal that more than 5 million patients are admitted annually to these ICU departments. Most often patients presenting to the ICU have high acuity diagnoses such as respiratory insufficiency, sepsis, and heart failure, necessitating treatment from skilled clinicians and the need for expert care. Since 1991 treatment of patients presenting with serious conditions has become more frequent due in part, to a rise in the U.S. population of individuals aged 65 and older. In fact, in 2004, the number of patients age 85 and older, rose from 4.1% in 1991 to 6.9%.

With regard to the nursing staff in ICUs, the proportion of nurses with specialized and advanced training in critical care medicine is higher in larger medical centers—about 16% in hospitals with 100 beds or fewer, but 21% in hospitals with more than 500 beds.

Most pediatric ICUs have four to six beds per unit. The mortality rate in pediatric ICUs tends to increase in proportion to size, with larger units reporting more deaths (approximately 8% in the larger units). Eighty percent of pediatric ICUs have full-time medical directors.

Description

ICUs are highly regulated departments, typically limiting the number of visitors to the patient's immediate family even during visiting hours. The patient usually has several monitors attached to various parts of his or her body for real-time evaluation of medical stability. The intensivist will make periodic assessments of the patient's cardiac status, breathing rate, urinary output, and blood levels for nutritional and hormonal problems that may arise and require urgent attention or treatment. Patients who are admitted to the ICU for observation after surgery may have special requirements for monitoring. These patients may have catheters placed to detect hemodynamic (blood pressure) changes, or require **endotracheal intubation** to help their breathing, with the breathing tube connected to a mechanical ventilator.

In addition to the intensivist's role in direct patient care, he or she is usually the lead physician when multiple consultants are involved in an intensive care program. The intensivist coordinates the care provided by the consultants, which allows for an integrated treatment approach to the patient.

Nursing care has an important role in an intensive care unit. The nurse's role usually includes clinical assessment, diagnosis, and an individualized plan of expected treatment outcomes for each patient (implementation of treatment and patient evaluation of results). The ICU pharmacist evaluates all drug therapy, including dosage, route of administration, and monitoring for signs of allergic reactions. In addition to checking and supervising all levels of medication administration, the ICU pharmacist is also responsible for enteral and parenteral nutrition (tube feeding) for patients who cannot eat on their own. ICUs also have respiratory care therapists with specialized training in cardiorespiratory (heart and lung) care for critically ill patients. Respiratory therapists generally provide medications to help patients breathe as well as the care and support of mechanical ventilators. Respiratory therapists also evaluate all respiratory therapy procedures to maximize efficiency and cost-effectiveness.

Large medical centers may have more than one ICU. These specialized intensive care units typically include a CCU (coronary care unit); a pediatric ICU (PICU, dedicated to the treatment of critically ill children); a newborn ICU or NICU, for the care of premature and critically ill infants; and a surgical ICU (SICU, dedicated to the treatment of postoperative patients).

Preparation

Persons who are critically ill may be admitted to the ICU from the emergency room, a surgical ward, or from any other hospital department. ICUs are arranged around a central station so that patients can be seen either through the room windows or from a nursing station a few steps away. Patients are given 24-hour

assessments by the intensivist. Preparatory orders for the ICU generally vary from patient to patient since treatment is individualized. The initial workup should be coordinated by the attending ICU staff (intensivist and ICU nurse specialist), pharmacists (for medications and IV fluid therapy), and respiratory therapists for stabilization, improvement, or continuation of cardiopulmonary care. Well-coordinated care includes prompt consultation with other specialists soon after the patient is admitted to the ICU. The patient is connected to monitors that record his or her **vital signs** (pulse, blood pressure, and breathing rate). Orders for medications, laboratory tests, or other procedures are instituted upon arrival.

In general there are eight categories of diseases and disorders that are regarded as medical justification for admission to an ICU. These categories include disorders of the cardiac, nervous, pulmonary, and endocrine (hormonal) systems, together with postsurgical crises and **medication monitoring** for drug ingestion or overdose. Cardiac problems can include heart attacks (myocardial infarction), shock, cardiac arrhythmias (abnormal heart rhythm), heart failure (congestive heart failure or CHF), high blood pressure, and unstable angina (chest pain). Lung disorders can include acute respiratory failure, pulmonary emboli (blood clots in the lungs), hemoptysis (coughing up blood), and respiratory failure. Neurological disorders may include acute stroke (blood clot in the brain), coma, bleeding in the brain (intracranial hemorrhage), such infections as meningitis, and traumatic brain injury (TBI). Medication monitoring is essential, including careful attention to the possibility of seizures and other drug side effects.

When patients are transferred to the ICU from another hospital department, treatment orders and planning must be reviewed and new treatment plans written for the patient's current status. For example, a chronically ill inpatient may grow markedly worse within a few hours and may be transferred to the ICU, where the staff must reevaluate orders for his or her care.

Resources

BOOKS

Brenner, Matthew, MD, et al. *Critical Care Medicine*. Mission Viejo, CA :Current Clinical Strategies, 2006.

Marino, Paul, L. and Kenneth M. Sutin. *The ICU Book*, 3rd ed. New York: Lippincott Williams & Wilkins, 2006.

PERIODICALS

Brilli, R. J., A. Spevetz, R. D. Branson, et al. "Critical Care Delivery in the Intensive Care Unit: Defining Clinical Roles and the Best Practice Model." *Critical Care Medicine* 29 (October 2001): 2007-2019.

Ethics Committee, Society of Critical Care Medicine. "Consensus Statement of the SCCM Ethics Committee Regarding Futile and Other Possibly Inadvisable Treatments." *Critical Care Medicine* 25 (May 1997): 887-891.

Truog, R. D., A. F. Cist, S. E. Brackett, et al. "Recommendations for End-of-Life Care in the Intensive Care Unit: The Ethics Committee of the Society of Critical Care Medicine." *Critical Care Medicine* 29 (December 2001): 2332-2348.

ORGANIZATIONS

American Hospital Association. One North Franklin, Chicago, IL 60606-3421. (312) 422-3000. www.hospitalconnect.com

Joint Commission on Accreditation of Healthcare Organizations (JCAHO). One Renaissance Blvd., Oakbrook Terrace, IL 60181. (630) 792-5000 or (630) 792-5085. www.jcaho.org/.

Society of Critical Care Medicine (SCCM). 701 Lee Street, Suite 200, Des Plaines, IL 60016. (847) 827-6869; Fax: (847) 827-6869. www.sccm.org.

Laith Farid Gulli, MD, MS
Bilal Nasser, MD, MS
Uchechukwu Sampson, MD, MPH, MBA
Laura Jean Cataldo, RN, EdD

Intensive care unit equipment

Definition

Intensive care unit (ICU) equipment includes patient monitoring, respiratory and cardiac support, **pain management**, emergency resuscitation devices, and other life support equipment designed to care for patients who are seriously injured, have a critical or life-threatening illness, or have undergone a major surgical procedure, thereby requiring 24-hour care and monitoring.

Purpose

An ICU may be designed and equipped to provide care to patients with a range of conditions, or it may be designed and equipped to provide specialized care to patients with specific conditions. For example, a neuro-medical ICU cares for patients with acute conditions involving the nervous system or patients who have just had neurosurgical procedures and require equipment for monitoring and assessing the brain and spinal cord. A neonatal ICU is designed and equipped to care for infants who are ill, born prematurely, or have a condition requiring constant monitoring. A trauma/burn

ICU provides specialized injury and **wound care** for patients involved in auto accidents and patients who have gunshot injuries or burns.

Description

Intensive care unit equipment includes patient monitoring, life support and emergency resuscitation devices, and diagnostic devices.

Patient monitoring equipment

Patient monitoring equipment includes the following:

- Acute care physiologic monitoring system—Comprehensive patient monitoring systems that can be configured to continuously measure and display a number of parameters via electrodes and sensors that are connected to the patient. These may include the electrical activity of the heart via an EKG, respiration rate (breathing), blood pressure, body temperature, cardiac output, and amount of oxygen and carbon dioxide in the blood. Each patient bed in an ICU has a physiologic monitor that measure these body activities. All monitors are networked to a central nurses' station.

- Pulse oximeter—Monitors the arterial hemoglobin oxygen saturation (oxygen level) of the patient's blood with a sensor clipped over the finger or toe.

- Intracranial pressure monitor—Measures the pressure of fluid in the brain in patients with head trauma or other conditions affecting the brain (such as tumors, edema, or hemorrhage). These devices warn of elevated pressure and record or display pressure trends. Intracranial pressure monitoring may be a capability included in a physiologic monitor.

- Apnea monitor—Continuously monitors breathing via electrodes or sensors placed on the patient. An apnea monitor detects cessation of breathing in infants and adults at risk of respiratory failure, displays respiration parameters, and triggers an alarm if a certain amount of time passes without a patient's breath being detected. Apnea monitoring may be a capability included in a physiologic monitor.

Life support and emergency resuscitative equipment

Intensive care equipment for life support and emergency resuscitation includes the following:

- Ventilator (also called a respirator)—Assists with or controls pulmonary ventilation in patients who cannot breathe on their own. Ventilators consist of a flexible breathing circuit, gas supply, heating/ humidification mechanism, monitors, and alarms.

KEY TERMS

Apnea—Cessation of breathing.

Arterial line—A catheter inserted into an artery and connected to a physiologic monitoring system to allow direct measurement of oxygen, carbon dioxide, and invasive blood pressure.

Catheter—A small, flexible tube used to deliver fluids or medications. A catheter may also be used to drain fluid or urine from the body.

Central venous line—A catheter inserted into a vein and connected to a physiologic monitoring system to directly measure venous blood pressure.

Chest tube—A tube inserted into the chest to drain fluid and air from around the lungs.

Critical care—The multidisciplinary health care specialty that provides care to patients with acute, life-threatening illness or injury.

Edema—An abnormal accumulation of fluids in intercellular spaces in the body; causes swelling.

Endotracheal tube—A tube inserted through the patient's nose or mouth that functions as an airway and is connected to the ventilator.

Foley catheter—A catheter inserted into the bladder to drain urine into a bag.

Gastrointestinal tube—A tube surgically inserted into the stomach for feeding a patient unable to eat by mouth.

Heart monitor leads—Sticky pads placed on the chest to monitor the electrical activity of the heart. The pads are connected to an electrocardiogram machine.

Infectious disease team—A team of physicians who help control the hospital environment to protect patients against harmful sources of infection.

Life support—Methods of replacing or supporting a failing bodily function, such as using mechanical ventilation to support breathing. In treatable or curable conditions, life support is used temporarily to aid healing, until the body can resume normal functioning.

Nasogastric tube—A tube inserted through the nose and throat and into the stomach for direct feeding of the patient.

Sepsis—The body's response to infection. Normally, the body's own defense system fights infection, but in severe sepsis, the body "overreacts," causing widespread inflammation and blood clotting in tiny vessels throughout the body.

Swan-Ganz catheter—Also called a pulmonary artery catheter. This type of catheter is inserted into a large vessel in the neck or chest and is used to measure the amount of fluid in the heart and to determine how well the heart is functioning.

Tracheostomy tube—A breathing tube inserted in the neck, used when assisted breathing is needed for a long period of time.

They are microprocessor-controlled and programmable, and regulate the volume, pressure, and flow of patient respiration. Ventilator monitors and alarms may interface with a central monitoring system or information system.

- Infusion pump—Device that delivers fluids intravenously or epidurally through a catheter. Infusion pumps employ automatic, programmable pumping mechanisms to deliver continuous anesthesia, drugs, and blood infusions to the patient. The pump is hung on an intravenous pole placed next to the patient's bed.

- Crash cart—Also called a resuscitation or code cart. This is a portable cart containing emergency resuscitation equipment for patients who are "coding." That is, their vital signs are in a dangerous range. The emergency equipment includes a defibrillator, airway intubation devices, a resuscitation bag/mask, and medication box. Crash carts are strategically located

in the ICU for immediate availability for when a patient experiences cardiorespiratory failure.

- Intraaortic balloon pump—A device that helps reduce the heart's workload and helps blood flow to the coronary arteries for patients with unstable angina, myocardial infarction (heart attack), or patients awaiting organ transplants. Intraaortic balloon pumps use a balloon placed in the patient's aorta. The balloon is on the end of a catheter that is connected to the pump's console, which displays heart rate, pressure, and electrocardiogram (ECG) readings. The patient's ECG is used to time the inflation and deflation of the balloon.

Diagnostic equipment

The use of diagnostic equipment is also required in the ICU. Mobile x-ray units are used for bedside radiography, particularly of the chest. Mobile x-ray units use a battery-operated generator that powers an x-ray tube. Handheld, portable clinical laboratory devices, or point-of-care analyzers, are used for blood analysis at the bedside. A small amount of whole blood is required, and blood chemistry parameters can be provided much faster than if samples were sent to the central laboratory.

Other ICU equipment

Disposable ICU equipment includes urinary (Foley) catheters, catheters used for arterial and central venous lines, Swan-Ganz catheters, chest and endotracheal tubes, gastrointestinal and nasogastric feeding tubes, and monitoring electrodes. Some patients may be wearing a posey vest, also called a Houdini jacket for safety; the purpose is to keep the patient stationary. Spenco boots are padded support devices made of lamb's wool to position the feet and ankles of the patient. Support hose may also be placed on the patient's legs to support the leg muscles and aid circulation.

Operation

The ICU is a demanding environment due to the critical condition of patients and the variety of equipment necessary to support and monitor patients. Therefore, when operating ICU equipment, staff should pay attention to the types of devices and the variations between different models of the same type of device so they do not make an error in operation or adjustment. Although many hospitals make an effort to standardize equipment—for example, using the same manufacturer's infusion pumps or patient monitoring systems, older devices and nonstandardized equipment may still be used, particularly when the ICU is busy. Clinical staff should be sure to check all devices and settings to ensure patient safety.

Intensive care unit patient monitoring systems are equipped with alarms that sound when the patient's **vital signs** deteriorate—for instance, when breathing stops, blood pressure is too high or too low, or when the heart rate is too fast or too slow. Usually, all patient monitors connect to a central nurses' station for easy supervision. Staff at the ICU should ensure that all alarms are functioning properly and that the central station is staffed at all times.

For reusable patient care equipment, clinical staff make certain to properly disinfect and sterilize devices that have contact with patients. Disposable items, such as catheters and needles, should be disposed of in a properly labeled container.

Maintenance

Since ICU equipment is used continuously on critically ill patients, it is essential that equipment be properly maintained, particularly devices that are used for life support and resuscitation. Staff in the ICU should perform daily checks on equipment and inform biomedical engineering staff when equipment needs maintenance, repair, or replacement. For mechanically complex devices, service and preventive maintenance contracts are available from the manufacturer or third-party servicing companies, and should be kept current at all times.

Health care team roles

Equipment in the ICU is used by a team specialized in their use. The team usually comprises a critical care attending physician (also called an intensivist), critical care nurses, an infectious disease team, critical care respiratory therapists, pharmacologists, physical therapists, and dietitians. Physicians trained in other specialties, such as anesthesiology, cardiology, radiology, surgery, neurology, pediatrics, and orthopedics, may be consulted and called to the ICU to treat patients who require their expertise. Radiologic technologists perform mobile x ray examinations (bedside radiography). Either nurses or clinical laboratory personnel perform point-of-care blood analysis. Equipment in the ICU is maintained and repaired by hospital biomedical engineering staff and/or the equipment manufacturer.

Some studies have shown that patients in the ICU following high-risk surgery are at least three times as likely to survive when cared for by "intensivists," physicians trained in critical care medicine.

Training

Manufacturers of more sophisticated ICU equipment, such as ventilators and patient monitoring devices, provide clinical training for all staff involved in ICU treatment when the device is purchased. All ICU staff must have undergone specialized training in the care of critically ill patients and must be trained to respond to life-threatening situations, since ICU patients are in critical condition and may experience respiratory or cardiac emergencies.

Resources

BOOKS

Brenner, Matthew, MD, et al. *Critical Care Medicine*. Mission Viejo, CA: Current Clinical Strategies, 2006.

Marino, Paul, L. and Kenneth M. Sutin. *The ICU Book*, 3rd ed. New York: Lippincott Williams & Wilkins, 2006.

Griffiths, Mark. *Management of Cardiovascular Conditions of Adults in Acute Care*, 1st ed. Malden, MA: Blackwell Publishers, 2008.

Milford, Cheryl, and Gladys Purvis. "Cardiovascular Care." In *Nursing Procedures*, 3rd ed. Springhouse, PA: Springhouse Corporation, 2000.

Skeehan, Thomas, and Michael Jopling. "Monitoring the Cardiac Surgical Patient." In *A Practical Approach to Cardiac Anesthesia*, 3rd edition, edited by Frederick A. Hensley, Donald E. Martin, and Glenn P. Gravlee. Philadelphia, PA: Lippincott Williams & Wilkins, 2003.

Woods, Susan, Erika Sivarajan, Sandra Adams Motzer, and Elizabeth Bridges. *Cardiac Nursing*, 5th ed. Philadelphia: Lippincott, 2004.

PERIODICALS

Brilli, R. J., A. Spevetz, R. D. Branson, et al. "Critical Care Delivery in the Intensive Care Unit: Defining Clinical Roles and the Best Practice Model." *Critical Care Medicine* 29 (October 2001): 2007-2019.

Savino, Joseph S., C. William Hanson III, and Timothy J. Gardner. "Cardiothoracic Intensive Care: Operation and Administration." *Seminars in Thoracic and Cardiovascular Surgery* 12 (October 2000): 362–70.

ORGANIZATIONS

American Association of Critical Care Nurses (ACCN). 101 Columbia, Aliso Viejo, CA 92656-4109. (800) 889-AACN [(800) 889-2226] or (949) 362-2000. http://www.aacn.org.

National Association of Neonatal Nurses. 4700 West Lake Ave., Glenview, IL 60025-1485. (847) 375-3660 or (800) 451-3795. http://www.nann.org.

National Heart, Lung and Blood Institute. Information Center. P.O. Box 30105, Bethesda, MD 20824-0105. (301) 251-2222. http://www.nhlbi.nih.gov.

National Institutes of Health, U.S. Department of Health and Human Services, 9000 Rockville Pike, Bethesda, MD 20892. (301) 496-4000. http://www.nih.gov.

Society of Critical Care Medicine. 701 Lee St., Suite 200, Des Plaines, IL 60016. (847) 827-6869. E-mail: info@sccm.org. http://www.sccm.org.

OTHER

Advanced Cardiac Monitoring: Ventricular Ectopy vs. Aberrancy. Videotape. RamEx, Inc.

ICU Guide. 2002. http://www.waiting.com/waitingicu.html.

ICU-USA, Society of Critical Care Medicine, 2002. http://www.icu-usa.com/tour/.

"Intensive Care Unit (ICU)." 2008. http://www.painchannel.com/icu/index.shtml.

Jennifer E Sisk, MA
Angela M Costello
Laura Jean Cataldo, RN, EdD

Interpositional reconstruction *see* **Arthroplasty**

Intestinal anastomosis *see* **Ileoanal anastomosis**

▌Intestinal obstruction repair

Definition

An intestinal obstruction is a partial or complete blockage of the small or large intestine. Surgery is sometimes necessary to relieve the obstruction.

Purpose

The small intestine is composed of three major sections: the duodenum just below the stomach; the jejunum, or middle portion; and the ileum, which empties into the large intestine. The large intestine is composed of the colon, where stool is formed; and the rectum, which empties to the outside of the body through the anal canal. A blockage that occurs in the small intestine is called a small bowel obstruction, and one that occurs in the colon is a colonic obstruction.

There are numerous conditions that may lead to an intestinal obstruction. The three most common causes of small bowel obstruction are adhesions, which are bands of scar tissue that form in the abdomen following injury or surgery; hernias, which develop when a portion of the intestine protrudes through a weak spot in the abdominal wall; and cancerous tumors. Adhesions account for approximately 50% to 75% of all small bowel obstructions, hernias for about 25%, and tumors for about 5% to 10%. Other causes include volvulus, or formation of kinks or knots in the bowel; the presence of foreign bodies in the digestive tract; intussusception, which occurs when a portion of the intestine telescopes or pulls over another portion; infection; and congenital defects. While most small bowel blockages can be treated with the administration of intravenous (IV) fluids and decompression of the bowel by the insertion of a nasogastric (NG) tube, surgical intervention can be avoided in approximately 65% to 81% of patients with a partial obstruction, while early operation is recommended for all patients with a complete obstruction.

An obstruction of the large intestine is less common than blockages of the small intestine. Blockages of the large bowel are usually caused by colon cancer; volvulus; **diverticulitis** (inflammation of sac-like structures called diverticula that form in the intestines); ischemic colitis (inflammation of the colon resulting from insufficient blood flow); Crohn's disease (a disease that causes chronic inflammation of the intestines); inflammation due to radiation therapy; and the presence of foreign bodies. As in the case of small bowel obstruction, most patients with a blockage of the large intestine can be treated with IV fluids and bowel decompression.

KEY TERMS

Adhesion—A band of fibrous tissue forming an abnormal bond between two adjacent tissues or organs.

Anastomosis (plural, anastomoses)—A surgically created joining or opening between two organs or body spaces that are normally separate.

Congenital defect—A defect present at birth.

Gangrenous—Referring to tissue that is dead.

Intestinal perforation—A hole in the intestinal wall.

Intussusception—The telescoping of one part of the intestine inside an immediately adjoining part.

Lysis—The process of removing adhesions from an organ. The term comes from a Greek word that means "loosening."

Simple obstruction—A blockage in the intestine that does not affect the flow of blood to the area.

Stoma (plural, stomata)—A surgically created opening in the abdominal wall to allow digestive wastes to pass to the outside of the body.

Strangulation obstruction—A blockage in the intestine that closes off the flow of blood to the area.

Volvulus—An intestinal obstruction caused by a knotting or twisting of the bowel.

Demographics

Approximately 300,000 intestinal obstruction repairs are performed in the United States each year. Among patients who are admitted to the hospital for severe abdominal pain, 20% have an intestinal obstruction. While bowel obstruction can affect individuals of any age, different conditions occur at higher rates in certain age groups. Children under the age of two, for example, are more likely to present with intussusceptions or congenital defects. Elderly patients, on the other hand, have a higher rate of colon cancer.

Description

After the patient has been prepared for surgery and given **general anesthesia**, the surgeon usually enters the abdominal cavity by way of a laparotomy, which is a large incision made through the patient's abdominal wall. This type of surgery is sometimes referred to as open surgery. An alternative to laparotomy is **laparoscopy**, a surgical procedure in which a laparoscope (a thin tube with a built-in light source) and other instruments are inserted into the abdomen through small incisions. The internal operating field is then visualized on a video monitor that is connected to the scope. In some patients, the technique may be used for abdominal exploration in place of a laparotomy. Laparoscopy is associated with faster recovery times, shorter hospital stays, and smaller surgical scars, but requires advanced training on the part of the surgeon as well as costly equipment. Moreover, it offers a more limited view of the operating field.

Treating an intestinal obstruction depends on the condition causing the blockage. Some of the more common surgical procedures used to treat bowel obstructions include:

- Lysis of adhesions. The process of removing these bands of scar tissue is called lysis. After the abdominal cavity has been opened, the surgeon locates the obstructed area and delicately dissects the adhesions from the intestine using surgical scissors and forceps.

- Hernia repair. This procedure involves an incision placed near the location of the hernia through which the hernia sac is opened. The herniated intestine is placed back in the abdominal cavity and the muscle wall is repaired.

- Resection with end-to-end anastomosis. "Resection" means to remove part or all of a tissue or structure. Resection of the small or large intestine, therefore, involves the removal of the obstructed or diseased section. Anastomosis is the connection of two cut ends of a tubular structure to form a continuous channel; the anastomosis of the intestine is most often accomplished with sutures or surgical staples.

- Resection with ileostomy or colostomy. In some patients, an anastomosis is not possible because of the extent of the diseased tissue. After the obstruction and diseased tissue is removed, an ileostomy or colostomy is created. Ileostomy is a surgical procedure in which the small intestine is attached to the abdominal wall; waste then exits the body through an artificial opening called a stoma and collects in a bag attached to the skin with adhesive. Colostomy is a similar procedure with the exception that the colon is the part of the digestive tract that is attached to the abdominal wall.

Diagnosis/Preparation

To diagnose an intestinal obstruction, the physician first gives a **physical examination** to determine the severity of the patient's condition. The abdomen is examined for evidence of scars, hernias, distension, or pain. The patient's medical history is also taken, as certain factors increase a person's risk of developing a bowel obstruction (including previous surgery, older age, and a history of constipation). A series of x rays

WHO PERFORMS THE PROCEDURE AND WHERE IS IT PERFORMED?

Ileoanal anastomoses are usually performed in a hospital operating room. Surgery may be performed by a general surgeon or a colorectal surgeon, a medical doctor who focuses on the surgical treatment of diseases of the colon, rectum, and anus.

QUESTIONS TO ASK THE DOCTOR

- Why are you recommending intestinal obstruction repair?
- What diagnostic tests will be performed to determine if an obstruction is present?
- Will an ileostomy or colostomy be created? Will it be temporary or permanent?
- Are any nonsurgical treatments available?
- How soon after surgery may normal diet and activities be resumed?

may be taken of the abdomen, as a definitive diagnosis of obstruction can be made by x ray in 50–60% of patients. Computed tomography (CT; an imaging technique that uses x rays to produce two-dimensional cross-sections on a viewing screen) or ultrasonography (an imaging technique that uses high-frequency sounds waves to visualize structures inside the body) may also be used to diagnosis intestinal obstruction.

Unless a patient presents with symptoms that indicate immediate surgery may be necessary (high fever, severe pain, a rapid heart beat, etc.), a course of IV fluids, NG decompression, and antibiotic therapy is usually prescribed in an effort to avoid surgery.

Aftercare

After surgery, the patient's NG tube remains until bowel function returns. The patient is closely monitored for signs of infection, leakage from an anastomosis, or other complications.

Risks

Complications associated with intestinal obstruction repair include excessive bleeding; infection; formation of abscesses (pockets of pus); leakage of stool from an anastomosis; adhesion formation; paralytic ileus (temporary paralysis of the intestines); and reoccurrence of the obstruction.

Normal results

Most patients who undergo surgical repair of an intestinal obstruction have an uneventful recovery and do not experience a recurrence of the obstruction.

Morbidity and mortality rates

The mortality rate of strangulated small bowel obstruction is 100% in untreated patients. In patients who receive treatment within 6 hours, mortality drops to 8%. If treatment is delayed to over 36 hours, mortality rises again to 25%. Large bowel obstruction

carries a mortality rate of 2% for volvulus to 40% if part of the bowel is gangrenous.

Alternatives

Such nonsurgical techniques as the administration of IV fluids and bowel decompression with a NG tube are often successful in relieving an intestinal obstruction. Patients who present with more severe symptoms that are indicative of a bowel perforation or strangulation, however, require immediate surgery.

Resources

BOOKS

Bitterman, Robert A., and Michael A. Peterson. "Large Intestine." (Chapter 90), in *Rosen's Emergency Medicine*, 5th ed. St. Louis, MO: Mosby, Inc., 2002.

Evers, B. Mark. "Small Bowel." (Chapter 44), in *Sabiston Textbook of Surgery*. Philadelphia, PA: W. B. Saunders Company, 2001.

"Mechanical Intestinal Obstruction." Section 3, Chapter 25 in *The Merck Manual of Diagnosis and Therapy*, edited by Mark H. Beers, MD, and Robert Berkow, MD. Whitehouse Station, NJ: Merck Research Laboratories, 1999.

Torrey, Susan P., and Philip L. Henneman. "Small Intestine." (Chapter 87), in *Rosen's Emergency Medicine*, 5th ed. St. Louis, MO: Mosby, Inc., 2002.

PERIODICALS

Basson, Marc D. "Colonic Obstruction." eMedicine, September 26, 2001 [cited May 2, 2003]. http://www.emedicine.com/med/topic415.htm.

Khan, Ali Nawaz, and John Howat. "Small-Bowel Obstruction." eMedicine, April 18, 2003 [cited May 2, 2003]. http://www.emedicine.com/radio/topic781.htm.

ORGANIZATIONS

American Society of Colon and Rectal Surgeons. 85 W. Algonquin Rd., Suite 550, Arlington Heights, IL 60005. (847) 290-9184. www.fascrs.org.

United Ostomy Association, Inc. 19772 MacArthur Blvd., Suite 200, Irvine, CA 92612-2405. (800) 826-0826. www.uoa.org.

Stephanie Dionne Sherk

Intra-Operative Parathyroid Hormone Measurement

Definition

Intra-Operative Parathyroid Hormone (IOPTH) Measurement is a method of monitoring the blood for levels of parathyroid hormone (PTH) during surgery to remove abnormal parathyroid glands (**parathyroidectomy**). The blood level of PTH drops after the abnormal parathyroid glands are removed, and indicates to the surgeon that the diseased glands have all been found.

Demographic

IOPTH measurement can be done on any patient having a parathyroidectomy. This procedure is done because of one or more abnormal parathyroid glands. The surgical procedure and IOPTH measurement are usually performed on patients with parathyroid adenomas (benign tumors). Parathyroid cancer is considered extremely rare, and adenomas make up most of the demographic for IOPTH measurement during parathyroidectomy.

Description

IOPTH is measured to monitor the activity of hyperfunctional parathyroid glands during a parathyroidectomy. IOPTH measurement helps surgeons determine whether they have removed all pathological tissue (abnormal parathyroid glands).

Calcium and the Parathyroid Glands

The regulation of calcium is an important aspect of our physiology because it has significant impact on many body systems. Calcium is necessary for nervous system function. It is responsible for the electrical impulses that travel along our nerve endings. Calcium is also critical for muscle contraction, including the heart muscle. Additionally calcium stored in the bones increases their strength. Calcium levels are very tightly regulated in the body, because too much or too little may have a serious impact on health. For this reason calcium is the only mineral present in our bodies that

has its own set of glands to regulate blood levels called the parathyroid glands.

The parathyroid glands are located in the neck area usually behind or within the thyroid gland. There are usually four glands located in parallel pairs around the superior and inferior portion of the trachea. There may be up to six glands in an individual, but this is unusual and only one is necessary to maintain body physiology. The glands are tiny, usually between the size of a grain of rice and a pea. Parathyroid glands are part of the body's endocrine system, and release hormones necessary for modulation of calcium in normal physiological functioning. The sole function of the parathyroid glands is to keep calcium levels within a narrow, safe, and functional range in the blood. The parathyroid glands monitor present levels of blood calcium and use PTH to increase or decrease levels as necessary throughout the day. PTH impacts the release of calcium from the bones and the absorption of calcium back into the bones to modulate the blood level.

Normal Parathyroid Function

A normal blood calcium level is 8.4 to 10.2 mg/dl. Blood calcium levels are always kept in this narrow range by PTH. The parathyroid gland releases PTH in response to low blood calcium. Accordingly, PTH release is decreased in response to high blood calcium. PTH travels to the skeletal system and causes the release of calcium from bone, to supply the muscles and nervous system. PTH also travels to the intestine, where it influences the absorption of calcium from ingested food. A normal blood PTH level ranges from 14 to 65 pg/ml.

Abnormal Parathyroid Function

One form of abnormal parathyroid function is hyperparathyroidism. In this disorder, one or more of the parathyroid glands secretes too much PTH despite high blood calcium levels. The normal regulatory mechanisms have lost control, and calcium levels fluctuate wildly. The most common cause of hyperparathyroidism is a parathyroid adenoma. An adenoma is a benign tumor and is not cancerous. It is merely a group of cells that grows and behaves without the normal regulatory control mechanisms. Parathyroid adenomas may grow to the size of a walnut. With some parathyroid adenomas, blood levels may exceed 200 pg/ml, while others may be present with blood PTH still within the normal range. While hyperparathyroidism may present with levels of PTH within the normal range, the diseased glands do not down regulate their activity even when blood calcium levels are high. Hyperparathyroidism causes a variety of medical problems such as damage to the kidneys, liver, and skeletal system. Patients may develop kidney stones, osteoporosis, high blood pressure, depression, difficulty sleeping, fatigue, and irritability. The heart rhythm is also affected, and heart complications such as arrhythmias may ensue.

IOPTH Measurement and Scanning for Pathology

Parathyroid glands can be very difficult to locate. Approximately 85% of parathyroid glands are found behind the thyroid gland, but they can be located anywhere between the jaw and the chest (very rarely). Their variation in size, number, and location make them very difficult for surgeons to find for parathyroidectomy, with more experienced surgeons having a higher success rate. The preferred way to scan for a parathyroid adenoma is through a **sestamibi scan**. A sestamibi scan is a type of radioimaging used to visualize certain types of abnormal cells in the body. One of the uses for a sestamibi scan is identification of a parathyroid adenoma. Sestamibi scans identify overactive parathyroid glands rather than larger sized ones. Pre-operative identification of the abnormal gland allows for a less invasive surgical procedure than an exploratory one would have been.

While sestamibi scanning is an important part of finding the location of abnormal parathyroid glands that need parathyroidectomy, it is often coupled with IOPTH measurement for confirmation that no glands were missed during the procedure. IOPTH measurement is done during surgery because parathyroid adenomas release excessive amounts of PTH. The half-life (amount of time is takes for half the present hormone to be metabolized or excreted) of PTH is less than 5 minutes. Because it takes so little time for the hormone to be metabolized, when the original source of the PTH is taken away, the remaining PTH takes very little time to drop off. When an abnormal adenoma is removed during a parathyroidectomy, a drop in PTH is observed in 10 to 15 minutes. If the PTH does drop off, it is likely that the surgeon removed all the abnormal parathyroid tissue. If the PTH level does not drop off into the expected range, then there is an additional abnormal parathyroid gland present in the body. If an additional abnormal gland was missed during the sestamibi scan, the IOPTH measurement has identified the mistake. More invasive types of surgery may be necessary to find the remaining abnormal tissue. Since parathyroid adenomas are often singular, IOPTH measurement often prevents unnecessary exploratory surgical procedures. IOPTH measurement may be done until all the abnormal glands are found and removed.

How IOPTH Measurement is Performed

IOPTH measurement is done from blood drawn during the surgical procedure, and sent it to the hospital's lab for quick analysis. A response from the lab is called into the **operating room** in a timely manner, while the surgery is ongoing. The blood samples required for IOPTH assays are usually taken from an indwelling intravenous catheter. The concentration of PTH is relatively constant in most peripheral veins. Which vein the blood is drawn from does not matter, as long as the same location is used for all the blood draws. After the anesthesia is administered, the blood is tested for a baseline value of PTH to use as comparison to PTH levels after the abnormal tissue is removed. Additional blood samples are taken at 5,10, and 15 minutes post-removal. A decrease of greater than or equal to 50% of baseline within 10 to 15 minutes after removal is usually indicative of successful removal of the abnormal tissue.

IOPTH Measurement for Predicting Post-operative Hypoparathyroidism

IOPTH is also a useful tool in predicting the occurrence of symptomatic hypocalcemia following parathyroidectomy. In chronic hyperparathyroidism the normal parathyroid glands become inactive over time in response to the high levels of calcium in the blood caused by excretion of excessive of PTH from the parathyroid adenoma. When the parathyroid adenoma is removed, the remaining healthy glands do not immediately return to normal function and secretion of PTH. Because the abnormal hormone-secreting parathyroid gland has been removed and the remaining normal glands are relatively inactive, many patients experience

Intra-Operative Parathyroid Hormone Measurement

a temporary state of blood calcium deficiency. Having a level of calcium in the blood that is too low is called hypocalcemia. If the levels are low enough, it can cause medically adverse effects.

To predict whether a patient will have post-operative symptomatic hypocalcemia, an IOPTH measurement is done following skin closure at the end of the surgical procedure. Studies have shown that a post-operative PTH level less than 10 pg/ml is predictive of symptomatic hypocalcemia. Patients with PTH levels this low are immediately given calcium and vitamin D supplementation. This supplementation is continued until the normal parathyroid glands return to full function. Measuring blood calcium levels after parathyroidectomy may also correlate with symptomatic hypocalcemia. However, the high levels of calcium that may be present from the excised parathyroid adenoma take longer to decrease than the PTH. Blood calcium measurement is usually not useful until 12 to 24 hours after surgery, and such a delay in calcium therapy may be detrimental. IOPTH is an effective predictive tool that has provided the necessary information before the patient leaves the operating room.

Risks Associated with IOPTH Measurement

There is very little risk associated with having blood drawn for an IOPTH measurement. Most people have no side effects from a blood draw, or a small bruise. However, with any blood draw there is a small chance that the area around the punctured vein may develop phlebitis, the inflammation of a vein. Phlebitis may also involve a bacterial infection if the site of the blood draw was not appropriately cleaned before the needle was inserted. Phlebitis can be locally painful but usually resolves in a short period of time. Additionally, patients with disorders involving the inability of the blood to form normal blood clots should discuss their condition and their medications with the physician before the procedure is done.

Resources

BOOKS

Cecil Essentials of Medicine, Sixth Edition. Saunders, Elsevier 2004.

Chaundhry H., et al. *Fundamentals of Clincal Medicine.* Lippincott Williams & Wilkins 2004.

Costanzo, Linda S. *Physiology,* Third Edition. Elsevier Health Sciences, 2006.

Harrison's Principles of Internal Medicine, Sixteenth Edition. McGraw-Hill, 2005.

Kumar, Vinay, Nelson Fausto, and Abul Abbas. *Robbins & Cotran: Pathologic Basis of Disease,* Seventh Edition. Saunders, Elsevier, 2005.

Le T., et al. *First Aid for the Wards.* McGraw-Hill, 2003.

Maxwell Quick Medical Reference, Fourth Edition. Maxwell Publishing Company 2002.

PERIODICALS

Bergson, Eric J., Laura A. Sznyter, Sanford Dubner, Christopher J. Palestro, and Keith S. Heller. "Sestamibi Scans and Intraoperative Parathyroid Hormone Measurement in the Treatment of Primary Hyperparathyroidism." *Arch Otolaryngol Head Neck Surg.* 2004;130:87-91.

Yen, Tina W. F., Stuart D. Wilson, Elizabeth A. Krzywda, and Sonia L. Sugg. "The role of parathyroid hormone measurements after surgery for primary hyperparathyroidism." *Surgery* 2006;140:665-74.

ORGANIZATIONS

American Academy of Otolaryngology—Head and Neck Surgery, One Prince Street, Alexandria, Virginia, 22314-3357, (703)836-4444, http://www.entnet.org/contactus.cfm.

American Association of Endocrine Surgeons, 3550 Terrace Street, Pittsburgh, Pennsylvania, 15261, (412)647-0467, (412)648-9551, http://www.endocrinesurgery.org/contact/contact.html.

Maria Basile, PhD

Intracranial aneurysm repair *see* **Cerebral aneurysm repair**

Intravenous rehydration

Definition

Intravenous (IV) rehydration is a treatment for fluid loss in which a sterile water solution containing small amounts of salt or sugar is injected into the patient's bloodstream.

Purpose

Rehydration is usually performed to treat the symptoms associated with dehydration, or excessive loss of body water. Fever, vomiting, and diarrhea can cause a person to become dehydrated fairly quickly. Infants and children are especially vulnerable to dehydration. Patients can become dehydrated due to an illness, surgery, metabolic disorder, hot weather, or accident. Athletes who have overexerted themselves may also require rehydration with IV fluids. An IV for rehydration can be used for several hours to several days, and is generally used if a patient is unable to keep down oral fluids due to excessive vomiting.

Description

A basic IV rehydration solution consists of sterile water with small amounts of sodium chloride (NaCl; salt) and/or dextrose (sugar) added. It is supplied in bottles or thick plastic bags that can hang on a pole or rolling stand mounted next to a patient's bed. Additional electrolytes (i.e., potassium, calcium, bicarbonate, phosphate, magnesium, chloride), vitamins, or drugs can be added as needed either in a separate minibag or via an injection into the intravenous line.

Diagnosis/Preparation

Signs and symptoms of dehydration include:

- extreme thirst
- sunken eyes
- reduced urine output; urine that is dark in color
- weakness and fatigue
- rapid weight loss
- dry, warm skin
- skin that is wrinkled or has little elasticity
- rapid pulse
- dry mouth
- "tearless" crying
- muscle cramps
- headache

In infants, dehydration may also be indicated by a sunken fontanelle (the soft spot on the head).

A doctor orders the IV solution and any additional nutrients or drugs to be added to it. The doctor also specifies the rate at which the IV will be infused. The intravenous solutions are prepared under the supervision of a pharmacist using sanitary techniques that prevent bacterial contamination. Just like a prescription, the IV is clearly labeled to show its contents and the amounts of any additives. A nurse will examine the patient's arm to find a suitable vein for insertion of the intravenous line. Once the vein is located, the skin around the area is cleaned and disinfected. The needle is inserted and is taped to the skin to prevent it from moving out of the vein.

Patients receiving IV therapy must be monitored to ensure that the IV solutions are providing the correct amounts of fluids and minerals needed. People with kidney and heart disease are at increased risk for overhydration, so they must be carefully monitored when receiving IV therapy.

Aftercare

Patients must be able to take (and keep down) fluids by mouth before an IV rehydration solution is discontinued. After the needle is removed, the insertion site should be inspected for any signs of bleeding or infection.

Risks

As with any invasive procedure, there is a small risk of infection or bruising at the injection site. It is possible that the IV solution may not provide all of the nutrients needed, leading to a deficiency or an imbalance. If the needle becomes dislodged, the solution may flow into tissues around the injection site rather than into the vein, resulting in swelling.

Morbidity and mortality rates

According to the United Nations Children's Fund (UNICEF), over two million children die of diarrhea-related dehydration each year. Eighty percent of these children were two years of age or younger. In the United States, an estimated 300 people (children and adults) die of dehydration annually.

Alternatives

For patients who are able to tolerate fluids by mouth, oral rehydration therapy (ORT) with oral rehydration salts (ORS) in solution is the preferred treatment alternative. Another technique in which fluid replacement is injected subcutaneously (under the skin into tissues) rather than into a vein is called hypodermoclysis. Hypodermoclysis is easier to administer than IV therapy, especially in the home setting. It may be used to treat mild to moderate dehydration in patients who are unable to take in adequate fluids by mouth and who prefer to be treated at home (geriatric or terminally ill patients).

Resources

BOOKS

Cheever, Kerry. *I.V. Therapy Demystified*, 1st ed. New York: McGraw-Hill Professional, 2007.

Fulcher, Eugenia, M. *Intravenous Therapy: A Guide to Basic Principles*, 1st ed. St Louis, MO: Saunders, 2005.

Hankins, Judy, et al., eds. *Infusion Therapy in Clinical Practice*, 2nd ed. Philadelphia, PA: WB Saunders, 2001.

Otto, Shirlie. *Mosby's Pocket Guide to Intravenous Therapy*, 5th ed. St. Louis, MO: Mosby Inc., 2004.

Weinstein, Sharon, M. *Plumer's Principles and Practice of Intravenous Therapy*, 8th ed. New York: Lippincott Williams & Wilkins, 2006.

PERIODICALS

Suhayda, Rosemarie, and Jane C. Walton. "Preventing and Managing Dehydration." *MedSurg Nursing* 11 (December 2002): 267-78.

ORGANIZATIONS

Infusion Nurses Society. 315 Norwood Park South, Norwood, MA 02062. (781) 440.9408. http://www.ins1.org.

League Of Intravenous Therapy Education. Empire Building, Suite 3, 3001 Jacks Run Road. White Oak, PA 15131. (412) 678-5025. http://www.lite.org/.

OTHER

Rehydration Project. P. O. Box 1, Samara, 5235, Costa Rica. (506) 656-0504. www.rehydrate.org.

Altha Roberts Edgren
Paula Ford-Martin
Laura Jean Cataldo, RN, EdD

Intussusception reduction

Definition

Intussusception is a condition in which one portion of the intestine "telescopes" into or folds itself inside another portion. The term comes from two Latin words, *intus*, which means "inside" and *suscipere*, which means "to receive." The outer "receiving" portion of an intussusception is called the intussuscipiens; the part that has been received inside the intussuscipiens is called the intussusceptum. The result of an intussusception is that the bowel is obstructed and its blood supply gradually cut off. Surgery is sometimes necessary to relieve the obstruction.

Purpose

The purpose of an intussusception reduction is to prevent gangrene of the bowel, which may lead to perforation of the bowel, severe infection, and **death**.

Intussusception reduction

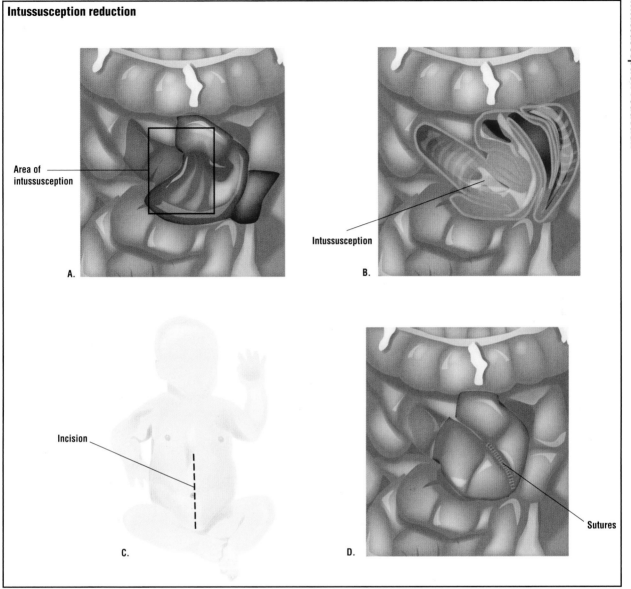

A.

B.

Incision

C.

Sutures

D.

Intussusception of the bowel results in the bowel telescoping onto itself (A and B). An incision is made in the baby's abdomen to expose the bowel (C). If the surgeon cannot manipulate the bowel into a normal shape manually, the area of intussusception wil be removed and remaining bowel sutured together (D). *(Illustration by GGS Information Services. Cengage Learning, Gale.)*

The cause of intussusception is idiopathic in most children diagnosed with the condition (88–99%). Idiopathic means that the condition has developed spontaneously or that the cause is unknown. In the remaining 1–12% of child patients, certain conditions called lead points have been associated with intussusception. These lead points include cystic fibrosis; recent upper respiratory or gastrointestinal illness; congenital abnormalities of the digestive tract; benign or malignant tumors; chemotherapy; or the presence of foreign bodies.

In contrast to children, there is a lead point in 90% of adults diagnosed with intussusception.

Demographics

About 95% of all cases of intussusception occur in children. Children under two years of age are most likely to be affected by the condition; the average age at diagnosis is seven to eight months. Among children, the rate of intussusception is one to four per 1,000. Conversely, only two to three adults out of every

KEY TERMS

Adhesion—A fibrous band of tissue that forms an abnormal connection between two adjacent organs or other structures.

Anastomosis—The connection of separate parts of a body organ or an organ system.

Benign tumor—A noncancerous growth that does not have the potential to spread to other parts of the body.

Congenital—Present at birth.

Gangrene—The death of a considerable mass of tissue, usually associated with loss of blood supply and followed by bacterial infection.

Idiopathic—Having an unknown cause or arising spontaneously. Most cases of intussusception in children are idiopathic.

Lead point—A well-defined abnormality in the area where the intussusception begins.

Malignant tumor—A cancerous growth that has the potential to spread to other parts of the body.

Stoma (plural, stomata)—A surgically created opening in the abdominal wall to allow digestive wastes to pass to the outside of the body.

Strangulation—A condition in which the blood circulation in a part of the body is shut down by pressure. Intussusception can lead to strangulation of a part of the intestine.

1,000,000 are diagnosed with intussusception each year. Intussusception is more likely to affect males than females in all age groups. Among children, the male to female ratio is three to two; in persons over the age of four, the male to female ratio is eight to one.

As of 2003, racial or ethnic differences do not appear to affect the occurrence of intussusception.

Description

Surgical correction of an intussusception is done with the patient under **general anesthesia**. The surgeon usually enters the abdominal cavity by way of a laparotomy, a large incision made through the abdominal wall. The intestines are examined until the intussusception is identified and brought through the incision for closer examination. The surgeon first attempts to reduce the intussusception by "milking" or applying gentle pressure to ease the intussusceptum out of the intussuscipiens; this technique is called

manual reduction. If manual reduction is not successful, the surgeon may perform a resection of the intussusception. Resect means to remove part or all of a tissue or structure; resection of the intussusception, therefore, involves the removal of the area of the intestine that has prolapsed. The two cut ends of the intestine may then be reconnected with sutures or surgical **staples**; this reconnection is called an end-to-end anastomosis.

More rarely, the segment of bowel that is removed is too large to accommodate an end-to-end anastomosis. These patients may require a temporary or permanent enterostomy. In this procedure, the surgeon creates an artificial opening in the abdomen wall called a stoma, and attaches the intestine to it. Waste then exits the body through the stoma and empties into a collection bag.

An alternative to the traditional abdominal incision is **laparoscopy**, a surgical procedure in which a laparoscope (a thin, lighted tube) and other instruments are inserted into the abdomen through small incisions. The internal operating field is then visualized on a video monitor that is connected to the scope. In some patients, the surgeon may perform a laparoscopy for abdominal exploration in place of a laparotomy. Laparoscopy is associated with speedier recoveries shorter hospital stays, and smaller surgical scars; on the other hand, however, it requires costly equipment and advanced training on the surgeon's part. In addition, it offers a relatively limited view of the operating field.

Diagnosis/Preparation

The diagnosis of intussusception is usually made after a complete **physical examination**, medical history, and series of imaging studies. In children, the pediatrician may suspect the diagnosis on the basis of such symptoms as abdominal pain, fever, vomiting, and "currant jelly" stools, which consist of blood-streaked mucus and pieces of the tissue that lines the intestine. When the doctor palpates (feels) the child's abdomen, he or she will typically find a sausage-shaped mass in the right lower quadrant of the abdomen. Diagnosis of intussusception in adults, however, is much more difficult, partly because the disorder is relatively rare in the adult population.

X rays may be taken of the abdomen with the patient lying down or sitting upright. Ultrasonography (an imaging technique that uses high-frequency sounds waves to visualize structures inside the body) and computed tomography (an imaging technique that uses x rays to produce two-dimensional cross-

WHO PERFORMS THE PROCEDURE AND WHERE IS IT PERFORMED?

Intussusception reduction is usually performed in a hospital operating room under general anesthesia. The operation may be performed by a general surgeon, a pediatric surgeon (in the case of pediatric intussusception), or a colorectal surgeon (a medical doctor who focuses on the surgical treatment of diseases of the colon, rectum, and anus).

QUESTIONS TO ASK THE DOCTOR

- What diagnostic tests will be needed to confirm the presence of an intussusception?
- Is there a lead point in this case?
- Can the intussusception be treated successfully without surgery?
- If resection becomes necessary, will an enterostomy be performed?
- How soon after surgery may normal diet and activities be resumed?

sections on a viewing screen) are also used to diagnose intussusception. A contrast enema is a diagnostic tool that has the potential to reduce the intussusception; during this procedure, x-ray photographs are taken of the intestines after a contrast material such as barium or air is introduced through the anus.

Children diagnosed with intussusception are started on intravenous (IV) fluids and nasogastric decompression (in which a flexible tube is inserted through the nose down to the stomach) in an effort to avoid surgery. An enema may also be given to the patient, as 40–90% of cases are successfully treated by this method. If these noninvasive treatments fail, surgery becomes necessary to relieve the obstruction.

There is some controversy among doctors about the usefulness of barium enemas in reducing intussusceptions in adults. In general, enemas are less successful in adults than in children, and surgical treatment should not be delayed.

Aftercare

After surgical treatment of an intussusception, the patient is given fluids intravenously until bowel function returns; he or she may then be allowed to resume a normal diet. Follow-up care may be indicated if the intussusception occurred as a result of a specific condition (e.g., cancerous tumors).

Risks

Complications associated with intussusception reduction include reactions to general anesthesia; perforation of the bowel; wound infection; urinary tract infection; excessive bleeding; and formation of adhesions (bands of scar tissue that form after surgery or injury to the abdomen).

Normal results

If intussusception is treated in a timely manner, most patients are expected to recover fully, retain normal bowel function, and have only a small chance of recurrence. The mortality rate is lowest among patients who are treated within the first 24 hours.

Morbidity and mortality rates

Intussusception recurs in approximately 1–4% of patients after surgery, compared to 5–10% after nonsurgical reduction. Adhesions form in up to 7% of patients who undergo surgical reduction. The rate of intussusception-related deaths in Western countries is less than 1%.

Alternatives

Such nonsurgical techniques as the administration of IV fluids, bowel decompression with a nasogastric tube, or a therapeutic enema are often successful in reducing intussusception. Patients whose symptoms point to bowel perforation or strangulation, however, require immediate surgery. If left untreated, gangrene of the bowel is almost always fatal.

Resources

BOOKS

"Congenital Anomalies: Gastrointestinal Defects." Section 19, Chapter 261 in *The Merck Manual of Diagnosis and Therapy*, edited by Mark H. Beers, MD, and Robert Berkow, MD. Whitehouse Station, NJ: Merck Research Laboratories, 1999.

Engum, Scott A., and Jay L. Grosfeld. "Pediatric Surgery: Intussusception." Chapter 67 in *Sabiston Textbook of Surgery*. Philadelphia: W. B. Saunders Company, 2001.

Wyllie, Robert. "Ileus, Adhesions, Intussusception, and Closed-Loop Obstructions." Chapter 333 in *Nelson*

Textbook of Pediatrics, 16th ed. Philadelphia, PA: W. B. Saunders Company, 2000.

PERIODICALS

Chahine, A. Alfred, MD. "Intussusception." *eMedicine*, April 4, 2002 [cited May 4, 2003]. www.emedicine.com/PED/topic1208.htm.

Irish, Michael, MD. "Intussusception: Surgical Perspective." *eMedicine*, April 29, 2003 [cited May 4, 2003]. www.emedicine.com/PED/topic2972.htm.

Waseem, Muhammad and Orlando Perales. "Diagnosis: Intussusception." *Pediatrics in Review* 22, no. 4 (April 1, 2001): 135-140.

ORGANIZATIONS

American Academy of Family Physicians. PO Box 11210, Shawnee Mission, KS 66207. (800) 274-2237. www.aafp.org.

American Academy of Pediatrics. 141 Northwest Point Blvd., Elk Grove Village, IL 60007-1098. (847) 434-4000. www.aap.org.

American College of Radiology. 1891 Preston White Dr., Reston, VA 20191-4397. (800) 227-5463. www.acr.org.

Stephanie Dionne Sherk

Iridectomy

Definition

An iridectomy is an eye surgery procedure in which the surgeon removes a small full-thickness piece of the iris, which is the colored circular membrane behind the cornea of the eye. An iridectomy is also known as a corectomy. In recent years, lasers have also been used to perform iridectomies.

Purpose

Today, an iridectomy is most often performed to treat closed-angle glaucoma or melanoma of the iris. An iridectomy performed to treat glaucoma is sometimes called a peripheral iridectomy, because it removes a portion of the periphery or root of the iris.

In some cases, an iridectomy is performed prior to cataract surgery in order to make it easier to remove the lens of the eye. This procedure is referred to as a preparatory iridectomy.

Closed-angle glaucoma

Closed-angle glaucoma is a condition in which fluid pressure builds up inside the eye because the fluid, or aqueous humor, that is produced in the anterior chamber at the front of the eye cannot leave the chamber through

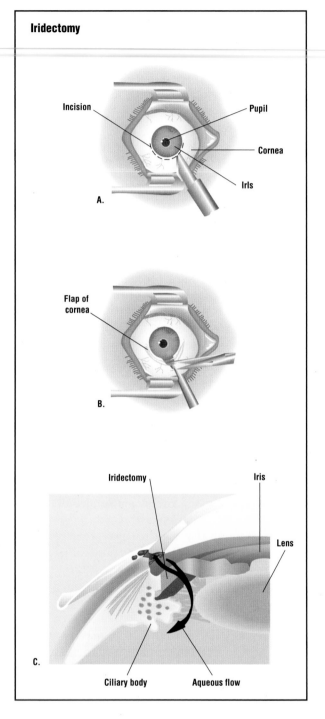

Iridectomy

For an iridectomy, an incision is made in the cornea just below the iris (A). A piece of the iris is removed (B). This allows fluid to flow between the areas to the front and rear of the iris (C). *(Illustration by GGS Information Services. Cengage Learning, Gale.)*

the usual opening. This opening lies at the angle where the iris meets the cornea, which is the clear front portion of the exterior cover of the eye. In closed-angle glaucoma, the fluid is blocked because a part of the iris has

Angle—The open point in the anterior chamber of the eye at which the iris meets the cornea. Blockage of the angle prevents fluid from leaving the anterior chamber, resulting in closed-angle glaucoma.

Aqueous humor—The watery fluid produced in the eye that ordinarily leaves the eye through the angle of the anterior chamber.

Corectomy—Another term for iridectomy.

Cornea—The transparent front portion of the exterior cover of the eye.

Enucleation—Surgical removal of the eyeball.

Glaucoma—A group of eye disorders characterized by increased fluid pressure inside the eye that eventually damages the optic nerve. As the cells in the optic nerve die, the patient gradually loses vision.

Gonioscopy—A technique for examining the angle between the iris and the cornea with the use of a special mirrored lens applied to the cornea.

Iridotomy—A procedure in which a laser is used to make a small hole in the iris to relieve fluid pressure in the eye.

Iris (plural, irides)—The circular pigmented membrane behind the cornea of the eye that gives the eye its color. The iris surrounds a central opening called the pupil.

Ocular melanoma—A malignant tumor that arises within the structures of the eye. It is the most common eye tumor in adults.

Ophthalmology—The branch of medicine that deals with the diagnosis and treatment of eye disorders.

Pupil—The opening in the center of the iris of the eye that allows light to enter the eye.

Tonometry—Measurement of the fluid pressure inside the eye.

Tunica (plural, tunicae)—The medical term for a membrane or piece of tissue that covers or lines a body part. The eyeball is surrounded by three tunicae.

Uvea—The middle of the three tunicae surrounding the eye, comprising the choroid, iris, and ciliary body. The uvea is pigmented and well supplied with blood vessels.

Uveitis—Inflammation of any part of the uvea.

Vitrectomy—Surgical removal of the vitreous body.

Vitreous body—The transparent gel that fills the inner portion of the eyeball between the lens and the retina. It is also called the vitreous humor or crystalline humor.

moved forward and closed off the angle. As a result, fluid pressure in the eye rises rapidly, which can damage the optic nerve and lead to blindness. About 10% of all cases of glaucoma reported in the United States is closed-angle. This type of glaucoma is also called angle-closure glaucoma, acute congestive glaucoma, narrow-angle glaucoma, and pupillary block glaucoma. It usually develops in only one eye at a time.

There are two major types of closed-angle glaucoma: primary and secondary. Primary closed-angle glaucoma most commonly results from pupillary block, in which the iris closes off the angle when the pupil of the eye becomes dilated. In some cases, the blockage happens only occasionally, as when the pupil dilates in dim light, in situations of high stress or anxiety, or in response to the drops instilled by a doctor during an eye examination. This condition is referred to as intermittent, subacute, or chronic open-angle glaucoma. In other cases, the blockage is abrupt and complete, leading to an attack of acute closed-angle glaucoma. In primary glaucoma, the difference between the chronic or intermittent forms and an acute attack is usually due to small variations in the anatomical structure of the eye. These include an unusually shallow anterior chamber; a lens that is thicker than average and situated further forward in the eye; or a cornea that is smaller in diameter than average. Any of these differences can narrow the angle between the iris and the cornea, which is about 45° in the normal eye. In addition, as people age, the lens tends to grow larger and thicker; this change may cause fluid pressure to build up behind the iris. Eventually, pressure from the aqueous humor may force the iris forward, blocking the drainage angle.

Secondary closed-angle glaucoma results from changes in the angle caused by disorders, medications, trauma, or surgery, rather than by the anatomy of the eye itself. In some cases, the iris is pulled up into the angle by scar tissue resulting from the abnormal formation of blood vessels in diabetes. Another common cause of secondary closed-angle glaucoma is uveitis, or inflammation of the uvea, which is the covering of the eye that includes the iris. Cases have been reported in which uveitis related to HIV infection has led to closed-angle glaucoma. Melanoma of the iris has also been associated with closed-angle glaucoma.

Any medication that causes the pupil of the eye to dilate, including antihistamines and over-the-counter cold preparations, may cause an acute attack of closed-angle glaucoma. Medications that are given to treat anxiety and depression, particularly the tricyclic antidepressants and the selective serotonin reuptake inhibitors (SSRIs), may trigger the onset of closed-angle glaucoma in some patients. In other instances, anesthesia for procedures on other parts of the body may produce an acute attack of closed-angle glaucoma.

In terms of trauma, a direct blow to the eye can dislocate the lens, bringing it forward and blocking the angle; overly vigorous **exercise** may have the same effect. Lastly, certain types of eye surgery performed to treat other conditions may result in secondary closed-angle glaucoma. These procedures include implantation of an intraocular lens; cataract surgery; **scleral buckling** to treat retinal detachment; and injection of silicone oil to replace the vitreous body in front of the retina following a vitrectomy.

Melanoma of the iris

Melanoma of the iris is a malignant tumor that develops within the pigmented cells of the iris; it is not a cancer that has developed elsewhere in the body and then spread to the eye. Melanoma of the iris can, however, enlarge and gradually destroy the patient's vision. If left untreated, it can also metastasize or spread to other organs—most commonly the liver—and eventually cause **death**.

Demographics

Closed-angle glaucoma affects between 350,000 and 400,000 people in the United States; in some Asian countries such as China, however, it is more common than open-angle glaucoma.

Risk factors for closed-angle glaucoma include:

- a family history of this type of glaucoma
- farsightedness
- small eyes
- age over 40
- scarring inside the eye from diabetes or uveitis
- a cataract in the lens that is growing
- Inuit or Asian heritage (Inuits have the highest rate of closed-angle glaucoma of any ethnic group.)

Melanoma of the iris is a relatively rare form of cancer, representing only about 10% of cases of intraocular melanoma. The American Cancer Society estimates that about 220 cases of melanoma of the iris are diagnosed in the United States each year. People over 50 are the most likely to develop this form of cancer, although it can occur at any age. It appears to affect men and women equally. Melanoma of the iris is more common in Caucasians and in people with light-colored irides than in people of Asian or African descent. Suspected causes include genetic mutations and exposure to sunlight.

Description

Laser iridotomy/iridectomy

A person who is at risk for an acute episode of closed-angle glaucoma or who has already had emergency medical treatment for an attack may be treated with a **laser iridotomy** to reduce the level of fluid pressure in the affected eye. The drawback of a laser iridotomy in treating closed-angle glaucoma is that the hole may not remain open, requiring repeated iridotomies, a laser iridectomy, or a surgical iridectomy. In addition, laser iridotomies have a higher rate of success when used preventively rather than after the patient has already had an acute attack.

To perform a laser iridotomy, the ophthalmologist uses a laser, usually an argon or an Nd:YAG laser, to burn a small hole into the iris to relieve fluid pressure behind the iris. If the procedure is an iridectomy, the laser is used to remove a full-thickness section of the iris. The patient sits in a special chair with his or her chin resting on a frame or support to prevent the head from moving. The ophthalmologist numbs the eye with anesthetic eye drops. After the anesthetic has taken effect, the doctor shines the laser beam into the affected eye. The entire procedure takes 10–30 minutes.

Conventional (surgical) iridectomy

Melanoma of the iris is usually treated by surgical iridectomy to prevent the tumor from causing secondary closed-angle glaucoma and from spreading to other parts of the body.

A surgical iridectomy is a more invasive procedure that requires an **operating room**. The patient lies on an operating table with a piece of sterile cloth placed around the eye. The procedure is usually done under **general anesthesia**. The surgeon uses a microscope and special miniature instruments to make an incision in the cornea and remove a section of the iris, usually at the 12 o'clock position. The incision in the cornea is self-sealing.

Diagnosis/Preparation

Closed-angle glaucoma

Closed-angle glaucoma may be diagnosed in the course of a routine eye examination or during emergency treatment for symptoms of an acute attack. A doctor who is performing a standard eye examination may notice that the patient's eye has a shallow anterior chamber or a narrow angle between the iris and the cornea. He or she may perform one or both of the following tests to evaluate the patient's risk of developing closed-angle glaucoma. One test, called tonometry, measures the amount of fluid pressure in the eye. It is a painless procedure that involves blowing a puff of pressurized air toward the patient's eye as the patient sits near a lamp and measuring the changes in the light reflections on the patient's corneas. Other methods of tonometry involve the application of a local anesthetic to the outside of the eye and touching the cornea briefly with an instrument that measures the fluid pressure directly. The second test, gonioscopy, involves the use of a special mirrored contact lens to evaluate the anatomy of the angle between the iris and the cornea. The doctor numbs the outside of the eye with a local anesthetic and touches the outside of the cornea with the gonioscopic lens. He or she can use a slit lamp to magnify what appears on the lens. Patients with subacute, intermittent, or chronic closed-angle glaucoma can then be treated before they develop acute symptoms.

If the patient is having a sudden attack of closed-angle glaucoma, he or she will feel intense pain, and is likely to be seen on an emergency basis with the following symptoms:

- nausea and vomiting
- severe pain in or above the eye
- visual disturbances that include seeing halos around lights and hazy or foggy vision
- headache
- redness and watering in the affected eye
- a dilated pupil that does not close normally in bright light

These symptoms are produced by the sharp rise in intraocular pressure (IOP) that occurs when the angle is completely blocked. This increase can occur in a matter of hours and cause permanent loss of vision in as little as two to five days. *An acute attack of closed-angle glaucoma is a medical emergency requiring immediate treatment.* Emergency treatment includes application of eye drops to reduce the pressure in the eye quickly, other eye drops to shrink the size of the pupil, and acetazolamide or a similar medication to stop the production of aqueous humor. In severe cases, the patient may be given drugs intravenously to lower the intraocular pressure. After the pressure has been relieved with medications, the eye will require surgical treatment.

Melanoma of the iris

Melanoma of the iris is usually discovered in the course of a routine eye examination because it will be visible to the ophthalmologist as he or she looks through the pupil in the center of the iris. A melanoma on the iris may look like a dark spot or ring, or it may resemble tapioca. The doctor can perform a gonioscopy, and use specialized imaging studies to rule out other possible eye disorders. An **ultrasound** study can be made by using a small probe placed on the eye that directs sound waves in the direction of the tumor. Another test is called fluorescein **angiography**, which involves injecting a fluorescent dye into a vein in the patient's arm. As the dye circulates throughout the body, it is carried to the blood vessels in the back of the eye. These blood vessels can be photographed through the pupil.

In a minority of patients, melanoma of the iris is discovered because the patient is experiencing eye pain resulting from a rise in IOP caused by tumor growth.

Preparation for treatment

Patients scheduled for a laser iridotomy or iridectomy are not required to fast or make other special preparations before the procedure. They may, however, be given a sedative to help them relax. Patients scheduled for a conventional iridectomy are asked to avoid eating or drinking for about eight hours before the procedure.

Aftercare

Short-term aftercare following laser iridectomy or iridotomy is minimal. Patients are asked to make arrangements for someone to drive them home after surgery, but can usually go to work the next day and resume other activities with no restrictions. They should not need any medication stronger than **aspirin** for discomfort.

Short-term aftercare following a surgical iridectomy includes wearing a patch over the affected eye for several days and using eye drops to minimize the risk of infection. The surgeon may also prescribe medication for discomfort. It will take about six weeks for vision to return to normal. Long-term aftercare following an iridectomy for closed-angle glaucoma usually involves taking medications to help control the fluid pressure in the eye and seeing the ophthalmologist for periodic checkups.

Aftercare for melanoma of the iris includes eye checkups to be certain that the tumor has not recurred. In addition, patients are advised to reduce their exposure to sunlight and other sources of ultraviolet light.

Risks

The risks of a laser iridotomy or iridectomy include the following:

- irritation in the eye for two to three days after the procedure
- bleeding
- scarring
- failure to relieve fluid pressure in the eye

The risks of a conventional iridectomy include:

- infection
- bleeding
- scarring in the area of the incision
- failure to relieve fluid pressure
- formation of a cataract

The risks of an iridectomy for melanoma of the iris include glaucoma resulting from the formation of new blood vessels near the angle; cataract formation; and recurrence of the tumor. In the event of a recurrence, the standard treatment is enucleation, or surgical removal of the entire eye.

Normal results

Normal results for a laser-assisted or conventional iridectomy are long-term lowering of IOP and/or complete removal of a melanoma on the iris.

Morbidity and mortality rates

About 60% of patients who have had conventional iridectomies consider the operation a success; 15%, on the other hand, maintain that their vision was better before the procedure.

Fortunately for patients, melanoma of the iris is a relatively slow-growing form of cancer; it metastasizes to the liver in only 2–4% of cases. If treated promptly, it has a high survival rate of 95–97% after five years.

Alternatives

Alternatives to a conventional iridectomy for the treatment of closed-angle glaucoma include repeated laser iridotomies or the long-term use of such medications as pilocarpine. Another surgical alternative, which is most commonly done when the size of the lens is a factor in pupillary block, is removal of the lens.

Alternatives to iridectomy in the treatment of melanoma of the iris include watchful waiting, periodic eye examinations, and the use of medication to control any symptoms of closed-angle glaucoma.

Resources

BOOKS

Albert, Daniel, M. and Mark J. Lucarelli, MD. *Clinical Atlas of Procedures in Ophthalmic Surgery*, 1st ed. Chicago, IL: American Medical Association Press, 2003.

"Angle-Closure Glaucoma." Section 8, Chapter 100 in *The Merck Manual of Diagnosis and Therapy*, edited by Mark H. Beers and Robert Berkow. Whitehouse Station, NJ: Merck Research Laboratories, 1999.

Azuara-Blanco, Augusto, M.D, Ph.D., et. al. *Handbook of Glaucoma*, 1st ed. London, England: Taylor & Francis, 2007.

Kanski, Jack J. M. D., et. al. *Glaucoma: A Colour Manual of Diagnosis and Treatment*. Oxford, England: Butterworth-Heinemann, 2003.

Ritch, Robert, M. D., et. al. *The Glaucomas*. St. Louis, MO: 1996.

PERIODICALS

Aung, T., and P. T. Chew. "Review of Recent Advancements in the Understanding of Primary Angle-Closure Glaucoma." *Current Opinion in Ophthalmology* 13 (April 2002): 89–93.

Chang, B. M., J. M. Liebmann, and R. Ritch. "Angle Closure in Younger Patients." *Transactions of the American Ophthalmological Society* 100 (2002): 201–212.

Goldberg, D. E., and W. R. Freeman. "Uveitic Angle Closure Glaucoma in a Patient with Inactive Cytomegalovirus Retinitis and Immune Recovery Uveitis." *Ophthalmic Surgery and Lasers* 33 (September–October 2002): 421–425.

Jackson, T. L., et al. "Pupil Block Glaucoma in Phakic and Pseudophakic Patients After Vitrectomy with Silicone Oil Injection." *American Journal of Ophthalmology* 132 (September 2001): 414–416.

Jacobi, P. C., et al. "Primary Phacoemulsification and Intraocular Lens Implantation for Acute Angle-Closure Glaucoma." *Ophthalmology* 109 (September 2002): 1597–1603.

Jiminez-Jiminez, F. J., M. Orti-Pareja, and J. M. Zurdo. "Aggravation of Glaucoma with Fluvoxamine." *Annals of Pharmacotherapy* 35 (December 2001): 1565–1566.

Kumar, A., S. Kedar, V. K. Garodia, and R. P. Singh. "Angle Closure Glaucoma Following Pupillary Block in an Aphakin Perfluoropropane Gas-Filled Eye." *Indian Journal of Ophthalmology* 50 (September 2002): 220–221.

Lentschener, C., et al. "Acute Postoperative Glaucoma After Nonocular Surgery Remains a Diagnostic Challenge." *Anesthesia and Analgesia* 94 (April 2002): 1034–1035.

Schwartz, G. P., and L. W. Schwartz. "Acute Angle Closure Glaucoma Secondary to a Choroidal Melanoma." *CLAO Journal* 28 (April 2002): 77–79.

Shields, C. L., et al. "Factors Associated with Elevated Intraocular Pressure in Eyes with Iris Melanoma." *British Journal of Ophthalmology* 85 (June 2001): 666–669.

Shields, C. L., et al. "Iris Melanoma: Risk Factors for Metastasis in 169 Consecutive Patients." *Ophthalmology* 108 (January 2001): 172–178.

Wang, N., H. Wu, and Z. Fan. "Primary Angle Closure Glaucoma in Chinese and Western Populations." *Chinese Medical Journal* 115 (November 2002): 1706–1715.

ORGANIZATIONS

American Academy of Ophthalmology. P. O. Box 7424, San Francisco, CA 94120-7424. (415) 561-8500. http://www.aao.org.

Canadian Ophthalmological Society (COS). 610-1525 Carling Avenue, Ottawa ON K1Z 8R9 Canada. http://www.eyesite.ca.

National Eye Institute. 2020 Vision Place, Bethesda, MD 20892-3655. (301) 496-5248. http://nei.nih.gov.

Prevent Blindness America. 500 East Remington Road, Schaumburg, IL 60173. (800) 331-2020. http://www.prevent-blindness.org.

Wills Eye Hospital. 840 Walnut Street, Philadelphia, PA 19107. (215) 928-3000. http://www.willseye.org.

OTHER

National Cancer Institute (NCI) Physician Data Query (PDQ). Intraocular (Eye) Melanoma: Treatment, January 2, 2003 [cited April 2, 2003]. http://www.nci.nih.gov/cancerinfo/pdq/treatment/intraocularmelanoma/healthprofessional.

National Eye Institute (NEI). Facts About Glaucoma. 2008. NIH Publication No. 99–651.http://www.nei.nih.gov/health/glaucoma/glaucoma_facts.asp.

Tanasescu, I., and F. Grehn. "Advantage of Surgical Iridectomy Over Nd:YAG Laser Iridotomy in Acute Primary Angle Closure Glaucoma." Presentation on September 29, 2001, at the 99th annual meeting of the Deutsche Ophthalmologische Gesellschaft. http://www.dog.org/2001/mo_13.htm.

Waheed, Nadia K., and C. Stephen Foster. "Melanoma, Iris." eMedicine, July, 2005 [cited April 2, 2003]. http://www.emedicine.com/oph/topic405.htm.

Rebecca Frey, PhD
Laura Jean Cataldo, RN, EdD

Irodotomy *see* **Laser iridotomy**

Islet cell transplantation

Definition

Pancreatic islet cell transplantation involves taking the cells that produce insulin from a second source, such as a donor pancreas, and transplanting them into a patient.

Purpose

Once transplanted, the new islet cells make and release insulin. Islet cell transplantation is primarily a treatment method for type 1 diabetes, but it can also be used to treat patients who have had their pancreas

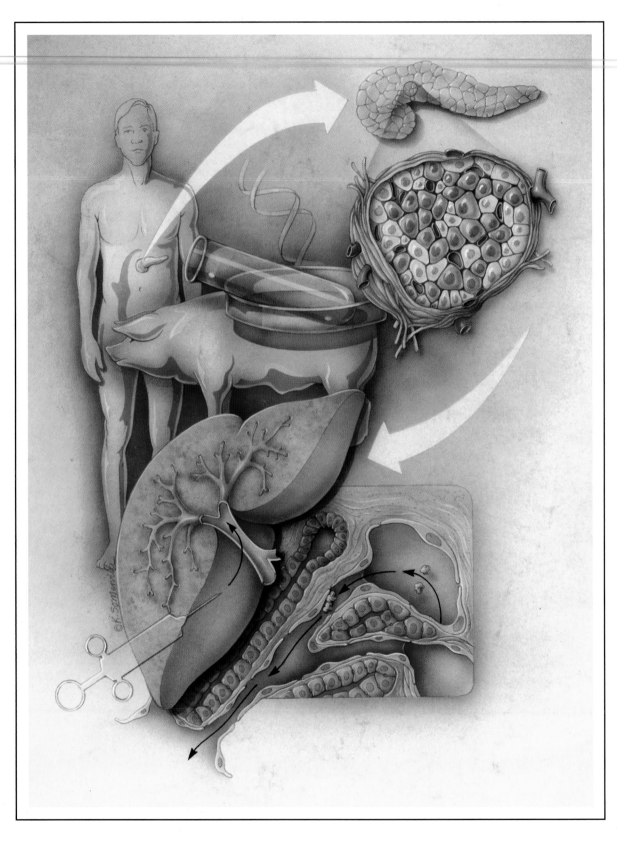

Islet cell transplantation. *(Kevin A. Somerville/Phototake. Reproduced by permission.)*

Immunosuppression—A drug-induced state that prevents rejection of transplanted body parts.

Invasive—Used to describe a procedure that involves surgical cutting into the body.

Islet cell—The cell type within the pancreas that produces insulin.

Portal vein—The main vessel that carries blood to the liver.

Steroids—A component of commonly used immunosuppressive drugs that have negative effects on insulin production.

removed or damaged from other medical conditions or injuries.

Demographics

An estimated 120–140 million people worldwide suffer from type 1 diabetes and might possibly benefit from this procedure, however, islet cell transplantation remains highly experimental at this time and occurs only as part of a clinical trial. The latest available data from the International Islet Transplant Registry indicate that, as of December 2000, about 500 procedures had been performed.

Description

The transplantation procedure is very straightforward, relatively noninvasive, and takes less than an hour to complete. After the patient is given light sedation, the surgeon begins by using an **ultrasound** machine to guide the placement of a small plastic tube, known as a catheter, through the upper abdomen and into the liver. The liver is used as the site for transplantation because the portal vein of liver is large and therefore, easier to access than smaller veins that supply the pancreas. In addition, it is known that islet cells that grow in the liver closely mimic normal insulin secretion.

Once the catheter is in place, the surgeon takes the cells that have been extracted from the donor pancreas and infuses them into the liver. Extraction is done as close as possible to the time of transplantation because of the fragility of the islet cells. The extraction process uses specialized enzymes to isolate the islet cells from the other cell types found in the pancreas. During the infusion process, the cells travel through the portal vein and become lodged in the capillaries of the liver, where they remain to produce insulin as they normally would in the pancreas. Only 1–2% of the pancreas is made up of islet

cells, an average of two pancreases are needed for one successful transplant.

Recent study has shown that the use of perfluorocarbon in the solution that preserves the pancreas before transplant allows older organs to be used as islet cell donors. New techniques have also been developed that allow the organs to be transported before being used for transplantation. These developments are initial steps to relieving the extreme shortage of donor pancreases needed for the procedure.

Diagnosis/Preparation

To qualify as a candidate for islet cell transplantation, the patient must suffer from type 1 diabetes and current insulin treatment methods must be insufficient. For example, some participants suffer from hypoglycemic unawareness, a condition where low blood sugar will cause very dangerous, unpredictable blackouts that cannot be controlled with insulin injections. The potential patient must also undergo extensive medical and psychological tests to determine their physical and mental appropriateness for enrollment in the trial. If the results of these tests support the candidacy, then sufficient donor pancreas tissue in the patient's blood type must be located. The patient is placed on an organ donor list. Waiting for more than a year is common.

In response to this long wait, research is ongoing to provide alternative sources of donor islet cells such as animal cells, a process known as a xenograft. Pigs are a particularly advantageous source of islet cells because human and pig insulin proteins differ by only one amino acid, and there is an extensive amount of fresh pancreas organs available from the pork industry. Other potential sources of donor islets cells include embryonic stem cells and cell lines of islet beta cells.

Prior to the transplantation, the patient must undergo a drug regime that suppresses the immune system so that the new cells will be accepted. Although only cells are being transplanted, the amount of immunosuppression is the same as that required for a whole organ transplant. Current protocols for islet transplantation include a mixture of non-steroidal drugs, as those that include steroids have been shown to aggravate the diabetic condition of the patient and inhibit the insulin-producing function of the transplanted cells.

Future research in this area may include the use of monoclonal antibody therapy to induce tolerance in patients prior to transplantation.

Aftercare

Recovery time from the procedure itself is minimal. However, current technology requires that patients continuously remain on immunosuppressive drugs to avoid rejection of the new islet cells. Side effects from these drugs can increase the amount of time that the patient must remain hospitalized.

It takes some time for the cells to attach to the liver blood vessels and begin producing insulin. Until that occurs, numerous blood **glucose tests** are performed, and injected insulin is used to keep blood glucose levels within normal ranges.

Risks

Until recently, success rates for this procedure were not promising. With success being defined as not requiring insulin for a full year after transplantation, the success rate from 1998–2000 was only about 14% of patients transplanted. However, newer procedures have been achieving at least short-term success rates approaching 80–100%, making the possibility of widespread use of this procedure much more feasible in the near future.

Because of the newness of the procedure, the long-term success rate of these new protocols is not yet known. Graft death is a significant risk even years after a successful transplant. The longest reported successful graft using older protocols has been six years. Over time, the ability of grafts transplanted using new protocols and then sustained by the new immunosuppressive drug mixtures, will be determined.

The long-term use of immunosuppressive drugs by the patient poses an additional risk. There is relatively little experience and therefore, little data to date, pertaining to the long-term use of these drugs. It is difficult then, to predict what exact physical effects long-term immunosuppression may have. Some known side effects include high blood pressure, toxicity of the kidneys, and opportunistic infections.

Alternatives

One alternative to islet cell transplantation is transplantation of an entire pancreas, a much more invasive procedure. Whole organ transplant has historically had a better success rate than islet transplantation.

However, newer islet cell transplant protocols are approaching whole organ results, thus overcoming one of the most important differences between the two procedures.

Resources

BOOKS

Farney, Alan C., and David E. R. Sutherland. "Pancrease and Islet Transplantation." In *The Pancreas: Biology, Pathobiology, and Disease*, edited by Vay Liang W. Go, et al. New York: Raven Press, 1993.

Robertson, R. Paul. "Pancreas and Islet Transplantation." In *Endocrinology*, edited by Leslie J. DeGroot, et al. Philadelphia: W.B. Saunders Company, 2001.

Shapiro, A., et al. *Islet Transplantation and Beta Cell Replacement Therapy*, 1st ed. London: Informa Healthcare, 2007.

PERIODICALS

"Islet Cell Transplantation for Diabetes Turns Corner." *Science Daily Magazine* (August 28, 2002).

Perry, Patrick. "Zeroing in on a Cure for Diabetes." *The Saturday Evening Post* (January/February 2002): 38–43.

ORGANIZATIONS

American Diabetes Association. 1701 North Beauregard Street, Alexandria, VA 22311. (800) 342-2383. http://www.diabetes.org.

Immune Tolerance Network (ITN). 5743 South Drexel Avenue, Suite 200, Chicago, IL 60637. (773) 834-5341. http://www.immunetolerance.org.

International Pancreas Transplant Registry (IPTR). University of Minnesota Department of Surgery, Mayo Mail Code 280, 420 Delaware Street SE, Minneapolis, MN 55455-0392. http://www.iptr.umn.edu/.

Michelle Johnson, MS, JD
Laura Jean Cataldo, RN, EdD

IV rehydration *see* **Intravenous rehydration**

J

Joint radiography *see* **Arthrography**
Joint resection *see* **Arthroplasty**
Joint x rays *see* **Arthrography**

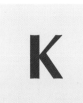

K

Keratoplasty *see* **Corneal transplantation**
Ketone test *see* **Urinalysis**

Kidney dialysis

Definition

Dialysis treatment replaces the function of the kidneys, which normally serve as the body's natural filtration system. Through the use of a blood filter and a chemical solution known as dialysate, the treatment removes waste products and excess fluids from the bloodstream, while maintaining the proper chemical balance of the blood. There are two types of dialysis treatment: hemodialysis and peritoneal dialysis.

Purpose

Dialysis is most commonly prescribed for patients with temporary or permanent kidney failure. People with end-stage renal disease (ESRD) have kidneys that are no longer capable of adequately removing fluids and wastes from their body or of maintaining the proper level of certain kidney-regulated chemicals in the bloodstream. For these individuals, dialysis is the only treatment option available outside of **kidney transplantation**. Dialysis may also be used to simulate kidney function in patients awaiting a transplant until a donor kidney becomes available. Also, dialysis may be used in the treatment of patients suffering from poisoning or overdose in order to quickly remove drugs from the bloodstream.

Demographics

As of 2003, in the United States, over 287,494 people were undergoing regular dialysis treatments to manage their ESRD. Diabetes mellitus is the leading single cause of ESRD: 40% of dialysis patients in the United States have ESRD caused by diabetes, 28%

by hypertension, 11.6% by glomerulonephritis, and 4.7% by cystic (bladder) or other urologic conditions.

Among children and young adults under 20 on dialysis, glomerulonephritis is the leading cause of ESRD (31%), and hereditary, cystic, and congenital diseases account for 37%. Pediatric patients typically spend less time on dialysis than adults; according to the USRDS the average waiting period for a kidney transplant for patients under age 20 is 10 months, compared to the adult wait of approximately two years.

Description

There are two types of dialysis treatment: hemodialysis and peritoneal dialysis.

Hemodialysis

Hemodialysis is the most frequently prescribed type of dialysis treatment in the United States. The treatment involves circulating the patient's blood outside of the body through an extracorporeal circuit (ECC), or dialysis circuit. Two needles are inserted into the patient's vein, or access site, and are attached to the ECC, which consists of plastic blood tubing, a filter known as a dialyzer (artificial kidney), and a dialysis machine that monitors and maintains blood flow and administers dialysate. Dialysate is a chemical bath that is used to draw waste products out of the blood.

Since the 1980s, the majority of hemodialysis treatments in the United States have been performed with hollow fiber dialyzers. A hollow fiber dialyzer is composed of thousands of tube-like hollow fiber strands encased in a clear plastic cylinder several inches in diameter. There are two compartments within the dialyzer (the blood compartment and the dialysate compartment).

The membrane that separates these two compartments is semipermeable. This means that it allows the passage of certain sized molecules across it, but prevents the passage of other, larger molecules. As blood

Access site—The vein tapped for vascular access in hemodialysis treatments. For patients with temporary treatment needs, access to the bloodstream is gained by inserting a catheter into the subclavian vein near the patient's collarbone. Patients in long-term dialysis require stronger, more durable access sites, called fistulas or grafts, that are surgically created.

Dialysate—A chemical bath used in dialysis to draw fluids and toxins out of the bloodstream and supply electrolytes and other chemicals to the bloodstream.

Dialysis prescription—The general parameters of dialysis treatment that vary according to each patient's individual needs. Treatment length, type of dialyzer and dialysate used, and rate of ultrafiltration are all part of the dialysis prescription.

Dialyzer—An artificial kidney usually composed of hollow fiber which is used in hemodialysis to eliminate waste products from the blood and remove excess fluids from the bloodstream.

Erythropoietin—A hormone produced by the kidneys that stimulates the production of red blood cells by bone marrow.

ESRD—End-stage renal disease; chronic or permanent kidney failure.

Extracorporeal circuit (ECC)—The path the hemodialysis patient's blood takes outside of the body. It typically consists of plastic tubing, a hemodialysis machine, and a dialyzer.

Glomerulonephritis—A disease of the kidney that causes inflammation and scarring and impairs the kidney's ability to filter waste products from the blood.

Hematocrit (Hct) level—A measure of red blood cells.

Glomerulonephritis—Kidney disease caused by scarring of the glomeruli, the small blood vessels in the nephrons, or filtering centers, of the kidneys.

Peritoneum—The abdominal cavity; the peritoneum acts as a blood filter in peritoneal dialysis.

---

is pushed through the blood compartment in one direction, suction or vacuum pressure pulls the dialysate through the dialysate compartment in a countercurrent, or opposite direction. These opposing pressures work to drain excess fluids out of the bloodstream and into the dialysate, a process called ultrafiltration.

A second process called diffusion moves waste products in the blood across the membrane and into the dialysate compartment, where they are carried out of the body. At the same time, electrolytes and other chemicals in the dialysate solution cross the membrane into the blood compartment. The purified, chemically balanced blood is then returned to the body.

Most hemodialysis patients require treatment three times a week, for an average of three to four hours per dialysis "run." Specific treatment schedules depend on the type of dialyzer used and the patient's current physical condition.

Blood pressure changes associated with hemodialysis may pose a risk for patients with heart problems. Peritoneal dialysis may be the preferred treatment option in these cases.

Peritoneal dialysis

In peritoneal dialysis, the patient's peritoneum, or lining of the abdomen, acts as a blood filter. A catheter is surgically inserted into the patient's abdomen. During treatment, the catheter is used to fill the abdominal cavity with dialysate. Waste products and excess fluids move from the patient's bloodstream into the dialysate solution. After a waiting period of six to 24 hours, depending on the treatment method used, the waste-filled dialysate is drained from the abdomen and replaced with clean dialysate.

There are three types of peritoneal dialysis:

- Continuous ambulatory peritoneal dialysis (CAPD). CAPD is a continuous treatment that is self-administered and requires no machine. The patient inserts fresh dialysate solution into the abdominal cavity, waits four to six hours, and removes the used solution. The solution is immediately replaced with fresh dialysate. A bag attached to the catheter is worn under clothing.

- Continuous cyclic peritoneal dialysis (CCPD). Also called automated peritoneal dialysis (APD), CCPD is an overnight treatment that uses a machine to drain and refill the abdominal cavity, CCPD takes 10 to 12 hours per session.

- Intermittent peritoneal dialysis (IPD). This hospital-based treatment is performed several times a week. A machine administers and drains the dialysate solution, and sessions can take 12 to 24 hours.

Peritoneal dialysis is often the treatment option of choice in infants and children, whose small size can make vascular (through a vein) access difficult to maintain. Peritoneal dialysis can also be done outside of a clinical setting, which is more conducive to regular school attendance.

Peritoneal dialysis is not recommended for patients with abdominal adhesions or other abdominal defects, such as a hernia, that might compromise the efficiency of the treatment. It is also not recommended for patients who suffer frequent bouts of **diverticulitis**, an inflammation of small pouches in the intestinal tract.

Diagnosis/Preparation

Patients are weighed immediately before and after each hemodialysis treatment to evaluate their fluid retention. Blood pressure and temperature are taken and the patient is assessed for physical changes since their last dialysis run. Regular blood tests monitor chemical and waste levels in the blood. Prior to treatment, patients are typically administered a dose of heparin, an anticoagulant that prevents blood clotting, to ensure the free flow of blood through the dialyzer and an uninterrupted dialysis run for the patient.

Aftercare

Both hemodialysis and peritoneal dialysis patients need to be vigilant about keeping their access sites and catheters clean and infection-free during and between dialysis runs.

Dialysis is just one facet of a comprehensive treatment approach for ESRD. Although dialysis treatment is very effective in removing toxins and fluids from the body, there are several functions of the kidney it cannot mimic, such as regulating high blood pressure and red blood cell production. Patients with ESRD need to watch their dietary and fluid intake carefully and take medications as prescribed to manage their disease.

Risks

Many of the risks and side effects associated with dialysis are a combined result of both the treatment and the poor physical condition of the ESRD patient. Dialysis patients should always report side effects to their healthcare provider.

Anemia

Hematocrit (Hct) levels, a measure of red blood cells, are typically low in ESRD patients. This deficiency is caused by a lack of the hormone erythropoietin, which is normally produced by the kidneys. The problem is elevated in hemodialysis patients, who may incur blood loss during hemodialysis treatments. Epoetin alfa, or EPO (sold under the trade name Epogen), a hormone therapy, and intravenous or oral iron supplements are used to manage anemia in dialysis patients.

Cramps, nausea, vomiting, and headaches

Some hemodialysis patients experience cramps and flu-like symptoms during treatment. These can be caused by a number of factors, including the type of dialysate used, composition of the dialyzer membrane, water quality in the dialysis unit, and the ultrafiltration rate of the treatment. Adjustment of the dialysis prescription often helps alleviate many symptoms.

Hypotension

Because of the stress placed on the cardiovascular system with regular hemodialysis treatments, patients are at risk for hypotension, a sudden drop in blood pressure. This can often be controlled by medication and adjustment of the patient's dialysis prescription.

Infection

Both hemodialysis and peritoneal dialysis patients are at risk for infection. Hemodialysis patients should keep their access sites clean and watch for signs of redness and warmth that could indicate infection. Peritoneal dialysis patients must follow the same precautions with their catheter. Peritonitis, an infection of the peritoneum, causes flu-like symptoms and can disrupt dialysis treatments if not caught early.

Infectious diseases

Because there is a great deal of blood exposure involved in dialysis treatment, a slight risk of contracting hepatitis B and hepatitis C exists. The hepatitis B vaccination is recommended for most hemodialysis patients. As of 2001, there has only been one documented case of HIV being transmitted in a United States dialysis unit to a staff member, and no documented cases of HIV ever being transmitted between dialysis patients in the United States. The strict standards of infection control practiced in modern hemodialysis units minimizes the chance of contracting one of these diseases.

Normal results

Because dialysis is an ongoing treatment process for many patients, a baseline for normalcy can be

WHO PERFORMS THE PROCEDURE AND WHERE IS IT PERFORMED?

The dialysis treatment prescription and regimen is usually overseen by a nephrologist (a doctor that specializes in the kidney). The hemodialysis treatment itself is typically administered by a nurse or patient care technician in outpatient clinics known as dialysis centers, or in hospital-based dialysis units. In-home hemodialysis treatment is also an option for some patients, although access to this type of treatment may be limited by financial and lifestyle factors. An investment in equipment is required and another person in the household should be available for support and assistance with treatments. Peritoneal dialysis is also performed at home by the patient, perhaps with the aide of a home health-care worker.

QUESTIONS TO ASK THE DOCTOR

- When and where will my dialysis treatments be scheduled?
- How should my diet change now that I'm on dialysis?
- What kind of vascular access will I get?
- Does my new dialysis center have a dialyzer reuse program? If so, what safety checks are in place to ensure I receive a properly treated dialyzer?
- What can I do to make dialysis more effective?
- Can you refer me to any ESRD patient support groups?
- Should I change my medication routine?

difficult to gauge. Puffiness in the patient related to edema, or fluid retention, may be relieved after dialysis treatment. The patient's overall sense of physical well being may also be improved.

Monthly blood tests to check the levels of urea, a waste product, help to determine the adequacy of the dialysis prescription. Another test, called Kt/V (dialyzer clearance multiplied by time of treatment and divided by the total volume of water in the patient's body), is also performed to assess patient progress. A urea reduction ratio (URR) of 65% or higher, and a Kt/V of at least 1.2 are considered the benchmarks of dialysis adequacy by the Kidney Disease Outcomes Quality Initiative (K/DOQI) of the National Kidney Foundation.

Morbidity and mortality rates

The USRDS reports that mortality rates for individuals on dialysis are also significantly higher than both kidney transplant patients and the general population, and expected remaining lifetimes of chronic dialysis patients are only one-fourth to one-fifth that of the general population. The hospitalization rates for people with ESRD are four times greater than that of the general population.

Alternatives

The only alternative to dialysis for ESRD patients is a successful kidney transplant. However, demand for donor kidneys has traditionally far exceeded supply. As of 2006, there were 70,000 patients on the United Network for Organ Sharing (UNOS) waiting list for a kidney transplant. In 2005, about 16,000 patients received a kidney.

For patients with diabetes, the number one cause of chronic kidney failure in adults, the best way to avoid ESRD and subsequent dialysis is to maintain tight control of blood glucose levels through diet, **exercise**, and medication. Controlling high blood pressure is also important.

Resources

BOOKS

Brenner, B. M., et al. *Brenner & Rector's The Kidney.* 7th ed. Philadelphia: Saunders, 2004.

Wein, A. J., et al. *Campbell-Walsh Urology.* 9th ed. Philadelphia: Saunders, 2007.

PERIODICALS

Eknoyan G., G. J. Beck, et al. "Effect of Dialysis Dose and Membrane Flux in Maintenance Hemodialysis." *New England Journal of Medicine* 347 (December 19, 2002): 2010–2019.

ORGANIZATIONS

American Association of Kidney Patients. 3505 E. Frontage Rd., Suite 315, Tampa, FL 33607. (800) 749-2257. http://www.aakp.org.

American Kidney Fund (AKF). Suite 1010, 6110 Executive Boulevard, Rockville, MD 20852. (800) 638-8299. http://www.akfinc.org.

National Kidney Foundation. 30 East 33rd St., Suite 1100, New York, NY 10016. (800) 622-9010. http://www.kidney.org.

United States Renal Data System (USRDS), Coordinating Center. The University of Minnesota, 914 South 8th Street, Suite D-206, Minneapolis, MN 55404. 1-888-99USRDS. http://www.usrds.org.

Paula Anne Ford-Martin

Kidney function tests

Definition

Kidney function tests include a variety of individual tests and procedures that can be done to evaluate how well the kidneys are functioning. A doctor who orders kidney function tests and uses the results to assess the functioning of the kidneys is called a nephrologist.

Purpose

The kidneys, the body's natural filtration system, perform many vital functions, including removing metabolic waste products from the bloodstream, regulating the body's water balance, and maintaining the pH (acidity/alkalinity) of the body's fluids. Approximately one and a half quarts of blood per minute are circulated through the kidneys, where waste chemicals are filtered out and eliminated from the body (along with excess water) in the form of urine. Kidney function tests help to determine if the kidneys are performing their tasks adequately.

Precautions

The doctor should take a complete history prior to conducting kidney function tests to evaluate the patient's food and drug intake. A wide variety of prescription and over-the-counter medications can affect blood and urine kidney function test results, as can some food and beverages.

Description

Many conditions can affect the ability of the kidneys to carry out their vital functions. Some conditions can lead to a rapid (acute) decline in kidney function; others lead to a gradual (chronic) decline in function. Both can result in a buildup of toxic waste substances in the blood. A number of clinical laboratory tests that measure the levels of substances normally regulated by the kidneys can help to determine the cause and extent of kidney dysfunction. Urine and blood samples are used for these tests.

The nephrologist uses these results in a number of ways. Once a diagnosis is made that kidney disease is present and what kind of kidney disease is causing the problem, the nephrologist may recommend a specific treatment. Although there is no specific drug therapy that will prevent the progression of kidney disease, the doctor will make recommendations for treatment to slow the disease as much as possible. For instance, the doctor might prescribe blood pressure medications, or treatments for patients with diabetes. If kidney disease

is getting worse, the nephrologist may discuss hemodialysis (blood cleansing by removal of excess fluid, minerals, and wastes) or **kidney transplantation** (surgical procedure to implant a healthy kidney into a patient with kidney disease or kidney failure) with the patient.

Laboratory tests

There are a number of urine tests that can be used to assess kidney function. A simple, inexpensive screening test—a routine urinalysis—is often the first test conducted if kidney problems are suspected. A small, randomly collected urine sample is examined physically for things like color, odor, appearance, and concentration (specific gravity); chemically, for substances such a protein, glucose, and pH (acidity/ alkalinity); and microscopically for the presence of cellular elements (red blood cells [RBCs], white blood cells [WBCs], and epithelial cells), bacteria, crystals, and casts (structures formed by the deposit of protein, cells, and other substances in the kidneys's tubules). If results indicate a possibility of disease or impaired kidney function, one or more of the following additional tests is usually performed to pinpoint the cause and the level of decline in kidney function.

- Creatinine clearance test. This test evaluates how efficiently the kidneys clear a substance called creatinine from the blood. Creatinine, a waste product of muscle energy metabolism, is produced at a constant rate that is proportional to the individual's muscle mass. Because the body does not recycle it, all creatinine filtered by the kidneys in a given amount of time is excreted in the urine, making creatinine clearance a very specific measurement of kidney function. The test is performed on a timed urine specimen—a cumulative sample collected over a two to 24-hour period. Determination of the blood creatinine level is also required to calculate the urine clearance.

- Urea clearance test. Urea is a waste product that is created by protein metabolism and excreted in the urine. The urea clearance test requires a blood sample to measure the amount of urea in the bloodstream and two urine specimens, collected one hour apart, to determine the amount of urea that is filtered, or cleared, by the kidneys into the urine.

- Urine osmolality test. Urine osmolality is a measurement of the number of dissolved particles in urine. It is a more precise measurement than specific gravity for evaluating the ability of the kidneys to concentrate or dilute the urine. Kidneys that are functioning normally will excrete more water into the urine as fluid intake is increased, diluting the urine. If fluid intake is decreased, the kidneys excrete less water and the urine becomes more concentrated. The test may be done on a urine sample collected first thing in the morning, on multiple timed samples, or on a cumulative sample collected over a 24-hour period. The patient will typically be prescribed a high-protein diet for several days before the test and be asked to drink no fluids the night before the test.

- Urine protein test. Healthy kidneys filter all proteins from the bloodstream and then reabsorb them, allowing no protein, or only slight amounts of protein, into the urine. The persistent presence of significant amounts of protein in the urine, then, is an important indicator of kidney disease. A positive screening test for protein (included in a routine urinalysis) on a random urine sample is usually followed up with a test on a 24-hour urine sample that more precisely measures the quantity of protein.

There are also several blood tests that can aid in evaluating kidney function. These include:

- **Blood urea nitrogen test (BUN).** Urea is a byproduct of protein metabolism. Formed in the liver, this waste product is then filtered from the blood and excreted in the urine by the kidneys. The BUN test measures the amount of nitrogen contained in the urea. High BUN levels can indicate kidney dysfunction, but because BUN is also affected by protein intake and liver function, the test is usually done together with a blood creatinine, a more specific indicator of kidney function.

- Creatinine test. This test measures blood levels of creatinine, a byproduct of muscle energy metabolism that, similar to urea, is filtered from the blood by the kidneys and excreted into the urine. Production of creatinine depends on a person's muscle mass, which usually fluctuates very little. With normal kidney function, then, the amount of creatinine in the blood remains relatively constant and normal. For this reason, and because creatinine is affected very little by liver function, an elevated blood creatinine level is a more sensitive indicator of impaired kidney function than the BUN.

- Other blood tests. Measurement of the blood levels of other elements regulated in part by the kidneys can also be useful in evaluating kidney function. These include sodium, potassium, chloride, bicarbonate, calcium, magnesium, phosphorus, protein, uric acid, and glucose.

Results

Normal values for many tests are determined by the patient's age and gender. Reference values can also vary by laboratory, but are generally within the following ranges:

Urine tests

- Creatinine clearance. For a 24-hour urine collection, normal results are 90 mL/min–139 mL/min for adult males younger than 40, and 80–125 mL/min for adult females younger than 40. For people over 40, values decrease by 6.5 mL/min for each decade of life.

- Urine osmolality. With restricted fluid intake (concentration testing), osmolality should be greater than 800 mOsm/kg of water. With increased fluid intake (dilution testing), osmolality should be less than 100 mOSm/kg in at least one of the specimens collected. A 24-hour urine osmolality should average 300–900 mOsm/kg. A random urine osmolality should average 500–800 mOsm/kg.
- Urine protein. A 24-hour urine collection should contain no more than 150 mg of protein.
- Urine sodium. A 24-hour urine sodium should be within 75–200 mmol/day.

Blood tests

- Blood urea nitrogen (BUN) should average 8–20 mg/dL.
- Creatinine should be 0.8–1.2 mg/dL for males, and 0.6–0.9 mg/dL for females.
- Uric acid levels for males should be 3.5–7.2 mg/dL and for females 2.6–6.0 mg/dL.

Low clearance values for creatinine indicate a diminished ability of the kidneys to filter waste products from the blood and excrete them in the urine. As clearance levels decrease, blood levels of creatinine, urea, and uric acid increase. Because it can be affected by other factors, an elevated BUN, alone, is suggestive, but not diagnostic for kidney dysfunction. An abnormally elevated plasma creatinine is a more specific indicator of kidney disease than is BUN.

Low clearance values for creatinine and urea indicate a diminished ability of the kidneys to filter these waste products from the blood and to excrete them in the urine. As clearance levels decrease, blood levels of creatinine and urea nitrogen increase. Since it can be affected by other factors, an elevated BUN alone is certainly suggestive for kidney dysfunction. However, it is not diagnostic. An abnormally elevated blood creatinine, a more specific and sensitive indicator of kidney disease than the BUN, is diagnostic of impaired kidney function.

The inability of the kidneys to concentrate the urine in response to restricted fluid intake, or to dilute the urine in response to increased fluid intake during osmolality testing, may indicate decreased kidney function. Because the kidneys normally excrete almost no protein in the urine, its persistent presence, in amounts that exceed the normal 24-hour urine value, usually indicates some type of kidney disease.

Patient education

Some kidney problems are the result of another disease process, such as diabetes or hypertension.

Doctors should take the time to inform patients about how their disease or its treatment will affect kidney function, as well as the different measures patients can take to help prevent these changes.

Resources

BOOKS

Brenner, Barry M., and Floyd C. Rector Jr., eds. *The Kidney, 6th Edition.* Philadelphia, PA: W. B. Saunders Company, 1999.

Burtis, Carl A. and Edward R. Ashwood. *Tietz Textbook of Clinical Chemistry.* Philadelphia, PA: W.B. Saunders Company, 1999.

Henry, J. B. *Clinical Diagnosis and Management by Laboratory Methods,* 20th ed. Philadelphia, PA: W. B. Saunders Company, 2001.

Pagana, Kathleen Deska. *Mosby's Manual of Diagnostic and Laboratory Tests.* St. Louis, MO: Mosby, Inc., 1998.

Wallach, Jacques. *Interpretation of Diagnostic Tests,* 7th ed. Philadelphia: Lippincott Williams & Wilkens, 2000.

ORGANIZATIONS

National Institute of Diabetes and Digestive and Kidney Diseases (NIDDK). National Institutes of Health, Building 31, Room 9A04, 31 Center Drive, MSC 2560, Bethesda, MD 208792-2560. (301) 496-3583. http://www.niddk.nih.gov/health/kidney/kidney.htm.

National Kidney Foundation (NKF). 30 East 33rd Street, New York, NY 10016. (800)622-9020. http://www.kidney.org.

OTHER

National Institutes of Health. [cited April 5, 2003] http://www.nlm.nih.gov/medlineplus/encyclopedia.html.

National Institutes of Health. [cited June 29, 2003] http://www.nlm.nih.gov/medlineplus/ency/article/003005.htm.

Paula Ann Ford-Martin
Mark A. Best, M.D.

Kidney removal *see* **Nephrectomy**

Kidney transplantation

Definition

Kidney transplantation is a surgical procedure to remove a healthy, functioning kidney from a living or brain-dead donor and implant it into a patient with non-functioning kidneys.

Kidney transplantation

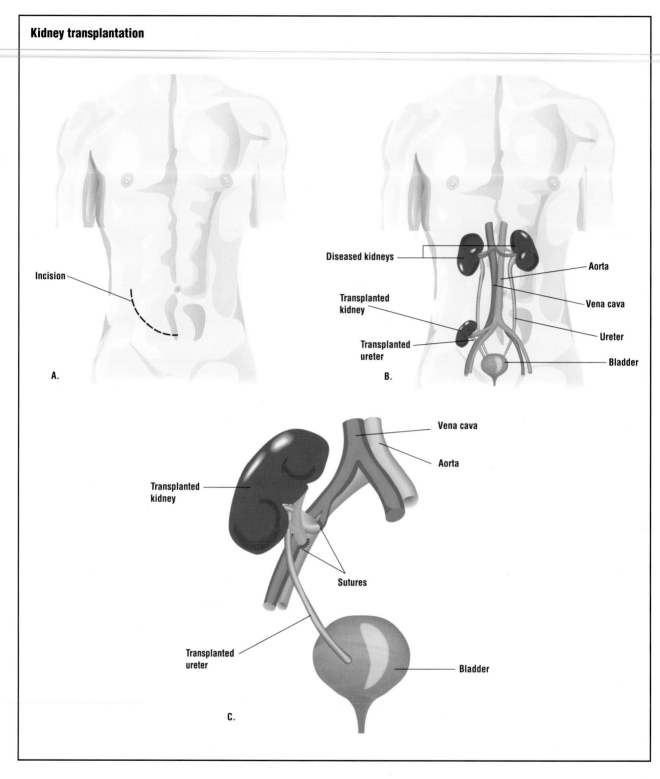

Incision

A.

Diseased kidneys

Transplanted kidney

Transplanted ureter

Aorta

Vena cava

Ureter

Bladder

B.

Vena cava

Aorta

Transplanted kidney

Sutures

Transplanted ureter

Bladder

C.

For a kidney transplant, an incision is made in the lower abdomen (A). The donor kidney is connected to the patient's blood supply lower in the abdomen than the native kidneys, which are usually left in place (B). A transplanted ureter connects the donor kidney to the patient's bladder (C). *(Illustration by GGS Information Services. Cengage Learning, Gale.)*

Purpose

Kidney transplantation is performed on patients with chronic kidney failure, or end-stage renal disease (ESRD). ESRD occurs when a disease, disorder, or congenital condition damages the kidneys so that they are no longer capable of adequately removing fluids and wastes from the body or of maintaining the proper level of certain kidney-regulated chemicals in the bloodstream. Without long-term dialysis or a kidney transplant, ESRD is fatal.

Demographics

Diabetes mellitus is the leading single cause of ESRD. Hypertension (high blood pressure) is the second leading cause of ESRD in adults, followed by glomerulonephritis. African Americans are more likely to develop hypertension-related ESRD than Caucasians and Hispanics. People of Native American and Hispanic descent are at an elevated risk for both kidney disease and diabetes.

Among children and young adults under 20 on dialysis, glomerulonephritis is the leading cause of ESRD, followed by hereditary, cystic, and congenital diseases account. According to USRDS, the average waiting period for a kidney transplant for patients under age 20 is 10 months, compared to the adult wait of approximately two years.

Description

Kidney transplantation involves surgically attaching a functioning kidney, or graft, from a brain-dead organ donor (a cadaver transplant) or from a living donor to a patient with ESRD. Living donors may be related or unrelated to the patient, but a related donor has a better chance of having a kidney that is a stronger biological match for the patient.

Open nephrectomy

The surgical procedure to remove a kidney from a living donor is called a **nephrectomy**. In a traditional, open nephrectomy, the kidney donor is administered **general anesthesia** and a 6–10-in (15.2–25.4-cm) incision through several layers of muscle is made on the side or front of the abdomen. The blood vessels connecting the kidney to the donor are cut and clamped, and the ureter is also cut and clamped between the bladder and kidney. The kidney and an attached section of ureter are removed from the donor. The vessels and ureter in the donor are then tied off and the incision is sutured together again. A similar procedure

---

is used to harvest cadaver kidneys, although both kidneys are typically removed at once, and blood and cell samples for tissue typing are also taken.

Laparoscopic nephrectomy

Laparoscopic nephrectomy is a form of minimally invasive surgery using instruments on long, narrow rods to view, cut, and remove the donor kidney. The surgeon views the kidney and surrounding tissue with a flexible videoscope. The videoscope and **surgical instruments** are maneuvered through four small incisions in the abdomen, and carbon dioxide is pumped into the abdominal cavity to inflate it for an improved visualization of the kidney. Once the kidney is freed, it is secured in a bag and pulled through a fifth incision, approximately 3 in (7.6 cm) wide, in the front of the abdominal wall below the navel. Although this surgical technique takes slightly longer than an open nephrectomy, studies have shown that it promotes a faster recovery time, shorter hospital stays, and less postoperative pain for kidney donors.

A modified laparoscopic technique called hand-assisted laparoscopic nephrectomy may also be used to remove the kidney. In the hand-assisted surgery, a small incision of 3–5 in (7.6–12.7 cm) is made in the patient's abdomen. The incision allows the surgeon to place his hand in the abdominal cavity using a special surgical glove that also maintains a seal for the inflation of the abdominal cavity with carbon dioxide. The technique gives the surgeon the benefit of using his or her hands to feel the kidney and related structures. The kidney is then removed through the incision by hand instead of with a bag.

Once removed, kidneys from live donors and cadavers are placed on ice and flushed with a cold preservative solution. The kidney can be preserved in this solution for 24–48 hours until the transplant takes place. The sooner the transplant takes place after harvesting the kidney, the better the chances are for proper functioning.

Kidney transplantation

During the transplant operation, the kidney recipient is typically under general anesthesia and administered **antibiotics** to prevent possible infection. A catheter is placed in the bladder before surgery begins. An incision is made in the flank of the patient, and the surgeon implants the kidney above the pelvic bone and below the existing, non-functioning kidney by suturing the kidney artery and vein to the patient's iliac artery and vein. The ureter of the new kidney is attached directly to the kidney recipient's bladder. Once the new kidney is attached, the patient's existing, diseased kidneys may or may not be removed, depending on the circumstances surrounding the kidney failure. Barring any complications, the transplant operation takes about three to four hours.

Since 1973, **Medicare** has picked up 80% of ESRD treatment costs, including the costs of transplantation for both the kidney donor and the recipient. Medicare also covers 80% of immunosuppressive medication costs for up to three years. To qualify for Medicare ESRD benefits, a patient must be insured or eligible for benefits under Social Security, or be a spouse or child of an eligible American. Private insurance and state **Medicaid** programs often cover the remaining 20% of treatment costs.

Patients with a history of heart disease, lung disease, cancer, or hepatitis may not be suitable candidates for receiving a kidney transplant.

Diagnosis/Preparation

Patients with chronic renal disease who need a transplant and do not have a living donor registered with United Network for Organ Sharing (UNOS) to be placed on a waiting list for a cadaver kidney transplant. UNOS is a non-profit organization that is under contract with the federal government to administer the Organ Procurement and Transplant Network (OPTN) and the national Scientific Registry of Transplant Recipients (SRTR).

Kidney allocation is based on a mathematical formula that awards points for factors that can affect a successful transplant, such as time spent on the transplant list, the patient's health status, and age. The most important part of the equation is that the kidney be compatible with the patient's body. A human kidney has a set of six antigens, substances that stimulate the production of antibodies. (Antibodies then attach to cells they recognize as foreign and attack them.) Donors are tissue matched for 0–6 of the antigens, and compatibility is determined by the number and strength of those matched pairs. Blood type matching is also important. Patients with a living donor who is a close relative have the best chance of a close match.

Before being placed on the transplant list, potential kidney recipients must undergo a comprehensive physical evaluation. In addition to the compatibility testing, radiological tests, urine tests, and a psychological evaluation will be performed. A panel of reactive antibody (PRA) is performed by mixing the patient's serum (white blood cells) with serum from a panel of 60 randomly selected donors. The patient's PRA sensitivity is determined by how many of these random samples his or her serum reacts with; for example, a reaction to the antibodies of six of the samples would mean a PRA of 10%. High reactivity (also called sensitization) means that the recipient would likely reject a transplant from the donor. The more reactions, the higher the PRA and the lower the chances of an overall match from the general population. Patients with a high PRA face a much longer waiting period for a suitable kidney match.

Potential living kidney donors also undergo a complete medical history and **physical examination** to evaluate their suitability for donation. Extensive blood tests are performed on both donor and recipient. The blood samples are used to tissue type for antigen matches, and confirm that blood types are compatible. A PRA is performed to ensure that the recipient antibodies will not have a negative reaction to the donor antigens. If a reaction does occur, there are some treatment protocols that can be attempted to reduce reactivity, including immunosuppresant drugs and plasmapheresis (a blood filtration therapy).

The donor's kidney function will be evaluated with a urine test as well. In some cases, a special dye that shows up on x rays is injected into an artery, and x rays are taken to show the blood supply of the donor kidney (a procedure called an arteriogram).

Once compatibility is confirmed and the physical preparations for kidney transplantation are complete, both donor and recipient may undergo a psychological or psychiatric evaluation to ensure that they are emotionally prepared for the transplant procedure and aftercare regimen.

Aftercare

A typical hospital stay for a transplant recipient is about five days. Both kidney donors and recipients will experience some discomfort in the area of the incision after surgery. Pain relievers are administered following the transplant operation. Patients may also experience numbness, caused by severed nerves, near or on the incision.

A regimen of immunosuppressive, or anti-rejection, medication is prescribed to prevent the body's immune system from rejecting the new kidney. Common immunosuppressants include cyclosporine, prednisone, tacrolimus, mycophenolate mofetil, sirolimus, baxsiliximab, daclizumab, and azathioprine. The kidney recipient will be required to take a course of **immunosuppressant drugs** for the lifespan of the new kidney. Intravenous antibodies may also be administered after **transplant surgery** and during rejection episodes.

Because the patient's immune system is suppressed, he or she is at an increased risk for infection. The incision area should be kept clean, and the transplant recipient should avoid contact with people who have colds, viruses, or similar illnesses. If the patient has pets, he or she should not handle animal waste. The transplant team will provide detailed instructions on what should be avoided post-transplant. After recovery, the patient will still have to be vigilant about exposure to viruses and other environmental dangers.

Transplant recipients may need to adjust their dietary habits. Certain immunosuppressive medications cause increased appetite or sodium and protein retention, and the patient may have to adjust his or her intake of calories, salt, and protein to compensate.

Risks

As with any surgical procedure, the kidney transplantation procedure carries some risk for both a living donor and a graft recipient. Possible complications include infection and bleeding (hemorrhage). A lymphocele, a pool of lymphatic fluid around the kidney that is generated by lymphatic vessels damaged in surgery, occurs in up to 20% of transplant patients and can obstruct urine flow and/or blood flow to the kidney if not diagnosed and drained promptly. Less

common is a urine leak outside of the bladder, which occurs in approximately 3% of kidney transplants when the ureter suffers damage during the procedure. This problem is usually correctable with follow-up surgery.

A transplanted kidney may be rejected by the patient. Rejection occurs when the patient's immune system recognizes the new kidney as a foreign body and attacks the kidney. It may occur soon after transplantation, or several months or years after the procedure has taken place. Rejection episodes are not uncommon in the first weeks after transplantation surgery, and are treated with high-dose injections of immunosuppressant drugs. If a rejection episode cannot be reversed and kidney failure continues, the patient will typically go back on dialysis. Another transplant procedure can be attempted at a later date if another kidney becomes available.

The biggest risk to the recovering transplant recipient is not from the operation or the kidney itself, but from the immunosuppressive medication he or she must take. Because these drugs suppress the immune system, the patient is susceptible to infections such as cytomegalovirus (CMV) and varicella (chickenpox). Other medications that fight viral and bacterial infections can offset this risk to a degree. The immunosuppressants can also cause a host of possible side effects, from high blood pressure to osteoporosis. Prescription and dosage adjustments can lessen side effects for some patients.

Normal results

The new kidney may start functioning immediately, or may take several weeks to begin producing urine. Living donor kidneys are more likely to begin functioning earlier than cadaver kidneys, which frequently suffer some reversible damage during the kidney transplant and storage procedure. Patients may have to undergo

PERIODICALS

Waller, J. R., et al. "Living Kidney Donation: A Comparison of Laparoscopic and Conventional Open Operations." *Postgraduate Medicine Journal* 78, no. 917 (March 2002): 153.

ORGANIZATIONS

American Association of Kidney Patients. 3505 E. Frontage Rd., Suite 315, Tampa, FL 33607. (800) 749-2257. E-mail: info@aakp.org. http://www.aakp.org.

American Kidney Fund (AKF). Suite 1010, 6110 Executive Boulevard, Rockville, MD 20852. (800) 638-8299. E-mail: helpline@akfinc.org. http://www.akfinc.org.

National Kidney Foundation. 30 East 33rd St., Suite 1100, New York, NY 10016. (800) 622-9010. http://www.kidney.org.

United Network for Organ Sharing (UNOS). 700 North 4th St., Richmond, VA 23219. (888) 894-6361. http://www.transplantliving.org.

United States Renal Data System (USRDS). USRDS Coordinating Center, 914 S. 8th St., Suite D-206, Minneapolis, MN 55404. (612) 347-7776. http://www.usrds.org.

OTHER

Infant Kidney Transplantation. Lucille Packard Children's Hospital. 725 Welch Road, Palo Alto, CA 94304. (650) 497-8000. http://www.lpch.org/clinicalSpecialtiesServices/COE/Transplant/KidneyTransplant/infantAdultToinfantKidneyTransplant.html.

A Patient's Guide to Kidney Transplant Surgery. University of Southern California Kidney Transplant Program. http://www.kidneytransplant.org/patientguide/index.html.

Paula Anne Ford-Martin

> ### QUESTIONS TO ASK THE DOCTOR
>
> - How many kidney transplants have both you and the hospital performed?
> - What are your transplant success rates? How about those of the hospital?
> - Who will be on my transplant team?
> - Can I get on the waiting list at more than one hospital?
> - Will my transplant be performed with a laparoscopic or an open nephrectomy?
> - What type of immunosuppressive drugs will I be on post-transplant?

dialysis for several weeks while their new kidney establishes an acceptable level of functioning.

Studies have shown that after they recover from surgery, kidney donors typically have no long-term complications from the loss of one kidney, and their remaining kidney will increase its functioning to compensate for the loss of the other.

Morbidity and mortality rates

Survival rates for patients undergoing kidney transplants are 89–98% one year post-transplant, and 67.4–91.4% five years after transplant. About 4,000 patients on the transplant waiting list die annually while awaiting a kidney. The success of a kidney transplant graft depends on the strength of the match between donor and recipient and the source of the kidney. Transplantations using living donor kidneys have a higher rate of success than do cadaver kidney transplantations.

Alternatives

Patients who develop chronic kidney failure must either go on dialysis treatment or receive a kidney transplant to survive.

Resources

BOOKS

Brenner, B. M., et al. *Brenner & Rector's The Kidney.* 7th ed. Philadelphia: Saunders, 2004.

Khatri, V. P. and J. A. Asensio. *Operative Surgery Manual.* 1st ed. Philadelphia: Saunders, 2003.

Townsend, C. M., et al. *Sabiston Textbook of Surgery.* 17th ed. Philadelphia: Saunders, 2004.

Knee arthroscopic surgery

Definition

Knee **arthroscopic surgery** is a procedure performed through small incisions in the skin to repair injuries to tissues such as ligaments, cartilage, or bone within the knee joint area. The surgery is conducted with the aid of an arthroscope, which is a very small instrument guided by a lighted scope attached to a television monitor. Other instruments are inserted through three incisions around the knee. Arthroscopic surgeries range from minor procedures such as flushing or smoothing out bone surfaces or tissue fragments (lavage and **debridement**) associated with osteoarthritis, to the realignment of a dislocated knee and ligament grafting surgeries. The range of surgeries represents very different procedures, risks, and aftercare requirements.

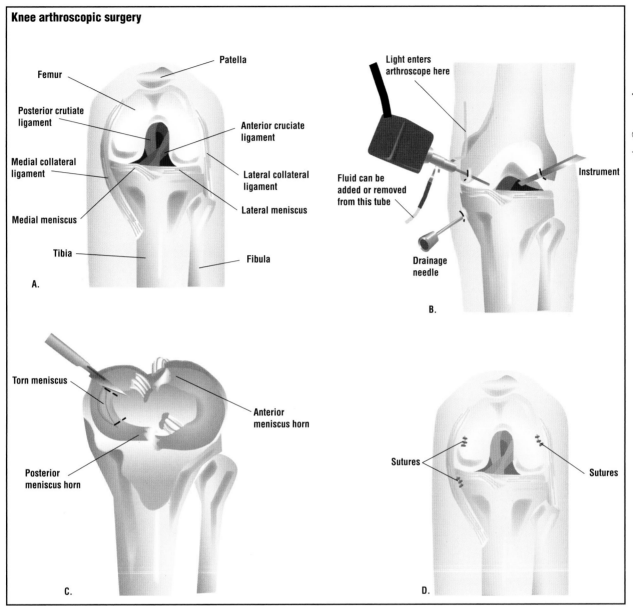

Knee arthroscopic surgery

A.
- Femur
- Patella
- Posterior crutiate ligament
- Anterior cruciate ligament
- Medial collateral ligament
- Lateral collateral ligament
- Medial meniscus
- Lateral meniscus
- Tibia
- Fibula

B.
- Light enters arthroscope here
- Instrument
- Fluid can be added or removed from this tube
- Drainage needle

C.
- Torn meniscus
- Anterior meniscus horn
- Posterior meniscus horn

D.
- Sutures
- Sutures

Step A shows the anatomy of the knee from the front with the leg bent. To repair a torn meniscus, three small incisions are made into the knee to admit laparoscopic instruments (B). Fluid is injected into the joint to aid in the operation. The injury is visualized via the instruments, and the torn area is removed (C). *(Illustration by GGS Information Services. Cengage Learning, Gale.)*

While the clear advantages of arthrocopic surgery lie in surgery with less anesthetic, less cutting, and less recovery time, this surgery nonetheless requires a very thorough examination of the causes of knee injury or pain prior to a decision for surgery.

Purpose

There are many procedures that currently fall under the general surgical category of knee arthroscopy. They fall into roughly two groups—acute injuries that destabilize the knee, and **pain management** for floating or displaced cartilage and rough bone. Acute injuries are usually the result of traumatic injury to the knee tissues such as ligaments and cartilage through accidents, sports movements, and some overuse causes. Acute injuries involve damage to the mechanical features, including ligaments and patella of the knee. These injuries can result in knee instability, severe knee dislocations, and complete lack of knee mobility. Ligament, tendon, and patella placements are key elements of the surgery. The type of

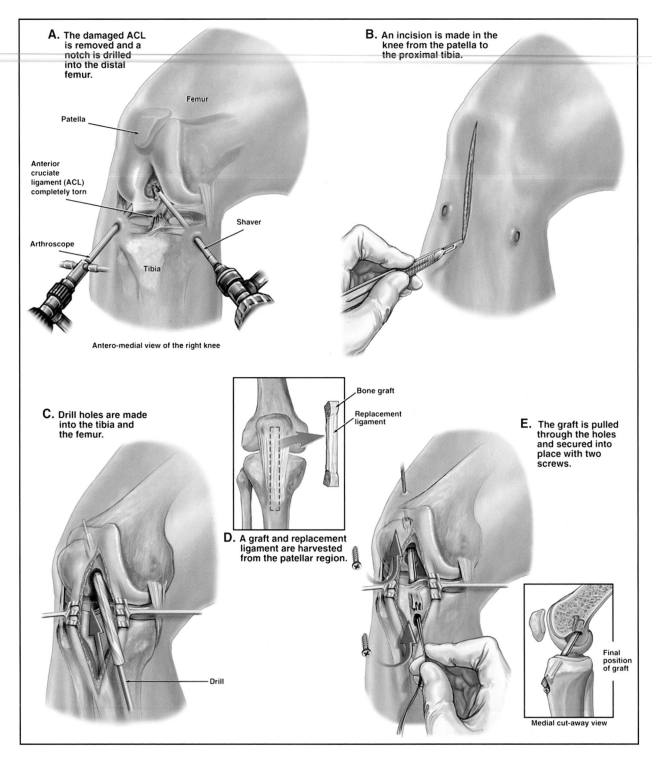

A. The damaged ACL is removed and a notch is drilled into the distal femur.

Femur

Patella

Anterior cruciate ligament (ACL) completely torn

Arthroscope

Shaver

Tibia

Antero-medial view of the right knee

B. An incision is made in the knee from the patella to the proximal tibia.

C. Drill holes are made into the tibia and the femur.

Bone graft

Replacement ligament

D. A graft and replacement ligament are harvested from the patellar region.

Drill

E. The graft is pulled through the holes and secured into place with two screws.

Final position of graft

Medial cut-away view

The surgical reconstruction of the anterior cruciate ligament of the knee. *(Nucleus Medical Art, Inc./Alamy)*

treatment for acute injuries depends in large part on a strict grading system that rates the injury. For instance, grades I and II call for rest, support by crutches or leg brace, pain management, and rehabilitation. Grades III and IV indicate the need for surgery. Acute injuries to the four stabilizing ligaments of the knee joint—the anterior

Anterior cruciate ligament (ACL)—A crossing ligament that attaches the femur to the tibia and stabilizes the knee against forward motion of the tibia.

Knee surgery—Refers primarily to knee repair, replacement or revision of parts of the knee, both tissue and bond, and includes both arthroscopic and open surgeries.

Lateral release surgery—Release of tissues in the knee that keep the kneecap from tracking properly in its groove (sulcus) in the femur; by realigning or tightening tendons, the kneecap can be forced to track properly.

Meniscus—The fibrous cartilage within the knee joint that covers the surfaces of the femur and the tibia as they join the patella.

cruciate ligament (ACL), the posterior cruciate ligament (PCL), the medial collateral ligament (MCL), and the lateral collateral ligament (LCL)—as well as to the "tracking," or seating of the patella, can be highly debilitating.

Treatment of these acute injuries include such common surgeries as:

• Repairs of a torn ligament or reconstruction of the ligament.

• Release of a malaligned kneecap. This involves tendon surgery to release and fit the patella better into its groove.

• Grafts to ligaments to support smoother tracking of the knee with the femur.

Pain management surgeries, on the other hand, are used to relieve severe discomfort of the knee due to osteoarthritis conditions. These treatments aim at relieving pain and instability caused by more chronic, "wear and tear" kinds of conditions and involve minor and more optional surgical procedures to treat cartilage and bone surfaces. These include arthroscopic techniques to remove detached or obtruding pieces of cartilage in the joint space such as the meniscus (a fibrous cushion for the patella), to smooth aged, rough surface bone, or to remove parts of the lining of the joint that are inflamed.

Treatment distinctions between arthroscopic surgery for acute injuries and those for pain management are important and should be kept in mind. They have implications for the necessity for surgery, risks of surgery, complications, aftercare, and expectations for improvement. Arthroscopic surgery for acute injuries is less controversial because clear dysfunction and/or severe instability are measurable indications for surgery and

easily identifiable. Surgery indications for pain management are largely for chronic damage and for the milder grades or stages of acute injuries (severity Grade I and II). These are controversial due to the existence of pain management and rehabilitation alternatives. Arthroscopic surgery for pain management is currently under debate.

Demographics

More than five and a half million people visit orthopedic surgeons each year because of knee problems. Over 650,000 arthroscopic surgeries are performed annually; 85% of them are for knee surgery. One very common knee injury is a torn anterior cruciate ligament (ACL) that often occurs in athletic activity. The most common source of ACL injury is skiing. Approximately 350,000 people in the United States sustain a torn or ruptured ACL each year. Research indicates that ACL injuries are on the rise in the United States due to the increase in sport activity.

The incidence of ACL injuries in women is two to eight times greater than in men. While the exact causes are not clear, differences in anatomy, strength, or conditioning are thought to play major roles. Women also seem to be more prone to patella-femoral syndrome (PFS), which is the inability of the patella to track smoothly with the femur. PFS is due primarily to development of tendons that influence the ways in which the knee tracks in movement. It can also be due to misalignments to other parts of the lower body like foot pronation. Other ligament surgeries can be caused by injury or overuse.

Knee dislocations are a focus of recent research because of their increasing frequency. Incidences range from 0.001% to 0.013% of all patients evaluated for orthopedic injuries. Many of these injuries heal without treatment and go undetected. Many people with multiple traumas in accidents have knee dislocations that go undiagnosed. Knee dislocations are of special concern, especially in traumatic injury, because their early diagnosis is required if surgery is to be effective. Knee dislocations in the morbidly obese individuals often occur spontaneously and may be associated with artery injury. This surgery involves complications related to the obesity. Finally, knee dislocations have been reported to occur in up to 6% of trampoline-associated accidents.

Description

Arthroscopic surgery for acute injuries

The knee bone sits between the femur and the tibia, attached by four ligaments that keep the knee stable as the leg moves. These ligaments can be damaged or torn through injuries and accidents. Once damaged, they do not offer stability to the knee and can cause buckling, or allow the knee to "give way." Ligaments can also "catch" and freeze the knee or make the knee track in a different direction than its leg movement, causing the knee to dislocate. Traumatic injuries such as automobile accidents may cause more than one ligament injury, necessitating multiple repairs to ligaments.

Four arthroscopic procedures relate to damage to each of the four ligaments that stabilize the knee joint movement. The four procedures are:

- Anterior cruciate ligament (ACL). A front-crossing ligament attaching the femur to the tibia through the knee; this ligament keeps the knee from hyperextension or being displaced back from the femur. The ACL is a rather large ligament that can withstand 500 lbs (227 kg) of pressure. If it is torn or becomes detached, it remains that way and surgery is indicated. In the most severe cases, a graft to the ligament is necessary to reattach it to the bone. The surgery can use tissue from the patient, called an autograft, or from a cadaver, called an allograft. The patella tendon, which connects the patella to the tibia, is the most commonly used autograft. ACL reconstructive surgery involves drilling a tunnel into the tibia and the femur. The graft is then pushed through the tunnels and secured by stapling or sutures.

- Posterior cruciate ligament (PCL). A back-crossing ligament that attaches the front of the femur to back of the tibia behind the knee that keeps the knee from hyperextension or being displaced backward. PCL injuries are not as frequent as ACL injuries. These injuries are largely due to falls directly on the knee or hitting the knee on the dashboard of a car in an accident. Both displace the tibia too far back and tear the ligament. Surgery to the PCL is rare, because the tear can usually be treated with rest and with rehabilitation. If surgery is required, it is usually to reattach the PCL to the tibia bone.

- Medial collateral ligament (MCL). This is an inside lateral ligament connecting the femur and tibia and stabilizing the knee against lateral dislocation to the left or to the right. The injury is usually due to external pressure against the inside of the knee. In the case of a grade I or II collateral ligament tear, doctors are likely to brace the knee for four to six weeks. A grade III tear may require surgery to repair ligament tear and is followed by three months of bracing. Physical therapy may be necessary before resuming full activity.

- Lateral collateral ligament (LCL). An outside lateral ligament connecting the femur and tibia and stabilizing the knee against lateral dislocation. In the case of a grade I or II collateral ligament tear, doctors are likely to brace the knee for four to six weeks. A Grade III tear may require surgery to reattach the ligament to bone. Surgery will be followed by three months of bracing. Physical therapy may be necessary before resuming full activity.

Patello-femoral syndrome (PFS)

The patella rests in a groove on the femur. Anything but a good fit can cause the patella to be unstable in its movement and very painful. Some individuals have chronic problems with the proper tracking of the patella with the femur. This may be associated with conditions related to physical features like foot pronation, or to types of body development in exercising or overuse of muscles. In the case of damage, an examination of the cartilage surrounding the patella can identify cartilage that increases friction as the patella moves. Smoothing the damaged cartilage can increase the ease of movement and eliminate pain. Finally, a tendon can occasionally make the patella track off center of the femur. By moving where the tendon is attached through lateral release surgery, the patella can be forced back into its groove.

Pain management with lavage and debridement

In addition to the ligament and patella surgeries that are largely required for traumatic injuries, arthroscopic surgery treats the wear and tear injuries related to a torn meniscus, which is the crescent-shaped cartilage that cushions the knee, as well as injuries to the surface of bone that makes joint movement painful. These are related to osteoarthritis and rheumatoid arthritis.

In lavage and debridement, the surgeon identifies floating or displaced tissue pieces and either flushes them out with a solution applied with arthroscopy or smoothes the surface of bone to decrease pain. These two surgical treatments are controversial because research has not indicated that alternatives to surgery are not as successful.

All of the above procedures are conducted through the visualization offered by the lighted arthroscope that allows the surgeon to follow the surgery on a television monitor. Instruments only about 0.15 in (4 mm) thick are inserted in a triangular fashion around the knee. The arthroscope goes in one incision, and instruments to cut and/or smooth and to engage in other maneuvers are put through the other incisions. In this fashion, the surgeon has magnification, perspective, and the ability to make tiny adjustments to the tissue without open surgery. The triangular approach is highly effective and safe.

Diagnosis/Preparation

Disease and injury can damage joints, ligaments, cartilage, and bone surfaces. Because the knee carries most of the weight of the body, this damage occurs almost inevitably as people age, due to sports injuries and through accidents.

The diagnosis of knee injuries or damage includes a medical history, **physical examination**, x rays, and the additional, more detailed imaging techniques with MRI or **CT scan**. Severe or chronic pain and/or knee instability initially brings the patient to an orthopedic physician. From there, the decision is made for surgery or for rehabilitation. Factors that influence the decision for surgery are the likelihood for repair and recovery of function, the patient's health and age, and, most importantly, the willingness of the patient to consider changes in lifestyle, especially as this relates to sport activity. Arthroscopic viewing is the most accurate tool for diagnosis, as well as for some repairs. The surgeon may provide only a provisional diagnosis until the actual surgery but will apprise the patient of the most likely course the surgery will take.

Arthroscopic surgery can be performed under local, regional, or general anesthetic. The type used depends largely upon the severity of damage, the level of pain after surgery, patient wishes, and patient health. The surgery is brief, less than two hours. After closing the incisions, the leg will be wrapped tightly and the patient is taken to recovery. For most same-day surgeries, individuals are allowed to leave once the anesthetic effects have worn off. Patients are not allowed to drive. Arrangements for pick up after surgery are mandated.

Unlike open surgery, arthroscopic surgery generally does not require a hospital stay. Patients usually go home the same day. Any crutches or canes required prior to surgery will be needed after surgery. Follow-up visits will be scheduled within about a week, at which point **dressings** will be removed.

Aftercare

Ligament- and patella-tracking surgeries

Arthroscopic surgery for severe ligament damage or knee displacement often involves ligament grafting. In some cases, this includes taking tissue from a tendon to use for the graft and drilling holes in the femur or tibia or both. Aftercare involves the use of crutches for six to eight weeks. A rehabilitation program for strengthening is usually suggested. Recovery times for resumed athletic activity are highly dependent on age and health. The surgeon often makes very careful assessments about recovery and the need for rehabilitation.

Patella-tracking surgeries offer about a 90% chance that the patella will no longer dislocate. However, many people have continued swelling and pain after surgery. These seem to be dependent upon how carefully the rehabilitation plan is developed and/or adhered to by the patient.

Lavage and debridement surgeries

Elevation of the leg after surgery is usually required for a short period. A crutch or knee immobilizer adds additional stability and assurance when walking. Physical therapy is usually recommended to strengthen the muscles around the knee and to provide extra support. Special attention should be paid to any changes to the leg a few days after surgery. Swelling and pain to the leg can mean a blood clot has been dislodged. If this occurs, the physician should be notified immediately. Getting out of bed shortly after surgery decreases the risk of blood clots.

Risks

The risks of arthroscopic surgery are much less than open surgery, but they are not nonexistent. The risk of any surgery carries with it danger in the use of anesthesia, including heart attacks, strokes, pneumonia, and blood clots. The risks are rare, but they increase with the age of the patient. Blood clots are the most common dangers, but they occur infrequently in arthroscopic surgery. Other risks include infections at the surgery site or at the skin level, bleeding, and skin scars.

Risks related specifically to arthroscopic surgery are largely ones related to injury at the time of surgery. Arteries, veins, and nerves can be injured, resulting in discomfort in minor cases and leg weakness or decreased sensation in more serious complications. These injuries are rare. One major risk of arthroscopic surgery to the knee for conditions related to tissue tears is that the pain may not be relieved by the operation; it may even become worse.

Normal results

Normal results of ligament surgery are pain, initial immobility and inflexibility, bracing of the leg, crutch dependence, with increasing mobility and flexibility with rehabilitation. Full recovery to the level of prior physical activity can take up to three months.

WHO PERFORMS THE PROCEDURE AND WHERE IS IT PERFORMED?

Surgery is performed by an orthopedic surgeon, a specialist in joint and bone surgery, trained in arthroscopic surgery. Arthoscopic surgery is usually performed in a general hospital with an outpatient operating suite.

QUESTIONS TO ASK THE DOCTOR

- Are there rehabilitation alternatives to this surgery?
- Will this surgery allow me to return to sports?
- How much success have you had with this surgery in eliminating pain?
- Is this injury one that I can live with if I pursue a change in lifestyle?
- How long will post-operative rehabilitation take and how can I help in moving it along faster?

With ACL surgery, pain in the front of the knee occurs in 10–20% of individuals. Limited range of motion occurs in less than 5% due to inadequate placement of the graft. A second surgery may be necessary.

Research indicates that the pain-relieving effects for arthroscopic partial menisectomy (removal of torn parts of cartilage) and debridement (the abrasion of cartilage to make it smooth) are not very reliable. Pain relief varies between 50% and 75%, depending upon the age, activity level, degree of damage, and extent of follow-up. One study indicates that the two surgical procedures, lavage and debridement, fared no better than no surgical procedure in relieving pain. The participants were divided into three groups for arthroscopic surgery: one third underwent debridement, a second third underwent lavage, and the remaining third likewise were anesthetized and had three incisions made in the knee area, though no procedure was performed. All three groups reported essentially the same results. Each had slightly less pain and better knee movement. The non-procedure had the best results. Debates about normal expectations from minor arthroscopic surgery continue with many surgeons believing that arthroscopic surgery of the knee should be restricted to acute injuries.

Morbidity and mortality rates

Complications occur in less than 1% of arthroscopic surgeries. Different procedures have different complications. In general, morbidity results mostly from medically induced nerve and vascular damage; **death** or amputations almost never occur. Graft infection may occur, along with other types of infection largely due to microbes introduced with instruments. The latter cases are becoming increasingly rare as the science of arthroscopic surgery develops.

Alternatives

Whether or not surgical treatment is the best choice depends on a number of factors and alternatives. Age and the degree of injury or damage are key to deciding whether to have surgery or rehabilitation. The physician calibrates the severity of acute injuries and either proceeds to a determined treatment plan immediately or recommends surgery. Alternatives for acute ligament injuries depend on the severity of injury and whether the patient can make lifestyle changes and is willing to move away from athletic activities. This decision becomes paramount for many people with collateral and cruciate injuries.

According to the American Association of Orthopedic Surgeons, conservative treatment for acute injuries involves RICE: Rest, Ice, Compression, Elevation, as well as a follow-up rehabilitation plan. The RICE protocol involves resting the knee to allow the ligament to heal, applying ice two or three times a day for 15–20 minutes, compression with a bandage or brace, and elevation of the knee whenever possible. Rehabilitation requires range-of-motion exercises to increase flexibility, braces to control joint immobility, **exercise** for quadriceps to support the front of the thigh, and upper thigh exercise with a bicycle.

For arthritis-related damage and pain management, anti-inflammatory medication, weight loss, and exercise can all be crucial to strengthening the knee to relieve pain. Evidence suggests that these alternatives work as well as surgery.

Resources

BOOKS

Canale, S. T., ed. *Campbell's Operative Orthopaedics*. 10th ed. St. Louis: Mosby, 2003.

DeLee, J. C. and D. Drez. *DeLee and Drez's Orthopaedic Sports Medicine*. 2nd ed. Philadelphia: Saunders, 2005.

PERIODICALS

Calvert, G. T. "The use of arthroscopy in the athlete with knee osteoarthritis." *Clinics in Sports Medicine* 24, no.1 (January 2005).

Day, B. "The indications for arthroscopic debridement for osteoarthritis of the knee." *Orthopedic Clinics of North America* 36, no. 4 (October 2005).

Heges, M. S., M. W. Richardson, and M. D. Miller. "The Dislocated Knee." *Clinics in Sports Medicine* 19, no. 3 (July 2000).

Moseley, J. B, et al. "A Controlled Trial of Arthroscopic Surgery for Osteoarthritis of the Knee." *New England Journal of Medicine* 347, no. 2 (July 11, 2002): 81–88.

ORGANIZATIONS

American Academy of Orthopaedic Surgeons (AAOS). 6300 North River Rd. Suite 200, Rosemont, IL 60018. (847) 823-7186 or (800) 346-2267; Fax: (847) 823-8125. http://www.aaos.org.

Arthritis Foundation. P.O. Box 7669, Atlanta, GA 30357-0669. (800) 283-7800. www.arthritis.org.

National Institute of Arthritis and Musculoskeletal and Skin Diseases Information Clearinghouse. 1 AMS Circle, Bethesda, MD 20892-3675. (301) 495-4484 or (877) 226-4267; Fax: (301) 718-6366; TTY: (301) 565-2966. http://www.nih.gov/niams.

OTHER

"Arthroscopic Knee Surgery No Better Than Placebo Surgery." *Medscape Medical News,* July 11, 2002. http://www.medscape.com.

"Arthroscopic Surgery." *Harvard Medical School Consumer Health.* http://www.intelihealth.com.

"Knee Arthroscopy Summary." Patient Education Institute. *National Library of Medicine, MedlinePlus.* http://www.nlm.nih.gov/medlineplus/tutorials/kneearthroscopy.

Nancy McKenzie, PhD

Knee osteotomy

Definition

Knee osteotomy is surgery that removes a part of the bone of the joint of either the bottom of the femur (upper leg bone) or the top of the tibia (lower leg bone) to increase the stability of the knee. Osteotomy redistributes the weight-bearing force on the knee by cutting a wedge of bone away to reposition the knee. The angle of deformity in the knee dictates whether the surgery is to correct a knee that angles inward, known as a varus procedure, or one that angles outward, called a valgus procedure. Varus osteotomy involves the medial (inner) section of the knee at the top of the tibia. Valgus osteotomy involves the lateral (outer) compartment of the knee by shaping the bottom of the femur.

Purpose

Osteotomy surgery changes the alignment of the knee so that the weight-bearing part of the knee is shifted off diseased or deformed cartilage to healthier tissue in order to relieve pain and increase knee stability. Osteotomy is effective for patients with arthritis in one compartment of the knee. The medial compartment is on the inner side of the knee. The lateral compartment is on the outer side of the knee. The primary uses of osteotomy occur as treatment for:

- Knee deformities such as bowleg in which the knee is varus-leaning (high tibia osteotomy, or HTO) and knock-knee (tibial valgus osteotomy), in which the knee is valgus leaning.
- A torn anterior cruciate ligament (ACL), which is a set of ligaments that connects the femur to the tibia behind the patella and offers stability to the knee on the left-right or medial-lateral axis. If this ligament is injured, it must be repaired by surgery. Many ACL injuries cause inflammation of the cartilage of the knee and result in bones extrusions, as well as instability of the knee due to malalignment. Osteotomy is performed to cut cartilage and increase the fit and alignment of the ends of the femur and tibia for smooth articulation. As one very common knee injury that often occurs in athletic activity, HTO is often performed when ACL surgery is used to repair the ligament. The combination of the two surgeries occurs primarily in young people who wish to return to a highly athletic life.
- Osteoarthritis that includes loss of range of motion, stiffness, and roughness of the articular cartilage in the knee joint secondary to the wear and tear of motion, especially in athletes, as well as cartilage breakdown resulting from traumatic injuries to the knee. Surgery for progressive osteoarthritis or injury-induced arthritis is often used to stave off total joint replacement.

Demographics

According to "Healthy People 2000, Final Review," published by the Centers for Disease Control and Prevention, the various forms of arthritis "the leading cause of disability in the United States" affect more than 15% of the total U.S. population (43 million persons) and more than 20% of the adult population. Osteoarthritis (OA) is the most common form of knee arthritis and involves a slowly progressive degenerative disease in which the joint cartilage gradually wears away. It most often affects middle-aged and older people. The most common source of ACL injury is skiing. Approximately 250,000 people sustain a torn or ruptured ACL in the United States each year. Research indicates that ACL injuries are on the rise in the United States due to the increase in sport activity.

Description

Osteotomy is performed as open surgery to the knee assisted by pre-operative arthropscopic diagnostic techniques. Surgery takes place on the tibia end or the femoral end at the knee according to whether the malalignment to be corrected is varus, or inward leaning, or valgus, outward leaning. The surgery involves the gaping or wedging of a piece of bone and its removal to change the pressure points of weight-bearing activity. The cut surfaces of the bone are held together with two **staples**, or a plate and screws. Other devices may be used, especially in tibial osteotomy where a fracture is involved. After surgery, a small plastic suction drain is left in the wound during recovery and early postoperative hospitalization.

Diagnosis/Preparation

Severe or chronic pain and/or knee instability brings the patient to an orthopedic physician. From there, the decision is made for surgery or for rehabilitation. Patients will undergo an examination and history with their physician. Once rehabilitation or other treatments are ruled out and surgery is indicated, the physician must assess for three factors: pain, instability, and knee alignment. Osteotomy is indicated if malalignment is a factor. **Debridement**, or the shaving of cartilage on the articulate femur or tibia, can usually resolve pain with instability problems. It must be determined whether the instability is related to malalignment and not to other sources such as ACL injury. Since the goal of osteotomy is to shift weight from a symptomatic cartilage to an asymptomatic area to relieve both an instability and pain due to excessive contact, alignment of the knee is assessed for pressure distribution along the mechanical axis and the loading axis. This requires an analysis of gait pattern, range of motion, localized areas of pain, and neurological factors, as well as other technical tests for anterior instability. A diagnostic arthroscopy—examination of the knee joint with a long tube attached to a video camera—is usually indicated before all knee osteotomies. Cartilage surfaces are examined for degenerative or late-stage arthritis. **Magnetic resonance imaging** (MRI) is useful in evaluating any intra-articular pathology such as bone chips, padding tears, or injuries to ligaments.

Aftercare

After surgery, patients are placed in a hinged brace. Toe-touching is the only weight-bearing activity allowed for four weeks in order to allow the osteotomy to hold its place. Continuous passive motion is begun immediately after surgery and physical therapy is used to establish full range of motion, muscle strengthening, and gait training. After four weeks, patients can begin weight-bearing movement. The brace is worn for eight weeks or until the surgery site is healed and stable. X rays are performed at intervals of two weeks and eight weeks after surgery.

Risks

The usual general surgical risks of thrombosis and heart attack are possible in this open surgery. Osteotomy surgery itself involves some risk of infection or injury during the procedure. Combined surgery for ACL and osteotomy has higher morbidity rates.

Normal results

Varus malalignment correction with osteotomy through the high tibia (HTO) is a proven and satisfactory operation. Success rates are high when the patient has a small angle deformity ($<10°$). Knees with more severe deformity have less satisfactory results. Tibial osteotomy for the less common valgus deformity is less satisfactory. Research indicates that only a few individuals are able to return to their previous level of high sports activity after a knee osteotomy, whether done with an ACL repair or not. However, more than half of patients in one study were able to return to leisure sports activities. Reports also indicate that those individuals who had osteotomy without ACL reconstruction had no differences in results with respect to measures of stability. It may take up to a year for the knee to be fully aligned and adapted to its new position after surgery. Most patients, more than 50%, gain

WHO PERFORMS THE PROCEDURE AND WHERE IS IT PERFORMED?

An orthopedic surgeon specializing in knee reconstruction surgery performs a knee osteotomy. Surgery takes place in a general hospital.

stability and are able to walk further than they could walk before osteotomy. However, according to one report, 13% of patients had severe pain or needed a total **knee replacement** after five years. In one European review, the results were better. Osteoarthritis was arrested in 105 cases (69%), with 47 cases showing deterioration. The main factors associated with further deterioration were insufficient correction and persistence of malalignment.

Morbidity and mortality rates

Morbidity rates include bleeding, inflammation of joint tissues, nerve damage, and infection.

Alternatives

For those individuals suffering from osteoarthritis, muscle-strengthening **exercise**, weight loss, and rehabilitation can be helpful in relieving pain and gaining stability. Anti-inflammatory medications can also be effective in helping pain and stability. For severe varus or valgus deformities, osteotomy or knee replacement may be indicated. For those with severe ACL injury with secondary trauma to knee cartilage, complete knee replacement may be suggested.

Resources

BOOKS

Canale, S. T. *Campbell's Operative Orthopedics*. St. Louis: Mosby, 2003.

Dutton, Mark. *Orthopaedic Examination, Evaluation, and Intervention*. New York: McGraw-Hill, 2004.

Ruddy, Shaun, et al., eds. *Kelly's Textbook of Rheumatology*, 6th ed. Philadelphia: WB Saunders Publishing, 2001.

Skinner, Harry. *Current Diagnosis & Treatment in Orthopedics*. New York: McGraw-Hill, 2006.

PERIODICALS

Alleyne, K. R., and M. T. Galloway. "Management of Osteochrondral Injuries of the Knee." *Clinics in Sports Medicine* 20, no. 2 (April 2001).

Shubin Stein, B. E., R. J. William, and T. L. Wickiewicz. "Arthritis and Osteotomies in Anterior Cruciate Ligament Reconstruction." *Orthopedic Clinics of North America* 34, no. 1 (January 2003).

QUESTIONS TO ASK THE DOCTOR

- Are there lifestyle changes, weight, diet, or rehabilitative factors that can help avoid this surgery?
- How many of your patients have been able to return to normal activities such as walking, running, and climbing stairs after surgery?
- How many of your patients have been able to return to exercise and to other athletic activities?
- Is this surgery just putting off my need for knee replacement surgery?
- How many of these surgeries have you performed?

ORGANIZATIONS

American Academy of Orthopaedic Surgeons. 6300 North River Road, Rosemont, IL 60018-4262. (847) 823-7186 or (800) 346-2267. http://www.aaos.org/wordhtml/home2.htm.

American College of Surgeons. 633 North Saint Claire Street, Chicago, IL 60611. (312) 202-5000. http://www.facs.org/.

American Society for Bone and Mineral Research. 2025 M Street, NW, Suite 800, Washington, DC 20036-3309. (202) 367-1161. http://www.asbmr.org/.

Arthritis Foundation. P.O. Box 7669, Atlanta, GA 30357-0669. (800) 283-7800. http://www.arthritis.org.

National Institute of Arthritis and Musculoskeletal and Skin Diseases Information Clearinghouse. 1 AMS Circle, Bethesda, MD 20892-3675. (301) 495-4484, Toll-Free (877) 226-4267. Fax: (301) 718-6366. TTY: (301) 565-2966. www.nih.gov/niams.

OTHER

"Osteotomy for Osteoarthritis." *WebMD Health*. http://www.webmd.com.

Nancy McKenzie, PhD
Laura Jean Cataldo, RN, EdD

Knee prosthesis surgery *see* **Knee revision surgery**

Knee replacement

Definition

Knee replacement is a procedure in which the surgeon removes damaged or diseased parts of the patient's knee joint and replaces them with new

Knee replacement

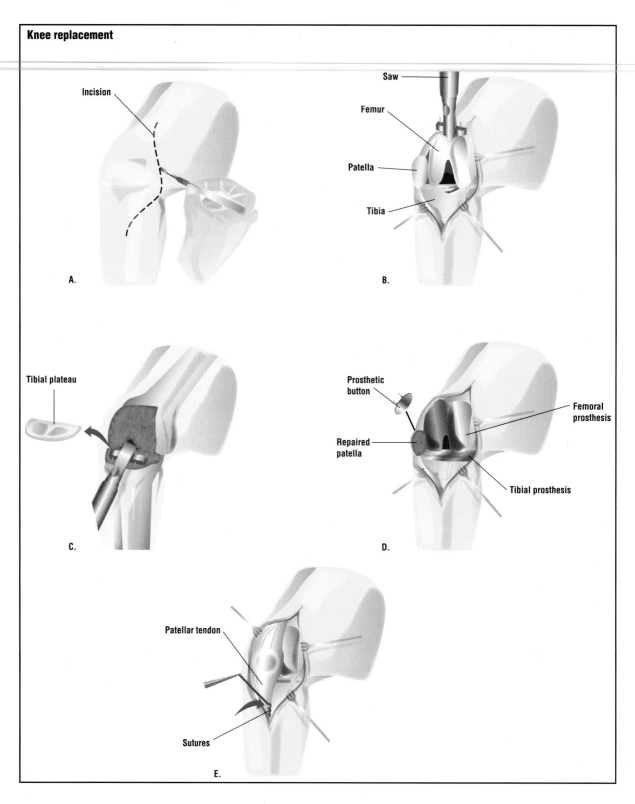

In a total knee replacement, an incision is made to expose the knee joint (A). The surfaces of the femur are cut with a saw to receive the prosthesis (B). The tibia is cut to create a plateau (C). The prostheses for the femur, tibia, and patella are put in place (D). The incision is closed (E). *(Illustration by GGS Information Services. Cengage Learning, Gale.)*

Analgesic—A medication given to relieve pain.

Arthroplasty—The medical term for surgical replacement of a joint. Arthroplasty can refer to hip as well as knee replacement.

Arthroscope—An instrument that contains a miniature camera and light source mounted on a flexible tube. It allows a surgeon to see the inside of a joint or bone during surgery.

Autologous blood—The patient's own blood, drawn and set aside before surgery for use during surgery in case a transfusion is needed.

Biomechanics—The application of mechanical laws to the structures in the human body, such as measuring the force and direction of stresses on a joint.

Bursitis—Inflammation of a bursa, which is a sac-like cavity filled with fluid that protects the tissues around certain joints in the body from friction. Bursitis of the knee frequently develops as a result of activities requiring frequent bending and kneeling, such as housecleaning.

Cartilage—A whitish elastic connective tissue that allows the bones forming the knee joint to move smoothly against each other.

Cortisone—A steroid compound used to treat autoimmune diseases and inflammatory conditions. It is sometimes injected into a joint to relieve the pain of arthritis.

Debridement—Surgical removal of foreign material and dead or contaminated tissue from a wound or the area of an incision.

Disease-modifying antirheumatic drugs (DMARDs)—A group of medications that can be given to slow or stop the progression of rheumatoid arthritis. DMARDs include such drugs as oral or injectable gold, methotrexate, leflunomide, and penicillamine.

Fibula—The smaller of the two bones in the lower leg.

Ligament—A band of fibrous tissue that connects bones to other bones or holds internal organs in place.

Meniscus (plural, menisci)—One of two crescent-shaped pieces of cartilage attached to the upper surface of the tibia. The menisci act as shock absorbers within the knee joint.

Nonsteroidal anti-inflammatory drugs (NSAIDs)—A term used for a group of analgesics that also reduce inflammation when used over a period of time. NSAIDs are often given to patients with osteoarthritis.

Orthopedics (sometimes spelled orthopaedics)—The branch of surgery that treats deformities or disorders affecting the musculoskeletal system.

Orthotics—Shoe inserts that are intended to correct an abnormal or irregular gait or walking pattern. They are sometimes prescribed to relieve gait-related knee pain.

Patella—The medical term for the knee cap. The patella is a triangular bone located at the front of the knee.

Prosthesis (plural, prostheses)—An artificial device that substitutes for or supplements a missing or damaged body part. Prostheses may be either external or implanted inside the body.

Quadriceps muscles—A set of four muscles on each leg located at the front of the thigh. The quadriceps straighten the knee and are used every time a person takes a step.

Tibia—The larger of two leg bones that lie beneath the knee. The tibia is sometimes called the shin bone.

artificial parts. The operation itself is called knee **arthroplasty**. Arthroplasty comes from two Greek words, *arthros* or joint and *plassein*, "to form or shape." The artificial joint itself is called a prosthesis. Most knee prostheses have four components or parts, and are made of a combination of metal and plastic, or metal and ceramic in some newer models.

Purpose

Knee arthroplasty has two primary purposes: pain relief and improved functioning of the knee joint. Because of the importance of the knee to a person's ability to stand upright, improved joint functioning includes greater stability in the knee.

Pain relief

Total knee replacement, or TKR, is considered major surgery. Therefore, it is usually not considered a treatment option until the patient's pain cannot be managed any longer by more conservative treatment. Alternatives to surgery are described below.

Pain in the knee may be either a sudden or gradual development, depending on the cause of the pain. Knee pain resulting from osteoarthritis and other degenerative disorders may develop gradually over a period of years. On the other hand, pain resulting from an athletic injury or other traumatic damage to the knee, or from such conditions as infectious arthritis or gout, may come on suddenly. Because the structure of the knee is complex and many different disorders or conditions can cause knee pain, the cause of the pain must be diagnosed before joint replacement surgery can be discussed as an option.

Joint function

Restoration of joint function and stability is the other major purpose of knee replacement surgery. It is helpful to have a brief outline of the major structures in the knee joint in order to understand the types of disorders and injuries that can make joint replacement necessary as well as to understand the operation itself.

The knee is the largest joint in the human body, as well as one of the most vulnerable. Unlike the hip joint, which is partly protected by the bony structures of the pelvis, the knee joint is not shielded by any other parts of the skeleton. In addition, the knee joint must bear the weight of the upper body as well as the stresses and shocks carried upward through the feet when a person walks or runs. Moreover, the knee is essentially a hinge joint, designed to move primarily backwards and forwards; it is not a ball-and-socket joint like the hip, which can swivel and rotate in a variety of directions. Many knee injuries result from stresses caused by twisting or turning movements, particularly when the foot remains in one position while the upper body changes direction rapidly, as in basketball, tennis, or skiing.

The normal knee joint consists of a bone, the patella or kneecap, and a set of tendons, ligaments, and cartilage disks that connect the femur, or thighbone, to the lower leg. There are two bones in the lower leg, the tibia, which is sometimes called the shinbone; and the fibula, a smaller bone on the outside of the lower leg. There are two collateral ligaments on the outside of the knee joint that connect the femur to the tibia and fibula respectively. These ligaments help to control the stresses of side-to-side movements on the knee. The patella—a triangular bone at the front of the knee—is attached by tendons to the quadriceps muscles of the thigh. This tendon allows a person to straighten the knee. Two additional tendons inside the knee stretch between the femur and the tibia to prevent the tibia from moving out of alignment with the femur. Cartilage, which is a whitish elastic tissue that allows bones to glide smoothly against each other, covers the ends of the femur, tibia, and fibula as well as the surfaces of the patella. In addition to the cartilage that covers the bones, the knee joint also contains two crescent-shaped disks of cartilage known as menisci (singular, meniscus), which lie between the lower end of the femur and the upper end of the tibia and act as shock absorbers or cushions. The entire joint is surrounded by a thick layer of protective tissue known as the joint capsule.

Disorders and conditions that may lead to knee replacement surgery include:

- Osteoarthritis (OA). Osteoarthritis is a disorder in which the cartilage in the knee joint gradually breaks down, allowing the surfaces of the bones to rub directly against each other. The patient experiences swelling, pain, inflammation, and increasing loss of mobility. OA most often affects adults over age 45, and is thought to result from a combination of wear and tear on the joint, lifestyle, and genetic factors. As of 2003, OA is the most common cause of joint damage requiring knee replacement.

- Rheumatoid arthritis (RA). Rheumatoid arthritis is a disease that begins earlier in life than OA and affects the whole body. Women are three times as likely as men to develop RA. Its symptoms are caused by the immune system's attacks on the body's own cells and tissues. Patients with RA often suffer intense pain even when they are not putting weight on the affected joints.

- Trauma. Damage to the knee from a fall, automobile accident, or workplace or athletic injury may trigger the process of cartilage breakdown inside the joint. Trauma is a common cause of damage to the knee joint. Some traumatic injuries are caused by repetitive motion or overuse of the knee joint; these types of injury include bursitis, or housemaid's knee, and so-called runner's knee. Other traumatic injuries are caused by sudden twisting of the knee, a direct blow to a bent knee, or being tackled from the side in football.

There are several factors that increase a person's risk of eventually requiring knee replacement surgery. While some of these factors cannot be avoided, others can be corrected through lifestyle changes:

- Genetic. Both OA and RA tend to run in families. One study done in France reported that the genetic factors affecting osteoarthritis in the knee can be traced back almost 8,000 years. Both OA and RA, however, are polygenic disorders, which means that more than one gene is involved in transmitting susceptibility to these forms of arthritis.

- Age. Knee cartilage becomes thinner and weaker with age, even in people who have no family history of arthritis.

- Sex. Women athletes have three times as many knee injuries as men. At present, orthopedic specialists are conducting studies to determine the cause(s) of this difference. Some doctors think it is related to the fact that most women have wider hips than most men, which results in a different pattern of stresses on the knee joint. Others think that the ligaments in women's knees tend to loosen more easily.

- Biomechanical. Biomechanics refers to the study of body structures in terms of the laws of mechanics, such as measuring the forces that affect the operation of a joint. Biomechanical studies have shown that people with certain types of leg or foot deformities, such as bowlegs or difference in leg length, are at increased risk of knee disorders because the stresses on the knee joint are not distributed normally.

- Gait-related factors. Gait refers to a person's pattern of motion when walking or running. Some people walk with their feet turned noticeably outward or inward; others tend to favor either the heel or the toe when they walk, which makes their gait irregular. Any of these factors can increase strain on the knee joint.

- Shoes. Poorly fitted or worn-out shoes contribute to knee strain by increasing the force transmitted upward to the knee when the foot strikes the sidewalk or other hard surface. They also introduce or increase irregularities in gait. Women's high-heeled shoes are particularly harmful to the knee joint because they do not cushion the foot; and they cause prolonged tightening and fatigue of the leg muscles.

- Work or other activities that involve jumping, jogging, or squatting. Jogging tends to loosen the ligaments that hold the parts of the knee joint in alignment, while jumping increases the shock on the knee joint and the risk of twisting or tearing the knee joint when the person lands. Squatting can increase the forces on the knee joint as much as eight times body weight.

Demographics

According to the American Academy of Orthopaedic Surgeons (AAOS), there are about 300,000 knee replacement operations performed each year in the United States. Although about 70% of these operations are performed in people over the age of 65, a growing number of knee replacements are being done in younger patients. Most surgeons expect to see the proportion of knee arthroplasties performed in younger patients continue to rise. One reason for this trend is improvements in surgical technique, as well as the design and construction of knee prostheses since the first knee replacement was performed in 1968. Minimaly invasive surgical techniques are allowing knee replacements to be performed with shorter recovery times, fewer complications, and less pain. A second reason is people's changing attitudes toward aging and their expectations of an active life after retirement. Fewer are willing to endure years of discomfort or resign themselves to a restricted level of activity.

In terms of gender and racial differences, women are slightly more likely to seek knee replacement surgery than men, and Caucasians in the United States are more likely to have the operation than African Americans. Researchers have suggested that one reason for the racial difference is a difference in social networks. People in general are influenced in their health care decisions by the experiences and opinions of friends or family members, and Caucasians are more likely than African Americans to know someone who has had knee replacement surgery.

Description

The length and complexity of a total knee replacement operation depend in part on whether both knee joints are replaced during the operation or only one. Such disorders as osteoarthritis usually affect both knees, and some patients would rather not undergo surgery twice. Replacement of both knees is known as bilateral TKR, or bilateral knee arthroplasty. Bilateral knee replacement seems to work best for patients whose knees are equally weak or damaged. Otherwise most surgeons recommend operating on the more painful knee first so that the patient will have one strong leg to help him or her through the recovery period following surgery on the second knee. The disadvantages of bilateral knee replacement include a longer period of time under anesthesia; a longer hospital stay and recovery period at home; and a greater risk of severe blood loss and other complications during surgery.

If the operation is on only one knee, it will take two to four hours. The patient may be given a choice of general, spinal, or epidural anesthesia. An epidural anesthetic, which is injected into the space around the spinal cord to block sensation in the lower body, causes less blood loss and also lowers the risk of blood clots or breathing problems after surgery. After the patient is anesthetized, the surgeon will make an incision in the skin over the knee and cut through the joint capsule. A standard incision may be used, or minimally invasive surgical techniques may dictate a more limited incision be utilized. In either case, the surgeon must be careful in working around the tendons and ligaments inside the joint. Knee replacement is a more complicated operation than **hip replacement** because the hip joint does not depend as much on ligaments for stability. The next step is cutting away the damaged cartilage and bone at the ends of the femur and tibia. The surgeon reshapes the end of the femur to receive the femoral component, or shell, which is usually made of metal and attached with bone cement.

After the femoral part of the prosthesis has been attached, the surgeon inserts a metal component into the upper end of the tibia. This part is sometimes pressed rather than cemented in place. If it is a cementless prosthesis, the metal will be coated or textured so that new bone will grow around the prosthesis and hold it in place. A plastic plate called a spacer is then attached to the metal component in the tibia. The plastic allows the femur and tibia to move smoothly against each other.

Lastly, another plastic component is glued to the rear of the patella, or kneecap. This second piece of plastic prevents friction between the kneecap and the other parts of the prosthesis. After all the parts of the prosthesis have been implanted, the surgeon will check them for proper positioning, make certain that the tendons and ligaments have not been damaged, wash out the incision with sterile saline solution, and close the incision.

Diagnosis/Preparation

Patient history

The first part of a diagnostic interview for knee pain is the careful taking of the patient's history. The doctor will ask not only for a general medical history, but also about the patient's occupation, **exercise** habits, past injuries to the knee, and any gait-related problems. The doctor will also ask detailed questions about the patient's ability to move or flex the knee; whether specific movements or activities make the pain worse; whether the pain is sharp or dull; its location in the knee; whether the knee ever buckles or catches; and whether there are clicking or popping sounds inside the joint.

Diagnostic tests

PHYSICAL EXAMINATION OF THE KNEE. Following the history, the doctor will examine the knee itself. The knee will be checked for swelling, reddening, bruises, breaks in the skin, lumps, or other unusual features while the patient is standing. The doctor will also make note of the patient's posture, including whether the patient is bowlegged or knock-kneed. The patient may be asked to walk back and forth so that the doctor can check for gait abnormalities.

In the second part of the **physical examination**, the patient lies on an examining table while the doctor palpates (feels) the structures of the knee and evaluates the strength or tightness of the tendons and ligaments. The patient may be asked to flex one knee and straighten the leg or turn the knee inward and outward so that the doctor can measure the range of motion in the joint. The doctor will also ask the patient to lie still while he or she moves the knee in different directions.

IMAGING STUDIES. The doctor will order one or more imaging studies in order to narrow the diagnosis. A radiograph or x ray is the most common, but is chiefly useful in showing fractures or other damage to bony structures. X-ray studies are usually supplemented by other imaging techniques in diagnosing knee disorders. A computed tomography, or CAT scan, which is a specialized type of x ray that uses computers to generate three-dimensional images of the knee joint, is often helpful in evaluating malformations of the joint. **Magnetic resonance imaging** (MRI) uses a large magnet, radio waves, and a computer to generate images of the knee joint. The advantage of an MRI is that it reveals injuries to ligaments, tendons, and menisci as well as damage to bony structures.

ASPIRATION. Aspiration is a procedure in which fluid is withdrawn from the knee joint by a needle and sent to a laboratory for analysis. It is done to check for infection in the joint and to draw off fluid that is causing pain. Aspiration is most commonly done when the knee has swelled up suddenly, but may be performed at any time. Blood in the fluid usually indicates a fracture or torn ligament; the presence of bacteria indicates infection; the presence of uric acid crystals indicates gout. Clear, straw-colored fluid suggests osteoarthritis.

ARTHROSCOPY. Arthroscopy can be used to treat knee problems as well as diagnose them. An arthroscope consists of a miniature camera and light source mounted on a flexible fiberoptic tube. It allows the surgeon to look into the knee joint. To perform an arthroscopy, the surgeon will make two to four small incisions known as ports. One port is used to insert the arthroscope; the second port allows insertion of miniaturized **surgical instruments**; the other ports drain fluid from the knee. Sterile saline fluid is pumped into the knee to enlarge the joint space and make it easier for the surgeon to view the knee structures and to cut, smooth, or repair damaged tissue.

Preoperative preparation

Knee replacement surgery requires extensive and detailed preparation on the patient's part because it affects so many aspects of life.

LEGAL AND FINANCIAL CONSIDERATIONS. In the United States, physicians and hospitals are required to verify the patient's insurance benefits before surgery and to obtain precertification from the patient's insurer or from **Medicare**. Without health insurance, the total cost of a knee replacement as of early 2003 can run as high as $38,000. In addition to insurance documentation, patients are legally required to sign an **informed consent** form prior to surgery. Informed consent signifies that the patient is a knowledgeable participant in making healthcare decisions. The doctor will discuss all of the following with the patient before he or she signs the form: the nature of the surgery; reasonable alternatives to the surgery; and the risks, benefits, and uncertainties of each option. Informed consent also requires the doctor to make sure that the patient understands the information that has been given.

MEDICAL CONSIDERATIONS. Patients are asked to do the following in preparation for knee replacement surgery:

- Get in shape physically by doing exercises to strengthen or increase flexibility in the knee joint. Specific exercises are described in the books listed below. Many clinics and hospitals also distribute illustrated pamphlets of preoperation exercises.
- Lose weight if the surgeon recommends it.
- Quit smoking. Smoking weakens the cardiovascular system and increases the risks that the patient will have breathing difficulties under anesthesia.
- Make donations of one's own blood for storage in case a transfusion is necessary during surgery. This procedure is known as autologous blood donation; it has the advantage of avoiding the risk of transfusion reactions or transmission of diseases from infected blood donors.
- Check the skin of the knee and lower leg for external infection or irritation, and check the lower leg for signs of swelling. If either is noted, the surgeon should be contacted for instructions about preparing the skin for the operation.
- Have necessary dental work completed before the operation. This precaution is necessary because small numbers of bacteria enter the bloodstream whenever a dentist performs any procedure that causes the gums to bleed. Bacteria from the mouth can be carried to the knee area and cause an infection.

- Discontinue taking birth control pills and any anti-inflammatory medications (aspirin or NSAIDs) two weeks before surgery. Most doctors also recommend discontinuing any alternative herbal preparations at this time, as some of them interact with anesthetics and pain medications.

LIFESTYLE CHANGES. Knee replacement surgery requires a long period of **recovery at home** after leaving the hospital. Since the patient's physical mobility will be limited, he or she should do the following before the operation:

- Arrange for leave from work, help at home, help with driving, and similar tasks and commitments.
- Obtain a handicapped parking permit.
- Check the house or apartment thoroughly for needed adjustments to furniture, appliances, lighting, and personal conveniences. People recovering from knee replacement surgery must avoid kneeling, and minimize bending, squatting, and any risk of falling. There are several good guides available that describe household safety and comfort considerations in detail.
- Stock up on nonperishable groceries, cleaning supplies, and similar items in order to minimize shopping.
- Have a supply of easy-care clothing with elastic waistbands and simple fasteners in front rather than complicated ties or buttons in the back. Women may find knit dresses that pull on over the head or wraparound skirts easier to put on than slacks or skirts that must be pulled up over the knees. Shoes should be slip-ons or fastened with Velcro.

Many hospitals and clinics now have "preop" classes for patients scheduled for knee replacement surgery. These classes answer questions about the operation and what to expect during recovery, but in addition they provide an opportunity for patients to share concerns and experiences. Studies indicate that patients who have attended preop classes are less anxious before surgery and generally recover more rapidly.

Aftercare

Aftercare following knee replacement surgery begins while the patient is still in the hospital. Most patients will remain there for five to 10 days after the operation. During this period the patient will be given fluids and antibiotic medications intravenously to prevent infection. Medications for pain will be given every three to four hours, or through a device known as a PCA (patient-controlled anesthesia). The PCA is a small pump that delivers a dose of medication into the IV when the patient pushes a button. To get the lungs back to normal functioning, a respiratory therapist will ask the patient to cough several times a day or breathe into blow bottles.

Aftercare during the hospital stay is also intended to lower the risk of a venous thromboembolism (VTE), or blood clot in the deep veins of the leg. Prevention of VTE involves medications to thin the blood; exercises for the feet and ankles while lying in bed; and wearing thromboembolic deterrent (TED) or deep vein thrombosis (DVT) stockings. TED stockings are made of nylon (usually white) and may be knee-length or thigh-length; they help to reduce the risk of a blood clot forming in the leg vein by putting mild pressure on the veins.

Physical therapy is also begun during the patient's hospital stay, often on the second day after the operation. The physical therapist will introduce the patient to using a cane or crutches and explain how to manage such activities as getting out of bed or showering without dislocating the new prosthesis. In most cases the patient will spend some time each day on a continuous passive motion (CPM) machine, which is a device that repeatedly bends and straightens the leg while the patient is lying in bed. In addition to increasing the patient's level of physical activity each day, the physical therapist will help the patient select special equipment for recovery at home. Commonly recommended devices include tongs or reachers for picking up objects without bending too far; a sock cone and special shoehorn; and bathing equipment.

Following **discharge from the hospital**, the patient may go to a skilled nursing facility, rehabilitation center, or home. Patients who have had bilateral knee replacement are unlikely to be sent directly home. Ongoing physical therapy is the most important part of recovery for the first four to five months following surgery. Most HMOs in the United States allow home visits by a home health aide, visiting nurse, and physical therapist for three to four weeks after surgery. Some hospitals allow patients to borrow a CPM machine for use at home for a few weeks. The physical therapist will monitor the patient's progress as well as suggest specific exercises to improve strength and range of motion. After the home visits, the patient is encouraged to take up other forms of low-impact physical activity in addition to the exercises; swimming, walking, and pedaling a stationary bicycle are all good ways to speed recovery. The patient may take a mild medication for pain (usually **aspirin** or ibuprofen) 30–45 minutes before an exercise session if needed.

The patient will be instructed to notify his or her dentist about the knee replacement so that extra precautions can be taken against infection resulting from bacteria getting into the bloodstream during dental work. Some surgeons ask patients to notify them whenever the dentist schedules a **tooth extraction**, root canal, or periodontal work.

Risks

Serious risks associated with TKR include the following:

- Loosening or dislocation of the prosthesis. The risk of dislocation varies, depending on the type of prosthesis used, the patient's level of activity, and the previous condition of the knee joint.
- Deep vein thrombosis (DVT). There is some risk (about 1.5% in the United States) of a clot developing in the deep vein of the leg after knee replacement surgery because the blood supply to the leg is cut off by a tourniquet during the operation. The blood-thinning medications and TED stockings used after surgery are intended to minimize the risk of DVT.
- Infection. The risk of infection is minimized by storing autologous blood for transfusion and administering intravenous antibiotics after surgery. The rate of infection following knee replacement is about 1.89%. Factors that increase the risk of infection after TKR include poor nutritional status, diabetes, obesity, a weakened immune system, and a history of smoking.
- Heterotopic bone. Heterotopic bone is bone that develops at the lower end of the femur after knee replacement surgery. It is most likely to develop in patients whose knee joints developed an infection. Heterotopic bone can cause stiffness and pain, and usually requires revision surgery.

Normal results

Normal results include relief of chronic pain in the knee and greater range of motion in the knee joint. Realistically, however, the patient should not expect complete restoration of function in the knee, and will usually be advised to avoid contact sports, skiing, jogging, or other athletic activities that strain the knee joint.

Mild swelling of the leg may occur for as long as three to six months after surgery. It can be treated by elevating the leg, applying an ice pack, and wearing compression stockings.

One commonplace side effect of TKR is that knee prostheses sometimes set off metal detectors in airports and high-security buildings because of their large metal content. Patients who fly frequently or whose occupations require security clearance should ask their doctor for a wallet card certifying that they have a knee prosthesis.

The patient can expect a cemented knee prosthesis to last about 10–15 years, although many still function well as long as 20 years later. Cementless prostheses have not been in use long enough for reliable evaluations of their long-term durability. When the prosthesis wears out or becomes loose, it is replaced in a procedure known as **knee revision surgery**.

Morbidity and mortality rates

A study published in 2002 reported that the 30-day mortality rate following total knee arthroplasty was 0.5%. The overall frequency of serious complications in this time period was 2.2%. This figure included 0.4% heart attack; 0.7% pulmonary embolism; and 1.5% deep venous thrombosis. The rate of complications was highest in patients over 70, and male patients were more likely to have heart attacks than women.

A 2001 study published by the Mayo Clinic reviewed the records of 22,540 patients who had had knee replacements between 1969 and 1997. The mortality rate within 30 days of surgery was 0.21%, or 47 patients. Forty-three of the 47 patients had had preexisting cardiovascular or lung disease. Patients who had had bilateral knee operations had a higher mortality rate than those who had not.

Alternatives

Nonsurgical alternatives

MEDICATION. The most common conservative alternatives to knee replacement surgery are **analgesics**, or painkilling medications. Most patients who try medication for knee pain begin with an over-the-counter NSAID such as ibuprofen (Advil). If the pain cannot be controlled by nonprescription analgesics, the doctor may give the patient cortisone injections, which relieve the pain of arthritis by reducing inflammation. Unfortunately, the relief provided by cortisone tends to diminish with each injection; moreover, the drug can produce serious side effects.

If the knee pain is caused by rheumatoid arthritis, a group of medications known as disease-modifying antirheumatic drugs, or DMARDs, may help to slow or stop the progress of the disease. They work by suppressing or interfering with the immune system. DMARDs include such drugs as penicillamine, methotrexate, oral or injectable gold, hydroxychloroquine, leflunomide, and sulfasalazine. DMARDs are

not suitable for all patients with RA, however, as they sometimes have serious side effects. In addition, some of them are slow-acting and may take several months to work before the patient feels some relief.

LIFESTYLE CHANGES. A second alternative to knee surgery is lifestyle changes. Losing weight helps to reduce stress on the knee joint. Giving up specific sports or other activities that damage the knee, such as jogging, tennis, high-impact aerobics, or stair-climbing exercise machines, may control the pain enough to make surgery unnecessary. Wearing properly fitted shoes and avoiding high heels and other extreme styles can also help to control pain and minimize further damage to the knee.

BRACES AND ORTHOTICS. Some patients with unstable knees are helped by functional braces or knee supports that are designed to keep the kneecap from slipping out of place. Orthotics, which are inserts placed inside shoes, are often helpful to patients whose knee problems are related to their gait. Orthotics are designed either to correct the position of the foot in order to keep it from turning too far outward or inward, or to correct problems in the arch of the foot. Some orthotics are made of soft material that cushions the foot and are particularly helpful for patients with osteoarthritis or diabetes.

Complementary and alternative (CAM) approaches

Complementary and alternative therapies are not substitutes for arthroscopy or joint replacement surgery, but some have been shown to relieve physical pain before or after surgery, or to help patients cope more effectively with the emotional and psychological stress of a major operation. Acupuncture, chiropractic, hypnosis, and mindfulness meditation have been used successfully to relieve the pain of osteoarthritis as well as postoperative discomfort. According to Dr. Marc Darrow, author of *The Knee Sourcebook*, a plant extract called RA-1, which is used in Ayurvedic medicine to treat arthritis, relieved pain and leg swelling in patients participating in a randomized trial. Alternative approaches that have helped patients maintain a positive mental attitude include meditation, **biofeedback**, and various relaxation techniques.

Alternative surgical procedures

Arthroscopy is the most common surgical alternative to knee replacement. It should be understood, however, as a way to postpone TKR rather than avoid it completely. The arthroscopic procedure most often used to treat knee pain from osteoarthritis is **debridement**, in which the surgeon cuts or scrapes away damaged structures or tissues until healthy tissue is reached. Most patients who have had arthroscopic debridement have been able to postpone TKR for three to five years.

Cartilage transplantation is a procedure in which small bone plugs with cartilage are removed from a part of the patient's knee where the cartilage is still healthy and transplanted to the area in which cartilage has been damaged. Another form of cartilage transplantation involves two operations, one to remove cartilage cells from the patient's knee for culture in a laboratory, and a second operation to place the new cells within the damaged part of the knee. The cultured cells are covered with a thin layer of tissue to hold them in place. After surgery, the cartilage cells multiply to form new cartilage inside the knee. Unfortunately, neither form of cartilage transplantation is usually beneficial to patients with osteoarthritis; transplantation has been most successful in treating patients whose knee cartilage was damaged by sudden trauma rather than by gradual degeneration.

Resources

BOOKS

Browner, B. D. et al. *Skeletal Trauma: Basic science, management, and reconstruction*. 3rd ed. Philadelphia: Elsevier, 2003.

Canale, S. T., ed. *Campbell's Operative Orthopaedics*. 10th ed. St. Louis: Mosby, 2003.

Darrow, Marc, MD, JD. *The Knee Sourcebook*. Chicago and New York: Contemporary Books, 2002.

DeLee, J. C. and D. Drez. *DeLee and Drez's Orthopaedic Sports Medicine*. 2nd ed. Philadelphia: Saunders, 2005.

Harris, E. D. et al. *Kelley's Textbook of Rheumatology*. 7th ed. Philadelphia: Saunders, 2005.

PERIODICALS

Alemparte, J., G. V. Johnson, R. L. Worland, et al. "Results of Simultaneous Bilateral Total Knee Replacement: A Study of 1208 Knees in 604 Patients." *Journal of the Southern Orthopaedic Association* 11 (Fall 2002): 153–156.

Blake, V. A., J. P. Allegrante, L. Robbins, et al. "Racial Differences in Social Network Experience and Perceptions of Benefit of Arthritis Treatments Among New York City Medicare Beneficiaries with Self-Reported Hip and Knee Pain." *Arthritis and Rheumatism* 47 (August 15, 2002): 366–371.

Chernajovsky, Y., P. G. Winyard, and P. S. Kabouridis. "Advances in Understanding the Genetic Basis of Rheumatoid Arthritis and Osteoarthritis: Implications for Therapy." *American Journal of Pharmacogenomics* 2 (2002): 223–234.

Crubezy, E., J. Goulet, J. Bruzek, et al. "Epidemiology of Osteoarthritis and Enthesopathies in a European Population Dating Back 7700 Years." *Joint, Bone, Spine: Revue du Rhumatisme* 69 (December 2002): 580–588.

Hasegawa, M., T. Ohashi, and A. Uchida. "Heterotopic Ossification Around Distal Femur After Total Knee Arthroplasty." *Archives of Orthopaedic and Trauma Surgery* 122 (June 2002): 274–278.

Mantilla, C. B., T. T. Horlocker, D. R. Schroeder, et al. "Frequency of Myocardial Infarction, Pulmonary Embolism, Deep Venous Thrombosis, and Death Following Primary Hip or Knee Arthroplasty." *Anesthesiology* 96 (May 2002): 1140–1146.

Parvisi, J., T. A. Sullivan, R. T. Trousdale, and D. G. Lewallen. "Thirty-Day Mortality After Total Knee Arthroplasty." *Journal of Bone and Joint Surgery*, American Volume 83-A (August 2001): 1157–1161.

Peersman, G., R. Laskin, J. Davis, and M. Peterson. "Infection in Total Knee Replacement: A Retrospective

Review of 6489 Total Knee Replacements." *Clinical Orthopaedics and Related Research* 392 (November 2002): 15–23.

Shah, S. N., D. J. Schurman, and S. B. Goodman. "Screw Migration from Total Knee Prostheses Requiring Subsequent Surgery." *Journal of Arthroplasty* 17 (October 2002): 951–954.

Silva, M., R. Tharani, and T. P. Schmalzried. "Results of Direct Exchange or Debridement of the Infected Total Knee Arthroplasty." *Clinical Orthopaedics and Related Research* 404 (November 2002): 125–131.

Wai, E. K., H. J. Kreder, and J. I. Williams. "Arthroscopic Debridement of the Knee for Osteoarthritis in Patients Fifty Years of Age or Older: Utilization and Outcomes in the Province of Ontario." *Journal of Bone and Joint Surgery*, American Volume 84-A (January 2002): 17–22.

ORGANIZATIONS

American Academy of Orthopaedic Surgeons (AAOS). 6300 North River Road, Rosemont, IL 60018. (847) 823-7186 or (800) 346-AAOS. http://www.aaos.org.

American Physical Therapy Association (APTA). 1111 North Fairfax Street, Alexandria, VA 22314. (703) 684-APTA or (800) 999-2782. http://www.apta.org.

Canadian Institute for Health Information/Institut canadien d'information sur la santé (CIHI). 377 Dalhousie Street, Suite 200, Ottawa, ON K1N 9N8. (613) 241-7860. http://secure.cihi.ca/cihiweb.

National Center for Complementary and Alternative Medicine (NCCAM) Clearinghouse. P.O. Box 7923, Gaithersburg, MD 20898. (888) 644-6226. TTY: (866) 464-3615. Fax: (866) 464-3616. http://www.nccam.nih.gov.

National Institute of Arthritis and Musculoskeletal and Skin Diseases (NIAMS) Information Clearinghouse. National Institutes of Health, 1 AMS Circle, Bethesda, MD 20892. (301) 495-4484. TTY: (301) 565-2966. http://www.niams.nih.gov.

Rush Arthritis and Orthopedics Institute. 1725 West Harrison Street, Suite 1055, Chicago, IL 60612. (312) 563-2420. http://www.rush.edu.

OTHER

American Academy of Orthopaedic Surgeons (AAOS) Patient Education Booklet #03057. *Total Knee Replacement*. Rosemont, IL: AAOS, 2001.

Canadian Institute for Health Information/Institut canadien d'information sur la santé (CIHI). *Total Hip and Total Knee Replacements in Canada, 2000/01*. Toronto, ON: Canadian Joint Replacement Registry, 2003.

Questions and Answers About Knee Problems. Bethesda, MD: National Institutes of Health, 2001. NIH Publication No. 01-4912.

University of Iowa Department of Orthopaedics. *Total Knee Replacement: A Patient Guide*. Iowa City, IA: University of Iowa Hospitals and Clinics, 1999.

Rebecca Frey, Ph.D.

Knee revision surgery

Definition

Knee revision surgery, which is also known as revision total knee **arthroplasty**, is a procedure in which the surgeon removes a previously implanted artificial knee joint, or prosthesis, and replaces it with a new prosthesis. Knee revision surgery may also involve the use of bone grafts. The bone graft may be an autograft, which means that the bone is taken from another site in the patient's own body; or an allograft, which means that the bone tissue comes from another donor.

Purpose

Knee revision surgery has three major purposes: relieving pain in the affected hip; restoring the patient's mobility; and removing a loose or damaged prosthesis before irreversible harm is done to the joint. Knee prostheses can come loose for one of two reasons. One is mechanical and is related to the fact that the knee joint bears a great deal of weight when a person is walking or running. It is unusual for the metal part of a knee prosthesis to simply break. This part, however, is inserted into the upper part of the tibia, the larger of the two bones in the lower leg, after the surgeon has removed the upper surface of the tibia. The bone tissue that receives the metal implant is softer than the bone that was removed, which means that the metal implant may sink into the softer bone and gradually loosen.

The second reason for loosening of a knee prosthesis is related to the development of inflammation in the knee joint. The plastic part of a knee prosthesis is made of a material called polyethylene, which can form small particles of debris as a result of wear on the prosthesis over time. If the patient has an uneven gait, or pattern of walking, the debris particles tend to form at a faster rate because one side of the prosthesis will tend to pull away from the bone and the other side will be pushed further into the bone. These tiny fragments of plastic are absorbed by tissue cells around the knee joint, which become inflamed. The inflammatory response begins to dissolve the bone around the prosthesis in a process known as osteolysis. As the osteolysis continues, bone loss accelerates and the prosthesis eventually comes loose.

A knee prosthesis that has become infected or completely dislocated must be removed and replaced to prevent permanent damage to the patient's knee.

KEY TERMS

Arthrodesis—A procedure that is sometimes used as an alternative to knee revision surgery, in which the joint is first fixed in place with a surgical nail and then fused as new bone tissue grows in.

Arthroscope—An instrument that contains a miniature camera and light source mounted on a flexible tube. It allows a surgeon to see the inside of a joint or bone during surgery.

Femur—The medical name for the thighbone.

Gait—A person's habitual pattern of walking. An irregular gait is a risk factor for knee revision surgery.

Heterotopic bone—Bone that develops as an excess growth around a joint following joint replacement surgery.

Impaction grafting—The use of crushed bone from a donor to fill in the central canal of the tibia during knee revision surgery.

Osteolysis—Dissolution and loss of bone resulting from inflammation caused by particles of polyethylene debris from a prosthesis.

Patella—The medical term for the knee cap. The patella is a triangular bone located at the front of the knee.

Prosthesis (plural, prostheses)—An artificial device that substitutes for or supplements a missing or damaged body part. Prostheses may be either external or implanted inside the body.

Tibia—The larger of two leg bones that lie beneath the knee. The tibia is sometimes called the shin bone.

Demographics

The demographics of knee revision surgery are somewhat difficult to evaluate because the procedure is performed much less frequently than total **knee replacement** (TKR). TKR itself is a relatively new operation; the first total knee replacement was performed in the United Kingdom in 1968 and the first TKR in the United States in 1970. Rates of prosthetic failure run at approximately 10% at 10 years, and 20% at 20 years post-surgery. Because of this high success rate, the number of patients who have had knee revision surgery yields a much smaller database than those who have had TKR. It is estimated that about 22,000 knee revision operations are performed in the United States each year; over half of them are done within two years of the patient's TKR.

Another difficulty in evaluating the demographics of knee revision surgery is the growing trend toward TKR in younger patients. As the number of knee replacement procedures done in younger patients continues to rise, the number of revision surgeries will increase as well. A study done in the United States in 1996 reported that women were almost twice as likely as men to have knee revision surgery, and that Caucasians were 1.5 times as likely as African Americans to have the procedure. This study, however, was limited to patients over the age of 65, so that its findings are not likely to be an accurate picture of younger patient populations.

Description

Most knee revision operations take about three hours to perform and are similar to knee replacement procedures. After the patient has been anesthetized, the surgeon opens the knee joint by cutting through the joint capsule. The first step in revision surgery is the removal of the old femoral component of the knee prosthesis. After the metal shell has been removed, the damaged bone at the end of the femur is scraped off and the femur is reshaped. If the bone is weak, the surgeon may decide to fill the cavity inside the femur with bone grafts. In some cases, metal wedges may be used to strengthen the attachment of the new femoral component.

After the new femoral component has been glued in place with bone cement, the old implant in the tibia is removed and the bone is reshaped to receive a new implant. If the old implant had loosened because it had moved downward into the softer tissue inside the tibia, the surgeon will pack the space with morselized bone from a donor before putting in the new implant. This technique is known as impaction grafting. The impaction grafting may be reinforced with wire mesh. If the tibia has been shortened by the removal of damaged bone, the surgeon will insert a wedge along with the new tibial implant and secure them to the end of the tibia with bone cement. A new plastic plate will be fastened to the tray at the top of the tibial implant so that the patient's femur can move smoothly over the tibia. If the patient's patella (kneecap) has been damaged, the surgeon will resurface its back surface and attach a plastic component to protect the patella from further bone loss. The tibial and femoral components of the prosthesis are then fitted together, the kneecap is replaced, and the knee tendons reattached with surgical wire. The knee joint is washed out with sterile saline fluid and the various layers of the incision closed.

Revision surgery on an infected knee requires two separate operations. In the first operation, the old prosthesis is taken out and a block of polyethylene cement known as a spacer block is inserted in the joint. The spacer block has been treated with **antibiotics** to fight the infection. The incision is closed and the spacer block remains inside the patient's knee for about six weeks. The patient is also given intravenous antibiotics during this period. After the infection has cleared, the knee is reopened and the new revision prosthesis is implanted.

Diagnosis/Preparation

In most cases, increasing pain, stiffness, and loss of mobility in the knee joint are early indications that the patient may benefit from revision surgery. The location of the pain may point to the part of the prosthesis that has been affected by osteolysis. Pain around or in the knee-cap is not always significant by itself because many TKR patients have occasional discomfort in that area after their knee replacement. If the pain is diffuse (felt throughout the knee rather than in only one part of the knee), it may indicate either an infection or loosening of the prosthesis. Pain felt throughout the knee accompanied by tissue fluid accumulating in the joint points to a problem with the polyethylene part of the prosthesis. Pain in the lower thigh or in the part of the leg just below the knee suggests that the metal plate attached to the femur or the metal implant in the tibia may have come loose.

The doctor may take risk factors into account in assessing the likelihood of a failed knee prosthesis. Six factors have been identified as increasing a patient's risk of needing revision surgery within two years of knee replacement surgery:

• age (Younger patients tend to be more active and to wear out knee prostheses more rapidly than older ones.)
• a long hospital stay for the original knee surgery
• concurrent diseases or disorders
• any type of arthritis
• surgical complications during the first knee operation
• having the first knee operation performed at an urban hospital

The doctor will then usually order a series of imaging tests to determine the location of the problem and the extent of bone loss. X-ray studies can be used to check for complete dislocation of the prosthesis as well as loosening. Computed tomography appears to be more effective in detecting the early stages of osteolysis than x-ray studies. If the doctor suspects that the knee prosthesis has become infected, he or she will aspirate the joint. Aspiration is a procedure in which fluid is withdrawn from a joint through a needle and

sent to a laboratory for analysis. The fluid will be cultured in order to identify the specific organism causing the infection.

Aftercare

Aftercare following knee revision surgery is essentially the same as for knee replacement, consisting of a combination of physical therapy, rehabilitation exercises, pain medication when necessary, and a period of home health care or assistance.

The length of recovery after revision knee surgery varies in comparison to the patient's first knee replacement. Some patients take longer to recover from revision surgery, but others recover more rapidly than they did from TKR, and they experience less discomfort. The reasons for this variation are not yet known.

Risks

The complications that may follow knee revision surgery are similar to those for knee replacement. They include:

• Deep vein thrombosis.
• Infection in the new prosthesis.
• Loosening of the new prosthesis. The risk of this complication is increased considerably if the patient is overweight.
• Formation of heterotopic bone. Heterotopic bone is bone that develops at the lower end of the femur following knee replacement or knee revision surgery. Patients who have had an infection in the joint have an increased risk of heterotopic bone formation.
• Bone fractures during the operation. These are caused by the force or pressure that the surgeon must sometimes apply to remove the old prosthesis and the cement that may be attached to it.
• Dislocation of the new prosthesis. The risk of dislocation is twice as great for revision surgery as for TKR.
• Difference in leg length resulting from shortening of the leg with the prosthesis.
• Additional or more rapid loss of bone tissue.

Normal results

Normal results of knee revision surgery are quite similar to those for TKR. Patients have less pain and greater mobility in the affected knee, but not complete restoration of the function of a normal knee. Between 5% and 20% of patients report some pain following either TKR or revision surgery for several years after their operation. Most patients, however, have considerably less discomfort in the knee after surgery than they did before the procedure. A recent British study found that revision knee surgery patients had the same positive results at six-month follow-up as patients who had had primary knee replacement surgery.

As with knee replacement surgery, patients who have had revision surgery may experience mild swelling of the leg for as long as three to six months after surgery. Swelling can be treated by elevating the leg, applying an ice pack, and wearing compression stockings.

Morbidity and mortality rates

The 30-day mortality rate following knee revision surgery is low, between 0.1% and 0.2%. The estimated rates of complications are as follows:

- deep infection: 0.97%
- loosening of the new prosthesis: 10–15%.
- dislocation of the new prosthesis: 2–5%.
- deep venous thrombosis: 1.5%

Alternatives

Nonsurgical alternatives

LIFESTYLE CHANGES. The American Association of Orthopaedic Surgeons (AAOS) has published a fact sheet about the effects of aging on the knee joint aimed at the baby boomer generation. Many adults in their 40s and 50s have been influenced by the contemporary emphasis on youthfulness to keep up athletic activities and forms of **exercise** that are hard on the knee joint. Some of them try to return to a high level of activity even after TKR. As a result, some surgeons are suggesting that adults in this age bracket scale back their athletic workouts or substitute low-impact forms of exercise. Good choices include water aerobics, tai chi, yoga, swimming, cycling, and walking.

COMPLEMENTARY AND ALTERNATIVE (CAM) APPROACHES. Complementary and alternative therapies are not substitutes for knee revision surgery, but some have been shown to relieve physical pain before or after surgery, or to help patients cope more effectively with the emotional and psychological stress of a major operation. Acupuncture, chiropractic, hypnosis, and mindfulness meditation have been used successfully to relieve postoperative discomfort following revision surgery. Alternative approaches that have helped patients maintain a positive mental attitude

WHO PERFORMS THE PROCEDURE AND WHERE IS IT PERFORMED?

Knee revision surgery is performed by an orthopedic surgeon, who is an MD and who has received advanced training in surgical treatment of disorders of the musculoskeletal system. Qualification for this specialty in the United States requires a minimum of five years of training after medical school. Most orthopedic surgeons who perform joint replacements and revision operations have had additional specialized training in these specific procedures.

In many cases, knee revision surgery is done by the surgeon who performed the original knee replacement operation. Some surgeons, however, refer patients to colleagues who specialize in revision procedures.

Knee revision surgery can be performed in a general hospital with a department of orthopedic surgery, but is also performed in specialized clinics or institutes for joint disorders.

include meditation, **biofeedback**, and various relaxation techniques.

Alternative surgical procedures

Arthroscopy is the most common surgical alternative to knee revision surgery. It is a procedure in which a surgeon makes three or four small incisions in the knee in order to insert a device that allows him or her to see the inside of the joint, insert miniaturized instruments to remove or repair damaged tissue, and drain fluid from the joint. Arthroscopy has been used successfully to treat stiffness in the knee following TKR and improve range of motion in the joint. It is not successful in treating infected prostheses unless it is used very early.

Other surgical alternatives to knee revision surgery include manipulation of the joint while the patient is under **general anesthesia**, and arthrodesis of the knee. Arthrodesis is a procedure in which the joint is fixed in place with a long surgical nail until the growth of new bone tissue fuses the knee. It is generally considered a less preferable alternative to knee revision surgery, but is sometimes used in the treatment of elderly patients with infected prostheses or weakened bone structure.

QUESTIONS TO ASK THE DOCTOR

- How many knee revision operations do you perform each year?
- Would I be likely to benefit from arthroscopy?
- What lifestyle changes can I make to extend the life of the new prosthesis?
- What are my chances of needing another revision operation in the future?

Resources

BOOKS

Browner, B. D. et al. *Skeletal Trauma: Basic science, management, and reconstruction.* 3rd ed. Philadelphia: Elsevier, 2003.

Canale, S. T., ed. *Campbell's Operative Orthopaedics.* 10th ed. St. Louis: Mosby, 2003.

Darrow, Marc, MD, JD. *The Knee Sourcebook.* Chicago and New York: Contemporary Books, 2002.

DeLee, J. C. and D. Drez. *DeLee and Drez's Orthopaedic Sports Medicine.* 2nd ed. Philadelphia: Saunders, 2005.

Harris, E. D. et al. *Kelley's Textbook of Rheumatology.* 7th ed. Philadelphia: Saunders, 2005.

PERIODICALS

Barrack, R. I., C. S. Brumfield, C. H. Rorabeck, et al. "Heterotopic Ossification After Revision Total Knee Arthroplasty." *Clinical Orthopaedics and Related Research* 404 (November 2002): 208–213.

Hartley, R. C., N. G. Barton-Hanson, R. Finley, and R. W. Parkinson. "Early Patient Outcomes After Primary and Revision Total Knee Arthroplasty. A Prospective Study." *Journal of Bone and Joint Surgery,* British Volume 84 (September 2002): 994–999.

Hasegawa, M., T. Ohashi, and A. Uchida. "Heterotopic Ossification Around Distal Femur After Total Knee Arthroplasty." *Archives of Orthopaedic and Trauma Surgery* 122 (June 2002): 274–278.

Incavo, S. J., J. W. Lilly, C. S. Bartlett, and D. L. Churchill. "Arthrodesis of the Knee: Experience with Intramedullary Nailing." *Journal of Arthroplasty* 15 (October 2000): 871–876.

Lonner, J. H., P. A. Lotke, J. Kim, and C. Nelson. "Impaction Grafting and Wire Mesh for Uncontained Defects in Revision Knee Arthroplasty." *Clinical Orthopaedics and Related Research* 404 (November 2002): 145–151.

Peersman, G., R. Laskin, J. Davis, and M. Peterson. "Infection in Total Knee Replacement: A Retrospective Review of 6489 Total Knee Replacements." *Clinical Orthopaedics and Related Research* 392 (November 2002): 15–23.

Shah, S. N., D. J. Schurman, and S. B. Goodman. "Screw Migration from Total Knee Prostheses Requiring Subsequent Surgery." *Journal of Arthroplasty* 17 (October 2002): 951–954.

Sharkey, P. F., W. J. Hozack, R. H. Rothman, et al. "Insall Award Paper: Why Are Total Knee Arthroplasties Failing Today?" *Clinical Orthopaedics and Related Research* 404 (November 2002): 7–13.

Teng, H. P., Y. C. Lu, C. J. Hsu, and C. Y. Wong. "Arthroscopy Following Total Knee Arthroplasty." *Orthopedics* 25 (April 2002): 422–424.

ORGANIZATIONS

American Academy of Orthopaedic Surgeons (AAOS). 6300 North River Road, Rosemont, IL 60018. (847) 823-7186 or (800) 346-AAOS. http://www.aaos.org.

American Physical Therapy Association (APTA). 1111 North Fairfax Street, Alexandria, VA 22314. (703)684-APTA or (800) 999-2782. http://www.apta.org.

Canadian Institute for Health Information/Institut canadien d'information sur la santé (CIHI). 377 Dalhousie Street, Suite 200, Ottawa, ON K1N 9N8. (613) 241-7860. http://secure.cihi.ca/cihiweb.

Center for Hip and Knee Replacement, Columbia University. Department of Orthopaedic Surgery, Columbia Presbyterian Medical Center, 622 West 168th Street, PH11-Center, New York, NY 10032. (212) 305-5974. www.hipnknee.org.

National Center for Complementary and Alternative Medicine (NCCAM) Clearinghouse. P.O. Box 7923, Gaithersburg, MD 20898. (888) 644-6226. TTY: (866) 464-3615. Fax: (866) 464-3616. http://www.nccam.nih.gov.

National Institute of Arthritis and Musculoskeletal and Skin Diseases (NIAMS) Information Clearinghouse. National Institutes of Health, 1 AMS Circle, Bethesda, MD 20892. (301) 495-4484. TTY: (301) 565-2966. http://www.niams.nih.gov.

Rothman Institute of Orthopaedics. 925 Chestnut Street, Philadelphia, PA 19107-4216. (215) 955-3458. http://www.rothmaninstitute.com.

OTHER

Questions and Answers About Knee Problems. Bethesda, MD: National Institutes of Health, 2001. NIH Publication No. 01-4912.

University of Iowa Department of Orthopaedics. *Total Knee Replacement: A Patient Guide.* Iowa City, IA: University of Iowa Hospitals and Clinics, 1999.

Rebecca Frey, Ph.D.

Kneecap removal

Definition

Kneecap removal, or patellectomy, is the partial or total surgical removal of the patella, commonly called the kneecap.

Purpose

Kneecap removal is performed under three circumstances:

- The kneecap is fractured or shattered.
- The kneecap dislocates easily and repeatedly.
- Degenerative arthritis of the kneecap causes extreme pain.

Demographics

A person of any age can break a kneecap in an accident. When the bone is shattered beyond repair, the kneecap has to be removed. No prosthesis or artificial replacement part is put in its place.

Dislocation of the kneecap is most common in young girls between the ages of 10–14. Initially, the kneecap will pop back into place of its own accord, but pain may continue. If dislocation occurs too often, or the kneecap does not go back into place correctly, the patella may rub the other bones in the knee, causing an arthritis-like condition. Some people are also born with birth defects that cause the kneecap to dislocate frequently.

Degenerative arthritis of the kneecap, also called patellar arthritis or chondromalacia patellae, can cause so much pain that it becomes necessary to remove the kneecap. As techniques of joint replacement have improved, arthritis in the knee is more frequently treated with total **knee replacement**.

People who have had their kneecap removed for degenerative arthritis and then later require a total knee replacement are more likely to have problems with the stability of their artificial knee than those who only have total knee replacement. This occurs because the realigned muscles and tendons provide less support once the kneecap is removed.

Description

General anesthesia is typically used for kneecap removal surgery, though in some cases a spinal or epidural anesthetic is used. The surgeon makes a linear incision over the front of the kneecap. The damaged kneecap is examined. If a part or the entire kneecap is

KEY TERMS

Degenerative arthritis, or osteoarthritis—A non-inflammatory type of arthritis, usually occurring in older people, characterized by degeneration of cartilage, enlargement of the margins of the bones, and changes in the membranes in the joints.

Patella—The knee cap; the quadriceps tendon attaches to it above and the patellar tendon below.

Patellectomy—Surgical removal of the patella, or kneecap removal.

so severely damaged that it cannot be repaired, it may be partially removed (partial patellectomy) or totally removed (full patellectomy). If kneecap removal is total, the muscles and tendons attached to the kneecap are cut and the kneecap is removed. However, the quadriceps tendon above the kneecap, the patellar tendon below, and the other soft tissues around the kneecap are preserved so that the patient may still be able to extend the knee after surgery. Next, the muscles are sewn back together, and the skin is closed with sutures or clips that stay in place for about two weeks.

Diagnosis/Preparation

Prior to surgery, x rays and other diagnostic tests are done on the knee to determine if removing the kneecap is the appropriate treatment. Preoperative blood and urine tests are also done.

Patients are asked not to eat or drink anything after midnight on the night before surgery. On the day of surgery, patients are directed to the hospital or clinic holding area where the final preparations are made. The knee area is usually shaved and the patient is asked to change into a hospital gown and to remove all jewelry, watches, dentures, and glasses.

Aftercare

Pain medication may be prescribed for a few days. The patient will initially need to use a cane or crutches to walk. Physical therapy exercises to strengthen the knee should start as soon as tolerated after surgery. Driving should be avoided for several weeks. Full recovery can take months.

Risks

Risks involved with kneecap removal are similar to those associated with any surgical procedure,

WHO PERFORMS THE PROCEDURE AND WHERE IS IT PERFORMED?

Kneecap removal surgery is usually performed in an outpatient setting and hospital stays, if any, are short, not exceeding more than a day. An orthopedic surgeon performs the surgery. Orthopedics is the medical specialty that focuses on the diagnosis, care, and treatment of patients with disorders of the bones, joints, muscles, ligaments, tendons, nerves, and skin.

QUESTIONS TO ASK THE DOCTOR

- How is the kneecap removed?
- What type of anesthesia will be used?
- How long will it take for the knee to recover from the surgery?
- When will I be able to walk without crutches?
- What are the risks associated with kneecap removal surgery?
- How many kneecap removal procedures do you perform in a year?

mainly allergic reaction to anesthesia, excessive bleeding, and infection.

Kneecap removal is very delicate surgery because the kneecap is part of the extensor mechanism of the leg, meaning the muscles and ligaments, the patella, the quadriceps tendon, and the patellar tendon; which all allow the knee to extend and remain stable when extended. When the kneecap is removed, the extensor assembly becomes more lax, and it may be impossible to ever regain full extension.

Normal results

People who undergo kneecap removal because of a broken bone or repeated dislocations have the best chance for complete recovery. Those who have this operation because of arthritis may have less successful results, and later need a total knee replacement.

Resources

BOOKS

Harner, C. D., K. G. Vince, and F. H. Fu, eds. *Techniques in Knee Surgery*. Philadelphia: Lippincott, Williams & Wilkins, 2001.

Winter Griffith, H., et al., eds. "Kneecap Removal." In *The Complete Guide to Symptoms, Illness and Surgery*, 3rd edition. New York: Berkeley Publishing, 1995.

PERIODICALS

Juni, P., et al. "Population Requirement for Primary Knee Replacement Surgery: A Cross-sectional Study." *Rheumatology* 42 (April 2003): 516–521.

Meijer, O. G., and Van Den Dikkenberg. "Levels of Analysis in Knee Surgery." *Knee Surgery Sports Traumatology Arthroscopy* 11 (January 2003): 53–54.

Petersen, W., C. Beske, V. Stein, and H. Laprell. "Arthroscopical Removal of a Projectile from the Intraarticular Cavity of the Knee Joint." *Archives of Orthopaedic Trauma Surgery* 122 (May 2002): 235–236.

ORGANIZATIONS

The American Academy of Orthopaedic Surgeons. 6300 North River Road, Rosemont, IL 60018-4262. (847) 823-7186, (800) 346-AAOS. http://www.aaos.org.

The American Association of Hip and Knee Surgeons (AAHKS). 704 Florence Drive, Park Ridge, IL 60068-2104. (847) 698-1200. <hhtp://www.aahks.org.

OTHER

"Patellectomy." *The Knee Guru Page*.http://www.kneeguru.co.uk/html/step_05_patella/step_05_patellectomy.html.

"Patellectomy or Partial Patellectomy." *Pro Team Physicians*. http://www.proteamphysicians.com/Patient/Treat/knee/kneefracture/patellectomy_procedure.asp.

Tish Davidson, AM
Monique Laberge, PhD